The Synthesis of Prostaglandins

THE SYNTHESIS OF PROSTAGLANDINS

ABHIJIT MITRA

Department of Chemistry
Columbia University, New York

Foreword by

PROFESSOR GILBERT STORK

A WILEY-INTERSCIENCE PUBLICATION

JOHN WILEY & SONS

New York • London • Sydney • Toronto

Library of Congress Cataloging in Publication Data:

Mitra, Abhijit.
The synthesis of prostaglandins.

"A Wiley-Interscience publication."
Includes indexes.
1. Prostaglandins. 2. Chemistry, Organic—Synthesis. I. Title. [DNLM: 1. Prostaglandins—Chemical synthesis. QU90 M684s]

QP801.P68M57 547'.43'7 77-23268
ISBN 0-471-02308-6

Printed in the United States of America

10 9 8 7 6 5 4 3 2 1

Dedicated to my mother

Mrs. Nira Mitra

Foreword

It is a pleasure to introduce this survey of prostaglandin synthesis that has been so clearly and effectively constructed by Abhijit Mitra. The prostaglandins have fired the imagination of "synthetic organic chemists" perhaps more than any other class of substances since the exciting era of steroid synthesis. It is surely not necessary to recall the great catalytic effect that the challenge of the steroid nucleus had on the development of many regio- and stereoselective methods of synthesis. They are now part of the tools routinely employed in solving problems of chemical architecture in contexts so diverse that their steroid origin is often no longer remembered

There are, of course, other arenas in which the challenge of a molecular target, the indole group alkaloids, to cite a conspicuous example, has led to considerable enrichment of the art and science of synthesis. But the prostaglandins, as the steroids before them, are unique in their combination of potential practical use, as such or in the form of related structures, together with the exciting scientific esthetic challenge of a complex—but not too complex—molecular array. These circumstances have resulted in much imaginative work in commercial as well as in academic research laboratories. As a result, it is difficult to overestimate the importance the prostaglandins have had and continues to have in the development of new synthetic tools, as well as in extending, or more precisely delineating, the scope of existing ones. The syntheses illustrated in the following pages give many examples to support this claim. Even more important, they emphasize the very large number of different strategies that can be employed to solve a specific problem in synthesis.

It would be surprising, indeed, if those who savor these pages from time to time, tyros and experienced molecular architects alike, do not find in this tribute to contemporary synthesis the inspiration to devise even more elegant and (or?) efficient methods of synthesis.

Columbia University
New York, New York
January, 1977

Gilbert Stork

Preface

The synthesis of prostaglandins has been a continuing challenge to the organic chemist. A multifaceted synthetic attack has shown that there are innumerable ways of constructing complex natural products such as the prostaglandins. This effort has led to the development of new synthetic methods and reactions characterized by stereoselectivity and stereospecificity.

In this book an effort has been made to present a comprehensive review of the subject. I hope it will serve as a useful reference book for practicing organic chemists and also for the student of organic chemistry.

It has been said that organic chemistry is pictorially like the Chinese language. It is in this spirit that the various syntheses have been presented as flow charts. *The Synthesis of Prostaglandins* aims to capture, by a predominantly pictorial language, a feeling for the adventure of organic chemistry. The important approaches have been arranged according to the major strategy, with the presentation of the synthetic strategy by an **antithetic** flow diagram.

New York, New York
January, 1977

Abhijit Mitra

Acknowledgment

This book would be incomplete without an acknowledgment of the help and encouragement of Professor Gilbert Stork, who kindly allowed me to work on this manuscript during the course of my graduate studies. I also wish to thank him for critically reading it in its entirety and for making valuable suggestions.

I am indebted to Professor Ronald Breslow for his enthusiastic support.

I am also indebted to Professors W. Clark Still, Jr. and Paul A. Grieco and Dr. Milan Uskokovic for reading the entire manuscript. I thank Professor Koji Nakanishi for reading the section on the biosynthesis of prostaglandins. I also thank all my friends and colleagues, in particular Professor George Kraus, Drs. J. E. Richman, Paul G. Williard, Ambrose Leong and Bruce Pearlman, and other members of Professor Stork's research group, for their helpful comments.

I thank Professor S. Ranganathan and Dr. Darshan Ranganathan for their encouragement. I also thank Mr. M. F. Schlecht and Dr. R. Cvetovich for proofreading the manuscript.

Most of all, I should like to thank my wife, Dr. Sudha Mitra, for her tolerance and help in preparing the manuscript.

Abhijit Mitra

Contents

The Synthesis of Prostaglandins

1

Introduction

HISTORICAL BACKGROUND

Prostaglandins are a group of closely related compounds that exert a diverse array of physiological effects in a variety of mammalian tissues. The discovery of prostaglandins as potent pharmaceutical agents has motivated a tremendous amount of research in synthetic organic chemistry, pharmacology, and clinical medicine. This has led to exciting developments and has prompted the reexamination of some respected theories of cell biochemistry.[1] The importance of the discovery of prostaglandins is equaled only by the earlier discovery of steroids and penicillins.

In 1930, Kurzrok and Leib[2] of Columbia University first observed that human seminal plasma induced contractions of uterine strips. Several years after their original observation, the presence of a vasodepressant and smooth muscle stimulant in extracts of human seminal plasma was demonstrated independently by Goldblatt[3,4] and von Euler.[5] Von Euler,[6,7,8] finding similar activity in the extracts of prostate glands of male sheep, demonstrated that the biological activity was associated with the fraction containing lipid soluble acids and coined[6] the name **Prostaglandin (PG)**. After 30 years, the prostaglandins were characterized and their structures elucidated by Samuelsson, Bergstrom, and their associates at the Karolinska Institute, Sweden.[9,10,11,12,13,14]

---

1. F. A. Kuehl, Jr., V. J. Cirillo, M. E. Zanetti, G. C. Beveridge & E. A. Ham, in *Advances in Prostaglandin and Thromboxane Research*, Vol. **I**, B. Samuelsson & R. Paoletti (Eds.), Raven, New York, 1976, p. 313. Prostaglandins like other hormones are believed to produce their intracellular effects through alterations in the level of the cyclic nucleotides, cAMP and cGMP. In a number of cases studied PGE_1 raises the level of cAMP and PGF that of cGMP, resulting in antagonistic effects. A plausible model for the mechanism of stimulation is as follows. The binding of PGE_1 and PGF to their specific receptors on the cell wall stimulates the corresponding membrane bound nucleotide cyclases and results in enhanced levels of cAMP and cGMP. CyclicAMP and cGMP have antagonistic regulatory influences in certain biological systems which can enter into a mutual interaction resulting in synthesis. This theory (G. Goldberg, *et al.*) of biological regulation based on dual opposing forces is embodied in the ancient oriental concept termed *Yin Yang*.
   N. D. Goldberg, M. K. Haddox, E. Dunham, C. Lopez & J. W. Hadden in "Control of Proliferation in Animal Cells," *Cold Spring Harbor Conferences On Cell Proliferation*, Vol. **I**, B. Clarkson & R. Baseraga (Eds.), 1974, p. 609.
2. R. Kurzrok & C. C. Leib, *Proc. Soc. Exp. Biol. Med.*, **26**, 268 (1930).
3. M. W. Goldblatt, *Chem. Ind. (Lond.)*, **52**, 1056 (1933).
4. M. W. Goldblatt, *J. Physiol. (Lond.)*, **84**, 208 (1935).
5. U. S. von Euler, *Arch. Exp. Pathol. Pharmakol. Nauyn-Schmiedebergs*, **175**, 78 (1934).
6. U. S. von Euler, *Klin. Wochenschr.*, **14**, 1182 (1935).
7. U. S. von Euler, *J. Physiol. (Lond.)*, **88**, 213 (1936).
8. U. S. von Euler, *Scand. Arch. Physiol.*, **81**, 65 (1939).
9. S. Bergstrom & J. Sjovall, *Acta. Chem. Scand.*, **14**, 1693 (1960).
10. S. Bergstrom, R. Ryhage, B. Samuelsson & J. Sjovall, *J. Biol. Chem.*, **238**, 3555 (1963).
11. S. Bergstrom, R. Ryhage, B. Samuelsson & J. Sjovall, *Arch. Kemi.*, **19**, 563 (1962).
12. B. Samuelsson, *J. Am. Chem. Soc.*, **85**, 1878 (1963).
13. S. Bergstrom & B. Samuelsson, *Annu. Rev. Biochem.*, **34**, 101 (1965).
14. B. Samuelsson, E. Granstrom, K. Green, M. Hamberg & S. Hamarstrom, *Annu. Rev. Biochem.*, **44**, 669 (1975).
15. N. A. Nelson, *J. Med. Chem.*, **17**, 911 (1974).

STRUCTURE AND NOMENCLATURE OF THE PROSTAGLANDINS[15]

The prostaglandins have been classified according to the general nomenclature shown below:

$$PGX_{n\alpha}$$

where X denotes the functionality in the cyclopentanone ring,
n denotes the number of double bonds in the side chains
and α denotes the stereochemistry of the C_9 hydroxyl group.

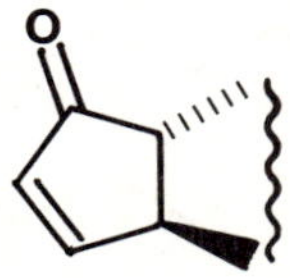

X = A

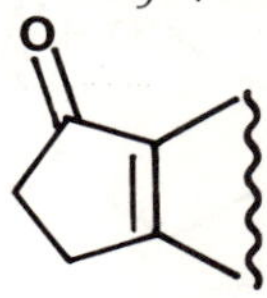

X = B

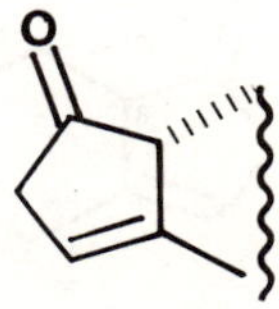

X = C

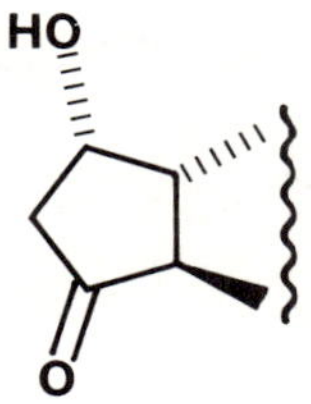

X = D

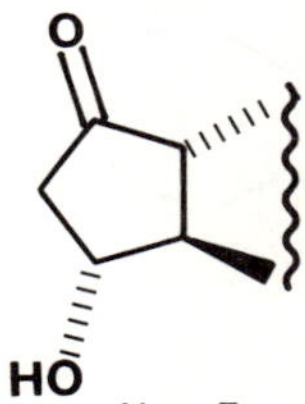

X = E

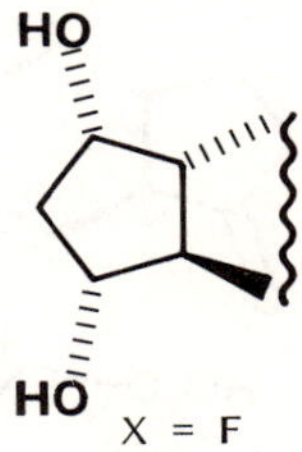

X = F

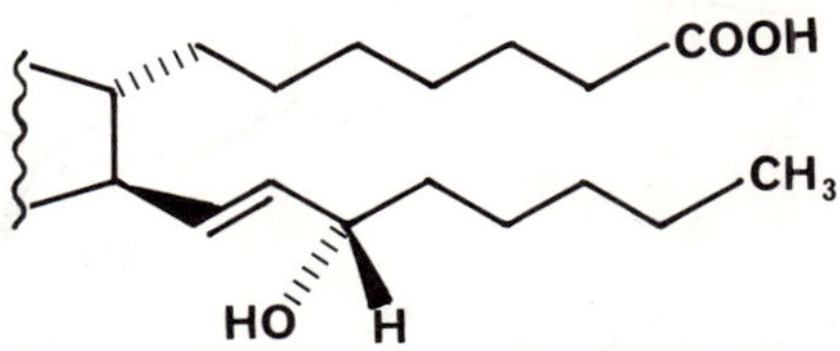

n = 1

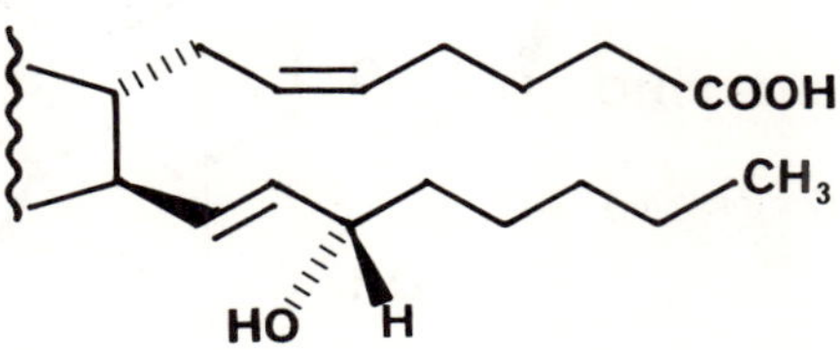

n = 2

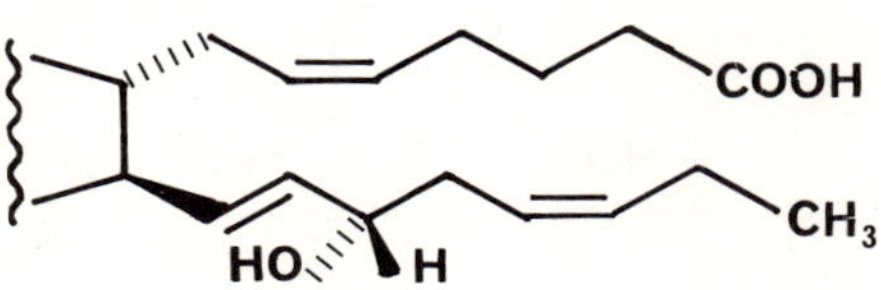

n = 3

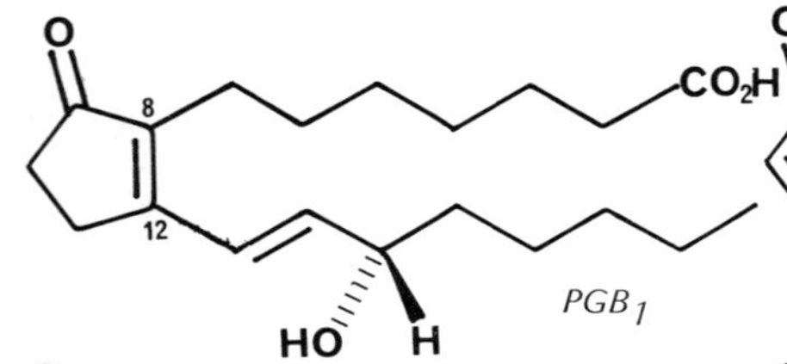

PGB₁

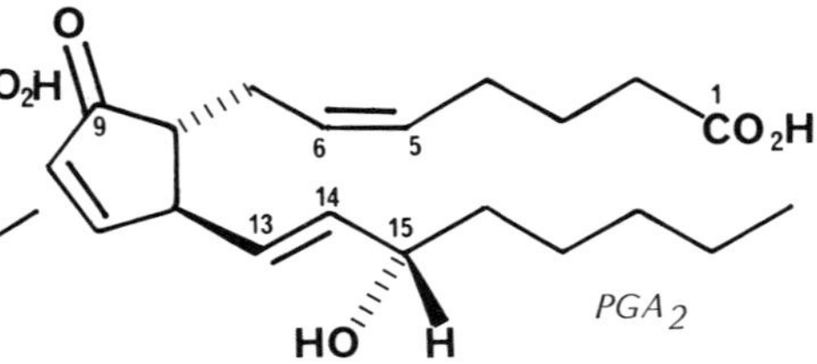

PGA_2

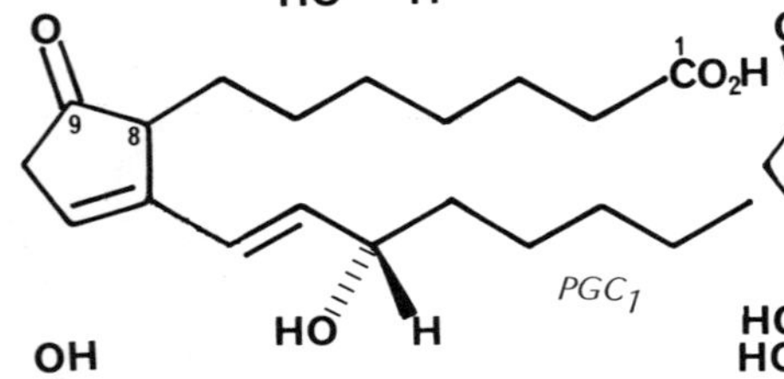

PGC_1

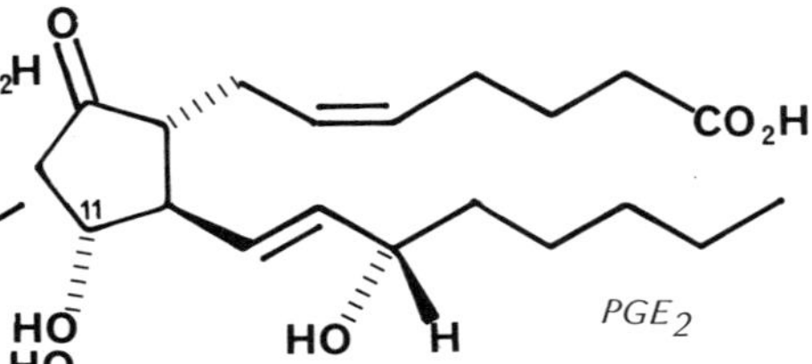

PGE_2

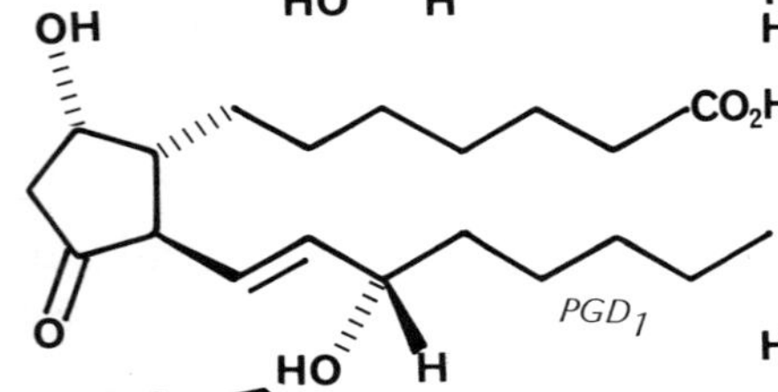

PGD_1

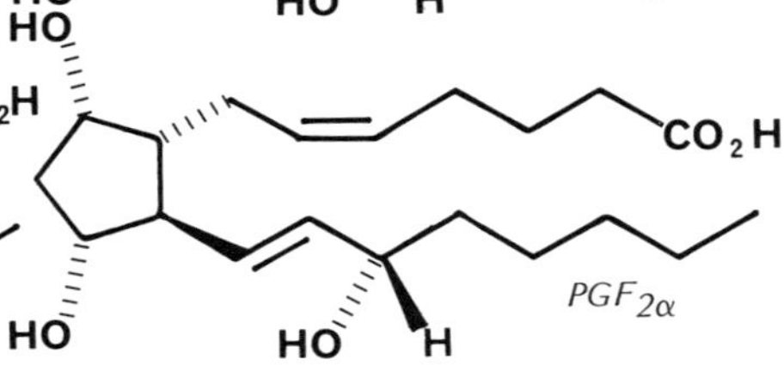

$PGF_{2\alpha}$

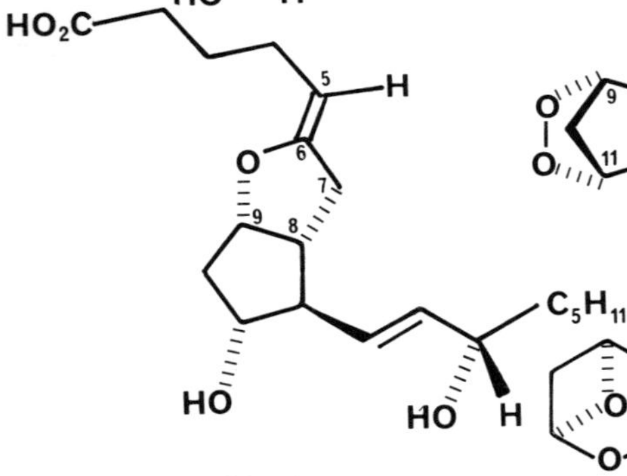

PGX (Prostacyclin)

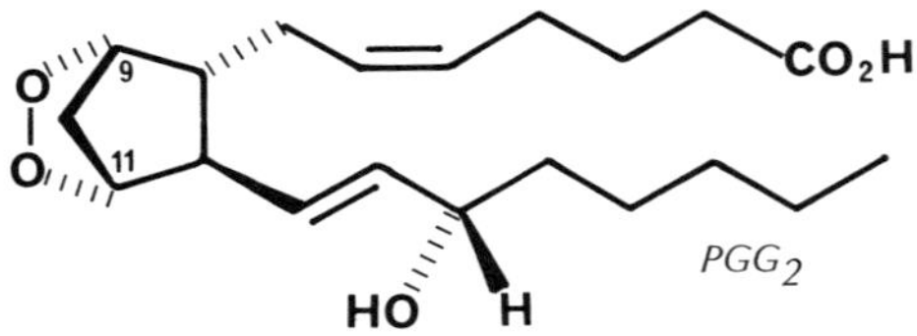

PGG_2

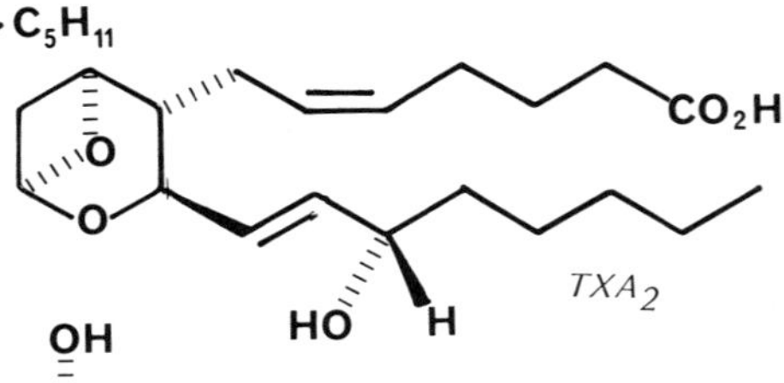

TXA_2

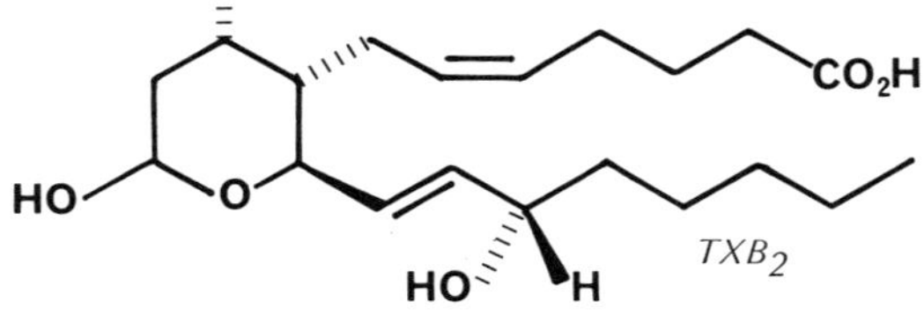

TXB_2

BIOSYNTHESIS

In 1964, it was first shown by Van Dorp, *et al.*[16] and Bergstrom, *et al.*[17] that essential fatty acids are precursors of prostaglandins. Homogenates of vesicular glands from sheep were incubated with tritium-labeled arachidonic acid, which resulted in the formation of radioactive PGE_2. Later it was also shown that PGE_1 and PGE_3 were biosynthesized from the corresponding essential fatty acids.[18,19]

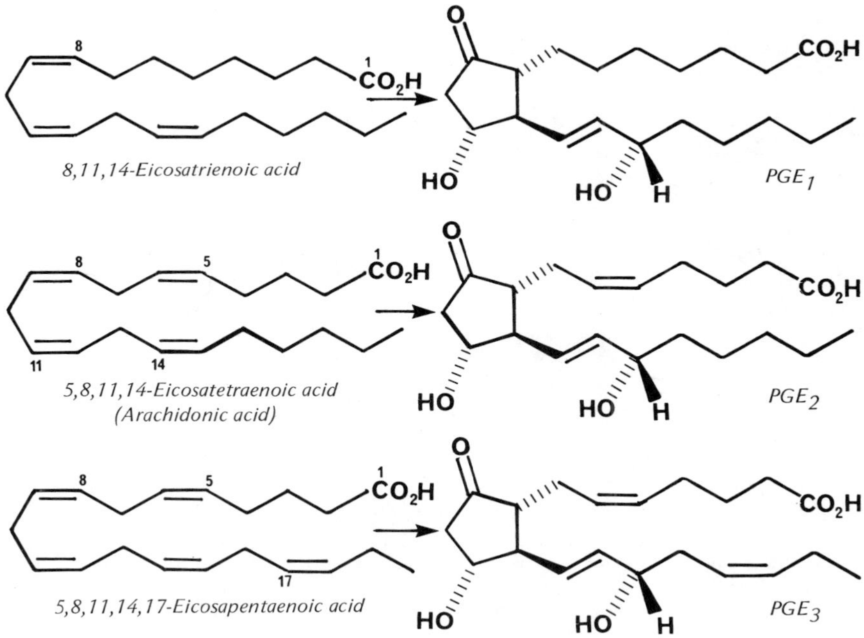

Fig. 1 Biosynthesis of prostaglandins from essential fatty acids.

16. D. A. Van Dorp, R. K. Beerthius, D. H. Nugteren & H. Vonkeman, *Biochim. Biophys. Acta.*, **90**, 204 (1964).
17. S. Bergstrom, H. Danielsson & B. Samuelsson, *Biochim. Biophys. Acta.*, **90**, 207 (1964).
18. S. Bergstrom, H. Danielsson, D. Klenberg & B. Samuelsson, *J. Biol. Chem.*, **239**, PC4006 (1964).
19. D. A. Van Dorp, R. K. Beerthius, D. H. Nugteren & H. Vonkeman, *Nature*, **203**, 839 (1964).

Using guinea pig lung homogenates, Anggard and Samuelsson[20] showed that arachidonic acid acts as a precursor to both PGE_2 and $PGF_{2\alpha}$, which are not interconvertible (**Fig. 2**). This finding was important in elucidating the mechanism of biosynthesis.

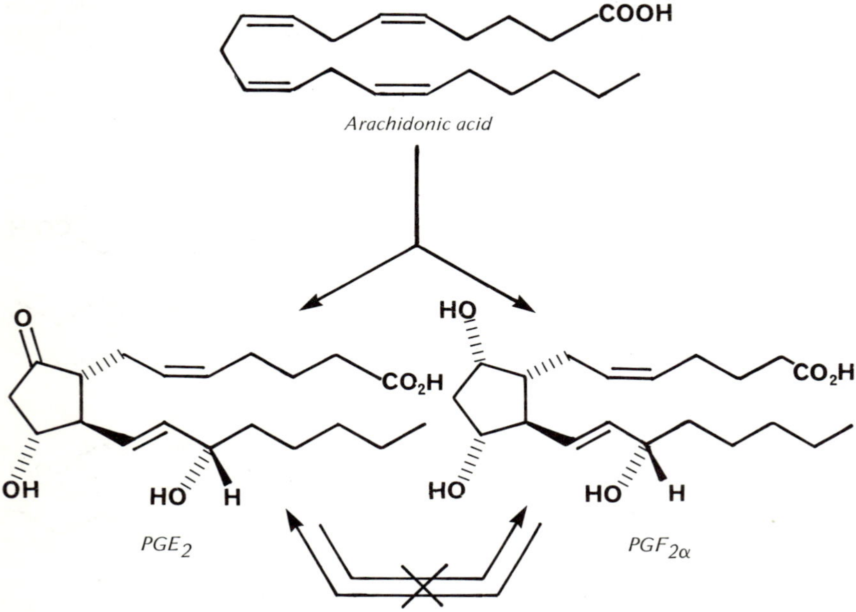

Fig. 2 Arachidonic acid acts as precursor to both PGE_2 and $PGF_{2\alpha}$

The transformation of 8,11,14-eicosatrienoic acid into PGE_1 involves the introduction of two hydroxyl groups and one keto group. Incubation of 8,11,14-eicosatrienoic acid in an atmosphere of $^{18}O_2$ showed that the C_9 and C_{11} oxygens originate from the same molecule of oxygen via a dioxygenase reaction and not a lipoxygenase reaction. This led to the suggestion that an *endo*-peroxide may be a possible intermediate in the biosynthetic pathway.[21] Extensive mechanistic studies have been done independently by Van Dorp, Samuelsson, and their associates.[22,23]

---

20. E. Anggard & B. Samuelsson, *J. Biol. Chem.*, **240**, 3518 (1965). Later it was observed that PGE-9 ketoreductase in microsomes of monkey and pigeon tissues can bring about this interconversion. S. C. Lee & L. Levine, *J. Biol. Chem.*, **249**, 1369 (1974).
21. B. Samuelsson, *J. Am. Chem. Soc.*, **87**, 3011 (1965).
22. B. Samuelsson, in *Progress in Biochemical Pharmacology*, R. Paoletti, (ed.), Krager, Basel, 1967, p. 59.
23. D. A. Van Dorp, in *Progress in Biochemical Pharmacology*, R. Paoletti, (Ed.), Krager, Basel, 1967, p. 71.

The proposal of Piper and Vane[24] that the *rabbit aorta contracting substance* (RCS) could be an *endo*-peroxide was confirmed by the isolation and characterization of the two *endo*-peroxides.[25,26] This led to suggestion of a plausible pathway for the prostaglandin biosynthesis (Fig. 3).[27]

Recent experimental results of Miyamoto[29,30] suggest the alternate reaction sequence shown in the following:

$$Precursor \rightarrow PGG_1 \rightarrow PGH_1 \rightarrow PGE_1$$

This finding does not rule out the original pathway proposed by Samuelsson and Hamberg[31] where the *endo*-peroxide isomerization precedes the hydroperoxide cleavage. Further studies by Samuelsson on the role of the *endo*-peroxide in platelet aggregation led to the isolation of two new compounds, Thromboxane A_2 and B_2.[32,33,34,35,36] (Fig. 4).

Yet another transformation of the endoperoxide (PGH_2) has been suggested by Vane[37] and Johnson[38] which gives rise to PGX (Prostacyclin). Thromboxanes and PGX play diametrically opposite roles in the body. Whereas thromboxanes cause platelets to aggregate and blood vessels to contract, prostacyclin inhibits platelet aggregation and causes dilation of blood vessels.

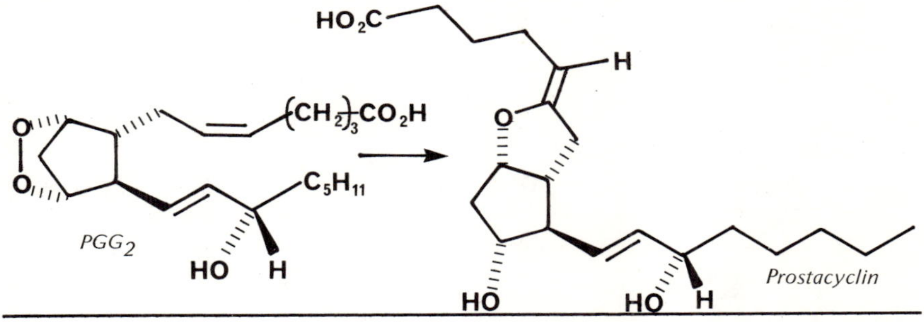

24. P. J. Piper & J. R. Vane, *Nature,* **223**, 29 (1969); *Nature* **231**, 232 (1971).
25. M. Hamberg & B. Samuelsson, *Proc. Natl. Acad. Sci. USA,* **70**, 899 (1973).
26. D. H. Nugteren & E. Hazelhof, *Biochim. Biophys. Acta.,* **326**, 448 (1973).
27. M. Hamberg, J. Svensson, T. Wakabayashi & B. Samuelsson, *Proc. Natl. Acad. Sci. USA,* **71**, 345 (1974).
28. The pro-S hydrogen is abstracted only. M. Hamberg & B. Samuelsson, *J. Biol. Chem.,* **242**, 5336 (1967).
29. T. Miyamoto, S. Yamamoto & O. Hayashi, *Proc. Natl. Acad. Sci. USA,* **71**, 364 (1974).
30. T. Miyamoto, N. Ogino, S. Yamamoto & O. Hayashi, *J. Biol. Chem.,* **251**, 2629 (1976).
31. M. Hamberg & B. Samuelsson, in *Prostaglandin Synthetase Inhibitors,* H. J. Robinson & J. R. Vane (Eds.), Raven, New York, 1974, p. 107.
32. M. Hamberg & B. Samuelsson, *Proc. Natl. Acad. Sci. USA,* **71**, 3400 (1974).
33. M. Hamberg, J. Svensson & B. Samuelsson, *Proc. Natl. Acad. Sci. USA,* **71**, 3824 (1974).
34. M. Hamberg, J. Svensson, B. Samuelsson, *Proc. Natl. Acad. Sci. USA,* **72**, 2994 (1975).
35. M. Hamberg, J. Svensson & B. Samuelsson, in *Advances in Prostaglandin & Thromboxane Research,* Vol. I, B. Samuelsson & R. Paoletti (Eds.), Raven, New York, 1976, p. 19.
36. Since this new class of compounds were originally found in thrombocytes, they were given the name thromboxane.
37. Dr. J. R. Vane of the Wellcome Research Laboratories reported the biological properties of PGX. S. Moncada, R. J. Gryglewski, S. Bunting & J. R. Vane, *Nature,* **263**, 663 (1976). S. Moncada, R. J. Gryglewski, S. Bunting & J. R. Vane, *Prostaglandins,* **12**, 685, 715 (1976).
38. Dr. R. A. Johnson of Upjohn revealed the structure of PGX to be (5*Z*)-9-deoxy-6,9α-epoxy-Δ^5-prostaglandin $F_{1\alpha}$.

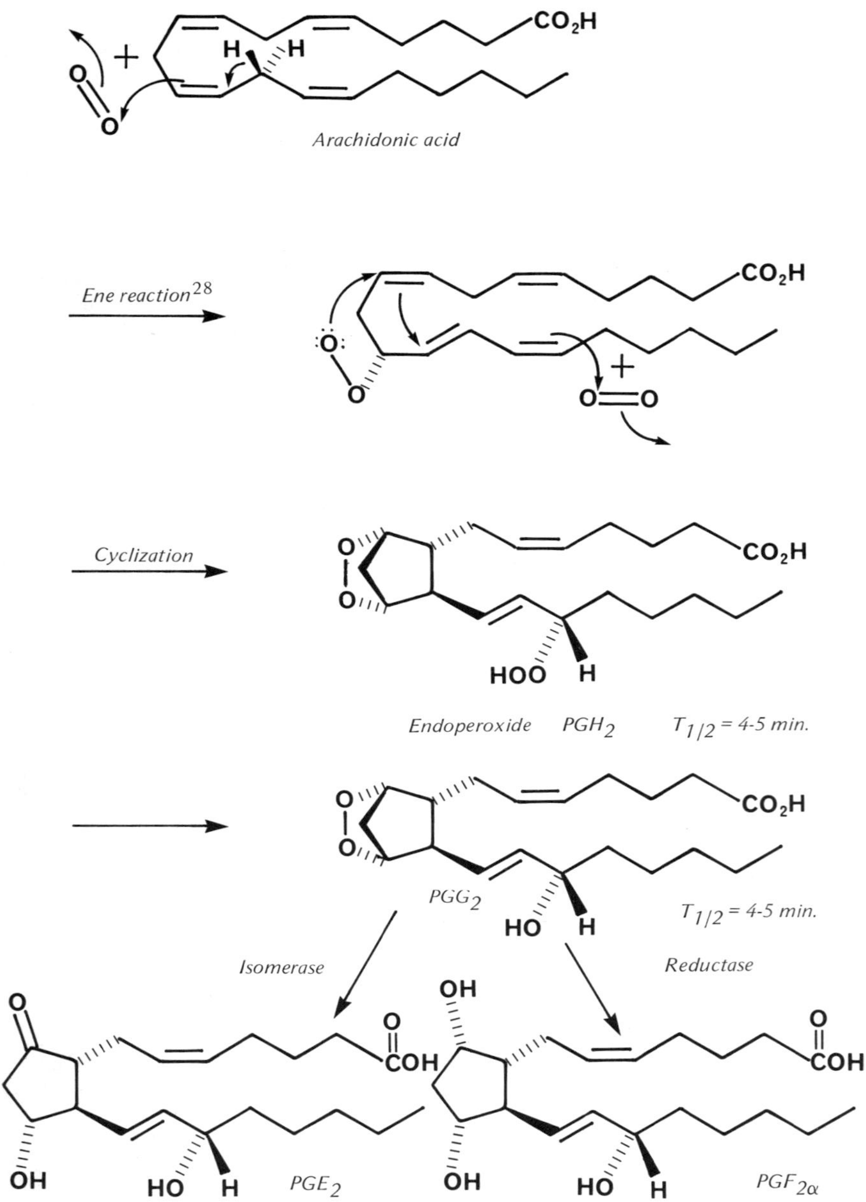

Fig. 3 A plausible biosynthetic pathway

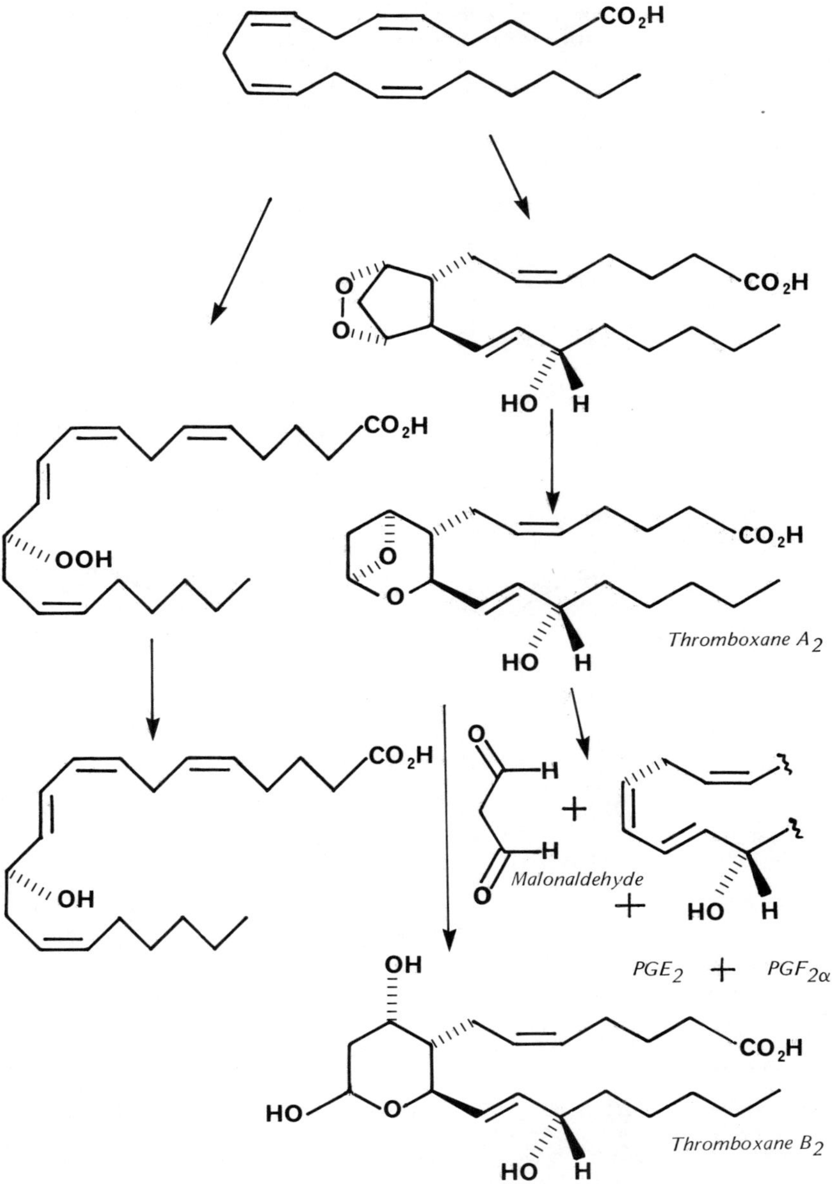

Fig. 4 The role of endoperoxide (PGG_2) in platelet aggregation.

Despite these facts, the precise nature of the biosynthetic pathway is not yet known. Also, it may be that different pathways are followed in other systems, for example, the corals.[39,40]

Some of the transformations that are carried out *in vivo* are very intriguing because such reactions have not yet been successfully carried out in the laboratory. Of these, the most interesting one is the formation of the *endo*-peroxide from the 1,4-diene. Attempts are being made to mimic this enzymatic reaction.[41] This reaction causes one to ponder the nature of the oxygen participating in the formation of the *endo*-peroxide: is the oxygen reacting in the singlet state, in the triplet state, or in some other activated form?[42]

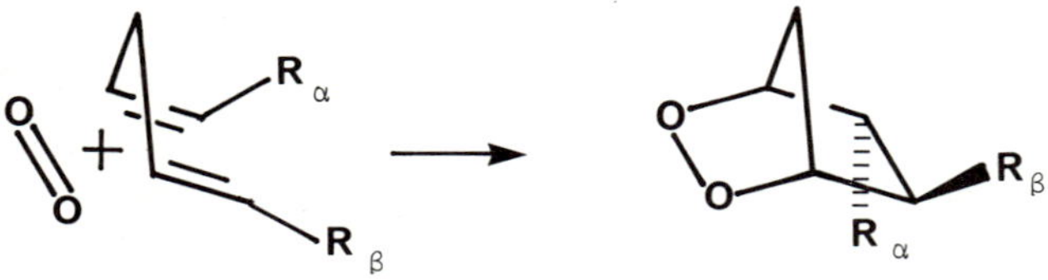

Another interesting *in vivo* reaction is the cleavage of the *endo*-peroxide in a retro $_{\sigma}2_s + {}_{\sigma}2_s + {}_{\sigma}2_s$ fashion to give malonaldehyde. Such a cleavage is not known even in the analogous carbocyclic system.

---

39. E. J. Corey, H. E. Ensley, M. Hamberg & B. Samuelsson, *Chem. Commun.*, 277 (1975).
40. E. J. Corey & W. N. Washburn, *J. Am. Chem. Soc.*, **96**, 934 (1974).
41. N. A. Porter & M. O. Funk, *J. Org. Chem.*, **40**, 3614 (1975).
42. Recent work shows that the *in vitro* fragmentation of the PG *endo*-peroxide, which is often pictured as a concerted bond shift process, may not be a simple unimolecular rearrangement. D. J. Coughlin & R. G. Salomon, *J. Am. Chem. Soc.*, **99**, 655 (1977).

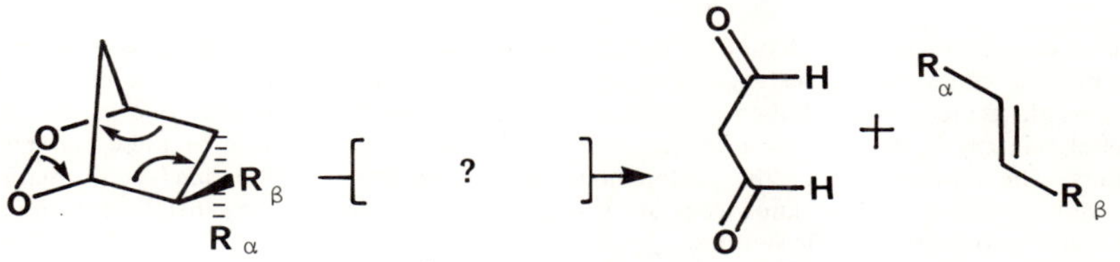

Malonaldehyde

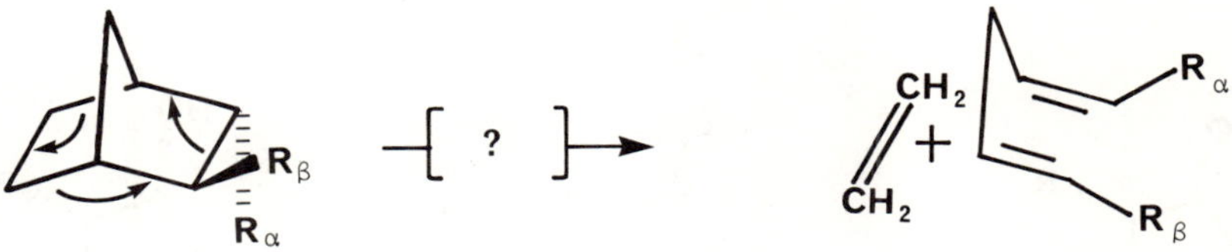

---

43. There are few examples of the cycloreversion reaction. One of them being the cycloreversion of diademane to triquinacene. A. de Meijere, D. Kaufmann & O. Schallner, *Angew. Chem. (Int. Ed. Engl.)*, **10**, 417 (1971); A. de Meijere, D. Kaufmann & O. Schallner, *Tet. Lett.*, 553 (1973).

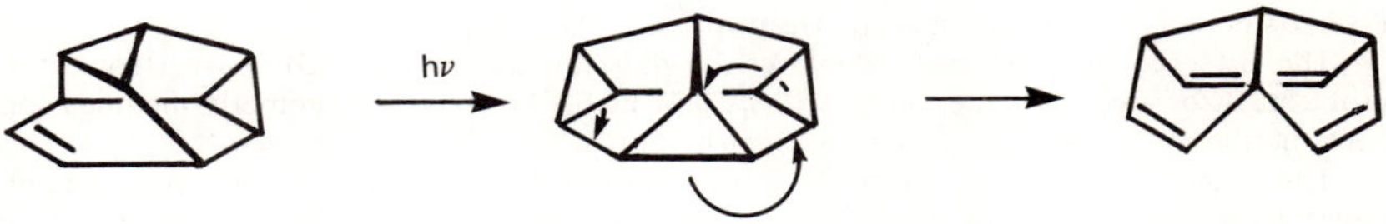

Diademane *Triquinacene*

44. For recent studies on the stereochemistry and mechanism of the $[\sigma 2 + \sigma 2 + \sigma 2]$ cycloreversion reaction see: J. A. Berson, S. S. Olon, E. W. Petrillo, Jr. & P. Bickart, *Tet.*, **30**, 1639 (1974).

THE SYNTHESIS OF PROSTAGLANDINS

Ever since the structure elucidation of the prostaglandins, the synthesis of this class of hormones has been a considerable challenge to synthetic chemists. With a maximum number of five asymmetric centers, four of them contiguous in the prostanoid nucleus and one in the allylic alcohol side chain, the primary problem is the stereospecific construction of these asymmetric centers. The recalcitrance of the cyclopentane system to follow well-defined conformational behavior, as well as a lack of knowledge of five-membered ring chemistry in general, contributes to the challenge of stereospecific synthesis.

Prostaglandins A, E, and F have been the main synthetic objectives because they contain the most complex array of functional groups.

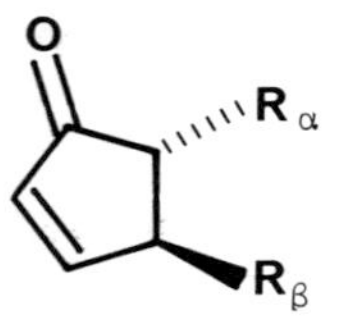

Less stable enone

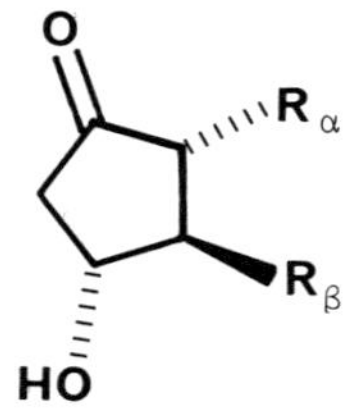

β-ketol

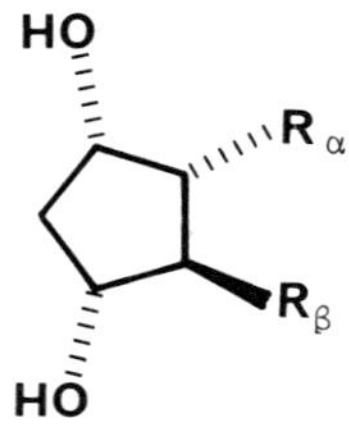

Cis-diol

The prostanoid nucleus of the PGE compounds contains a β-ketol function that is sensitive to acid and base. This requires its generation at a late stage of the synthetic sequence. The selective oxidation of the C_9 alcohol of the *cis*-1,3-diol of PGF_α, deprotection of the protected C_9 ketone or its generation from a latent carbonyl function are some of the various possible sequences for the generation of the β-ketol function.

The PGA nucleus, possessing the unsubstituted (less stable) enone function presents a different set of problems. The enone can be made by the dehydration of the β-ketol (PGE) but the problem then is to prevent the double bond from migrating to the tetra-substituted position (more stable PGB compounds) via the intermediate trisubstituted (PGC) olefin.

The presence of a relatively stable *cis*-1,3-diol function in the PGF nucleus obviates the problems associated with the ketones (PGA and PGE), but requires synthetic methods for the construction of the four contiguous asymmetric centers.

The generation of the chiral center at C_{15} is difficult because it is in an acyclic part of the molecule. The generation of the *cis*- and of the *trans*- olefin is easier. Wittig type olefin-forming reactions or reduction of suitable acetylenic precursors can be envisaged as leading to the *cis*- and *trans*- olefins.

The method by which the various workers have surmounted the problems inherent in these complex molecules, both in the development of new synthetic methods and in the application of existing methods, is the subject of this book.

2

Syntheses via Symmetric Intermediates

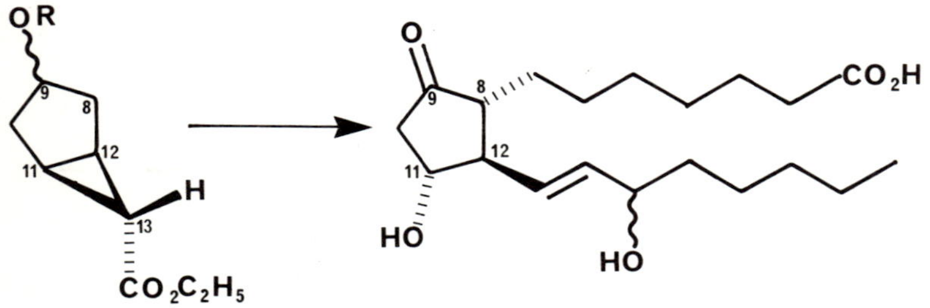

Sometimes a symmetric molecule is used to construct a dissymmetric molecule. This interesting concept was first demonstrated within the context of a prostaglandin synthesis by Just and Simonovitch,[1] and later by others.

The basic concept of G. Just and C. Simonovitch (of McGill University) was to generate the allylic alcohol system of the β-chain by the solvolysis of an appropriately substituted cyclopropylcarbinyl alcohol derivative. This concept was fully developed and modified by the Upjohn group.[2,3,11] These approaches go through the symmetric intermediate [1] and has been adapted to the syntheses of all known prostaglandins and a wide variety of analogs. Considerable stereochemical control could eventually be achieved by various more recent modifications *(vide infra)*.

---

1. G. Just & C. Simonovitch, *Tet. Lett.*, 2093 (1967).
2. W. P. Schneider, U. Axen, F. H. Lincoln, J. E. Pike & J. L. Thompson, *J. Am. Chem. Soc.*, **90**, 5895 (1968).
3. W. P. Schneider, U. Axen, F. H. Lincoln, J. E. Pike & J. L. Thompson, *J. Am. Chem. Soc.*, **91**, 5372 (1969).

SYNTHETIC STRATEGY

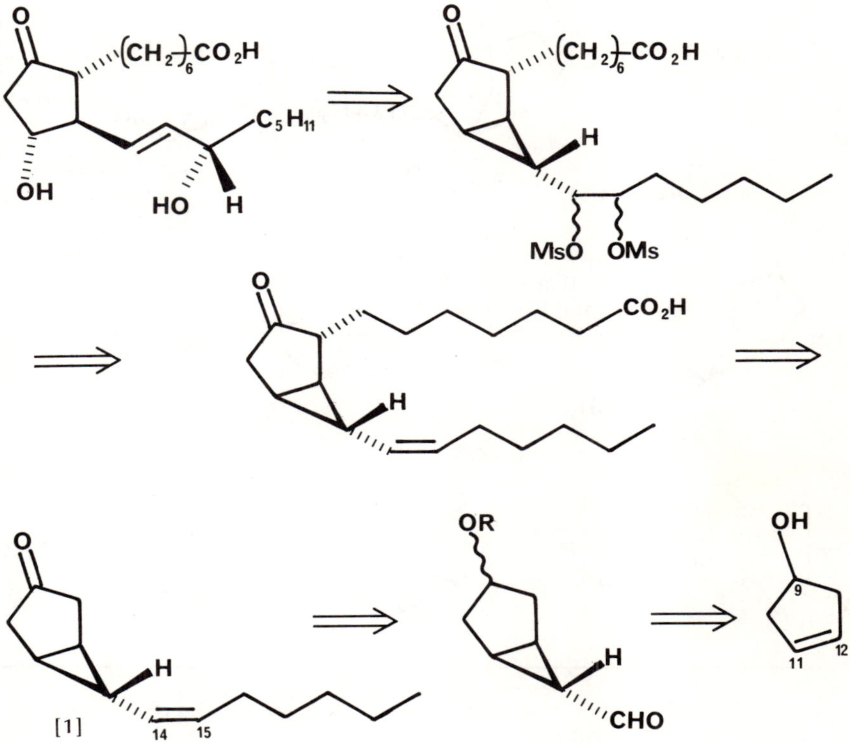

[1]

Symmetric intermediate

SYNTHETIC PLAN[2,3]

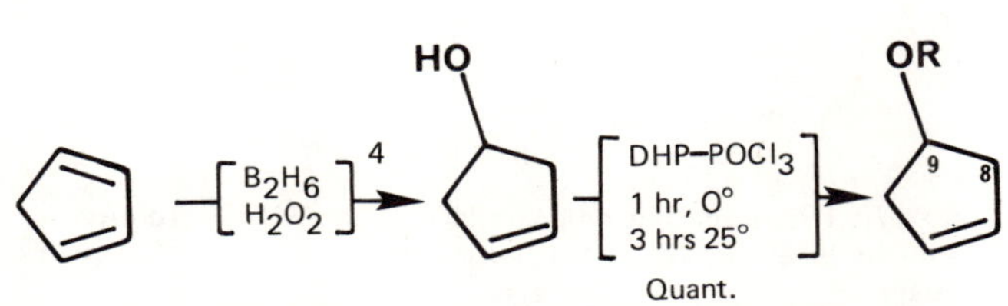

---

4. E. L. Allred, J. Sonnenberg & S. Winstein, *J. Org. Chem.*, 25, 26 (1960). Hydroboration 1,3-cyclohexadiene gives the allylic alcohol. See p. 243.

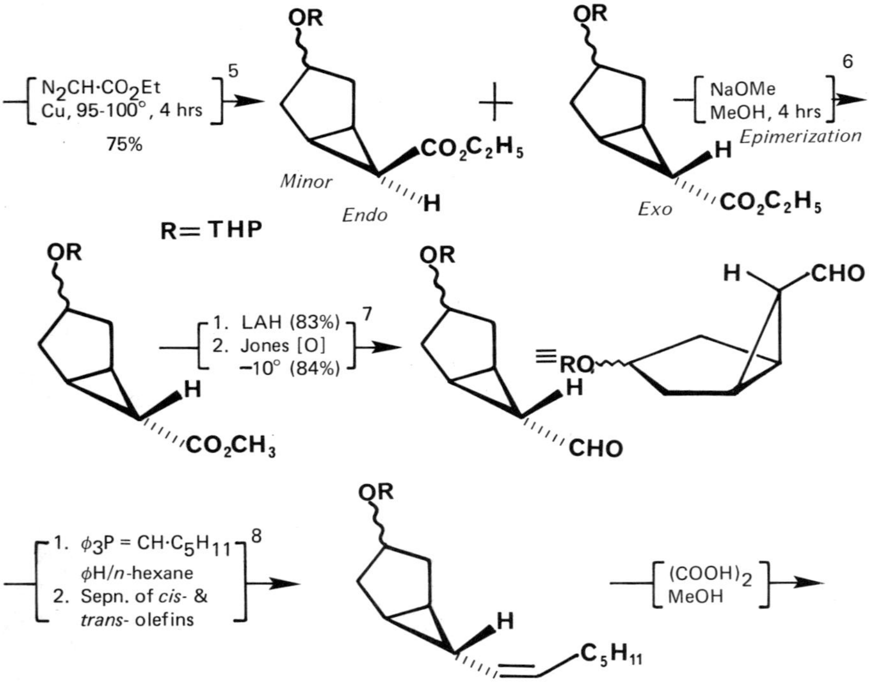

5. Cu catalyzed addition of diazoacetate to double bond has a strong preference for exocyclic addition. W. von E. Doering & T. Mole, *Tet.*, **10**, 65 (1960). For recent mechanistic studies on the Cu catalyzed addition of carbenes to olefins see: D. S. Wulfman, *et al.*, *Tet.*, **32**, 1257 (1976) and references cited therein.
6. The epimerization in the unsaturated system is more difficult. J. Warkentin, E. Singleton & J. F. Edgar, *Can. J. Chem.*, **43**, 3456 (1965).

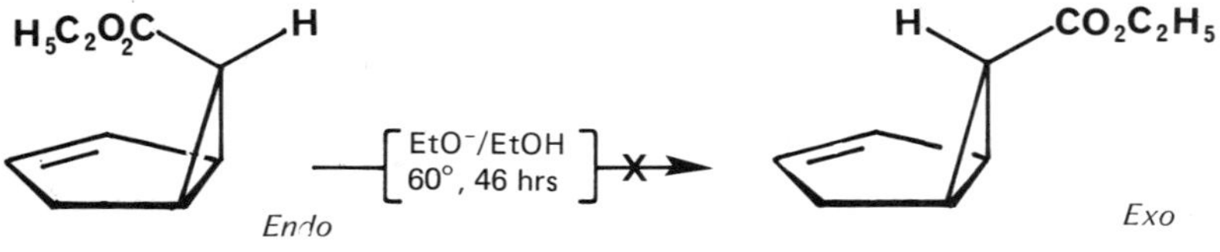

7. It is interesting to note that THP- protecting group of the C_9 alcohol is not hydrolyzed under the acidic conditions of the Jones oxidation. It is also interesting to note that the oxidation stops at the aldehyde stage.
8. 80-85% *cis*-olefin and 15-20% *trans*-olefin were formed when the reaction was carried out in benzene/*n*-hexane, whereas 1:1=*cis:trans* olefins were formed when THF was used as the solvent. In contrast, only the *cis* olefin was formed in the *endo* bicyclo[3.1.0] hexane system. For details see footnote 21, p. 24.

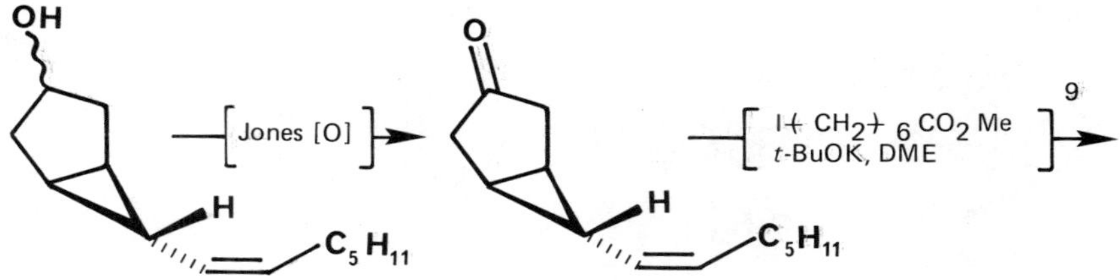

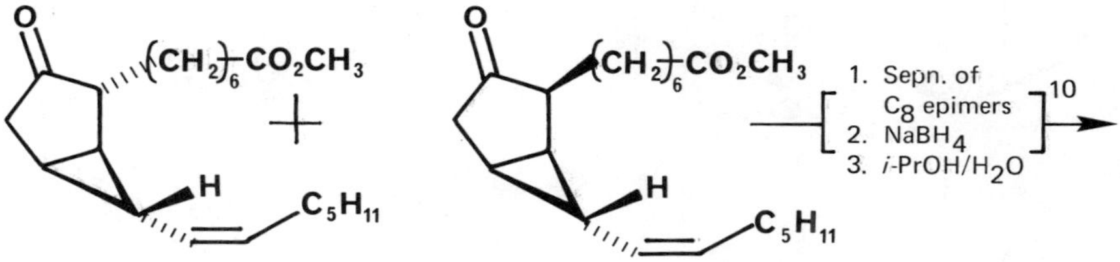

15% *and 21% Dialkylation* 17%

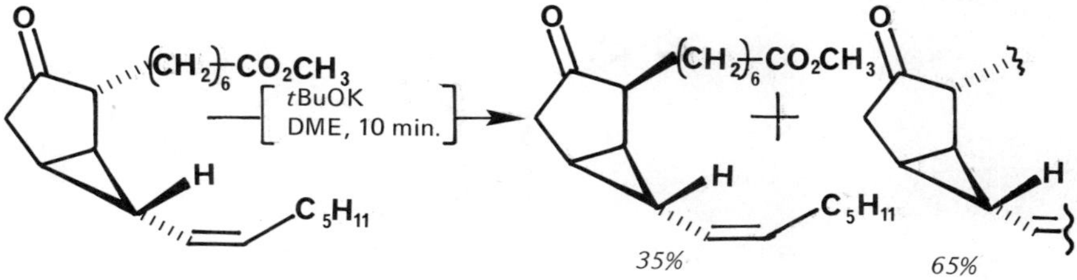

35% *65%*

9. The probable preference of the bicyclo[3.1.0]hexane system for a boat-like conformation makes the bulky carbomethoxyalkyl side chain assume the more stable equatorial orientation. H. E. Smith, J. C. D. Brand, E. H. Massey & L. J. Durham, *J. Org. Chem.*, 31, 690 (1966).

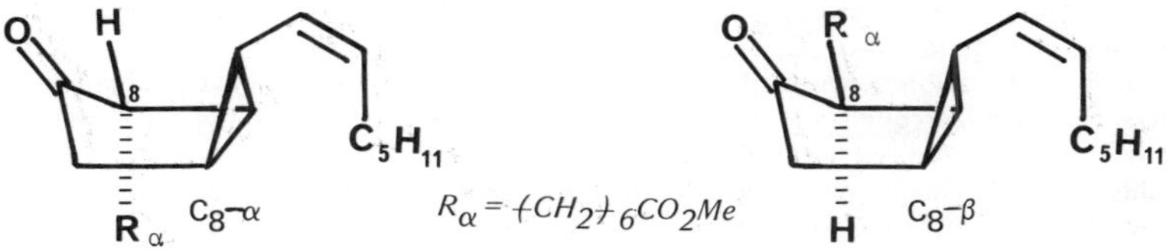

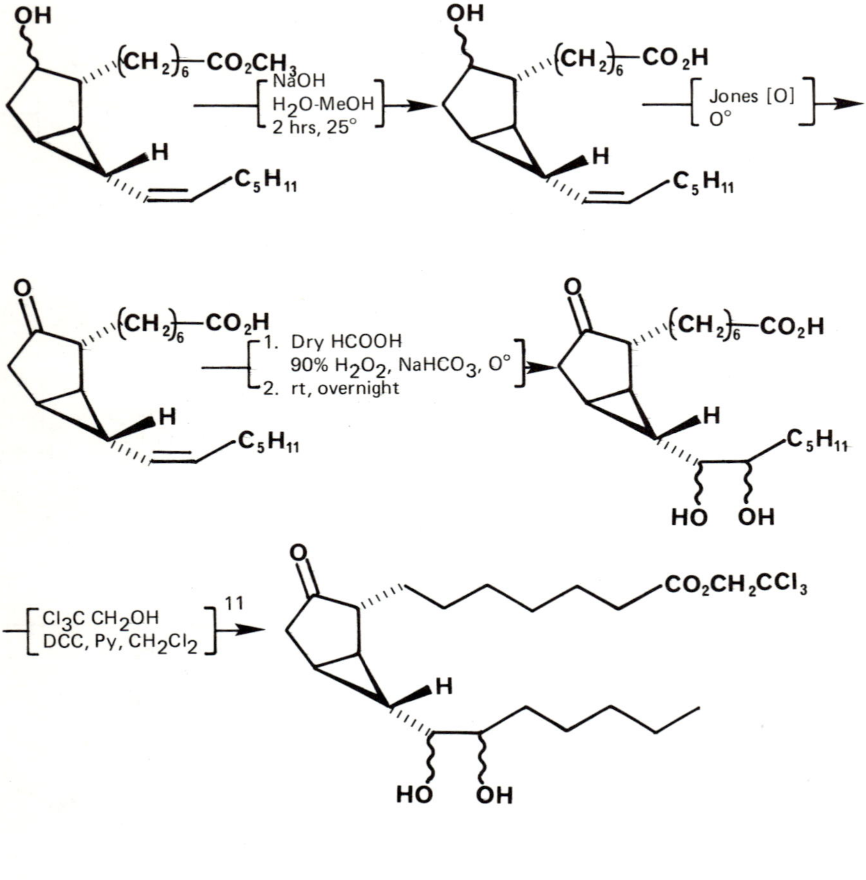

10. Hydrolysis of the keto-ester under basic conditions would epimerize the ω-carboxyhexyl side chain to the more stable undesired C_8-β epimer. This necessitates prior reduction and subsequent reoxidation of the C_9 function.

11. The facile dehydration of the 3-hydroxycyclopentanone (β-ketol) to 2-cyclopentanone (PGE to PGA) under basic conditions (required for the hydrolysis of the methyl ester) necessitates the use of trichloroethylester rather than the methyl-ester derivative. For the use of β, β, β-trichloroethyl protecting group see: R. B. Woodward, J. Gosteli, P. Naegeli, W. Oppolzer, R. Ramage, S. Ranganathan & H. Vorburggen, *J. Am. Chem. Soc.*, **88**, 852 (1966).

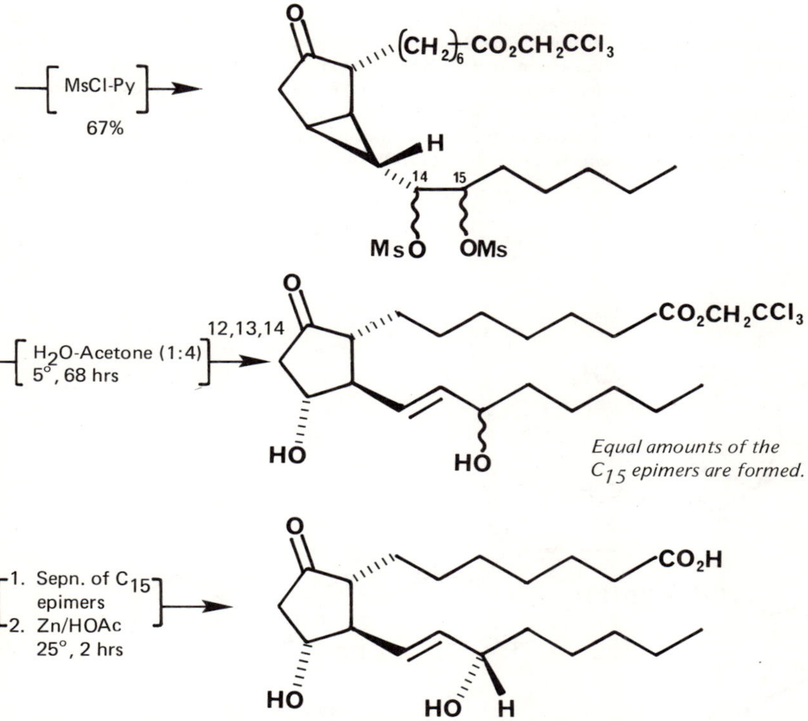

12. The major product of the solvolysis reaction is the hydroxy mesylate [2] [contrast to the observation of K. B. Wiberg & A. J. Ashe, *J. Am. Chem. Soc.*, **90**, 63 (1968), where with a simpler system the predominant reaction involves ring opening].

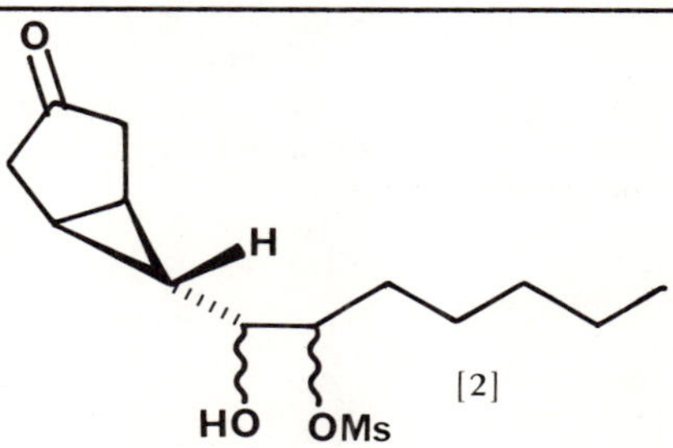

[2]

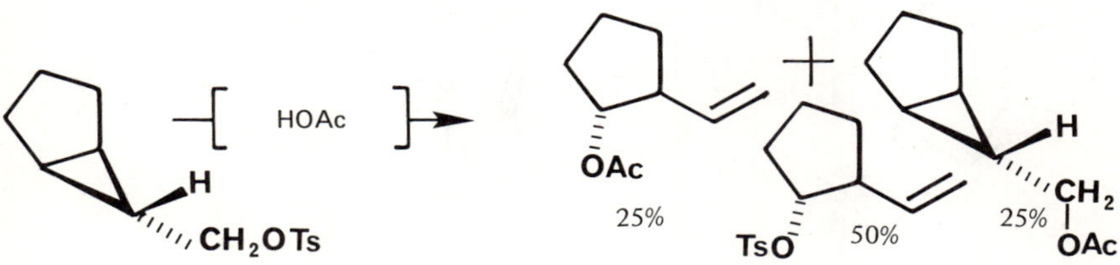

13. *Cis* hydroxylation, mesylation and solvolysis of the *cis* and *trans* olefinic compounds under identical conditions gave nearly the same product distribution: 4-8% (dl) PGE_1 Me-ester and none of the C_{13}-C_{14} olefinic compound. This has been interpreted to mean that the solvolysis of the cyclopropyl-carbinyl mesylate does not take place by a completely concerted mechanism, although Johnson has rationalized the streoselective formation of *trans*-olefin from cyclopropylcarbinyl systems on the basis of concerted process. S. F. Brady, M. A. Ilton & W. S. Johnson, *J. Am. Chem. Soc.*, **90**, 2882 (1968).

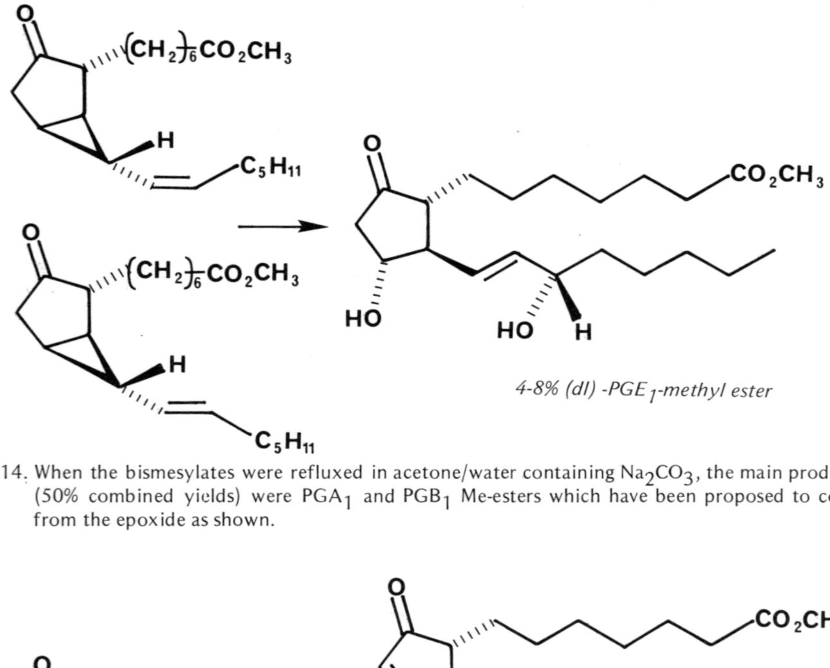

4-8% (dl) -PGE₁-methyl ester

14. When the bismesylates were refluxed in acetone/water containing Na_2CO_3, the main products (50% combined yields) were PGA_1 and PGB_1 Me-esters which have been proposed to come from the epoxide as shown.

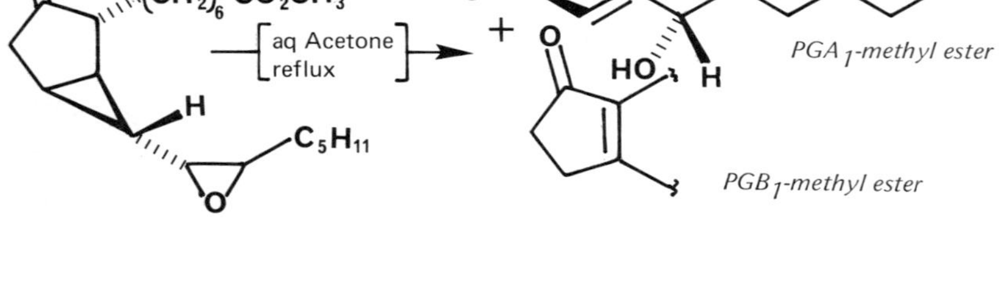

An earlier modification[15] was to synthesize the epoxide [3] and then solvolyze it as shown. This was successful only in low yields in the PGF series.

SYNTHETIC PLAN[15]

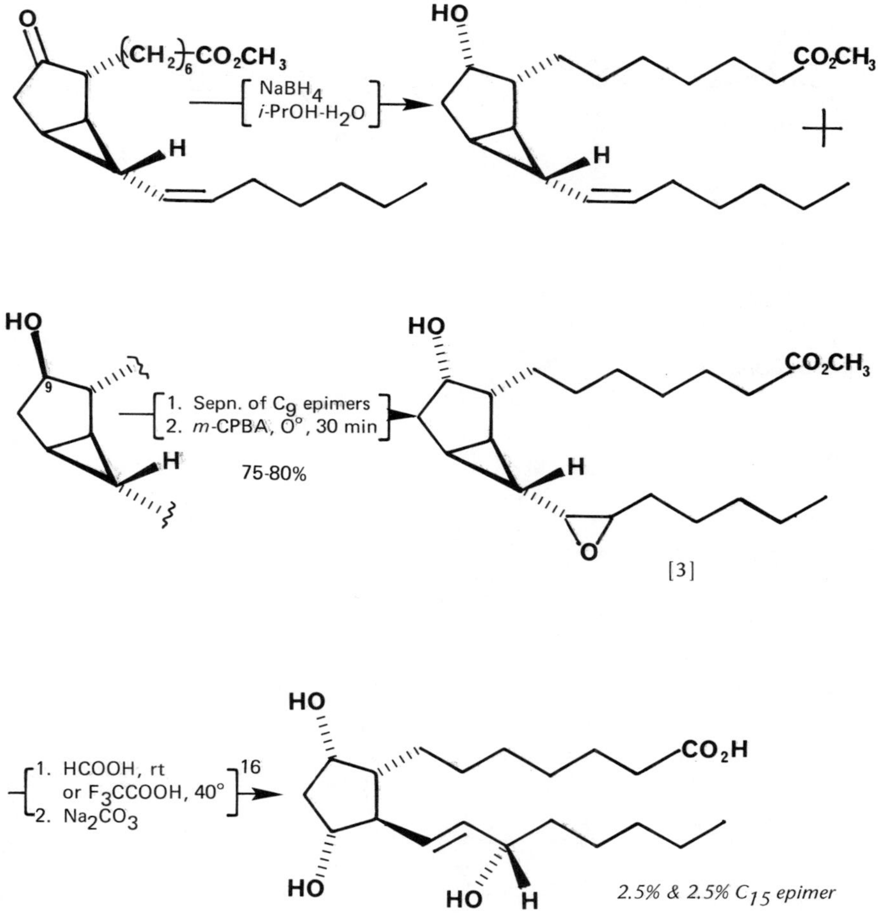

[3]

15. G. Just, C. Simonovitch, F. H. Lincoln, W. P. Schneider, U. Axen, G. B. Spero & J. E. Pike, *J. Am. Chem. Soc.*, **91**, 5364 (1969).
16. Solvolysis under various other conditions using different leaving groups were also tried. E. S. Ferdinandi & G. Just, *Can. J. Chem.*, **49**, 1070 (1971).

Of all the approaches which go through the bicyclo[3.1.0]hexane system, the best results were obtained by solvolyzing the *endo*-bismesylates.[17,22,25] Steric hindrance at C_{14} suppresses the competing hydrolysis to C_{14}-hydroxymesylate [2][18] without ring opening, thus increasing the yield of the ring opened products.

SYNTHETIC PLAN[17]

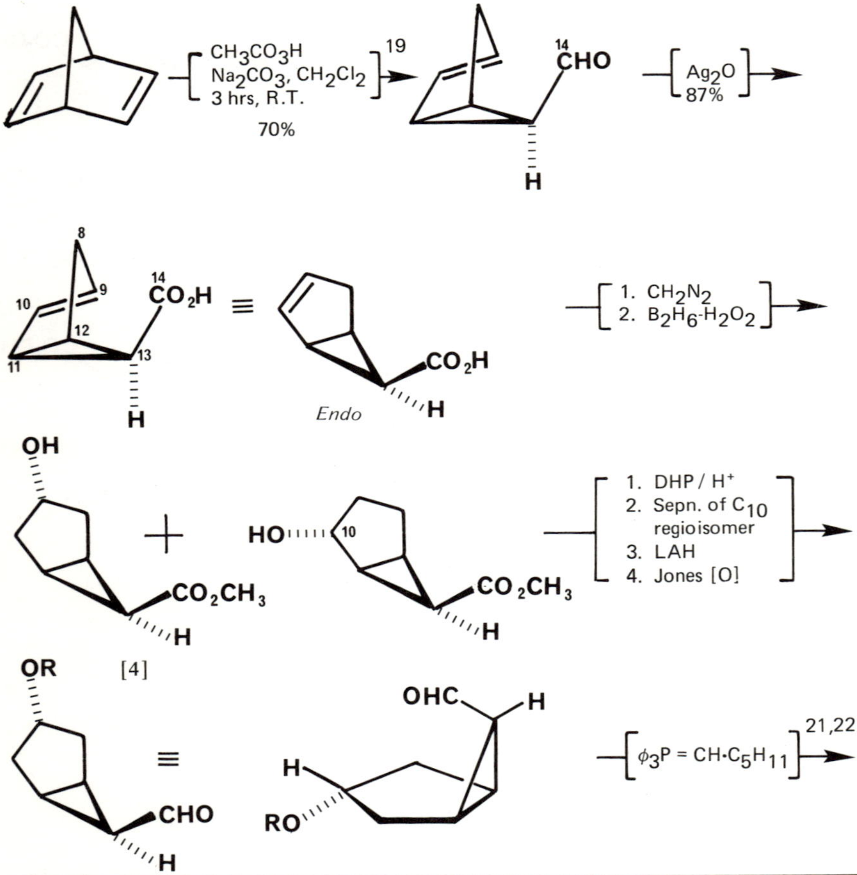

17. U. Axen, F. H. Lincoln & J. L. Thompson, *Chem. Commun.*, 303 (1969).
18. See ref. 12, p. 19.
19. J. Meinwald, S. S. Cabana & M. S. Chadha, *J. Am. Chem. Soc.*, **85**, 582 (1963).
20. The *endo*-bicyclo[3.1.0]hexane derivative [4] cannot be made by the Cu catalyzed diazoacetate addition to the protected cyclopentenol because it gives the less stable *endo* isomer as the minor product.

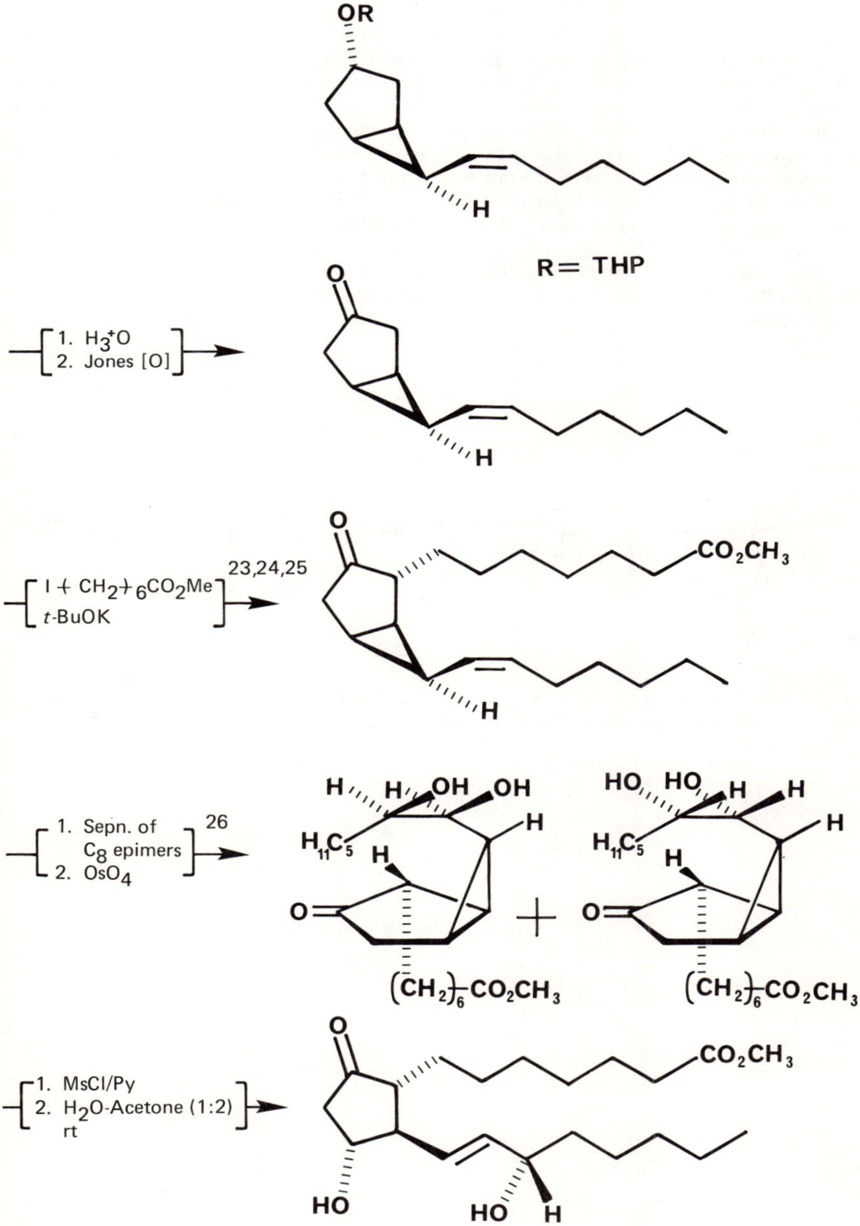
OR
H
R= THP
1. H_3^+O
2. Jones [O]
O
H
23,24,25
I ⟮ CH_2 ⟯ $_6CO_2Me$
t-BuOK
O
CO_2CH_3
H
1. Sepn. of C_8 epimers
2. OsO_4
26
H H OH OH
H
$H_{11}C_5$
H
O
$(CH_2)_6CO_2CH_3$
HO HO H H
H
$H_{11}C_5$
H
O
$(CH_2)_6CO_2CH_3$
1. MsCl/Py
2. H_2O-Acetone (1:2) rt
O
CO_2CH_3
HO
HO H

21. Only the *cis* olefin is obtained. This is in contrast to the *exo*-bicyclo (3.1.0)hexane system in which a mixture of *cis* and *trans* olefins are obtained (see ref. 8).
22. PGE_3 is obtained by using $Br^- \phi_3P^+(CH_2)_2$—C≡C—C_2H_5 as the Wittig reagent. U. Axen, J. L. Thompson & J. E. Pike, *Chem. Commun.*, 602 (1970).
23. Unlike the *exo* series, the *endo*-bicyclo[3.1.0]hexane system exhibits a thermodynamic equilibrium which favors the α-isomer at C_8 (α:β=4:1) (see ref. 8). This is presumably due to the *endo* substituent which forces the ring system into a chair-like conformation.
24. PGE_2 is obtained by using $BrCH_2$—C≡C—$(CH_2)_3$—OTHP as the alkylating agent.
25. $PGF_{2\alpha}$ has also been made by this *endo*-bicyclo(3.1.0)hexane route. W. P. Schneider, *Chem. Commun.*, 304 (1969).
26. An improved *cis*-hydroxylation procedure using catalytic amount of OsO_4 and a tertiary amine oxide as the oxidant has been developed. V. Van Rheenen, R. C. Kelly & D. Y. Cha, *Tet. Lett.*, 1973 (1976).

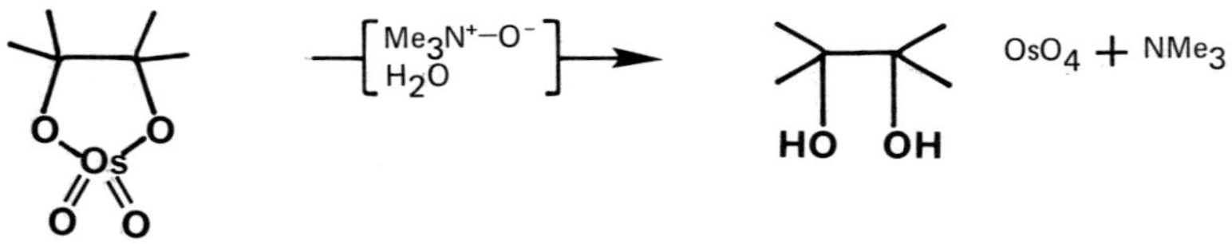

A similar method using catalytic OsO_4 and *t*-BuOOH as the oxidant has also been reported. K. Barry Sharpless, & K. Akashi, *J. Am. Chem. Soc.*, **98**, 1986 (1976).

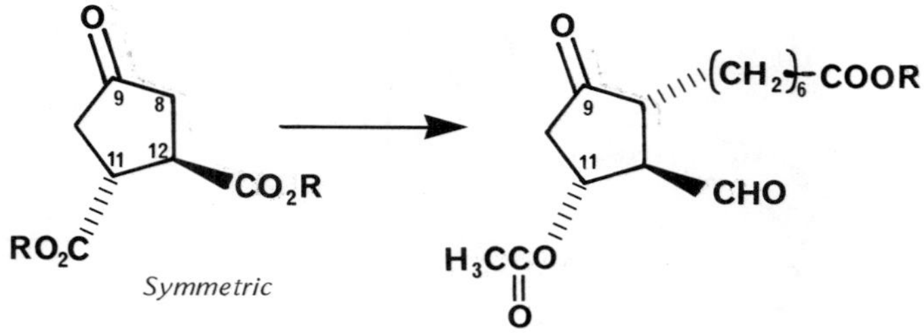

The Sakai synthesis [27] starts with the symmetric dicarboxylate ester of cyclopentanone [5]. Alkylation of the β-ketolactone gives the bicyclic intermediate [6]. Subsequent hydrolysis and decarboxylation gives the dissymmetric molecule [7] with the stable all *trans* orientation of the substituents around the cyclopentanone ring. The synthesis was then completed by known reaction sequences.

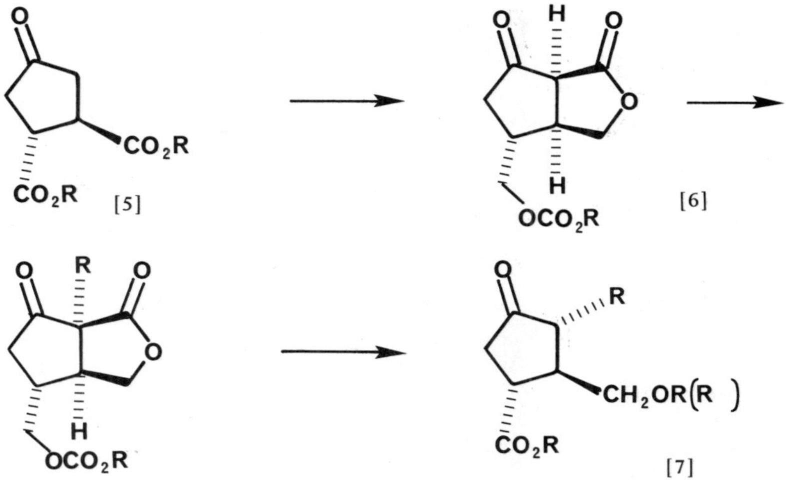

27. O. Oda & K. Sakai, *Tet. Lett.*, 3705 (1975).
O. Oda, K. Kojima & K. Sakai, *Tet. Lett.*, 3709 (1975).
K. Sakai, J. Ide & O. Oda, *Tet. Lett.*, 3021 (1975).

SYNTHETIC STRATEGY

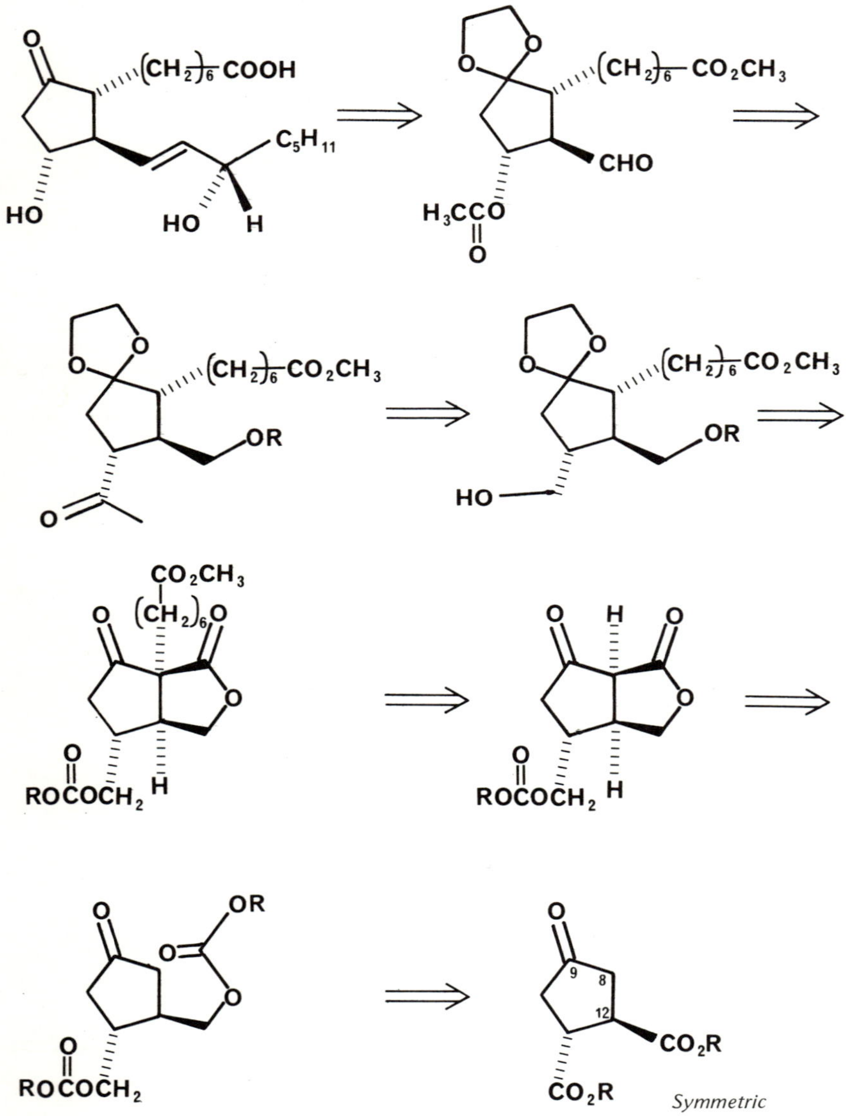

Symmetric intermediate

SYNTHETIC PLAN[27]

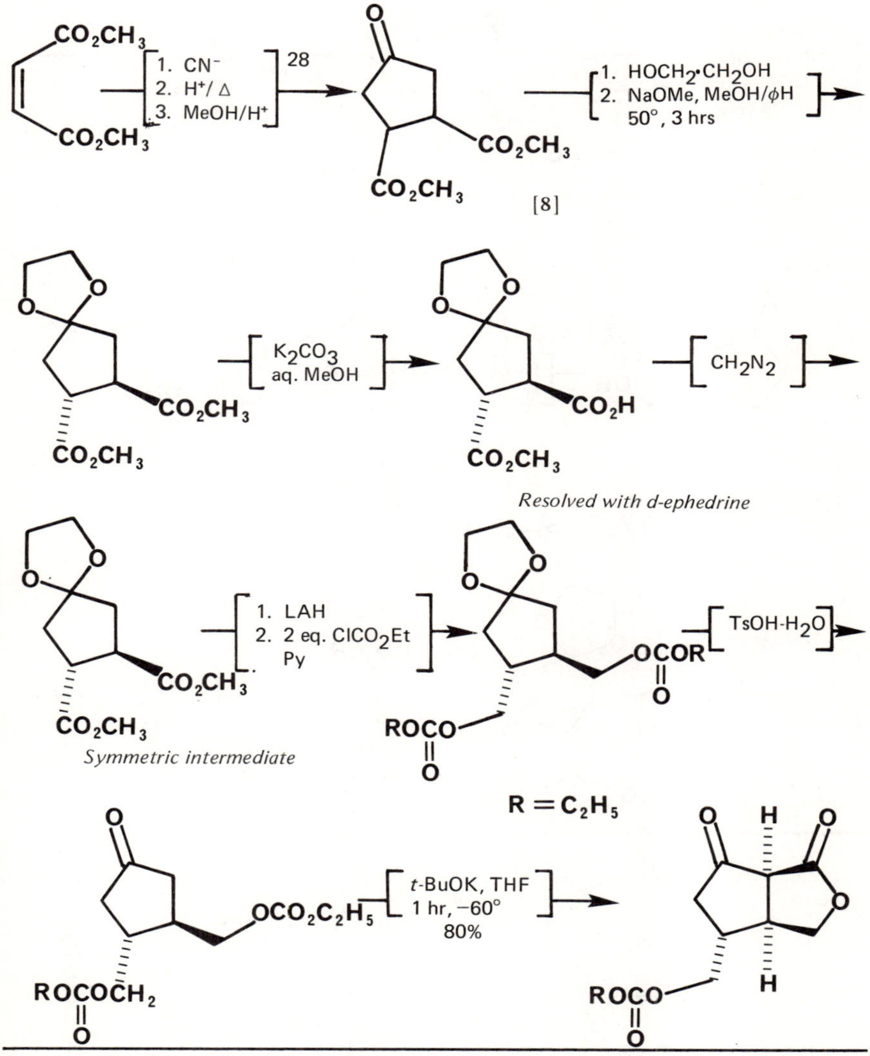

28. The cyclopentanone derivative [8] is obtained by the dimerization of dimethylmaleate by cyanide ion. S. Dolby, S. Esfandiari, C. Elliger & K. S. Marshall, *J. Org. Chem.*, **36**, 1277 (1971).

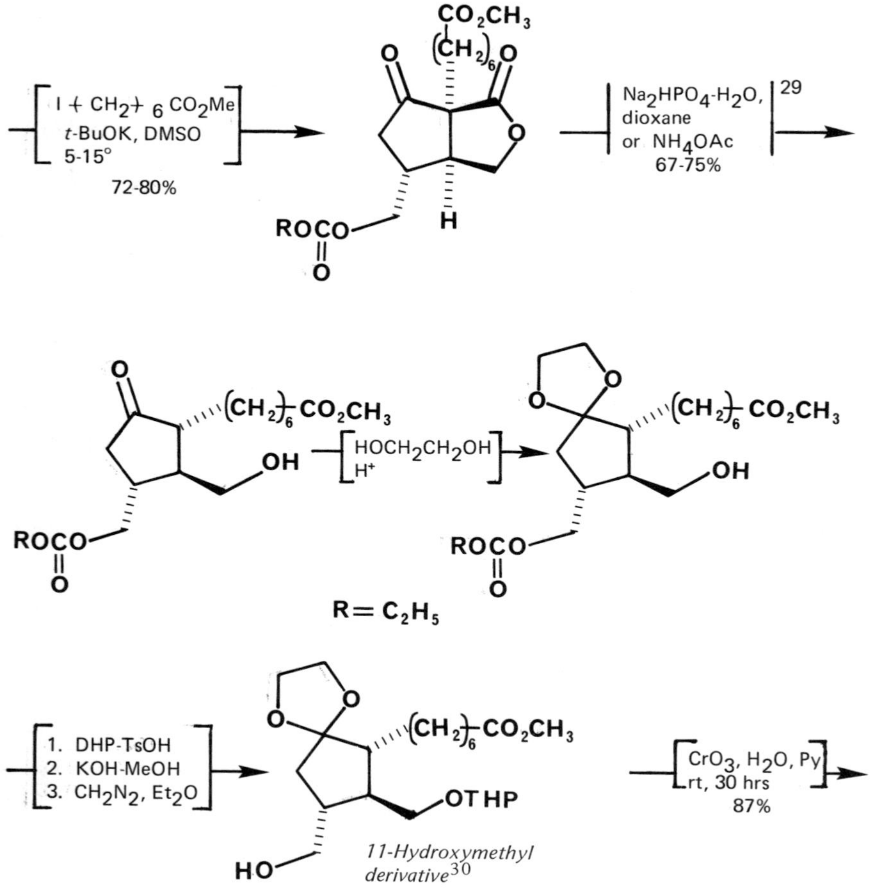

29. Comparatively stronger bases like K_2CO_3 or NaOMe in MeOH give undesired cleavage products.

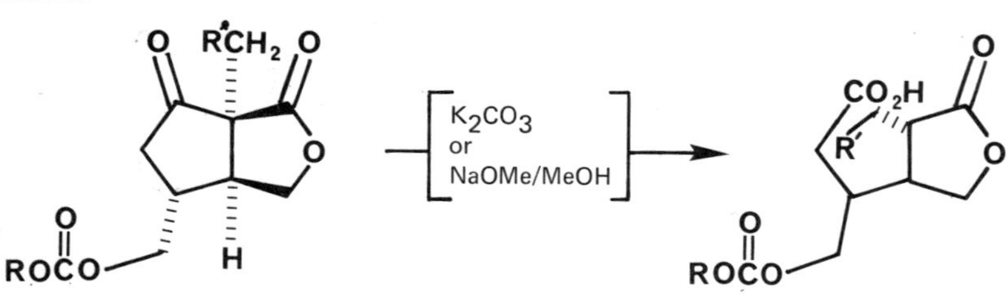

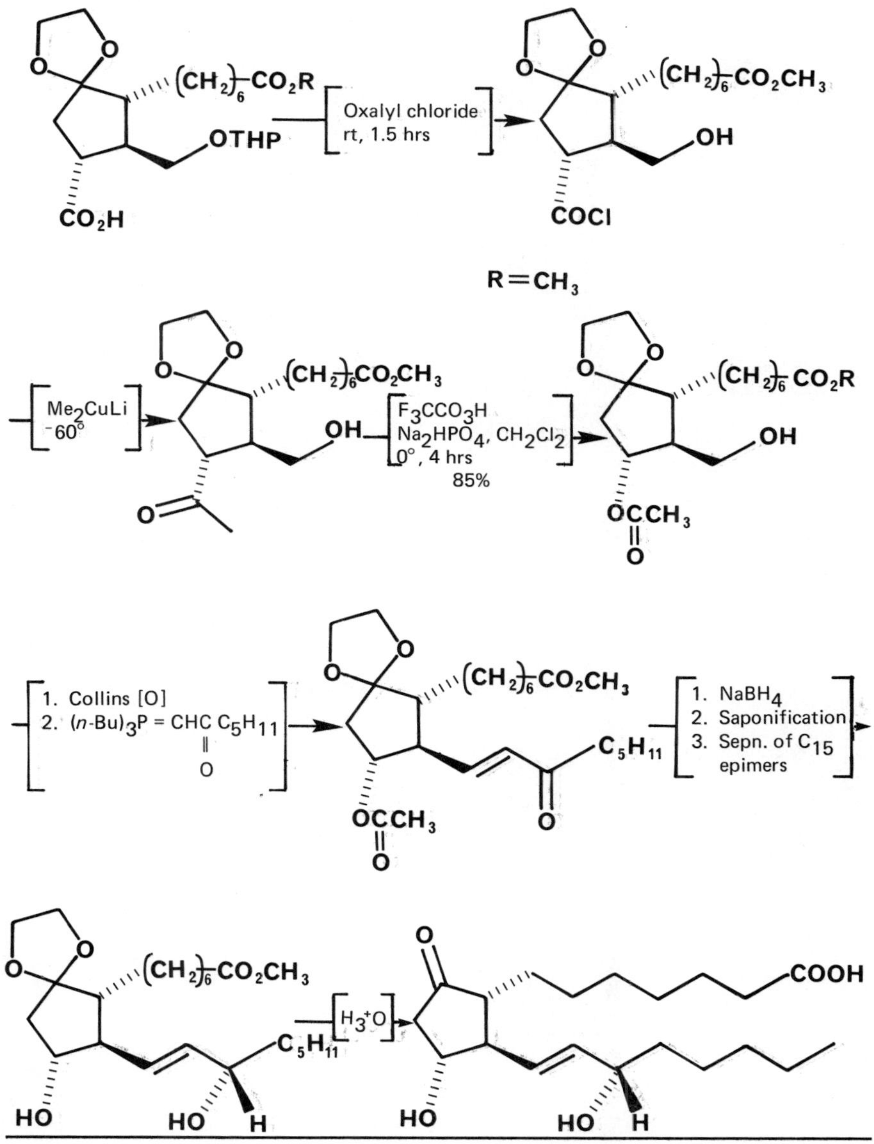

30. This intermediate has been converted to 11-hydroxymethyl PGs.

31. An alternative to this Baeyer-Villiger oxidation is the carboxyl inversion sequence used by Rosen. For details see p. 177.

3

Syntheses from Acyclic Precursors

C_{11}-C_{12} BOND FORMATION

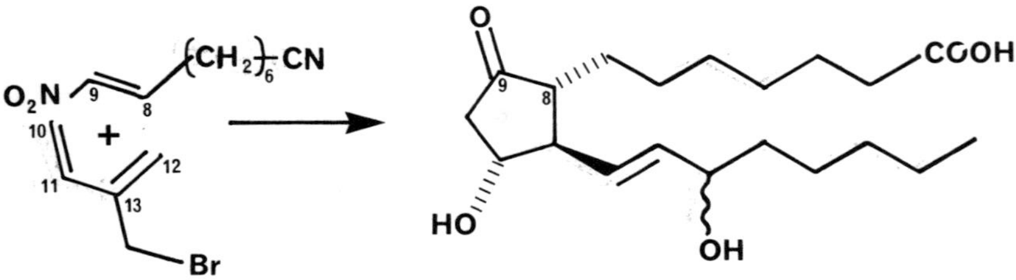

In the earlier nonstereospecific syntheses of PGE_1 the cyclopentane ring was constructed by aldol[1] or vinylogous aldol[2] condensation of the N protected amino- or nitro- aldehydes. The labile β-ketol (sensitive to both acid and base) was generated from the cyclized amino alcohol [**1**] under mild reaction conditions. This led to the desirable distinction between the C_9 and C_{11} functions, but required the development of newer methods for the amine to ketone conversation[3] shown in the following:

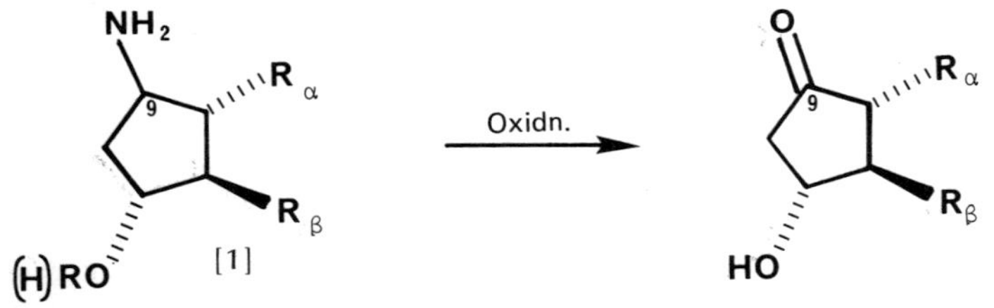

[1]

9-Amino prostanes *9-Keto prostanes*

1. E. J. Corey, N. H. Andersen, R. M. Carlson, J. Paust, E. Vedejs, I. Vlattas, R. E. K. Winter, *J. Am. Chem. Soc.*, **90**, 3245 (1968).
2. E. J. Corey, I. Vlattas & K. Harding, *J. Am. Chem. Soc.*, **91**, 535 (1969).
3. E. J. Corey, in *Proceedings of The Robert A. Welch Foundation on Chemical Synthesis*, 1968, p. 51.
4. H. Ruschig, W. Fritsch, J. Schmidt-Thome & W. Haade, *Ber.*, **88**, 883 (1955).

Methods for the Conversion of Primary Amines to Carbonyl Compounds

Ruschig-Type Oxidation[3,4]

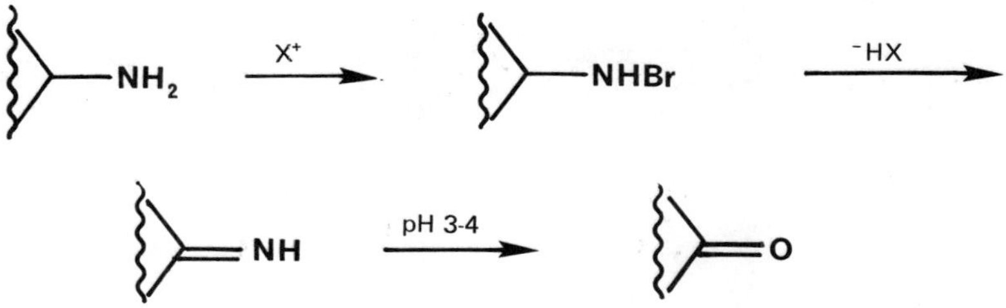

Schiff Base Tautomerization[3]

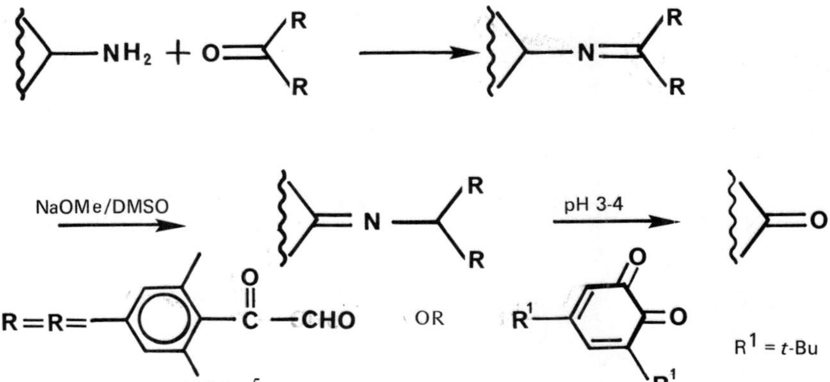

Oxidation by Argentic Salts:[5]

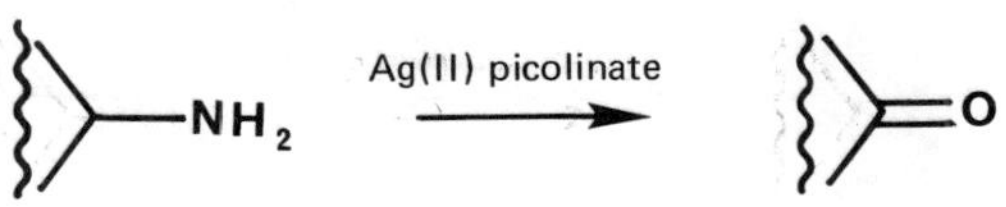

---

5. R. G. R. Bacon & W. J. N. Hanna, *J. Chem. Soc.*, 4962 (1965).

SYNTHETIC STRATEGY

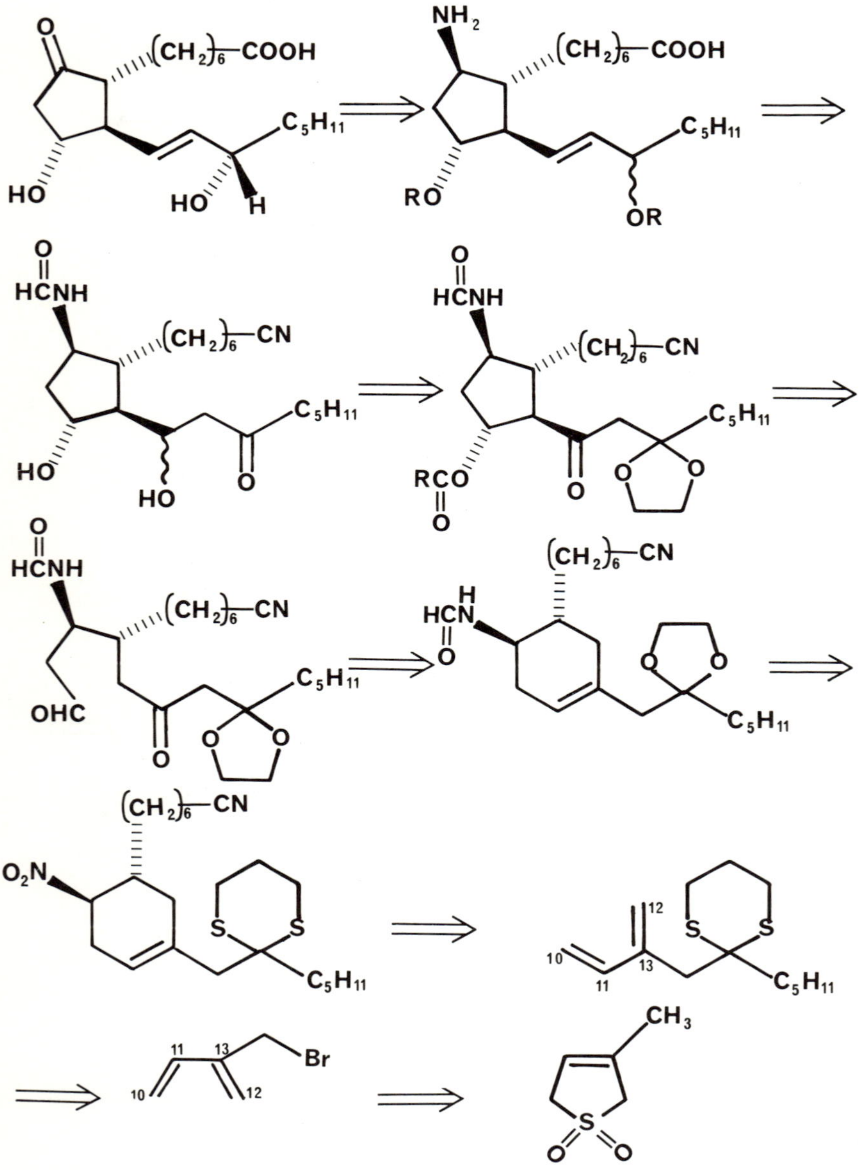

SYNTHETIC PLAN[1,3]

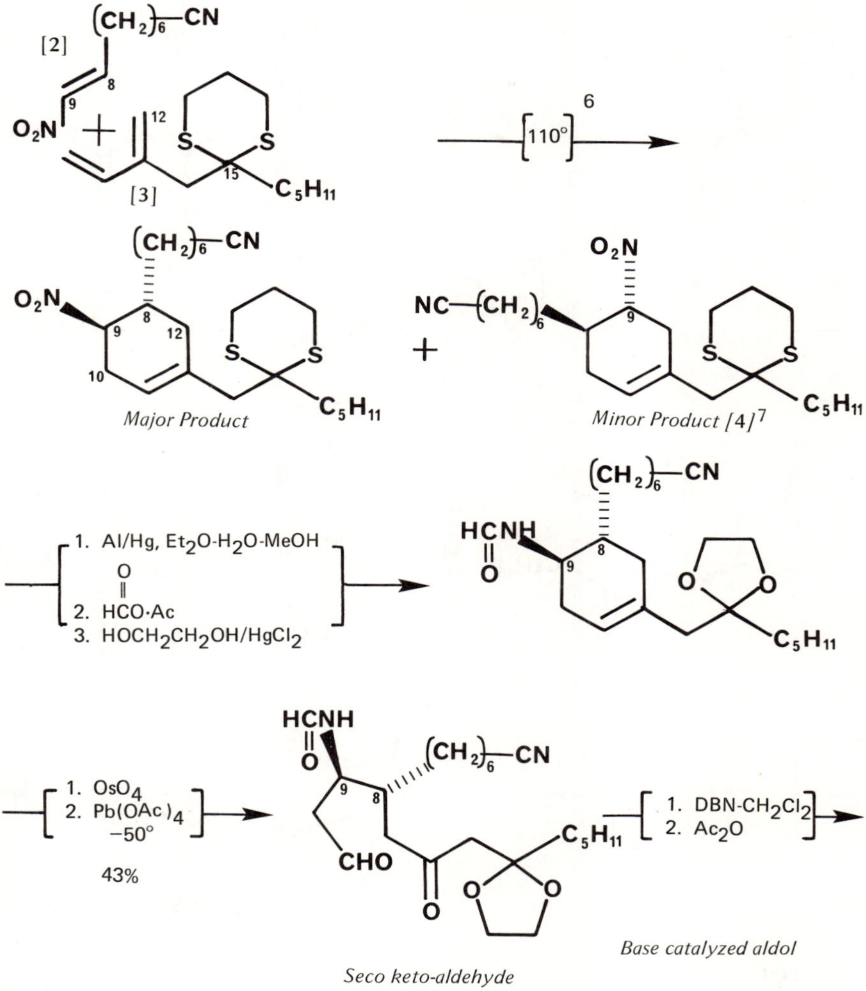

---

6. Lewis acid catalysis did not change the product composition.
7. The undesired isomer [4] was removed at the seco-aldehyde stage.

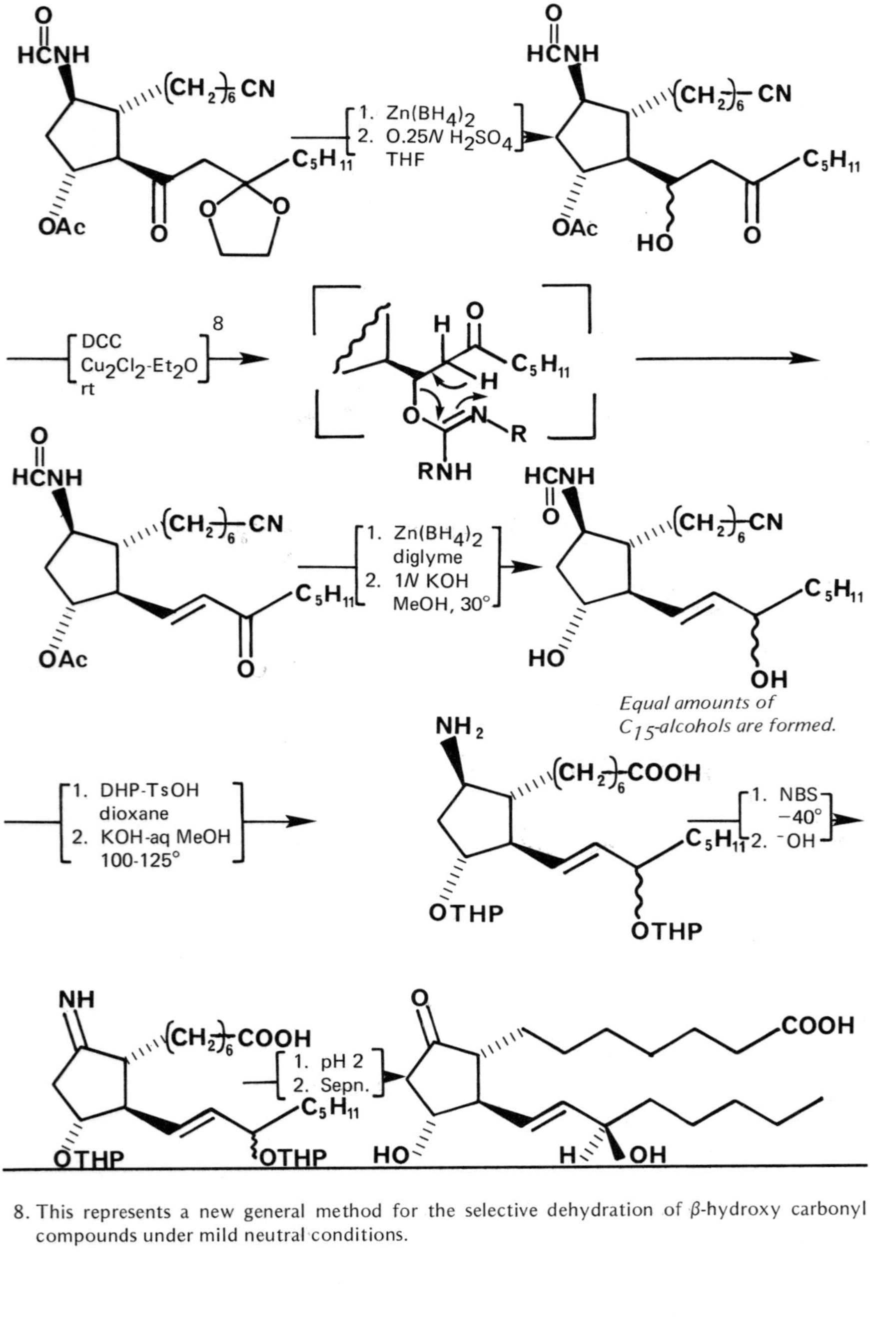

8. This represents a new general method for the selective dehydration of β-hydroxy carbonyl compounds under mild neutral conditions.

Synthesis of the Diene [3]

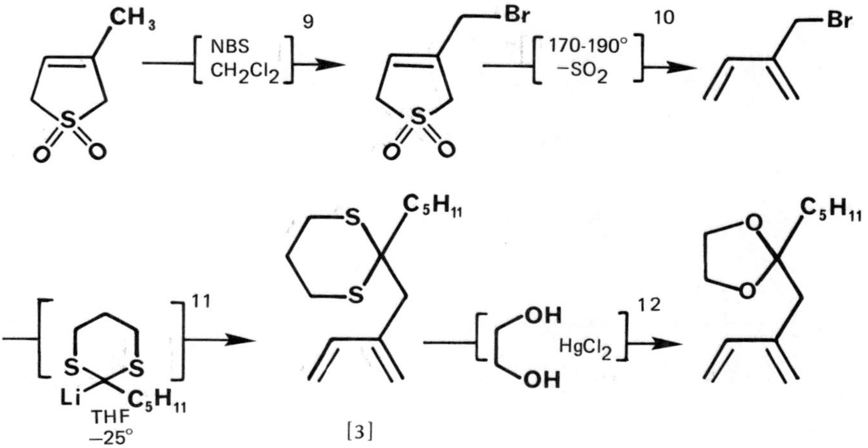

[3]

Synthesis of the Dienophile [2][13]

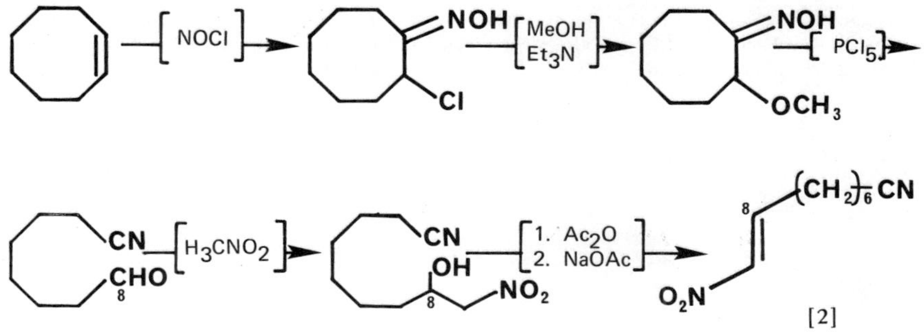

[2]

9. R. C. Krug & T. F. Yen, *J. Org. Chem.*, **21**, 1082 (1956).
10. This is a six electron linear cheletropic cycloreversion process. W. L. Mock, *J. Am. Chem. Soc.*, **88**, 2857 (1966) & S. D. McGregor & D. M. Lemal, *J. Am. Chem. Soc.*, **88**, 2858 (1966).
11. For a review on ACE (acyl carbanion equivalent) see D. Seebach, *Angew. Chem. [Int. Edit.]*, **8**, 639 (1969), and for recent examples and references see: J. E. Baldwin, G. A. Hofle, O. William Lever, Jr., *J. Am. Chem. Soc.*, **96**, 7125 (1974).
12. Even though both the dienes were available the use of the dithiane [3] seemed to be more satisfactory.
13. M. Ohno, N. Naruse, S. Torimitsu & I. Terasawa, *J. Am. Chem. Soc.*, **88**, 3168 (1966).

C_{11}-C_{12} BOND FORMATION

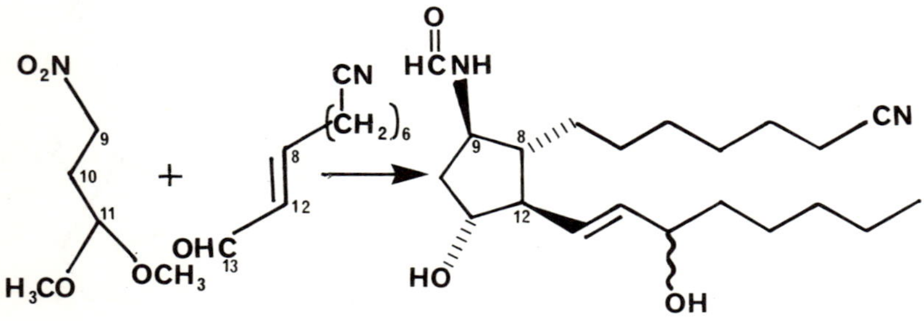

[6] [7] *Key Intermediate*

Vinylogous Aldol Route

The most important feature in the second synthesis of the key intermediate[14] is the use of a vinylogous aldol condensation for the construction of the cyclopentane ring. The acyclic unit [5] is made by the Michael addition of the nitro acetal [6] to the unsaturated aldehyde [7] with the remaining β-chain being introduced by the Horner-Emmons modification of the Wittig reaction.

---

14. E. J. Corey, I. Vlattas & K. Harding, *J. Am. Chem. Soc.*, **91**, 535 (1969).

SYNTHETIC STRATEGY

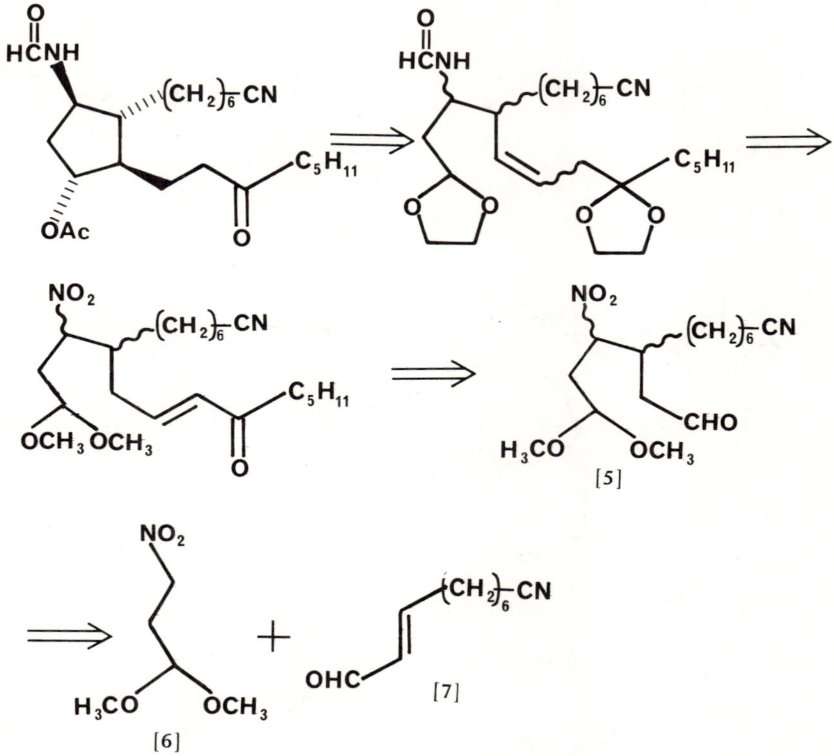

SYNTHETIC PLAN[14]

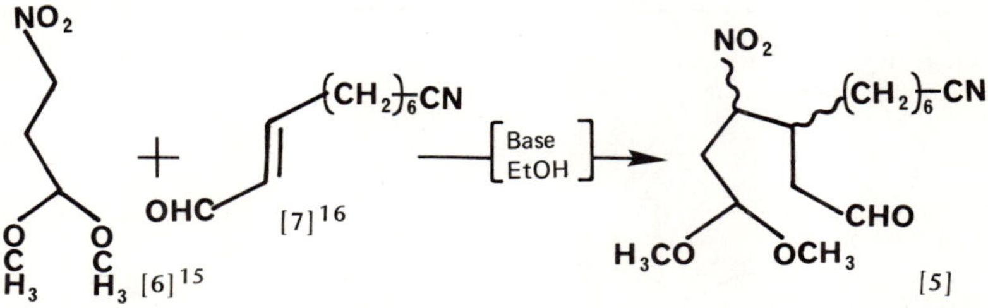

15. N. Kornblum, *et al.*, *J. Am. Chem. Soc.*, **78**, 1497 (1956).
16. W. Nagata & Y. Hayase, *Tet. Lett.*, 4359 (1968).

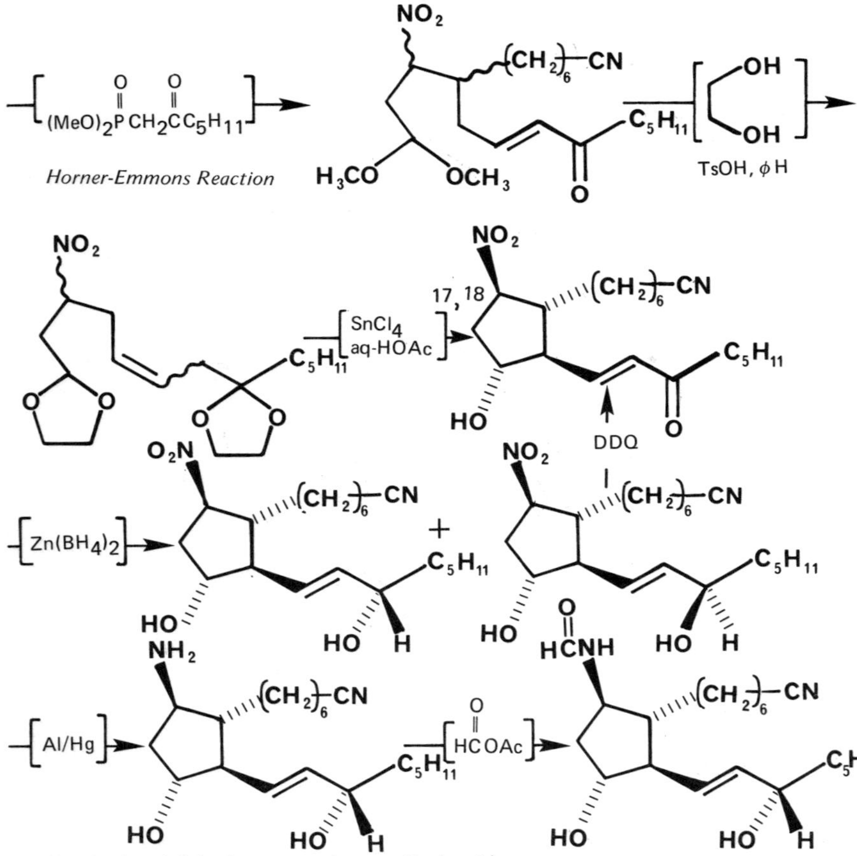

Resolved with (−)-α-bromocamphor-π-sulfonic acid

---

17. The amounts of C_{11} epimer formed depends on the experimental conditions.
18. Attempts to do a base-catalyzed aldol condensation led to the elimination of the -NO_2 group to give the α,β-unsaturated aldehyde [9].

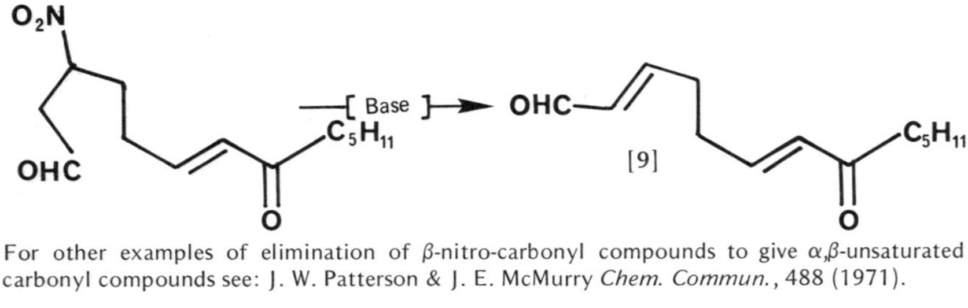

For other examples of elimination of β-nitro-carbonyl compounds to give α,β-unsaturated carbonyl compounds see: J. W. Patterson & J. E. McMurry *Chem. Commun.*, 488 (1971).

In an earlier approach[19] the vinylogous aldol condensation was done on the N-formylamino protected compound [8].

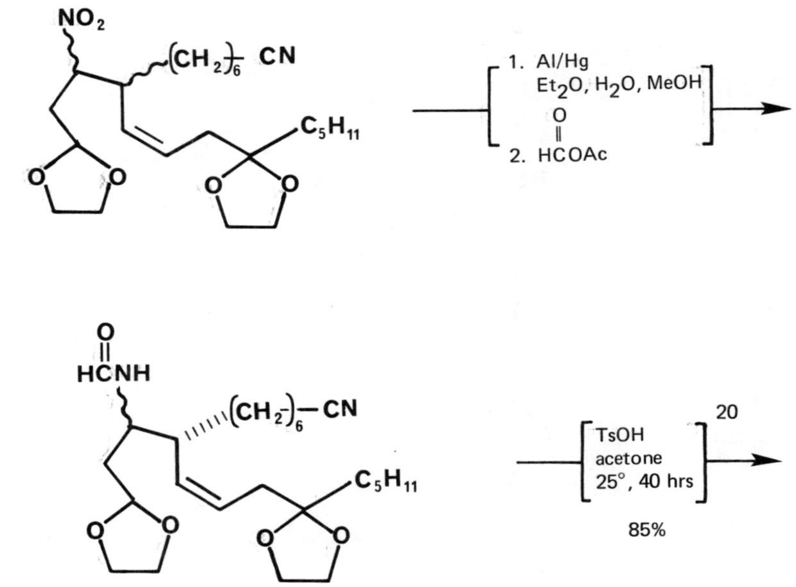

[8]

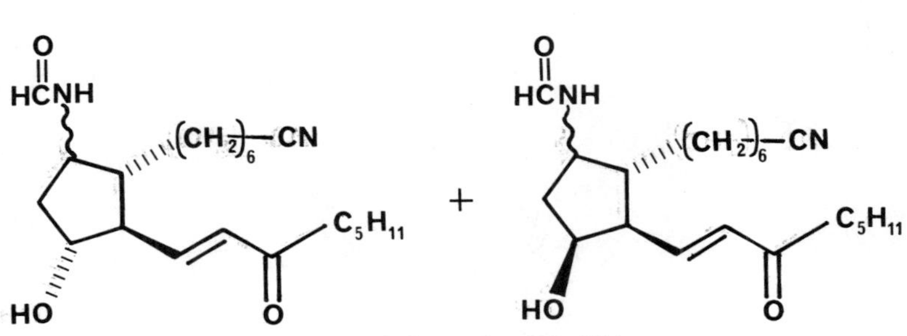

1 : 1 *85%*

19. E. J. Corey, I. Vlattas, N. H. Andersen & K. Harding, *J. Am. Chem. Soc.*, **90**, 3247 (1968).
20. Four percent H_2SO_4 in THF-H_2O (1:1) at 25° C and 24 hrs. gave twice as much of the undesired C_{11}-β epimer as the desired C_{11}-α product.

The third shorter synthesis of the intermediate [9] is limited by the low yield in the Wittig reaction.[21] In the first unusual step an ylid is used as the carbon electrophile rather than a nucleophile.

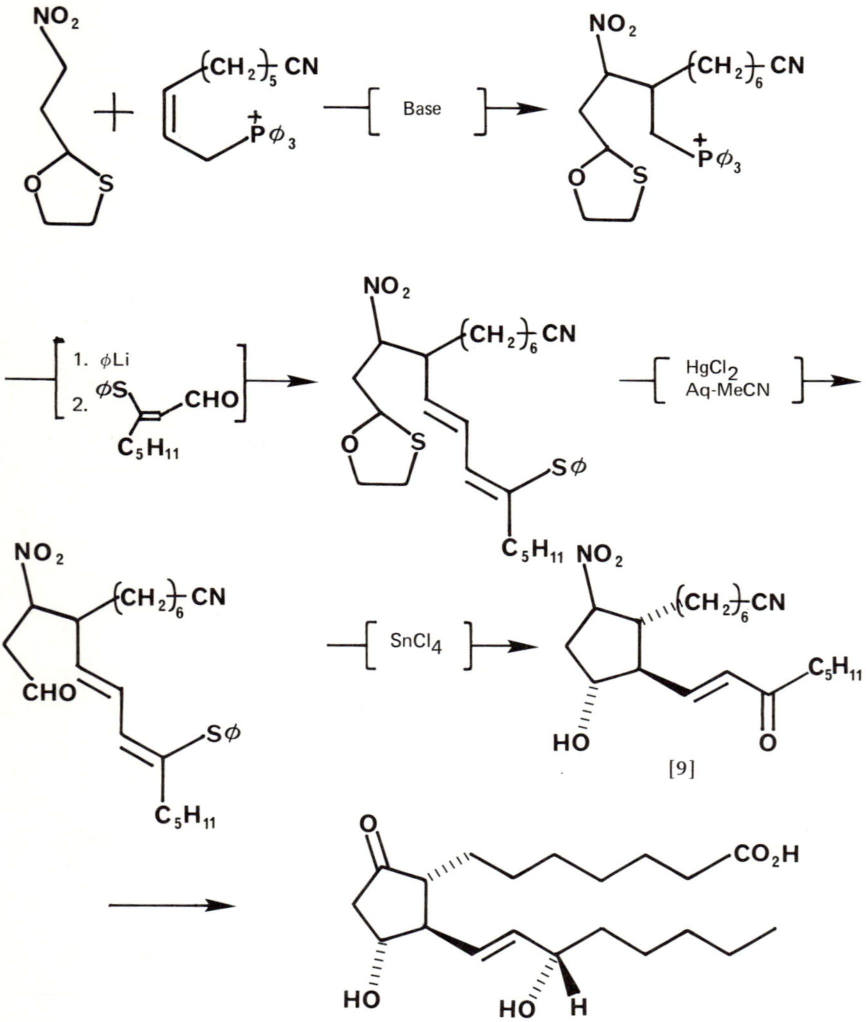

21. E. J. Corey in "Prostaglandins," *Annals of the New York Academy of Sciences*, P. Ramwell & J. E. Shaw (eds.), 1971, **180**, 24.

C_8-C_{12} BOND FORMATION

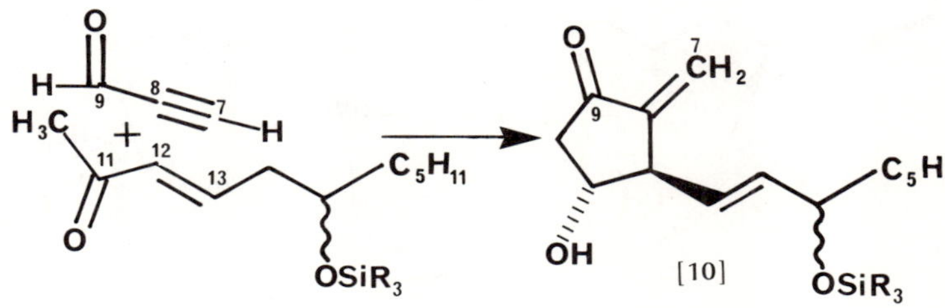

[10]

Of the various methods to construct the cyclopentane ring the Stork-Kraus approach[22] uses a novel application of the intramolecular ene reaction[23] to synthesize the enone [**10**] which has also been made by a different route.[24] Another interesting feature of the ene reaction is that it generates the C_{13}-C_{14} *trans* double bond.

---

22. G. Stork & G. Kraus, *J. Am. Chem. Soc.*, **98**, 6747 (1976).
23. Similar applications of the ene reaction are known.

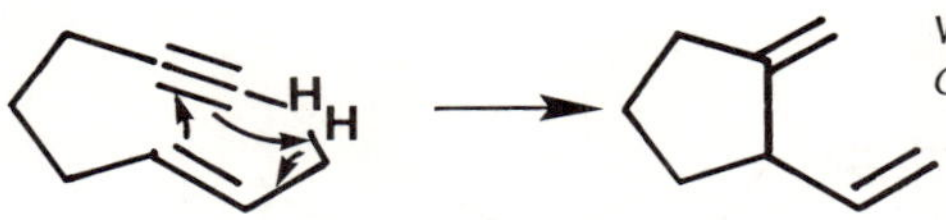

W. D. Huntsman & R. P. Hall, *J. Org. Chem.*, **27**, 1988 (1962).

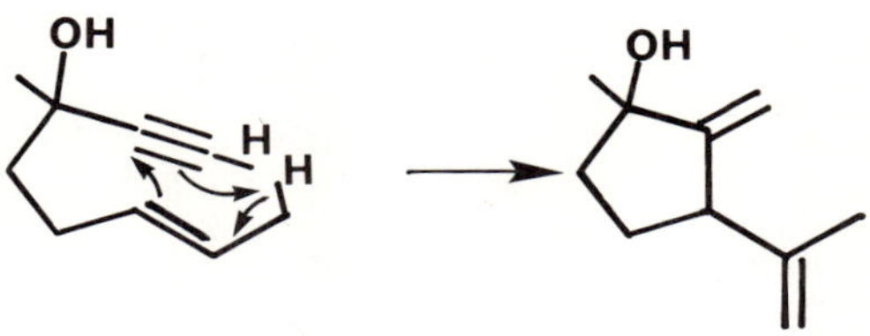

P. Naegli & R. Kaiser, *Tet. Lett.*, 2013 (1972).

24. G. Stork & M. Isobe, *J. Am. Chem. Soc.*, **97**, 4745 (1975); G. Stork & M. Isobe, *J. Am. Chem. Soc.*, **97**, 6260 (1975).

SYNTHETIC STRATEGY

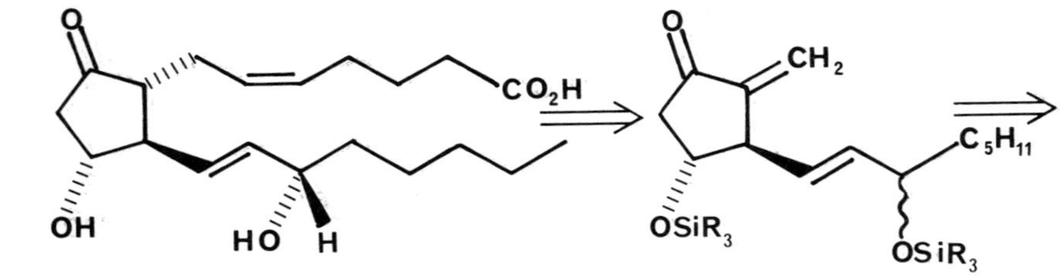

[10]

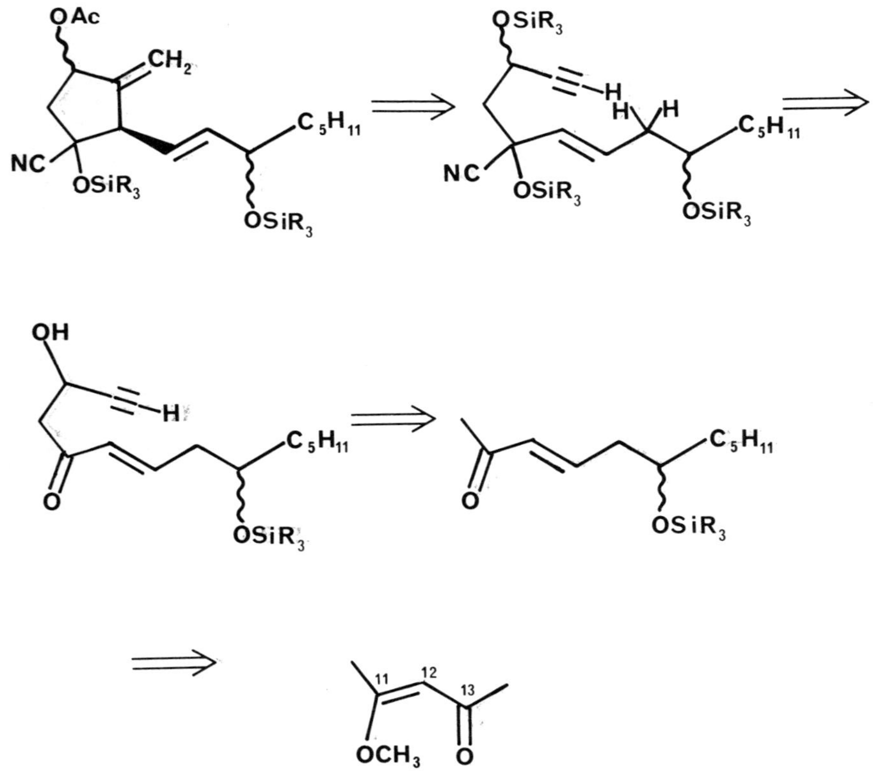

SYNTHETIC PLAN[22]

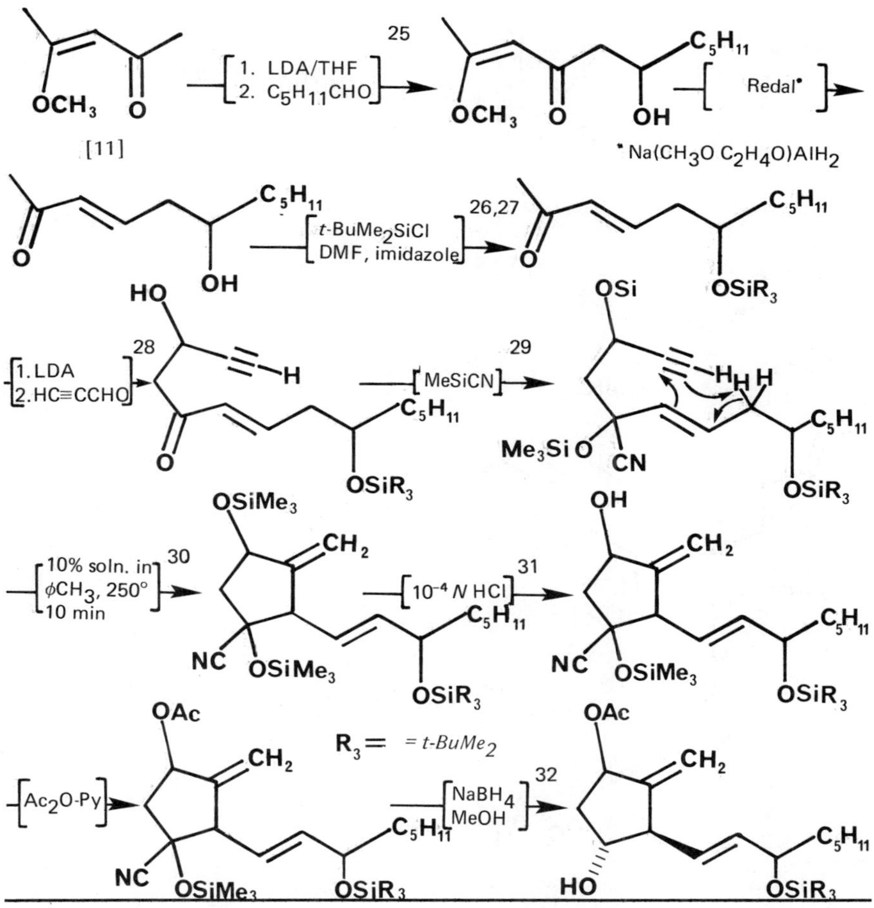

25. Trapping of kinetic enolates of vinylogous esters like [11] with carbonyl compounds was developed at Columbia University. G. Stork & G. Kraus, *J. Am. Chem. Soc.*, **98**, 2351 (1976).
26. E. J. Corey & A. Venkateswarlu, *J. Am. Chem. Soc.*, **94**, 6190 (1972).
27. The preservation of the C_{15} oxygen function during the thermal ene reaction necessitates the use of the bulky *tert*-butyldimethylsilyl protecting group rather than the trimethylsilyl protecting group.
28. G. Stork, G. Kraus & G. Garcia, *J. Org. Chem.*, **39**, 3459 (1974).
29. D. A. Evans, L. K. Truesdale & G. L. Carroll, *Chem. Commun.*, **55**, (1973).
30. For a review on the ene reaction, see H. M. R. Hoffmann, *Angew. Chem. [Int. Edit.]*, **8**, 556 (1969).

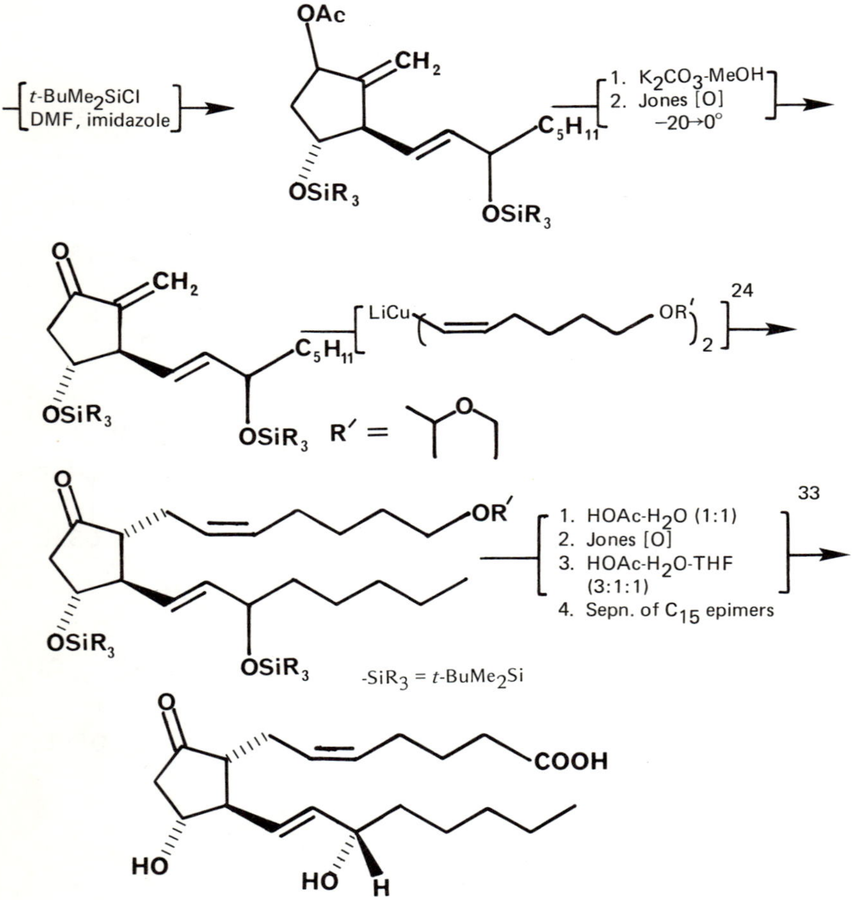

---

31. The C_9 silyl ether is selectively hydrolyzed. The slower rate of hydrolysis of the silylated cyanohydrin may be either due to steric hindrance to hydrolysis or a rate determining oxygen protonation step in this case or both.
32. The masking of the C_{11} carbonyl group as the O-trimethylsilyl protected cyanohydrin serves the important purpose of subsequent *in-situ* generation of the unstable β,γ-unsaturated ketone during the sodium borohydride reduction which stereoselectively produces the required *trans*-2-alkylcyclopentanol system. *Trans:cis* = 80:20. The separation is postponed to the last stage.
33. The C_{11} C_{12} *cis*-isomer is separated now.

C_8-C_{12} BOND FORMATION

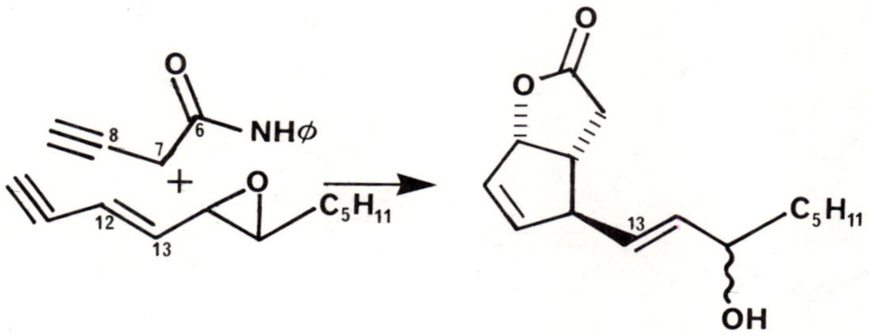

Corey's biogenetically related approach[34] to the synthesis of the PGA_2 precursor demonstrated the first application of the pentadienyl→cyclopentenyl cation process to the synthesis of a natural product.[35] The amide function is a potential neighboring group in the intermediate allylic cation [12] and stereospecifically delivers the C_9 oxygen *cis* to the C_8 substituent.

It has subsequently been shown that the epoxide does not give PGE_1 when treated with BSVM, as shown in the following: R. Sood, M. Nagasawa, & C. J. Sih, *Tet. Lett.*, 423 (1974).

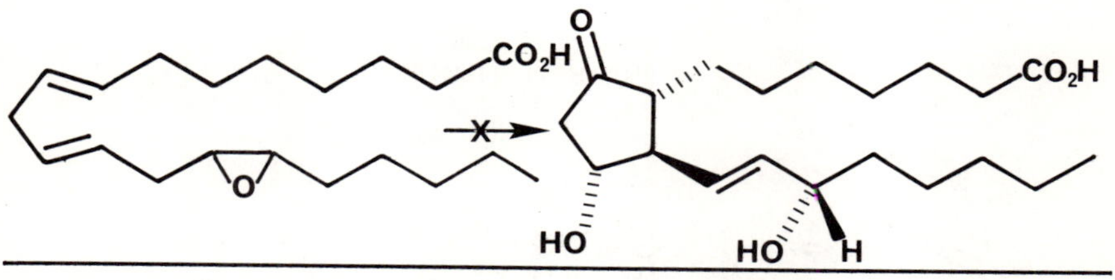

---

34. E. J. Corey, W. J. Fleet & M. Kato, *Tet. Lett.*, 3963 (1973).
35. N. C. Deno, C. U. Pittman, Jr. & J. O. Turner, *J. Am. Chem. Soc.*, **87**, 2153 (1965).

SYNTHETIC STRATEGY

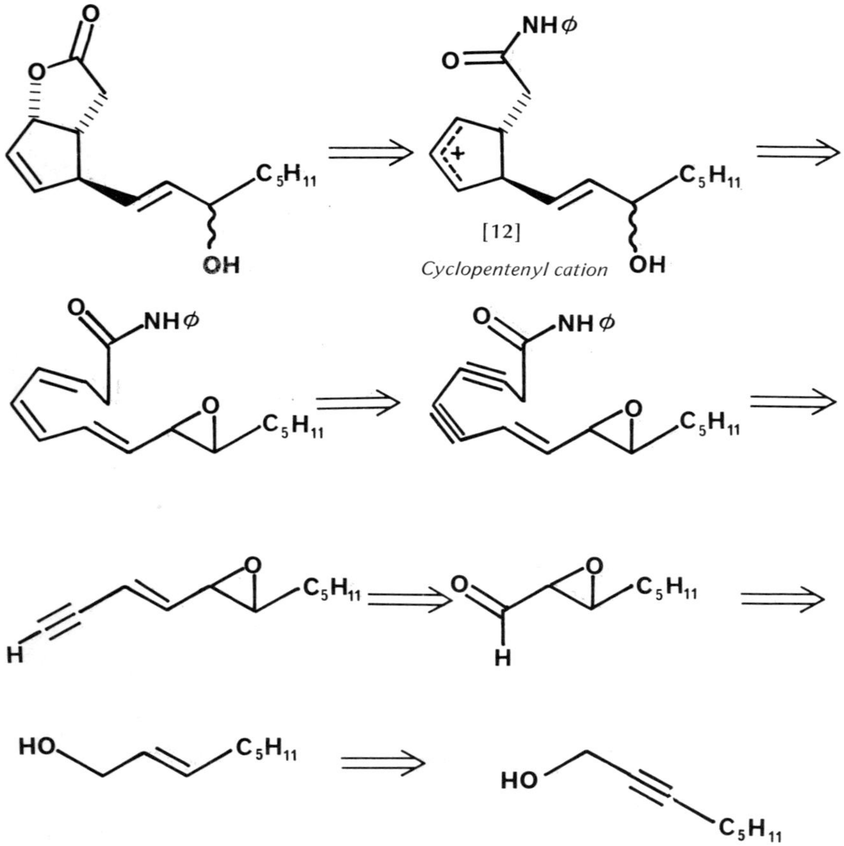

[12]
Cyclopentenyl cation

SYNTHETIC PLAN[34]

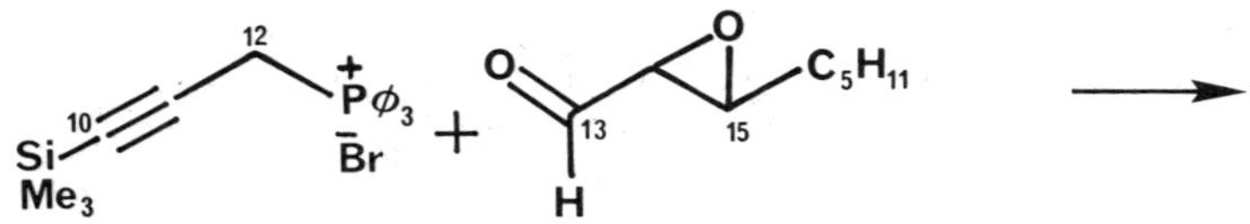

[13] [14]

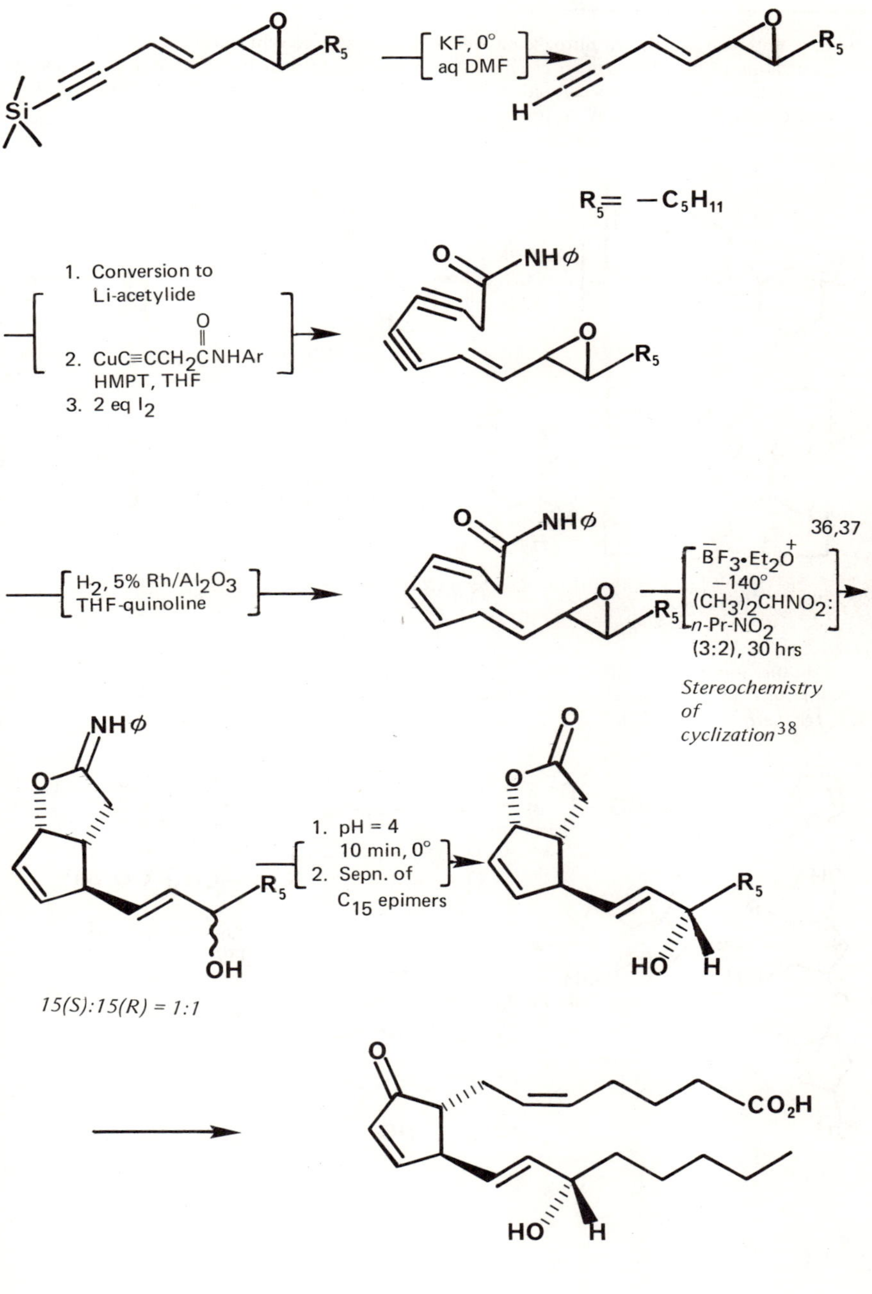

Si
KF, 0°
aq DMF
H
R5
R5 = —C5H11
1. Conversion to Li-acetylide
2. CuC≡CCH2CNHAr
HMPT, THF
3. 2 eq I2
NHφ
H2, 5% Rh/Al2O3
THF-quinoline
36,37
BF3•Et2O
−140°
(CH3)2CHNO2:
n-Pr-NO2
(3:2), 30 hrs
Stereochemistry of cyclization38
1. pH = 4
10 min, 0°
2. Sepn. of
C15 epimers
OH
HO H
15(S):15(R) = 1:1
CO2H

---

36. It is not clear whether a nitroalkane which is used as a solvent participates in the cationic cyclization or not. Johnson, *et al.*, have shown that the nitroalkane which is used as a solvent can trap an intermediary carbonium ion to give an oximino ether. D. R. Morton, M. B. Gravestock, R. J. Parry & W. S. Johnson, *J. Am. Chem. Soc.*, 95, 4417 (1973).

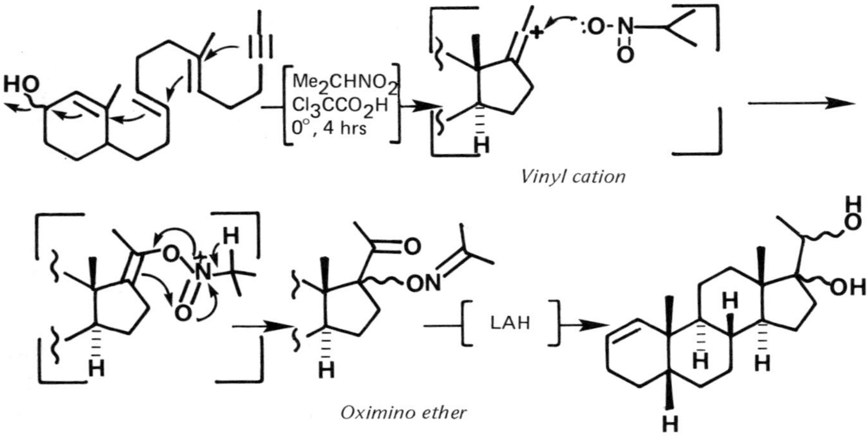

37. Another synthesis involving the pentadienyl cyclopentenyl process has been reported. The intermediate pentadienyl cation undergoes a conrotatory closure.[38] G. Piancatelli & A. Sceltri, *Tet. Lett.*, 1131 (1977).

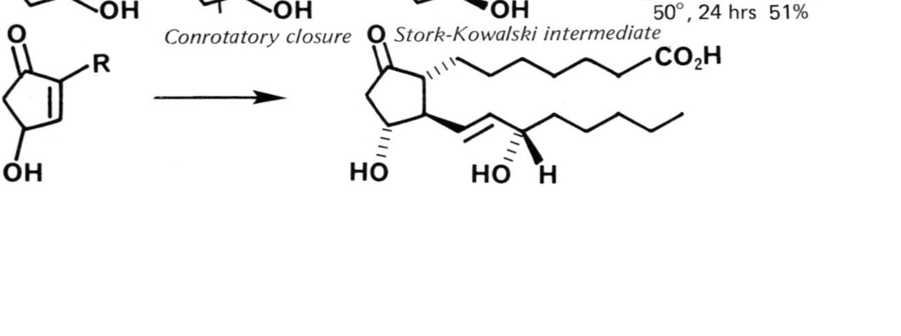

Synthesis of the Phosphonium Salt [13]

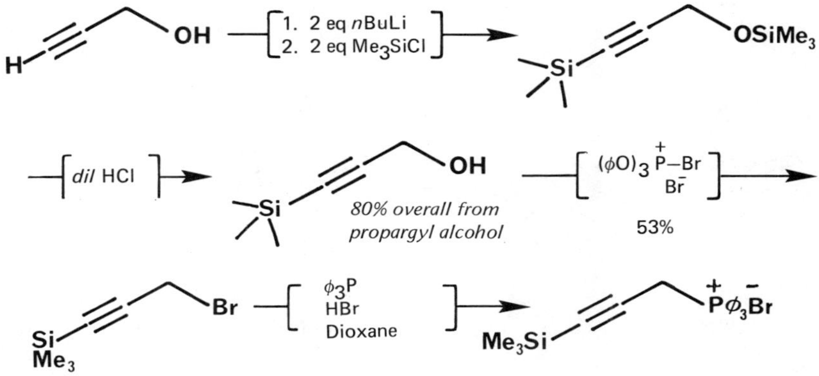

[13]

Synthesis of the Epoxy-aldehyde [14]

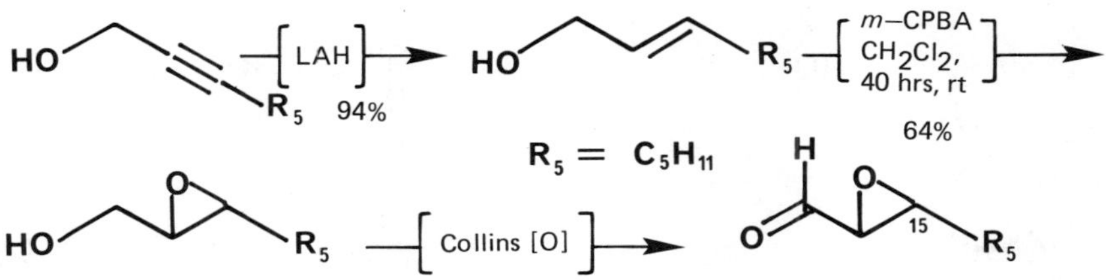

[14]

Stereochemistry of Cyclization[38]

If the reaction is concerted and controlled by orbital symmetry, only the conformation in which the C_{11}-C_{12} bond is S-*cis* should lead to the desired *trans* product. Apparently the more crowded conformation [15] must lead to a lower energy transition state (probably because it leads to the more stable product).

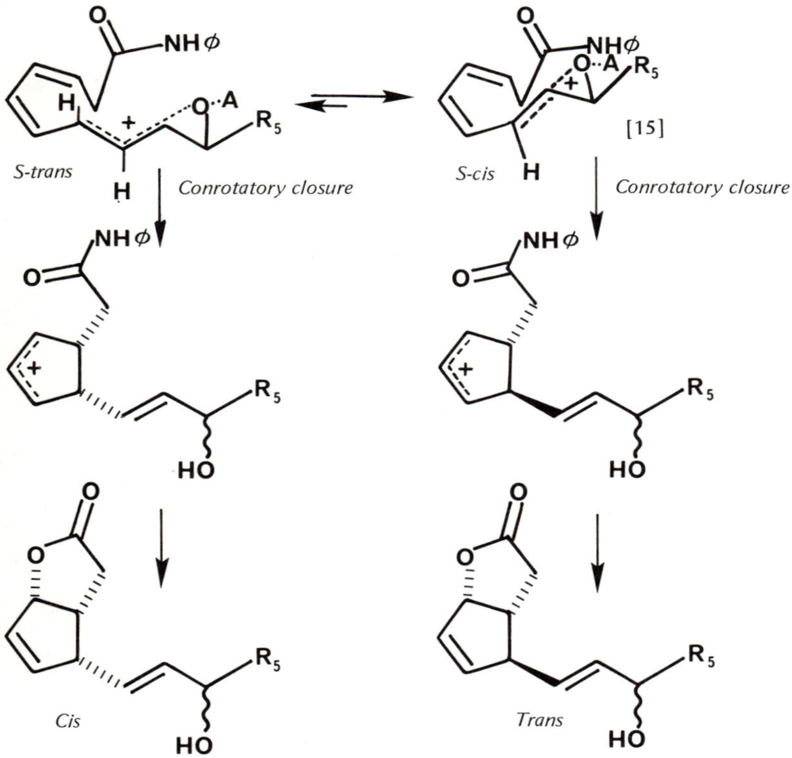

Conrotatory closure

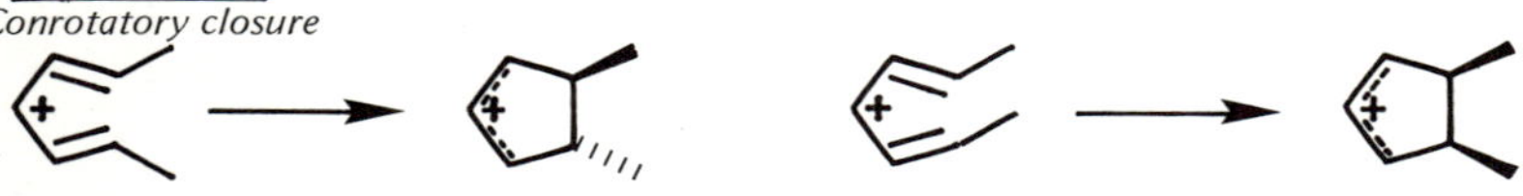

38. R. B. Woodward & R. Hoffmann in "The Conservation of Orbital Symmetry," Verlag Chemie GmbH, Weinheim 1970, p. 58.

C_8-C_{12} BOND FORMATION

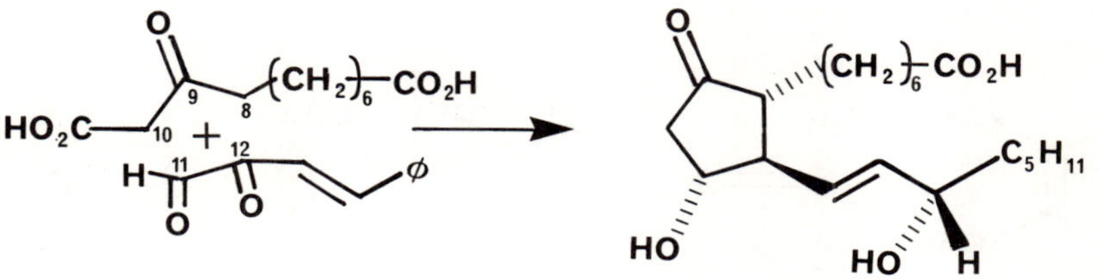

Adaptation of the classical cinerolone[39] synthesis to prostaglandin synthesis would lead to a 3-vinylcyclopentenone. The problem then becomes one of saturating the ring double bond while keeping the external one. A solution to this problem is illustrated in this synthesis.[40,41,42]

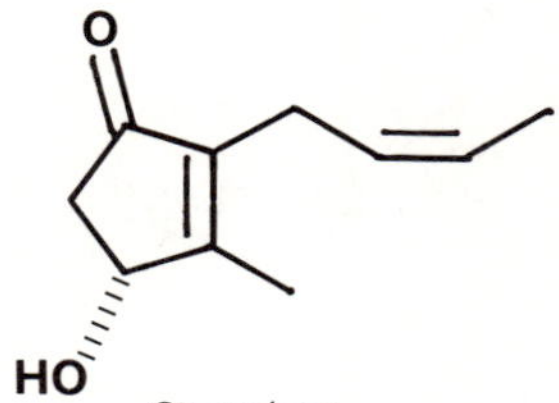

Cinerolone

---

39. "Chemistry of the Natural Pyrethrins" by L. Crombie & M. Eliot in L. Zeichmeister (ed.) *Progress in the Chemistry of Organic Natural Products*, **19**, 120 (1961).
    See also the references cited in: R. F. Romanet & R. H. Schlessinger, *J. Am. Chem. Soc.*, **96**, 3701 (1974).
40. M. Miyano & M. A. Stealey, *Chem. Commun.*, 180 (1973).
41. M. Miyano, C. R. Dorn & R. A. Mueller, *J. Org. Chem.*, **37**, 1810 (1972).
42. For a general review, see M. Miyano, R. A. Mueller & C. R. Dorn, *Intra-Science Chem. Rept.*, **6**, 43 (1972).

SYNTHETIC STRATEGY

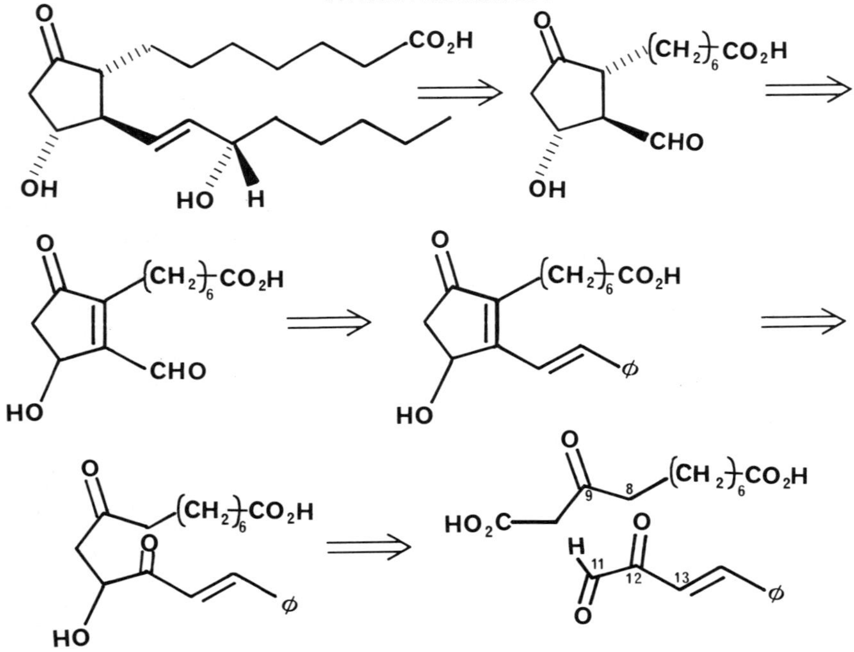

SYNTHETIC PLAN[40,41,42]

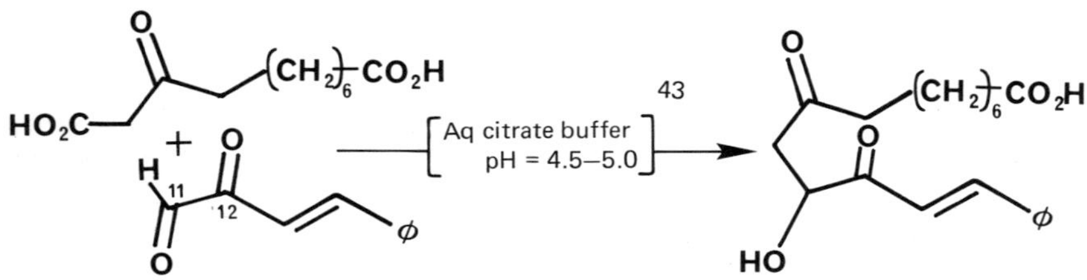

---

43. Similar condensations between pyruvic aldehyde and 3-keto acids are known. M. S. Schechter, N. Green & F. B. LaForge, *J. Am. Chem. Soc.*, 71, 3165 (1949).

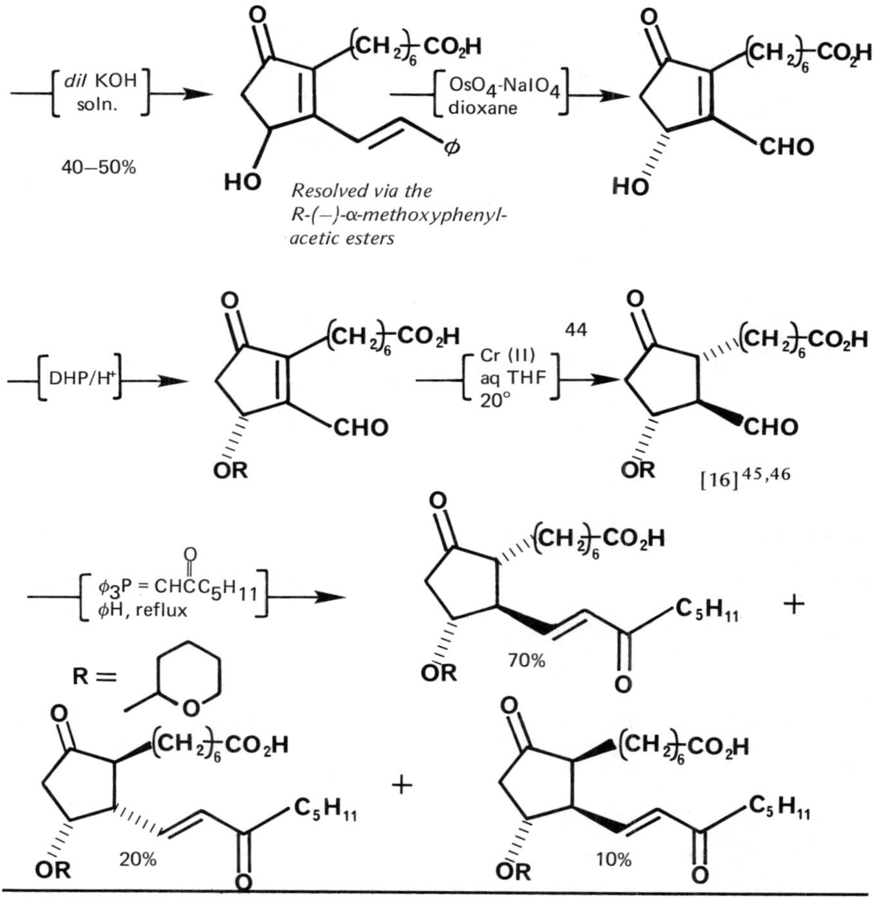

44. In the earlier approach [M. Miyano, C. R. Dorn & R. A. Mueller, *J. Org. Chem.*, 37, 1810 (1972)] Zn/HOAc was used, but gave poor results.

45. This aldehyde is assumed to exist as a mixture of cyclic hydrates like [17].

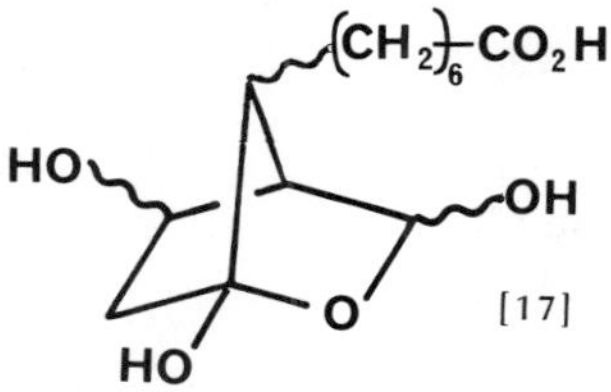

[17]

46. The 8-epi and 8, 12-bis epi compounds are also present as minor components.

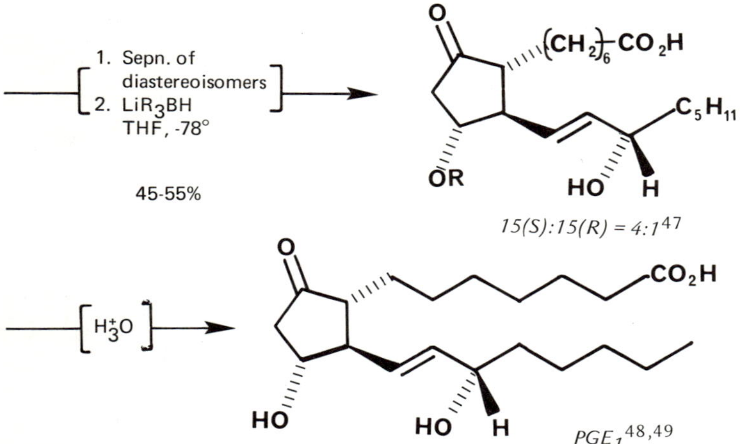

15(S):15(R) = 4:1[47]

PGE1[48,49]

LiR$_3$BH = Thexyltetrahydro limonyl lithium borohydride

47. E. J. Corey, S. M. Albonico, U. Koelliker, T. K. Schaaf & R. K. Varma, *J. Am. Chem. Soc.*, **93**, 1491 (1971).
48. For the synthesis of 15-dehydro PGB$_1$ see:
    M. Miyano, *J. Org. Chem.*, **35**, 2314 (1970); and
    M. Miyano, *Tet. Lett.*, 2771 (1969).
49. For the synthesis of 8,12-dehydro PGE$_1$ see:
    M. Miyano & C. R. Dorn, *J. Org. Chem.*, **37**, 1818 (1972).

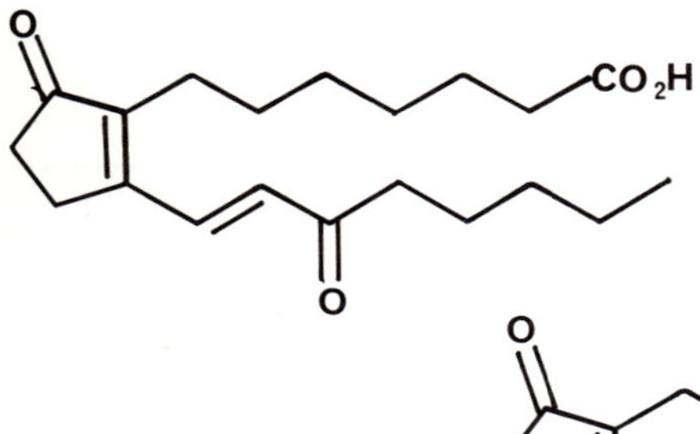

15-dehydro-PGB$_1$

8, 12-dehydro-PGE$_1$

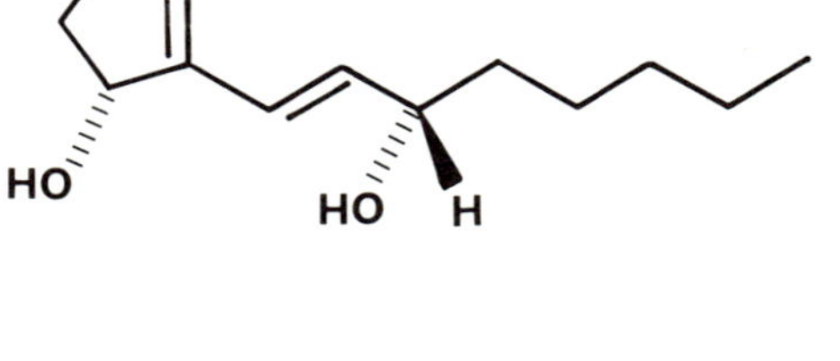

C_8-C_{12} BOND FORMATION

The Sakai approach[50] is based on the general synthesis of cinerelones.

SYNTHETIC STRATEGY

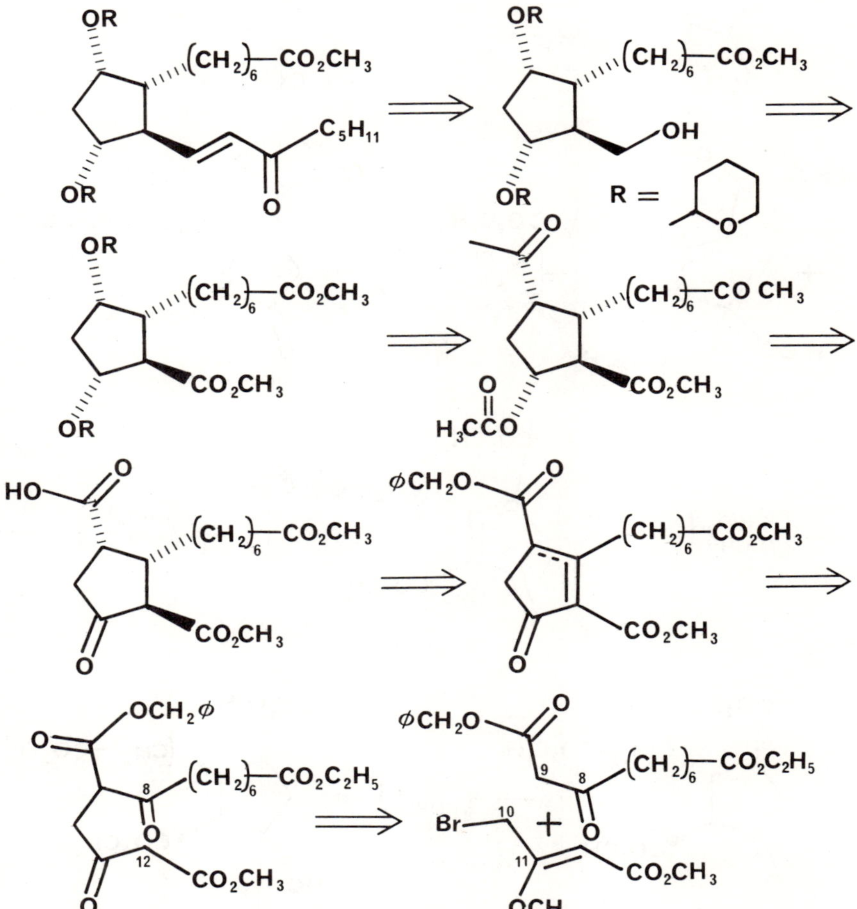

50. K. Kojima & K. Sakai, *Tet. Lett.*, 3333 (1972).

SYNTHETIC PLAN[50]

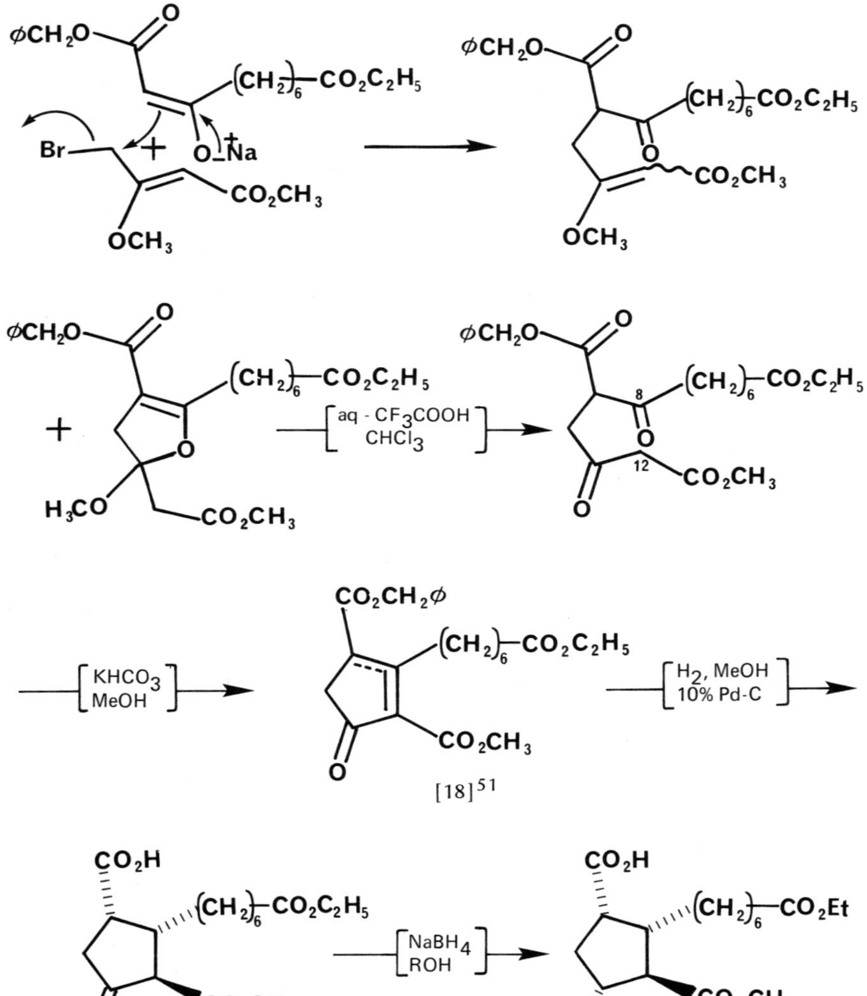

[18][51]

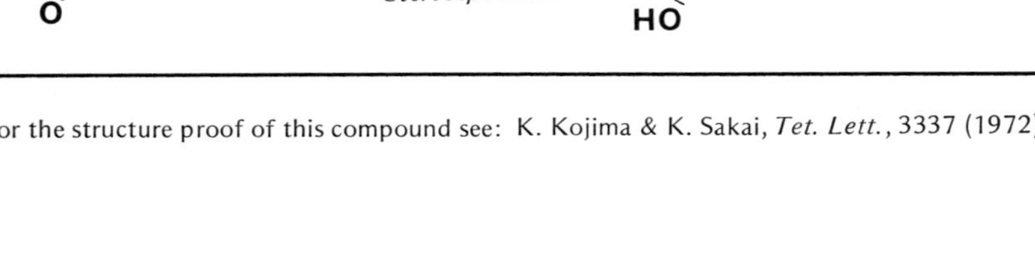

51. For the structure proof of this compound see: K. Kojima & K. Sakai, *Tet. Lett.*, 3337 (1972).

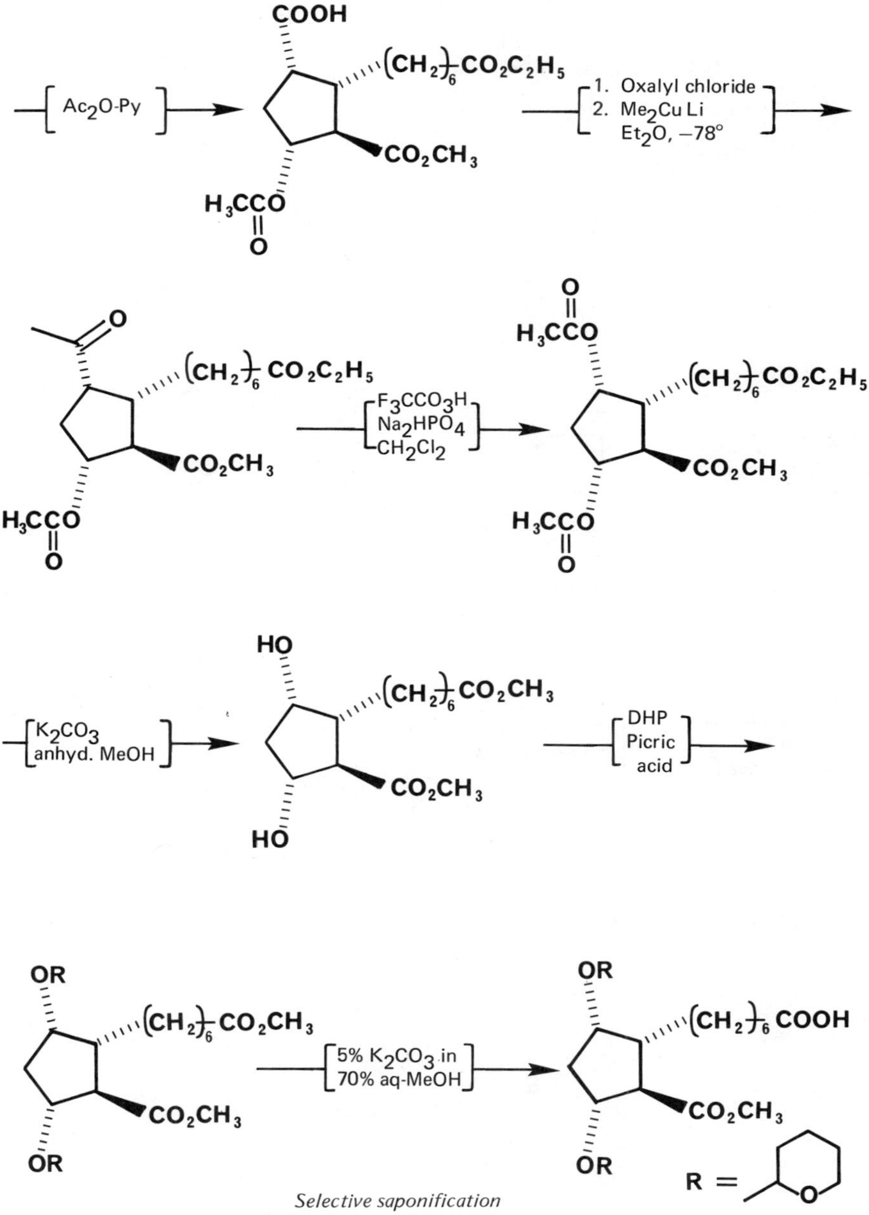

Selective saponification

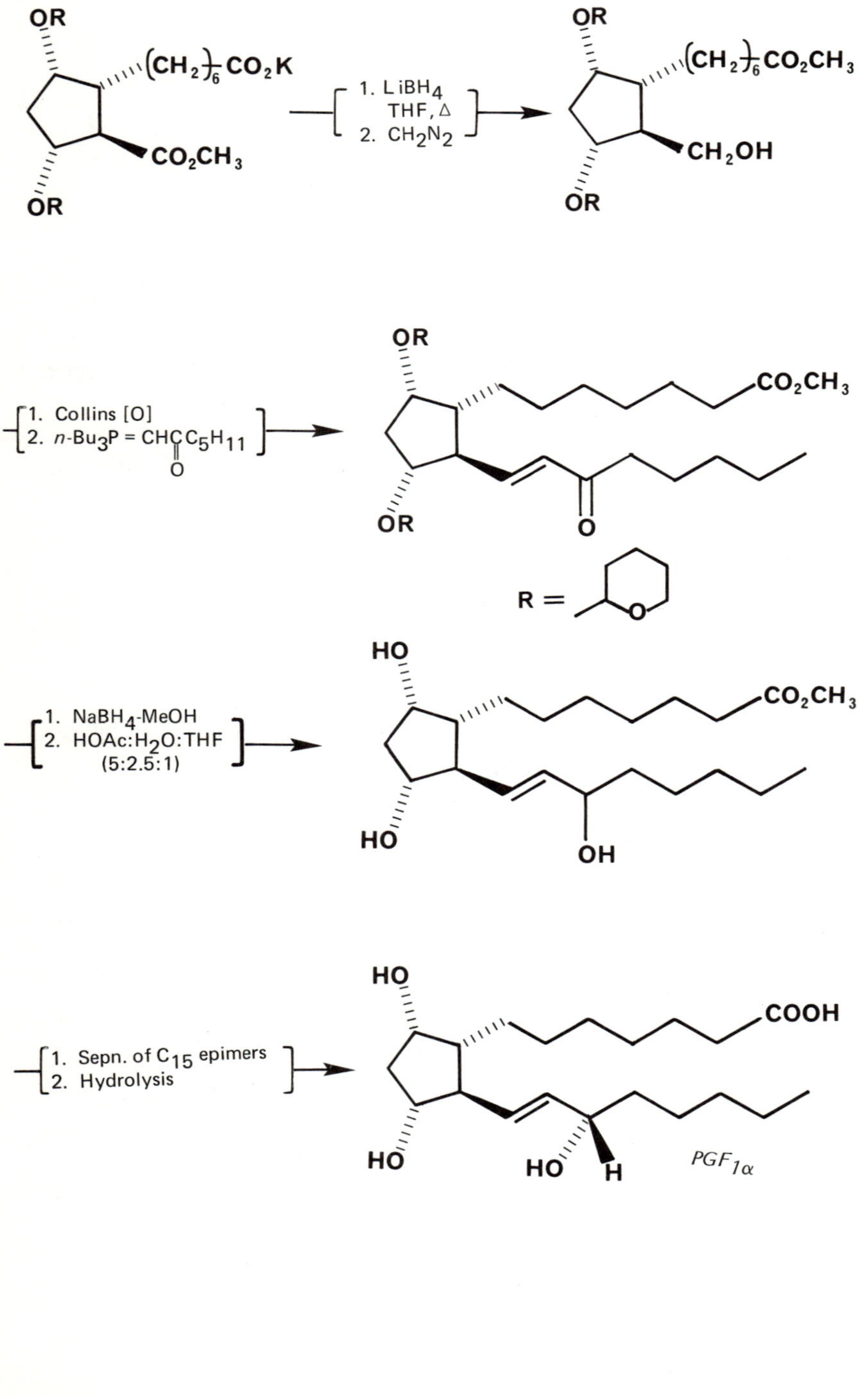
1. LiBH4
THF, Δ
2. CH2N2
1. Collins [O]
2. n-Bu3P = CHCC5H11
R =
1. NaBH4-MeOH
2. HOAc:H2O:THF
(5:2.5:1)
1. Sepn. of C15 epimers
2. Hydrolysis
PGF1α

C_8-C_{12} BOND FORMATION

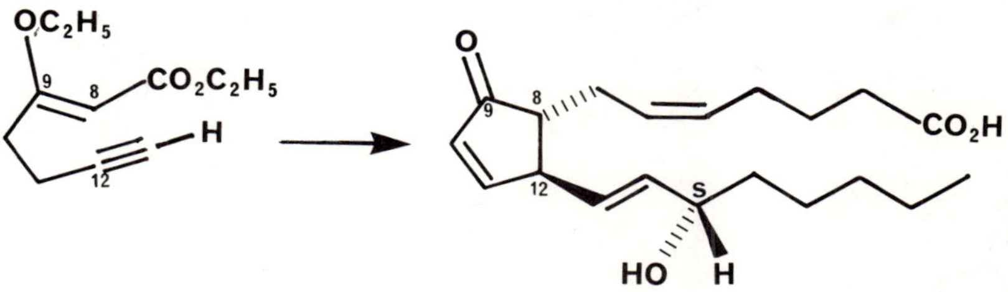

The Roussel-Uclaf approach[52] towards the prostanoid nucleus is conceptually one of the most interesting syntheses. The C_8 and C_{12} chiral centers are created simultaneously by a S_N2'-type intramolecular alkylation. The stereochemical outcome is based on the original observation of Stork and White[53] that the nucleophile comes in *syn* to the leaving group, although recent work[54,55] has cast doubt on the generality of the Stork-White hypothesis.[53]

---

52. J. Martel, E. Toromanoff, J. Mathieu & G. Nomine, *Tet. Lett.*, 1491 (1972).
53. G. Stork & W. N. White, *J. Am. Chem. Soc.*, **78**, 4609 (1956).
54. A. Kreft, Ph.D. Dissertation, Columbia University (1976).
55. F. G. Bordwell, *Accounts Chem. Res.*, **3**, 281 (1970).

SYNTHETIC STRATEGY

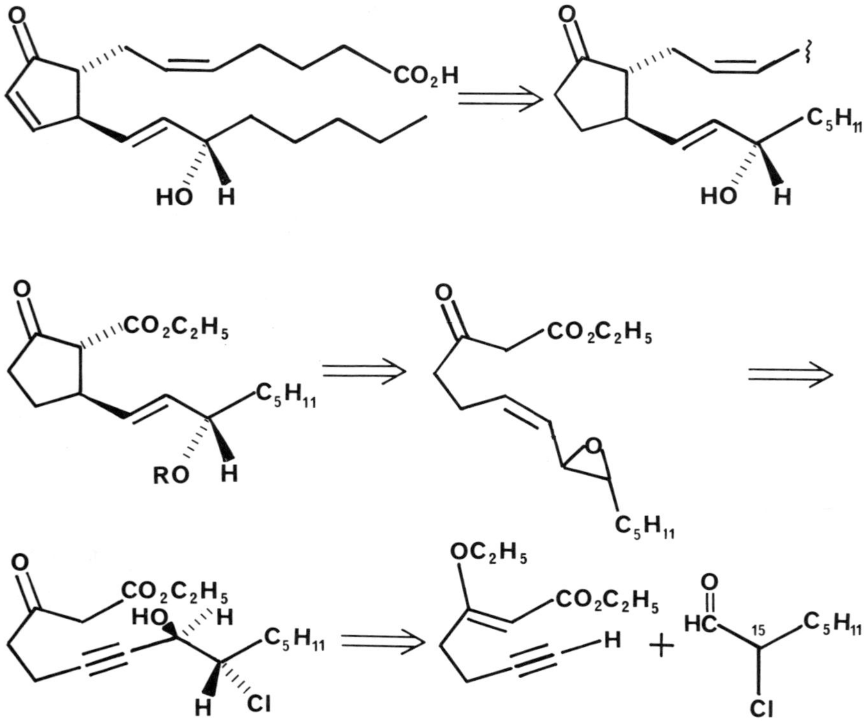

SYNTHETIC PLAN[52]

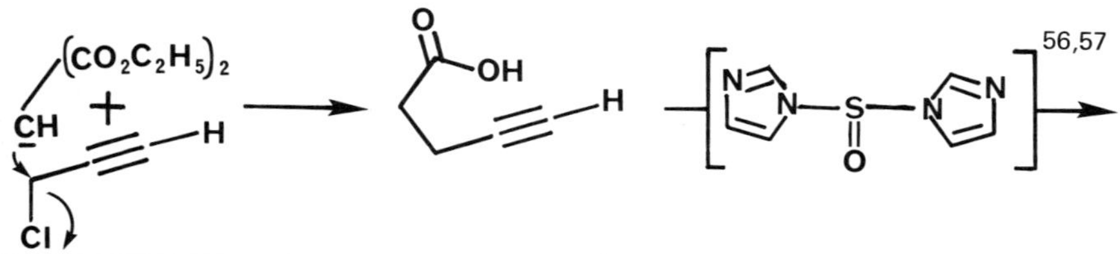

56. H. A. Staab & K. Wendel, *Angew. Chem.*, 73, 26 (1961).
57. For a review on the use of N,N'-carbonyldiimidazoles and N,N'-thionyldiimidazoles see "Syntheses Using Heterocyclic Amides (Azolides)" by H. A. Staab, *Angew. Chem., [Int. Ed.]*, 1, 351 (1962).

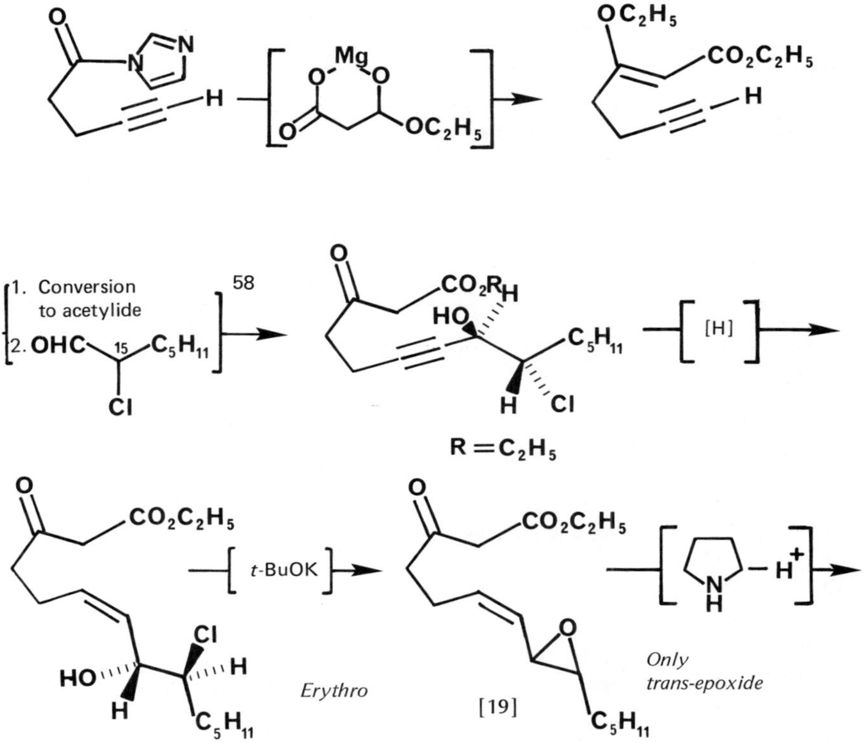

58. The Cornforth method was used to ensure the stereoselective formation of the *erythro* chlorohydrin which is then transformed into the desired *cis-trans* diene epoxide [19] J. Cornforth, R. H. Cornforth & K. K. Mathew, *J. Chem. Soc.*, 112 (1959).

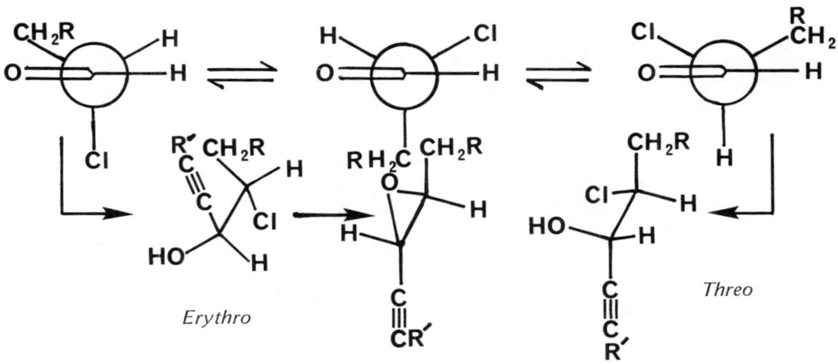

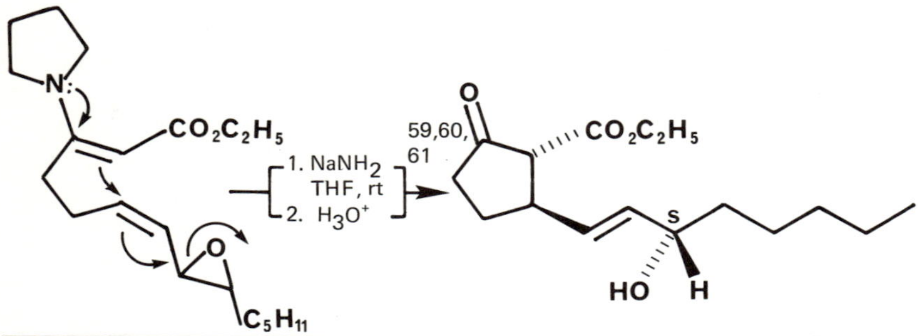

59. Other methods of alkylation give 0-alkylation product [20]:

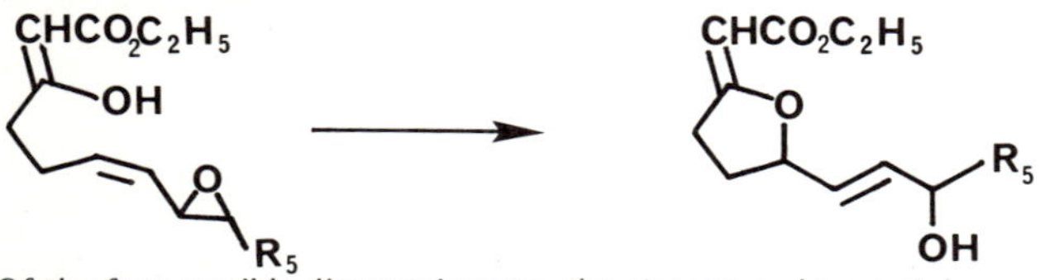

[20]

60. Of the four possible diastereoisomers, the *cis-trans* and *trans-cis* isomers gave the right relative C_{12}, C_{15} configuration.

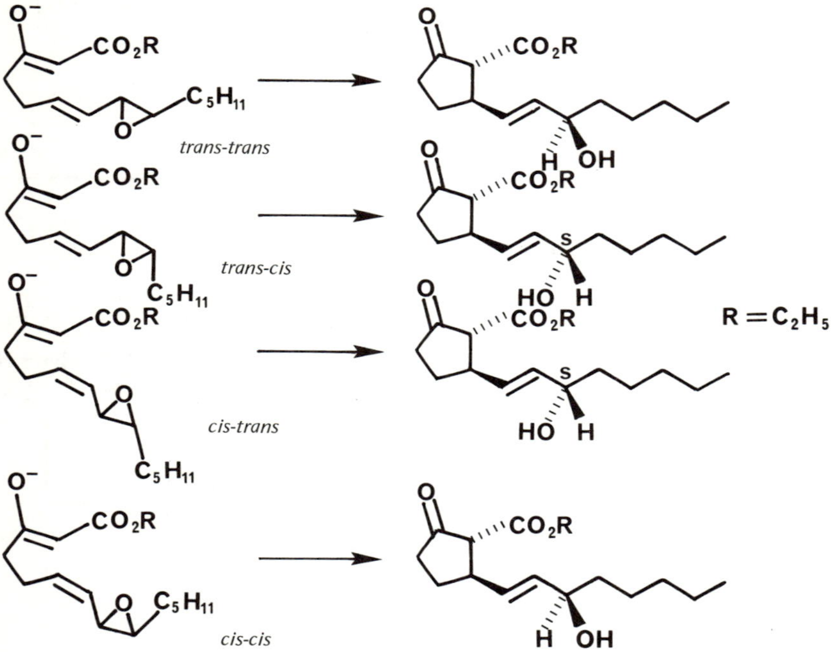

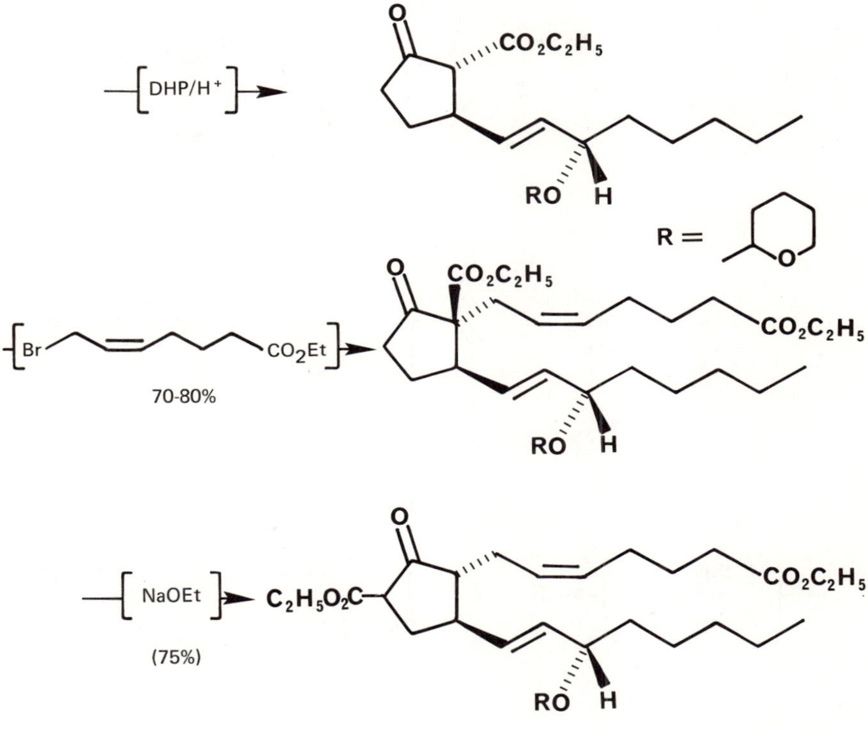

61. The ratio of cyclopentanone to cyclopropane formed depends on the reaction temperature. For example, at $-40°$ the ratio is 70:30, at $+30°$ only the cyclopentanone is formed.

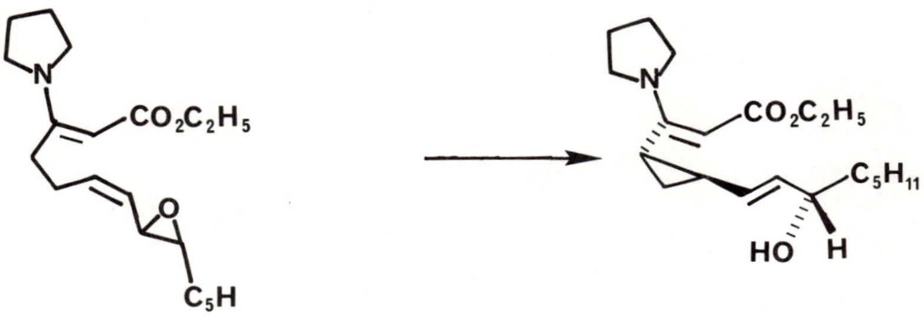

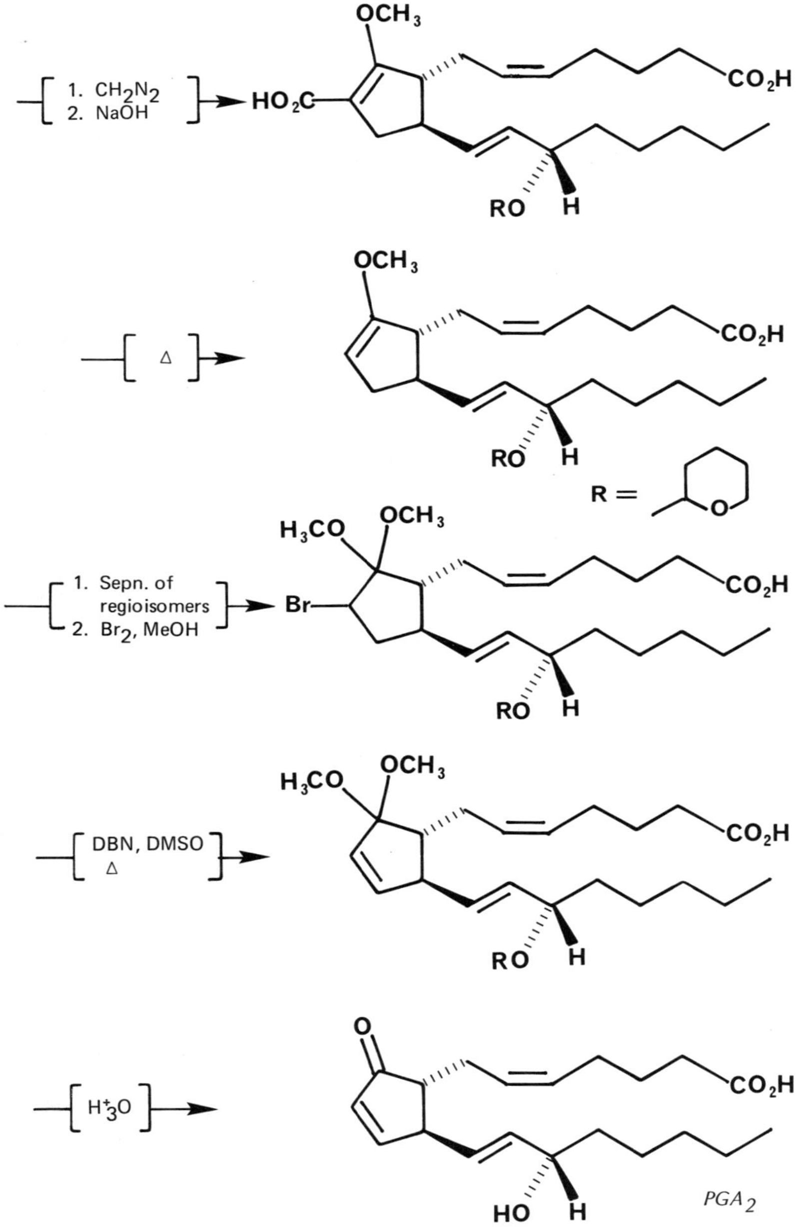
1. CH2N2
2. NaOH
OCH3
HO2C
CO2H
RO H
Δ
R =
O
1. Sepn. of regioisomers
2. Br2, MeOH
H3CO
Br
DBN, DMSO
Δ
H3+O
HO H
PGA2

C_{10}-C_{11} BOND FORMATION

The highly base-sensitive β-ketol function of PGE limits its synthesis by an aldol condensation. The limitations are:

1. The migration of the C_{13}-C_{14} double bond into conjugation; and

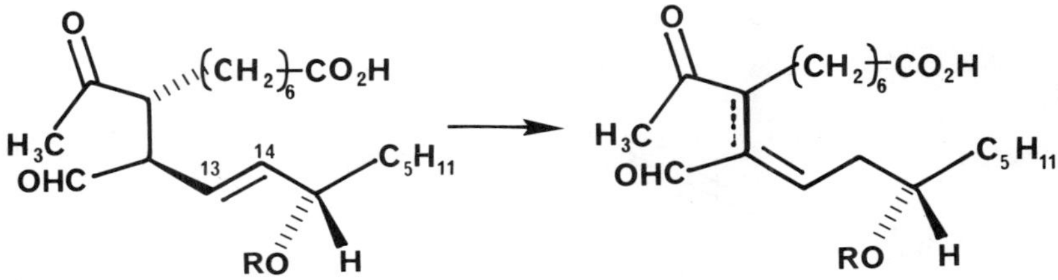

2. The dehydration of the initially formed aldol (β-ketol) to the enone, that is, PGE to PGA, followed by the migration of the double bond to the monosubstituted (PGC) and then to the disubstituted position (PGB).

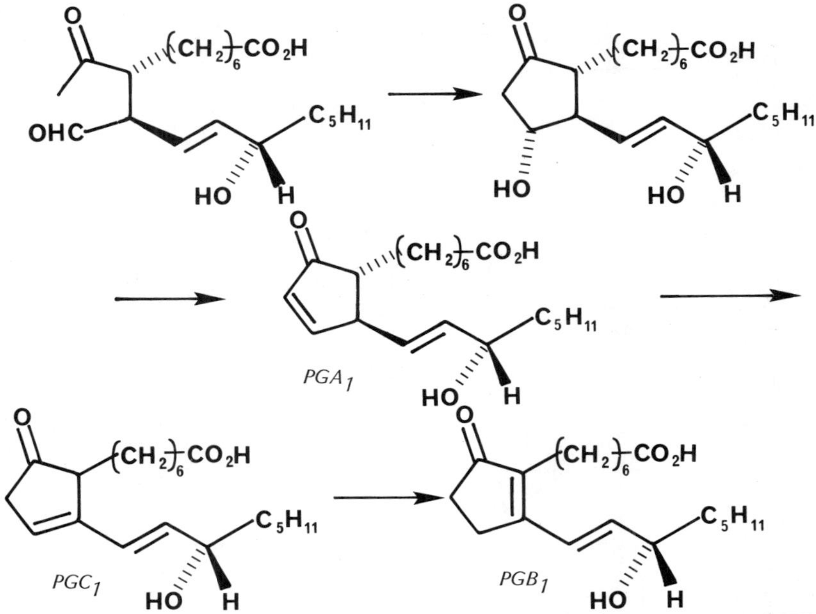

62. D. P. Strike & H. Smith, *Tet. Lett.*, 4393 (1970).
63. H. Smith in, "Prostaglandins," *Annals of the New York Academy of Sciences*, P. Ramwell & J. E. Shaw (eds.), **180**, 91 (1971).

Partial success along these lines has been attained by Strike and Smith[62,63] in the synthesis of 13,14-dihydro-PGE_1 [21].

SYNTHETIC PLAN[62,63]

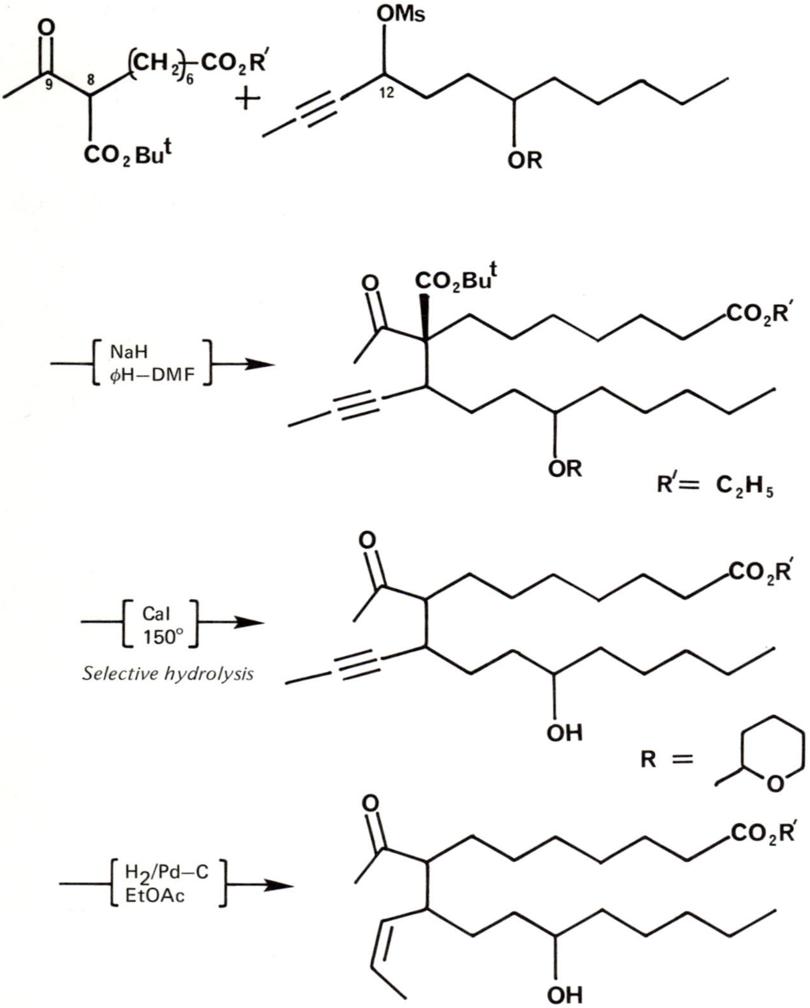

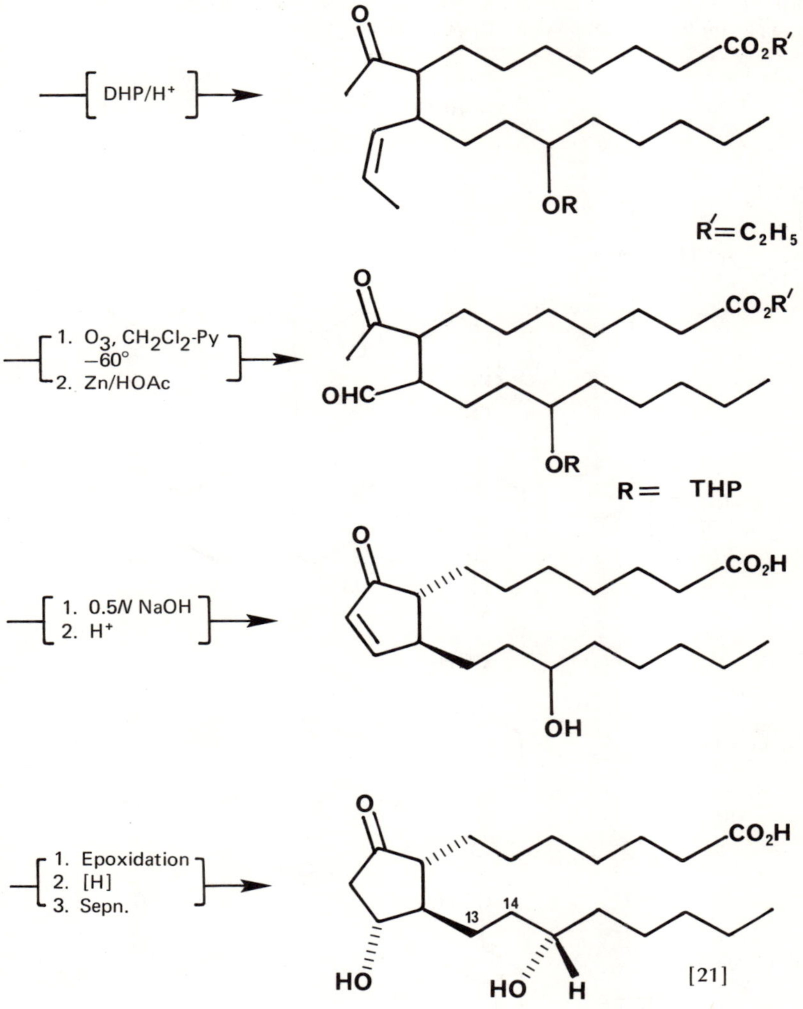

[21]

13, 14-Dihydro-PGE$_1$

A similar attempt (though unsuccessful) was made by Ireland,[64] by putting an extra methyl group at C_{12} to prevent the conjugation of the C_{13}-C_{14} double bond.

SYNTHETIC PLAN[64]

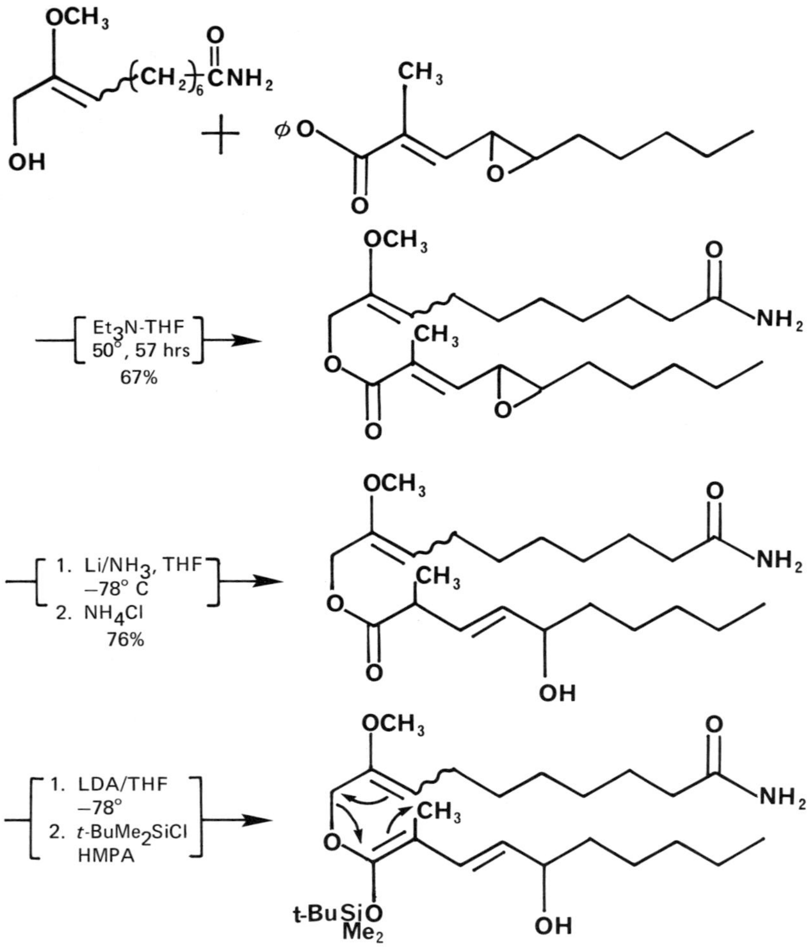

64. R. E. Ireland, R. H. Mueller & A. K. Willard, *J. Org. Chem.*, 41, 986 (1976).

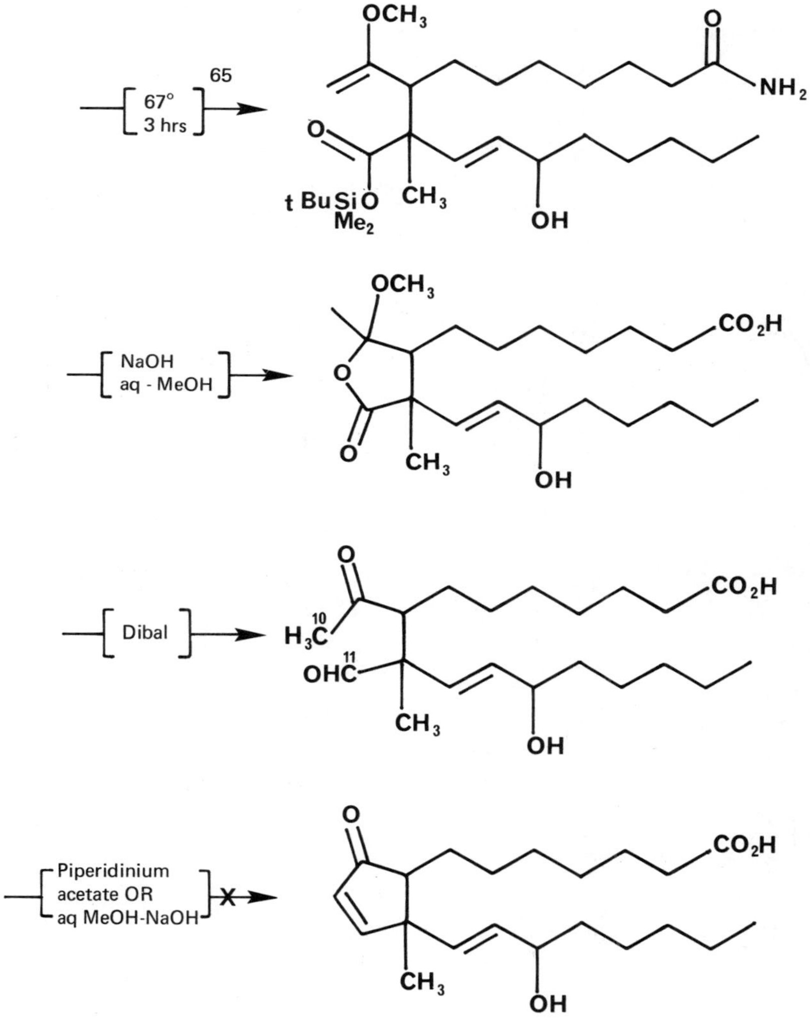

65. R. E. Ireland, R. H. Mueller & A. K. Willard, *J. Am. Chem. Soc.,* **98**, 2868 (1976). Other examples of the rearrangement of Zn-enolate anions of allyl esters has been reported. J. E. Baldwin & J. Walker, *Chem. Commun.*, 117 (1973).

Partial success along these lines has been attained by Schlessinger. The intermediate sulfide [22] was cyclized under mild basic conditions using phase transfer catalysis.[66]

SYNTHETIC PLAN[66]

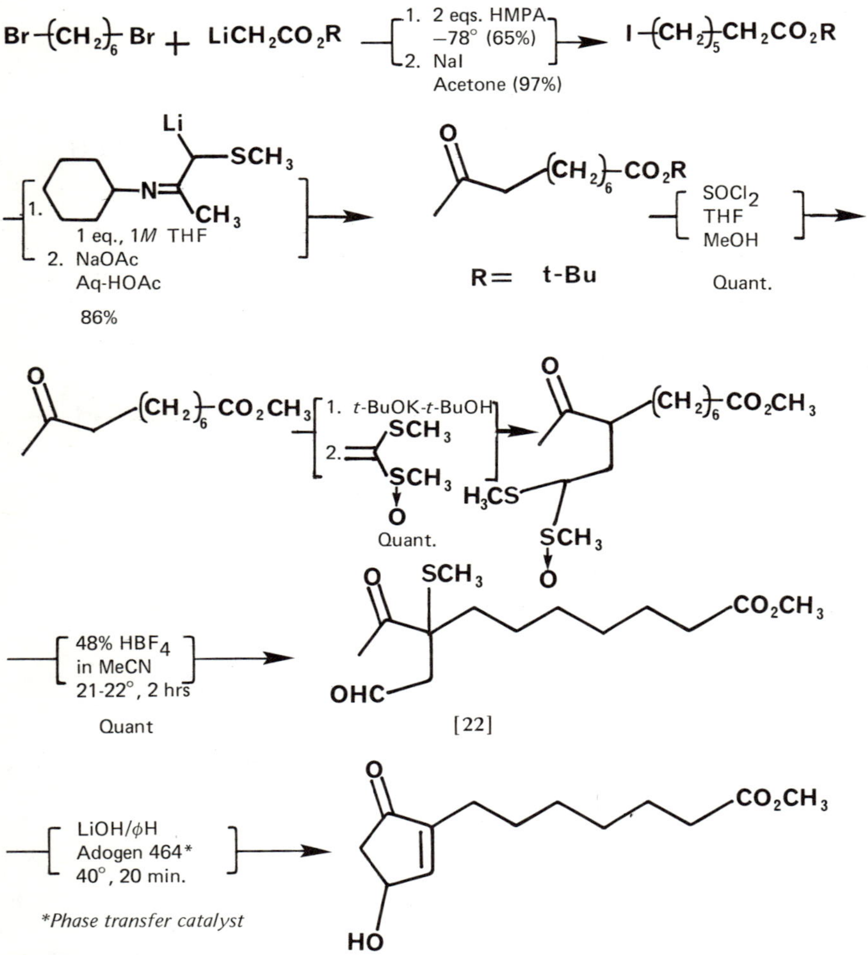

66. G. R. Kieczykowski, C. S. Pogonowski, J. E. Richman & R. H. Schlessinger, *J. Org. Chem.*, 42, 175 (1977).

C_9-C_{10} BOND FORMATION

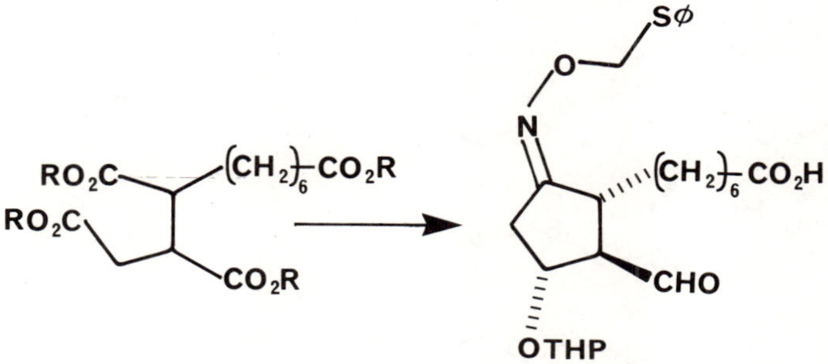

The Ciba approach to the synthesis of PGE_1 involves the protection of the C_9 carbonyl group (of the β-ketol) in the form of an oxime with a new hydroxylamine derivative and the selective borohydride reduction of an ester function.[67,68]

---

67. N. Finch & J. J. Fitt, *Tet. Lett.*, 4639 (1969).
68. N. Finch, L. Della Vecchia, J. J. Fitt, R. Stephani & I. Vlattas, *J. Org. Chem.*, 38, 4412 (1973).

SYNTHETIC STRATEGY

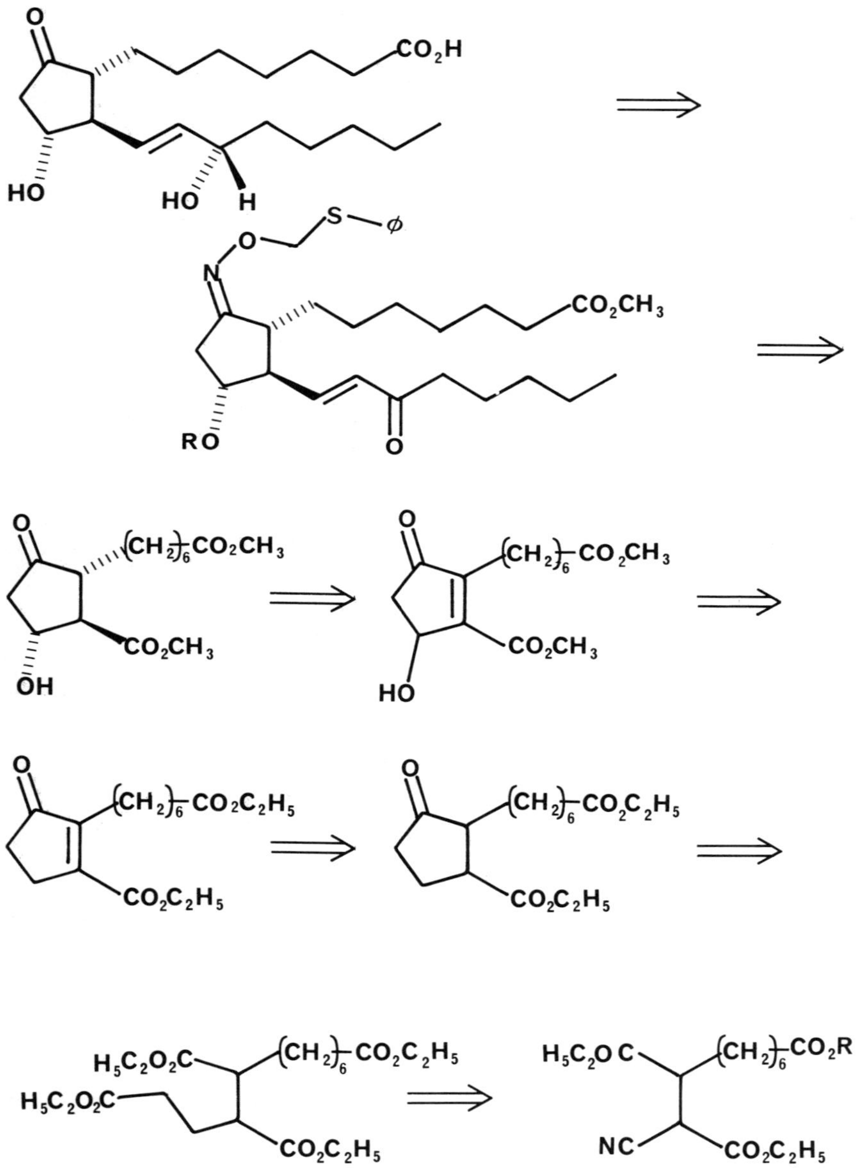

SYNTHETIC PLAN[67,68]

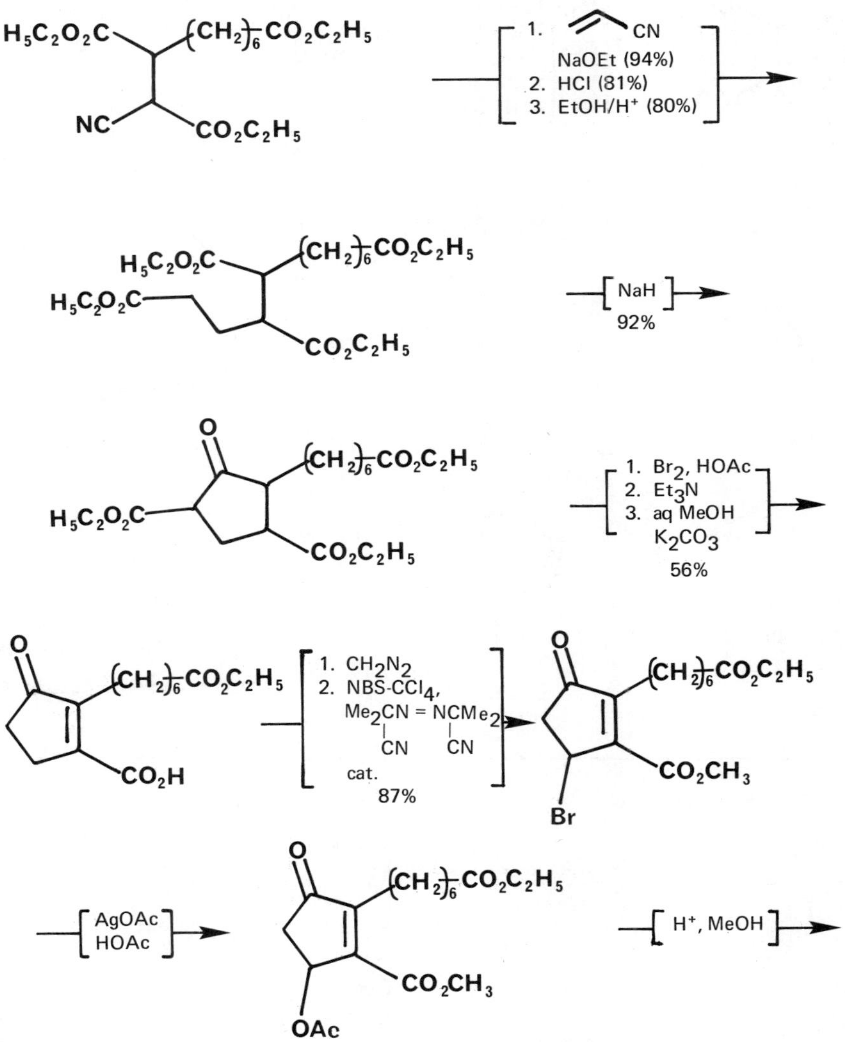

69. A similar enone has been reduced with chromous ion. For details see p. 55. M. Miyano & M. A. Stealey, *Chem. Commun.*, 180 (1973).

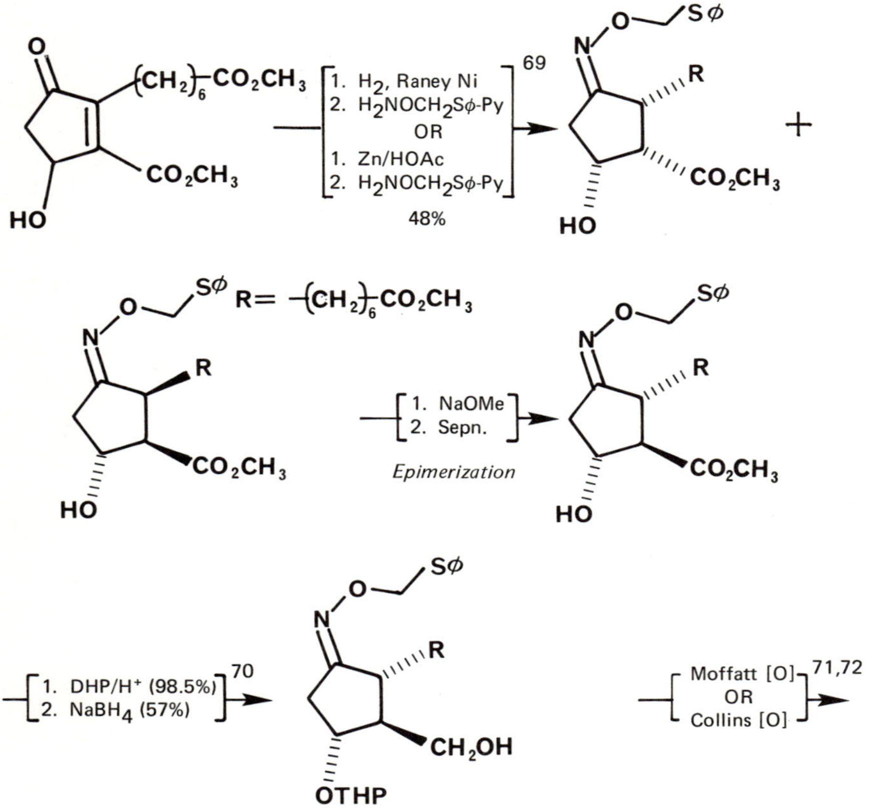

70. A different behavior is noticed in the case of the methyl oximes [23] and [24].

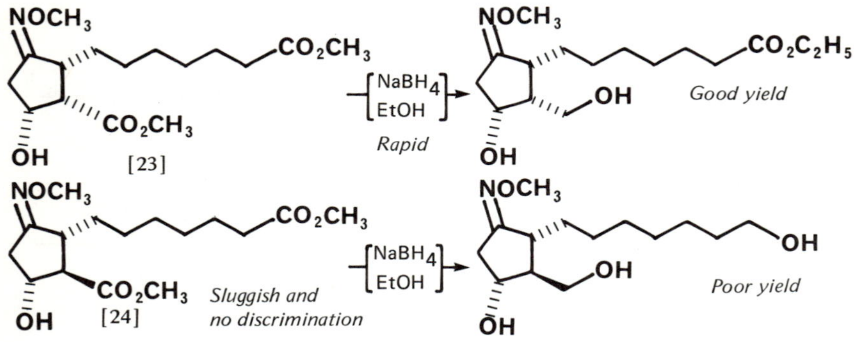

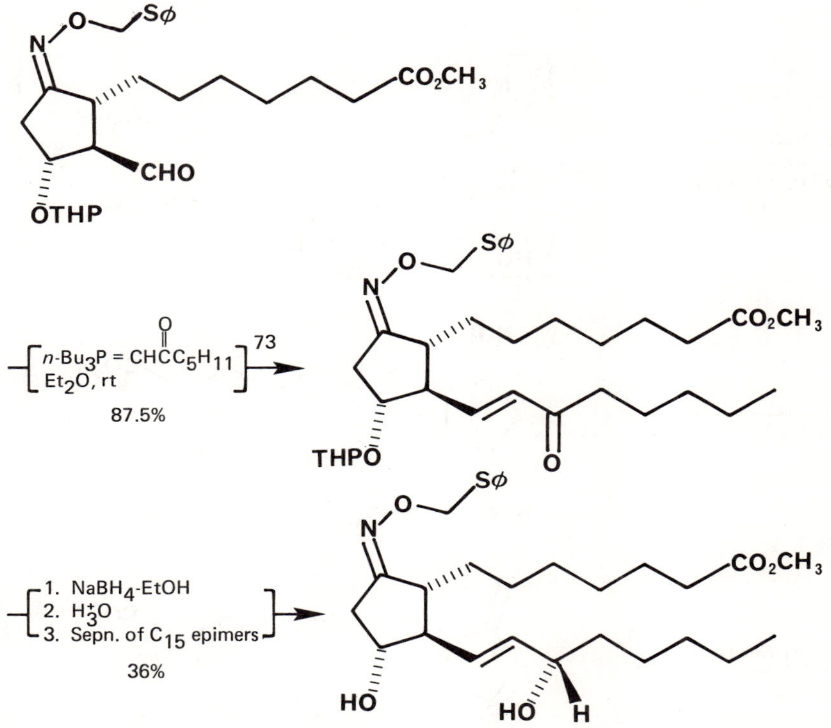

71. The water soluble carbodiimide derivative was used: 1-cyclohexyl-3-(2-morpholinoethyl)carbodiimide metho-*p*-toluenesulfonate.

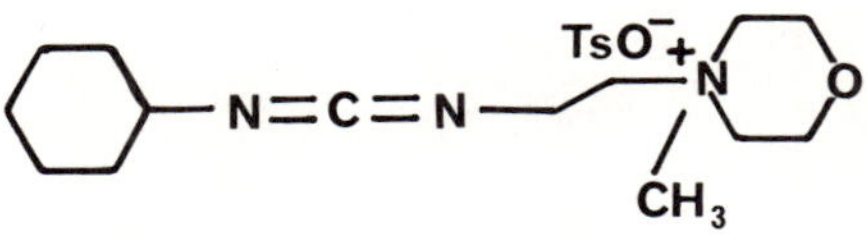

72. A polymer supported DCC derivative has also been shown to oxidize the alcohol in high yields.
N. M. Weinshenker & C. M. Shen, *Tet. Let.*, 3285 (1972).
G. A. Crosby, N. M. Weinshenker & H. S. Uh, *J. Am. Chem. Soc.*, **97**, 2232 (1975).

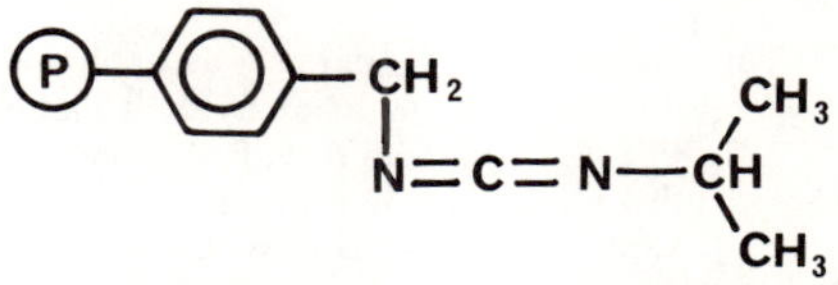

73. The instability of the aldehyde led to the development of the use of tributylphosphorane as the Wittig reagent. Tributyl phosphoranes are known to be more reactive than the conventional triphenyl phosphoranes.
A. J. Speziale & D. E. Bissing, *J. Am. Chem. Soc.*, **85**, 3878 (1963).

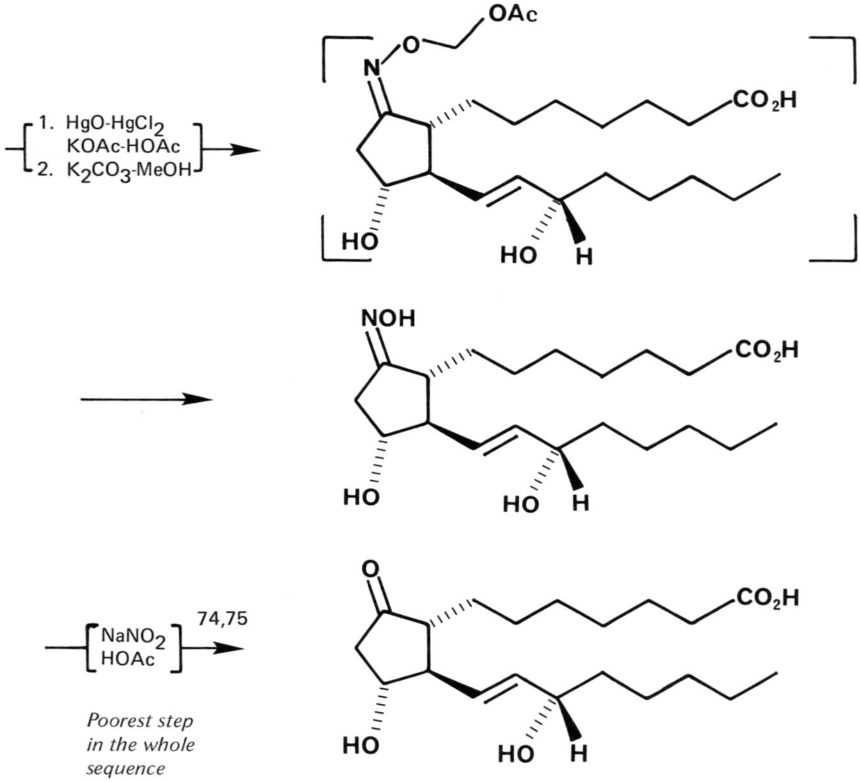

PGE$_1$[76]

---

74. The claim that the C_9-oxime was a suitable protecting group for the ketonic function of the β-ketol system was first made by the Upjohn group.
J. E. Pike, F. H. Lincoln & W. P. Schneider, *J. Org. Chem.*, 34, 3552 (1969).
75. For other methods of hydrolysis of oximes see:
E. J. Corey & J. E. Richman, *J. Am. Chem. Soc.*, **92**, 5276 (1970) and the references cited therein.
Also see:
G. H. Timms & E. Wildsmith, *Tet. Lett.*, 195 (1971); and
J. W. Bird & D. J. M. Diaper, *Can. J. Chem.*, **47**, 145 (1969).
76. A similar synthesis of PGE_1 going through the O-methyl oxime led to complications.

C_8-C_{12} BOND FORMATION

Like the Roussel-Uclaf approach,[77] Taber[78] has reported a synthesis where the relative stereochemistry of the C_{12} and C_{15} centers are stereospecifically controlled.[79,80]

SYNTHETIC STRATEGY

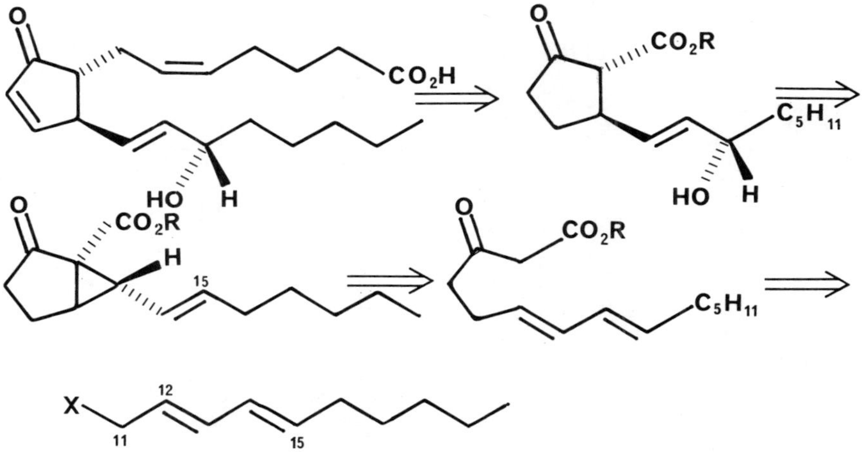

SYNTHETIC PLAN[78]

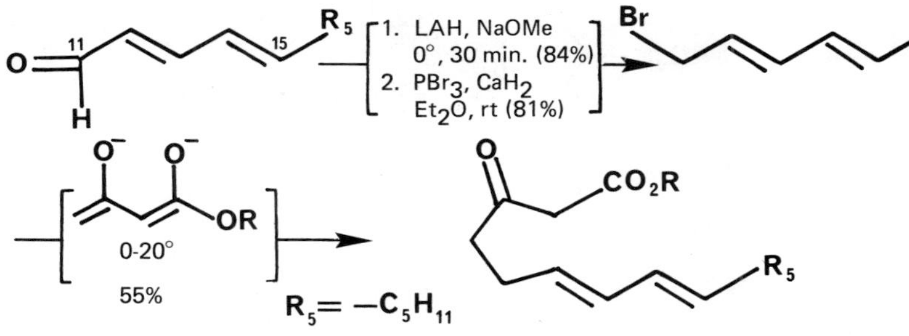

77. J. Martel, E. Toromanoff, J. Mathieu & G. Nomine, *Tet. Lett.*, 1491 (1972).
78. D. F. Taber, *J. Am. Chem. Soc.*, **99**, 3513 (1977).
79. A similar approach has also been published by K. Kondo, T. Umemoto, Y. Takahatake & D. Tunemoto, *Tet. Lett.*, 113 (1977).
80. The synthesis is based on the stereospecific opening of an activated cyclopropane by a nucleophile observed by B. Trost, *Tet. Lett.*, 3857 (1976).

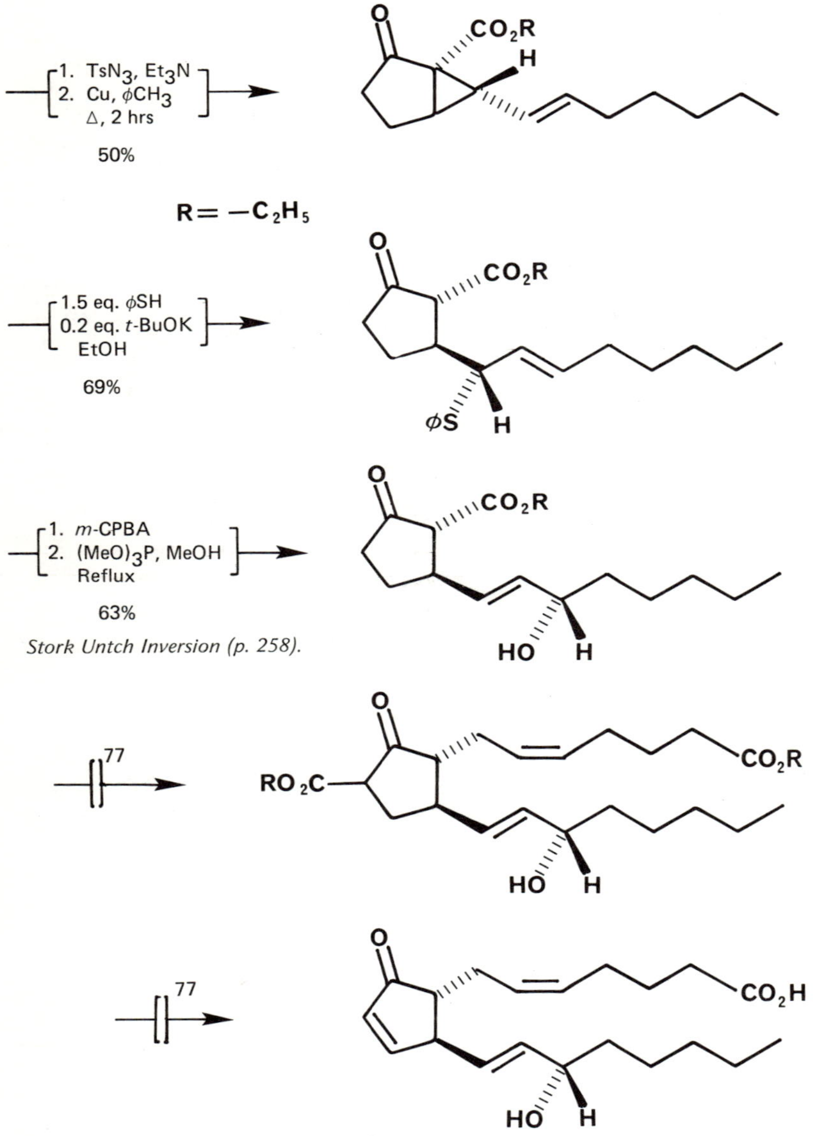

81. The corresponding *trans, cis* alcohol should give the opposite stereochemistry at C_{15} i.e., *R*.

4

Hydrindenone Approach

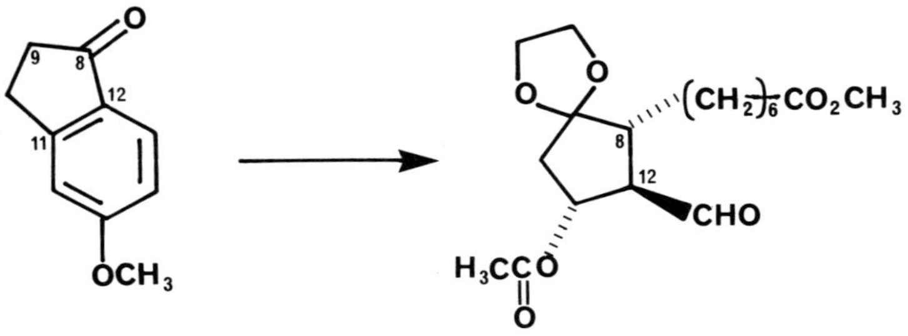

The lengthy (31 steps) hydrindenone approach to the synthesis of PGE_1 utilizes a four carbon degradation sequence which generates the all *trans* orientation of the substituents about the cyclopentanone ring by carefully planned equilibration at various points in the sequence.[1,2,3]

---

1. D. Taub, R. D. Hoffsommer, C. H. Kuo, H. L. Slates, Z. S. Zelawski & N. L. Wendler, *Chem. Commun.*, 1258 (1970).
2. D. Taub in "Prostaglandins," *Annals of the New York Academy of Sciences*, P. Ramwell & J. E. Shaw (Ed.) **180**, p. 101 (1971).
3. D. Taub, R. D. Hoffsommer, C. H. Kuo, H. L. Slates, Z. S. Zelawski & N. L. Wendler, *Tet.*, **30**, 819 (1974).

SYNTHETIC STRATEGY

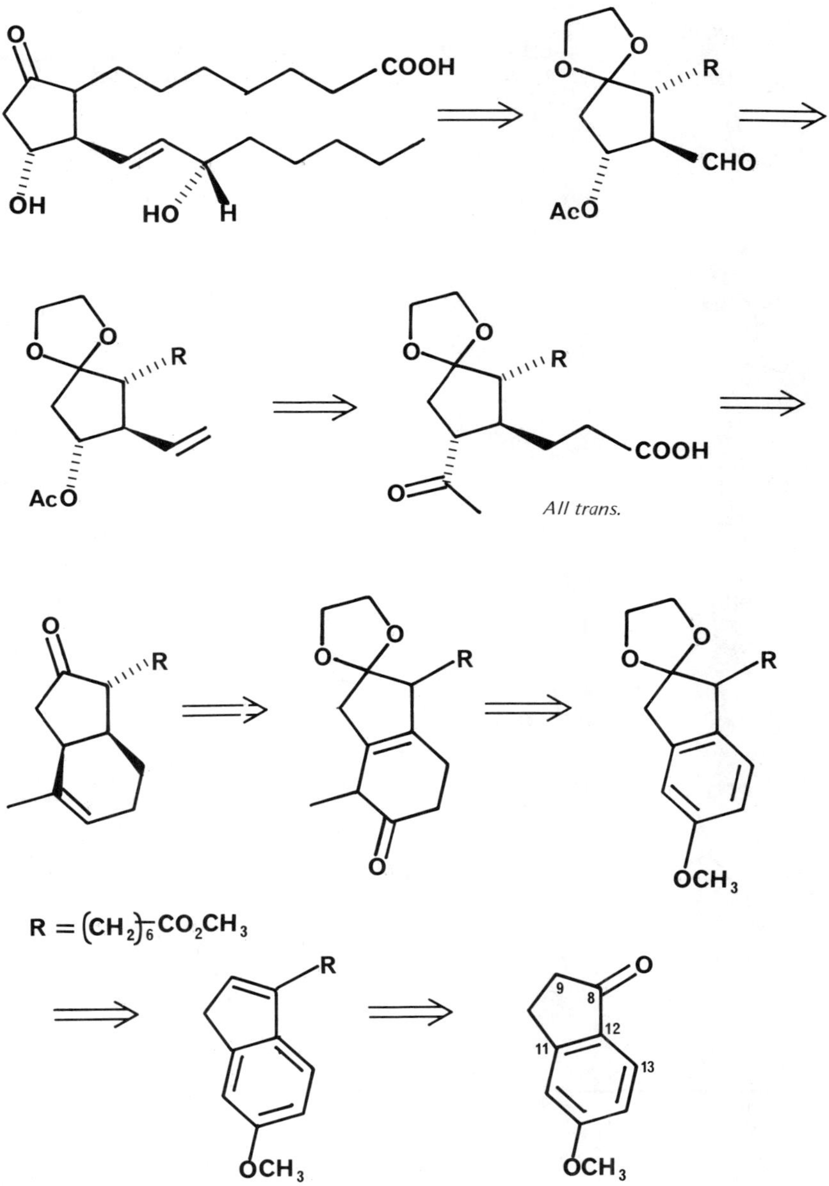

SYNTHETIC PLAN[1,2,3]

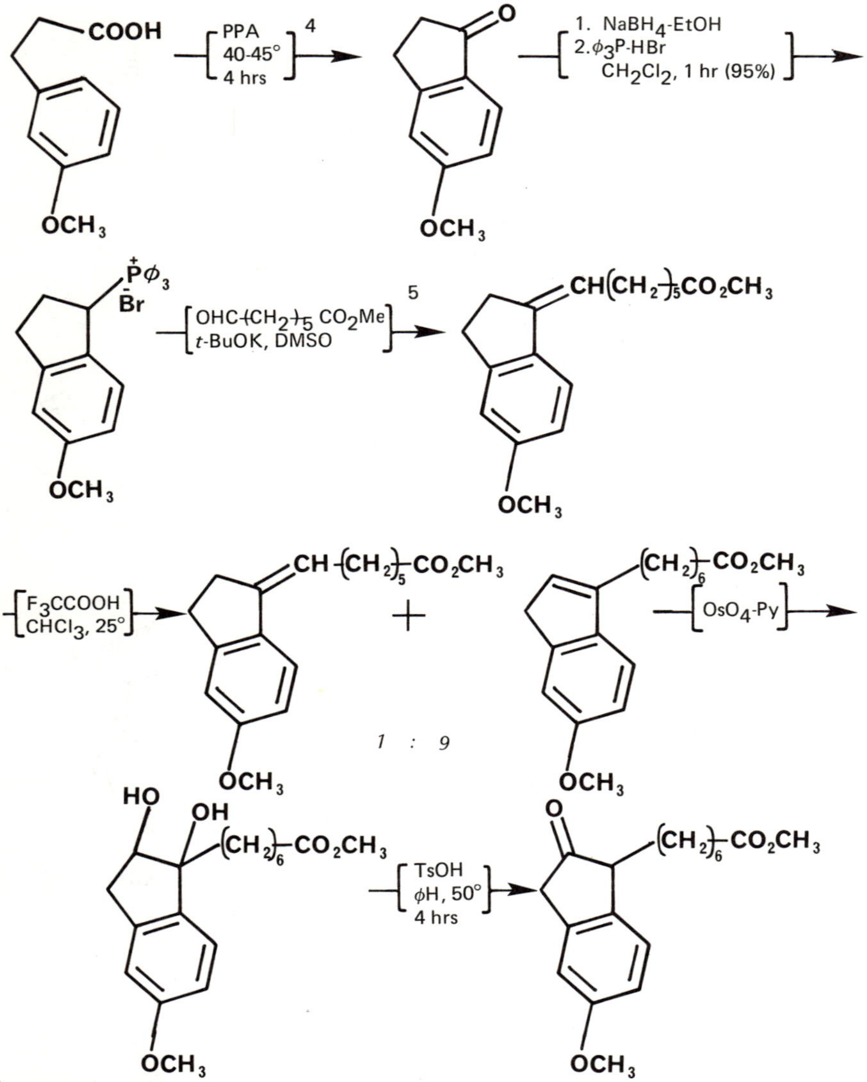

4. A. J. Birch, J. A. K. Quartey & H. Smith, *J. Chem. Soc.*, 1768 (1952).
5. Methyl-6-formylhexanoate was made from cycloheptanone.

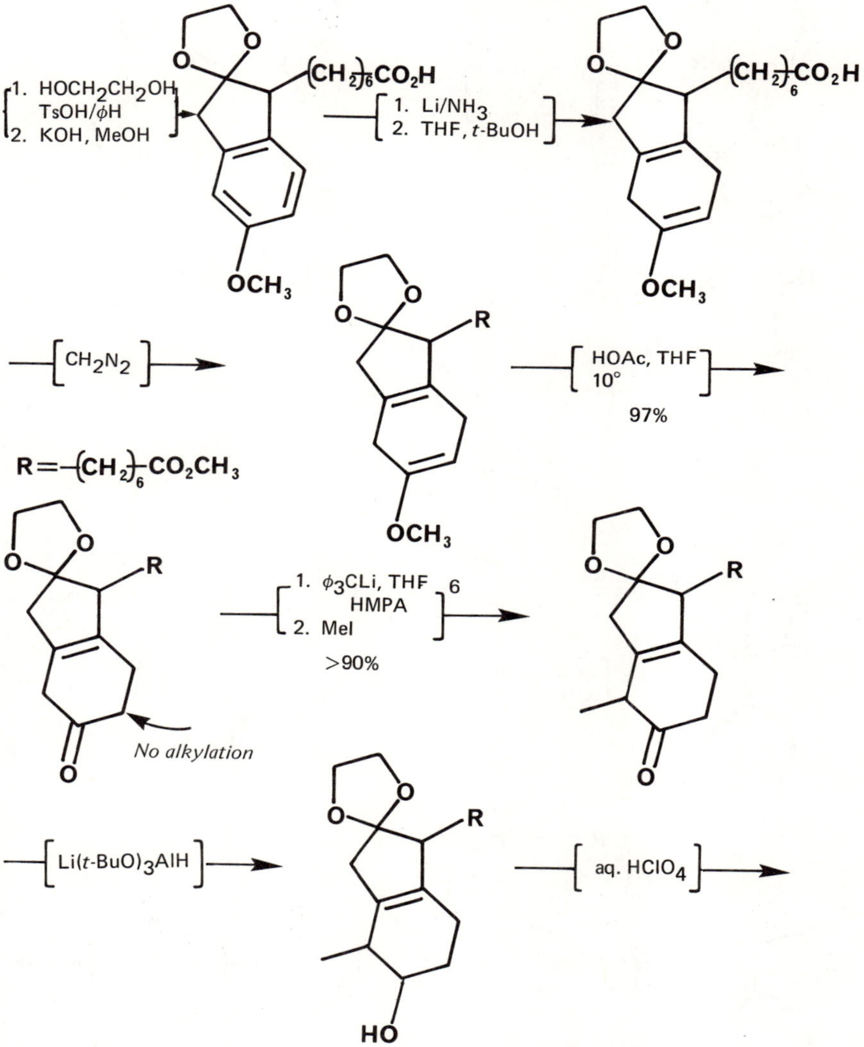

6. This alkylation serves a dual purpose. First, it drives the dehydration in the desired direction, and secondly, it forms the methylketone [1] and not the aldehyde upon oxidation. This methylketone is necessary for the subsequent Baeyer-Villiger oxidation. In a later modified synthesis this methyl group is introduced at the start of the synthesis by a different method. For details see p. 89

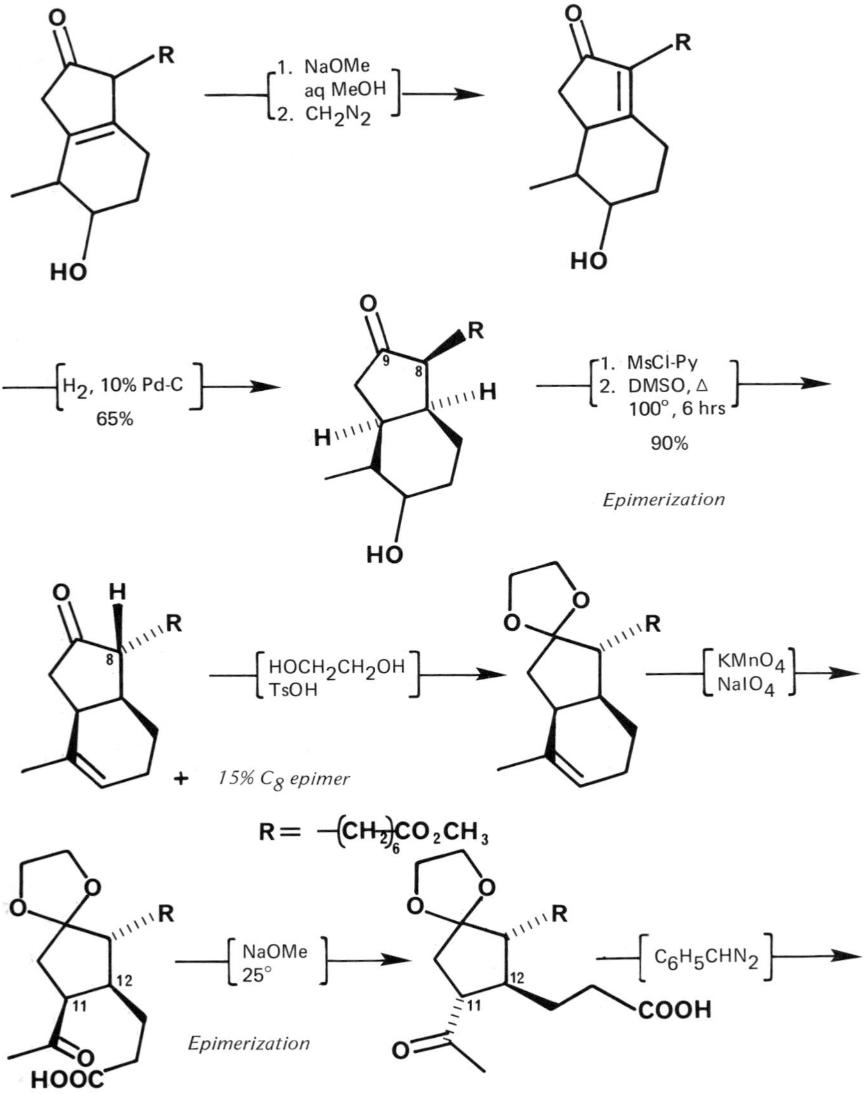

All trans.

[1]
Methylketone

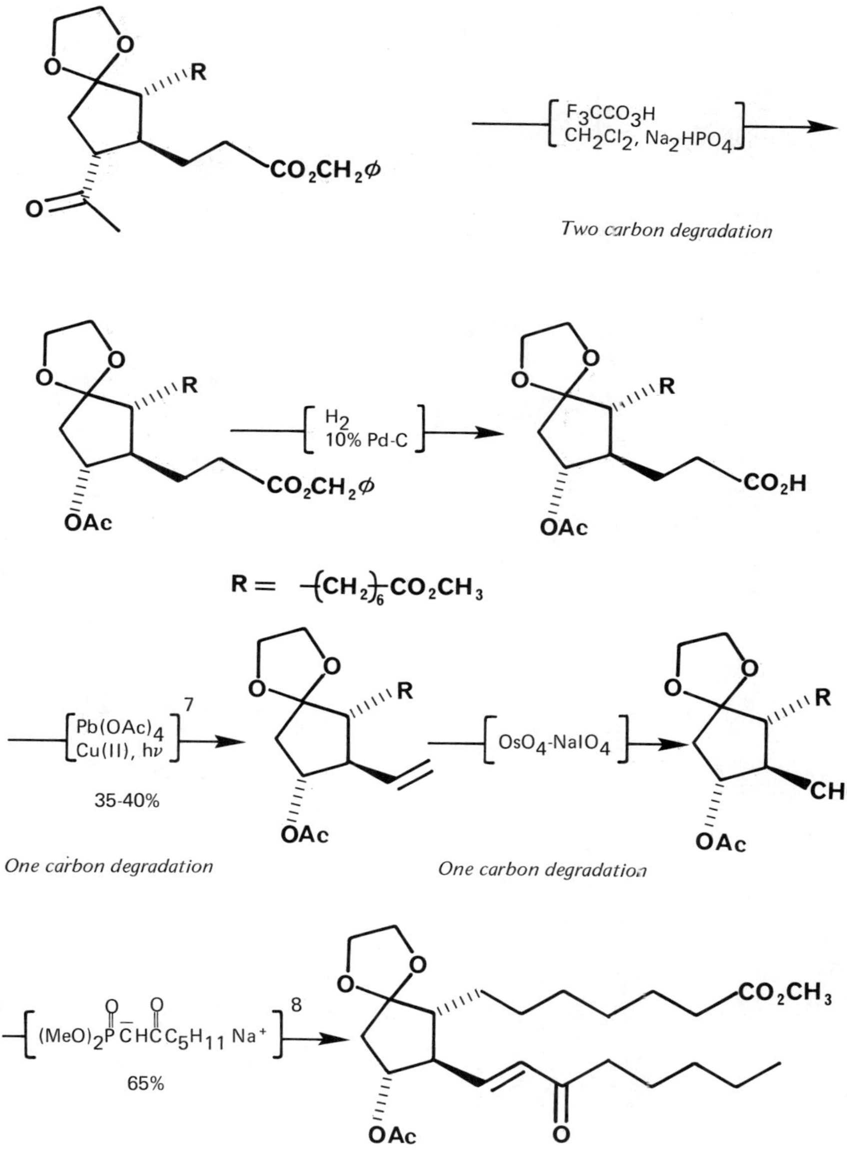

7. R. A. Sheldon & J. K. Kochi, *Organic Reactions*, 19, 279 (1972).

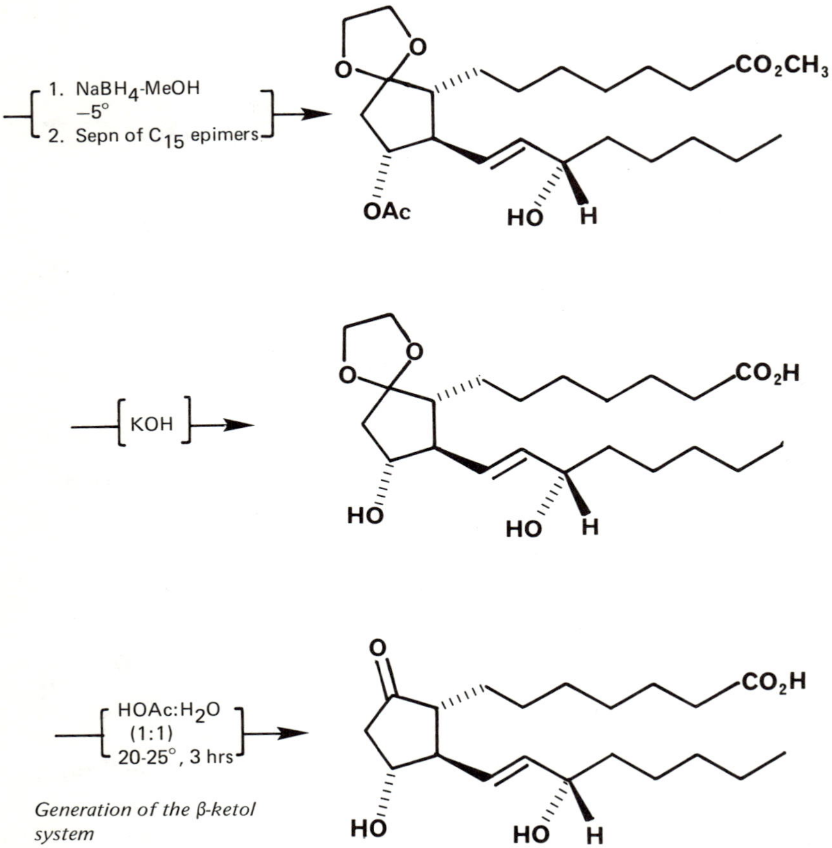

Generation of the β-ketol system

---

8. Some of the dienone [2] is formed as a by-product in Horner-Emmons reaction.

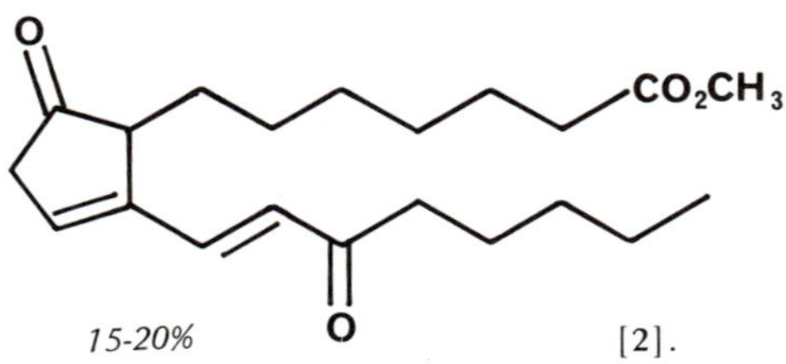

15-20% [2].

Dienone (PGC-derivative)

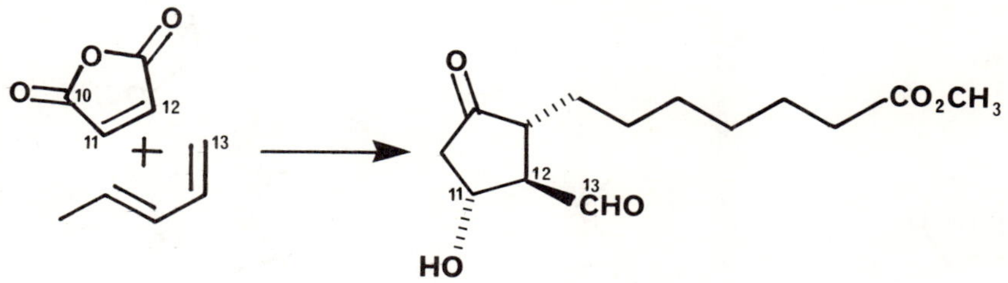

A desire to make improvements on the 5-methoxyindanone approach led to this modified hydrindenone route. The use of 1,3-pentadiene in the Diels-Alder reaction makes it a more convergent synthesis and serves a twofold purpose. First, it allows the introduction of the double bond in the desired (more stable) position. Second, the methyl ketone can undergo a Baeyer-Villiger Reaction (a two carbon degradation) which the aldehyde derived from butadiene cannot. The other two carbon degradation, via an enol acetate, circumvents the low yield oxidative decarboxylation reaction (Kochi reaction).[9,10,11]

---

9. H. L. Slates, Z. S. Zelawski, D. Taub & N. L. Wendler, *Chem. Commun.*, 304 (1972).
10. D. Taub, *Intra-Science Chem. Rept.*, **6**, 99 (1972).
11. H. L. Slates, Z. S. Zelawski, D. Taub & N. L. Wendler, *Tet.*, **30**, 819 (1974).

SYNTHETIC STRATEGY

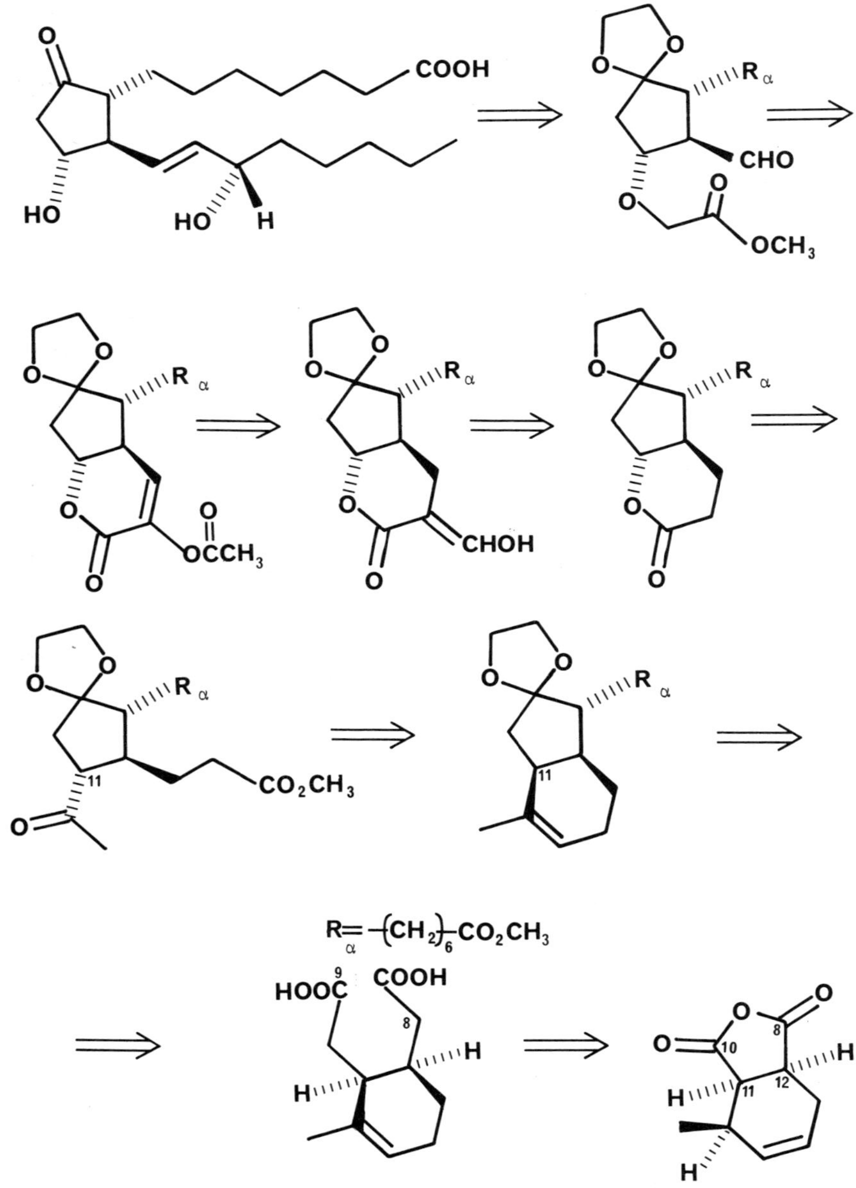

SYNTHETIC PLAN[9,10,11]

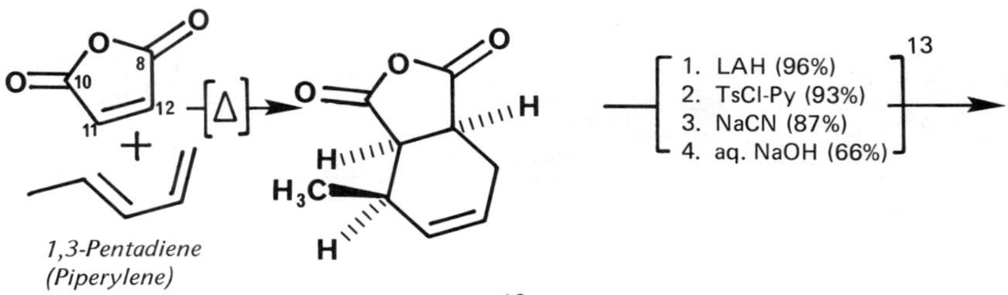

[3][12]

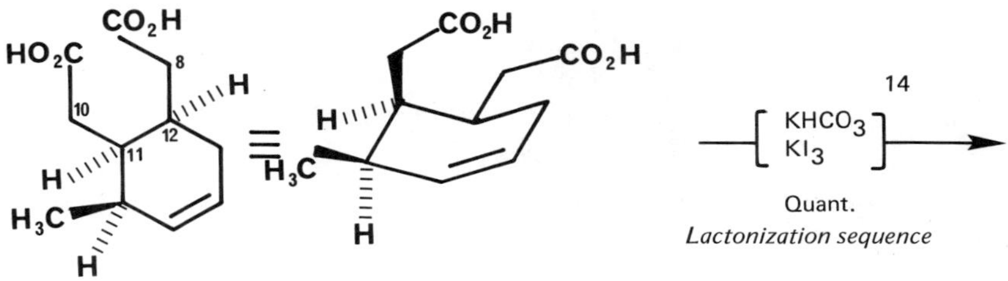

[5]

---

12. The half acid ester was resolved through its dehydroabietyl ammonium salt.

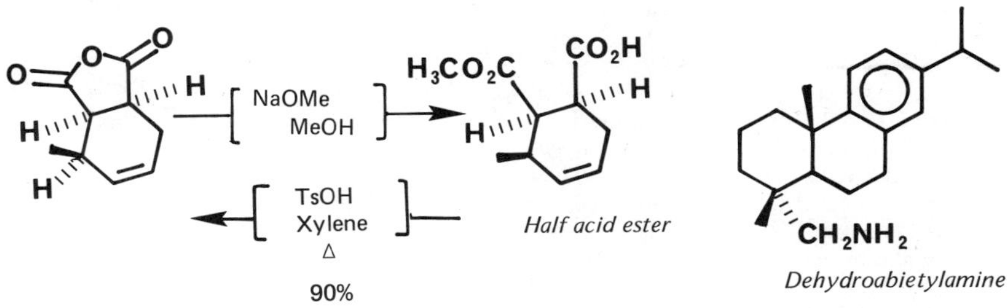

13. Tosylation at room temp. gives the cyclic ether [4]:

[4]

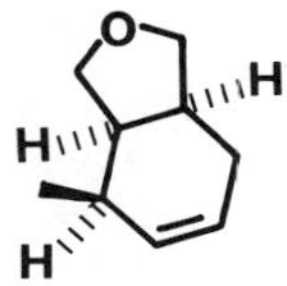

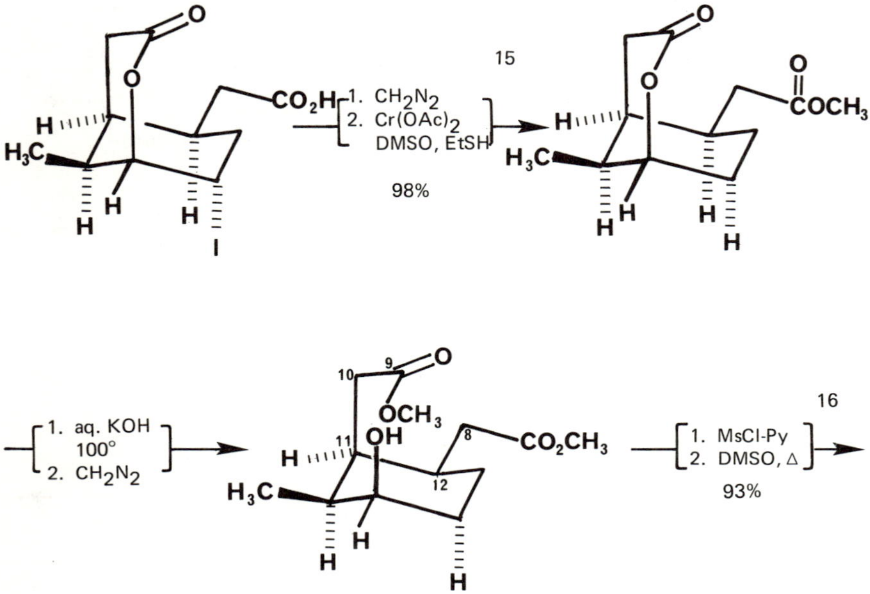

---

14. The highly strained nature of 1,3-diaxial groups presumably drives iodolactonization in the desired direction. The other iodolactone [6] is not formed.

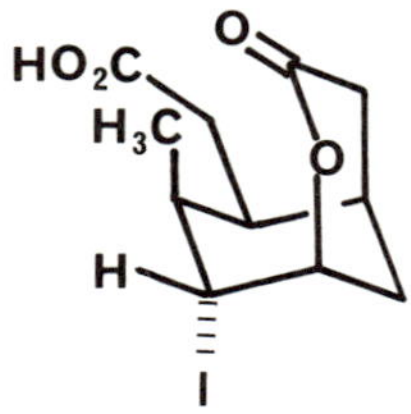

[6]

15. EtSH traps the intermediate radical, thus preventing elimination back to the olefin [5]. D. H. R. Barton, N. K. Basu, R. H. Hesse, F. S. Morehouse & M. M. Pechtet, *J. Am. Chem. Soc.*, **88**, 3016 (1966).
16. The purpose of the lactonization sequence is to move the position of the original double bond in [5].
17. Steric effects lead to the desired Dieckmann cyclization. The other cyclization product [7] is not formed.

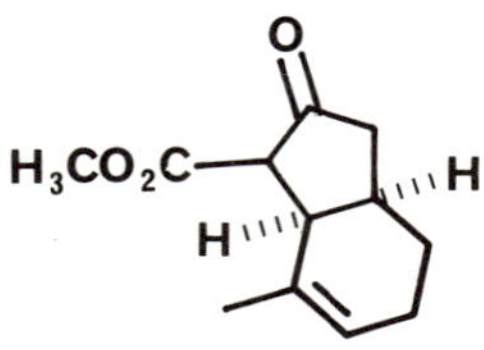

[7]

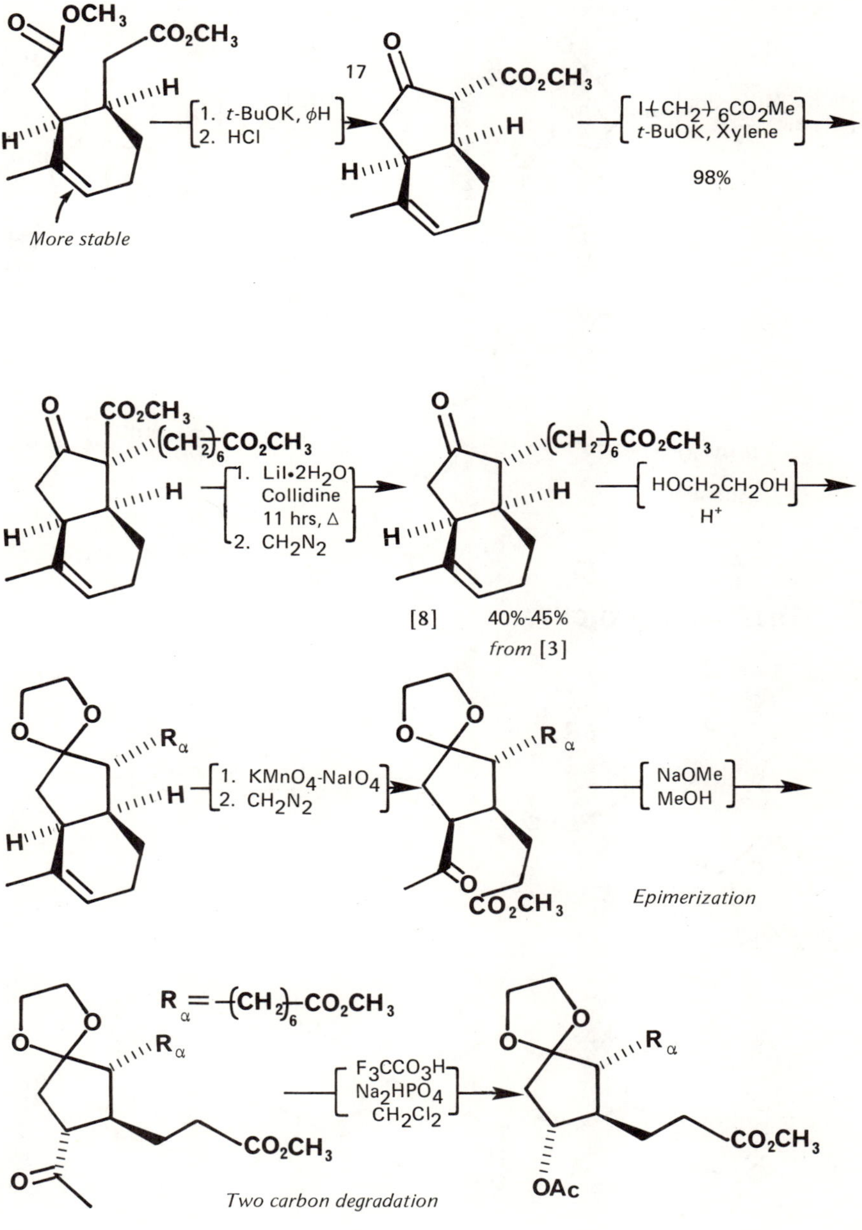
OCH3
CO2CH3
More stable
1. t-BuOK, ϕH
2. HCl
17
CO2CH3
I+CH2+6CO2Me
t-BuOK, Xylene
98%
CO2CH3
(CH2)6CO2CH3
1. LiI•2H2O
Collidine
11 hrs, Δ
2. CH2N2
(CH2)6CO2CH3
[8]
40%-45%
from [3]
HOCH2CH2OH
H+
Rα
1. KMnO4-NaIO4
2. CH2N2
Rα
CO2CH3
NaOMe
MeOH
Epimerization
Rα = (CH2)6 CO2CH3
Rα
CO2CH3
F3CCO3H
Na2HPO4
CH2Cl2
Rα
CO2CH3
OAc
Two carbon degradation

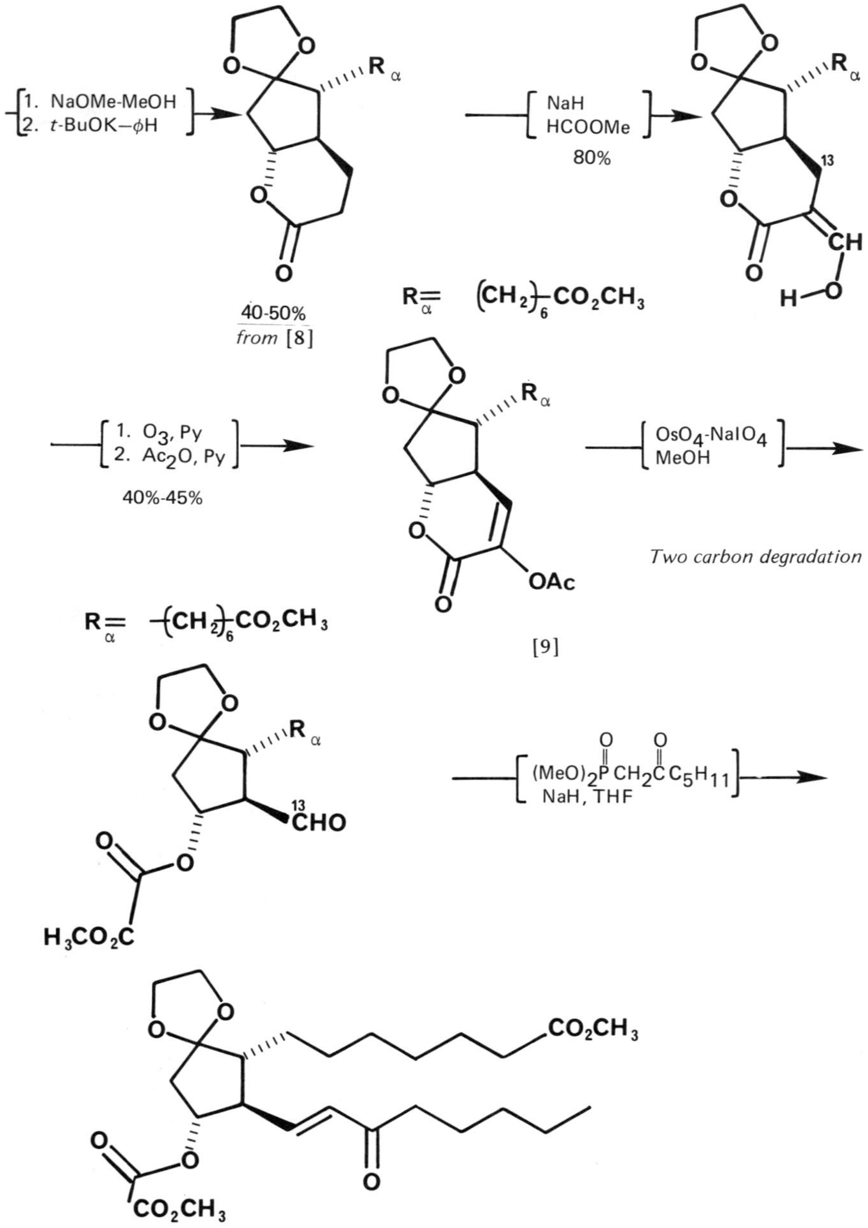
1. NaOMe-MeOH
2. t-BuOK–φH
40-50%
from [8]
NaH
HCOOMe
80%
R_α = (CH2)6CO2CH3
1. O3, Py
2. Ac2O, Py
40%-45%
OsO4-NaIO4
MeOH
Two carbon degradation
[9]
(MeO)2P(O)CH2C(O)C5H11
NaH, THF

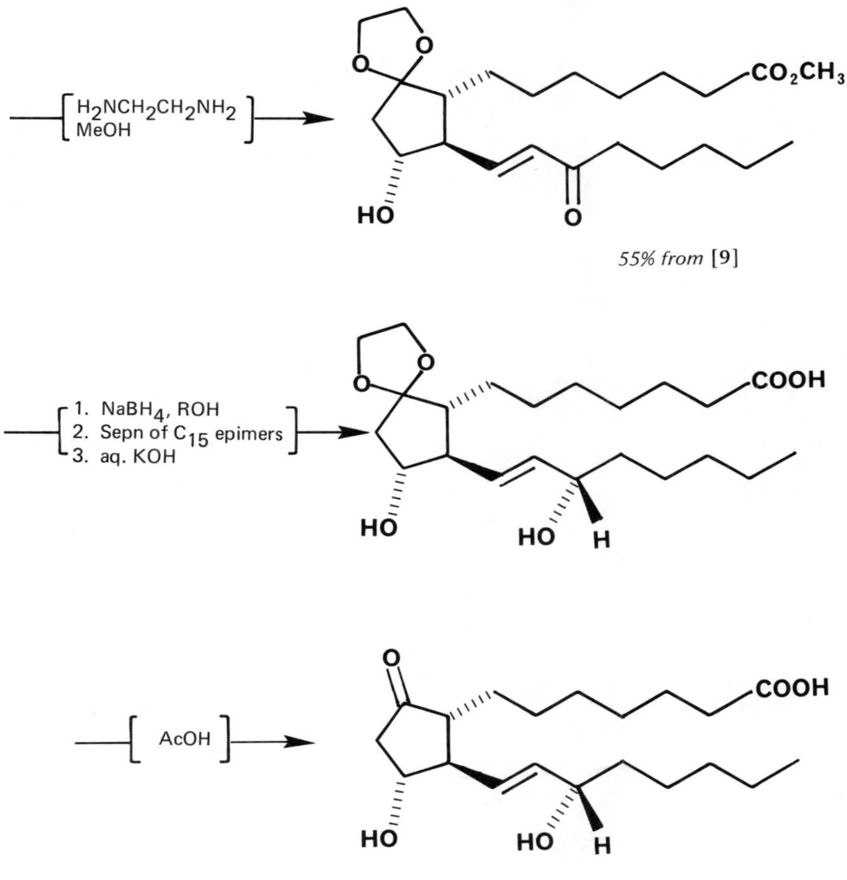

55% from [9]

PGE_1

5

Bicyclo[2.2.1]heptane Approach

After Corey's initial success in the synthesis of PGE_1,[1] an attempt was made to devise a short synthesis of a common intermediate that had the requisite stereochemistry at the four contiguous asymmetric centers and that could be converted to all the naturally occurring prostaglandins.

A retro synthetic analysis of $PGF_{2\alpha}$ with bond disconnections between C_5-C_6 and C_{13}-C_{14} leads to the bis-aldehyde [1]. The two aldehyde units can be differentiated in the subsequent elaborations via the hemiacetal [2] or via the bicyclic lactones [3] or [4]. Such an approach was conceived and executed successfully by E. J. Corey at Harvard University.

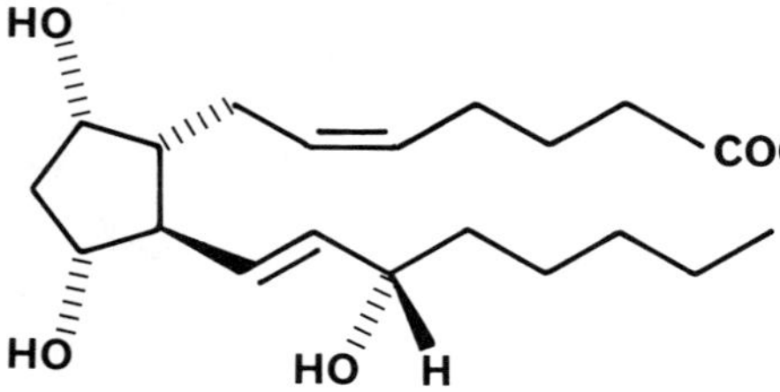

$PGF_{2\alpha}$

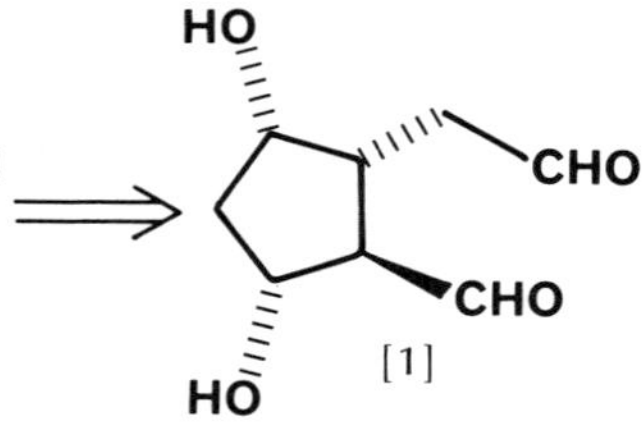

[1]

Turner type intermediate (p. 201)
Bis-aldehyde

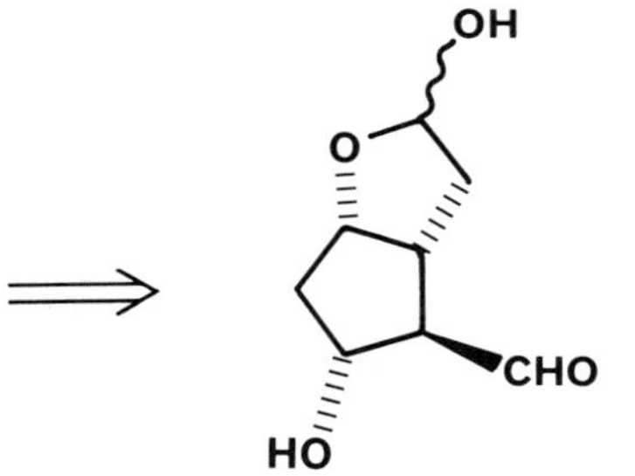

[2]
Hemiacetal

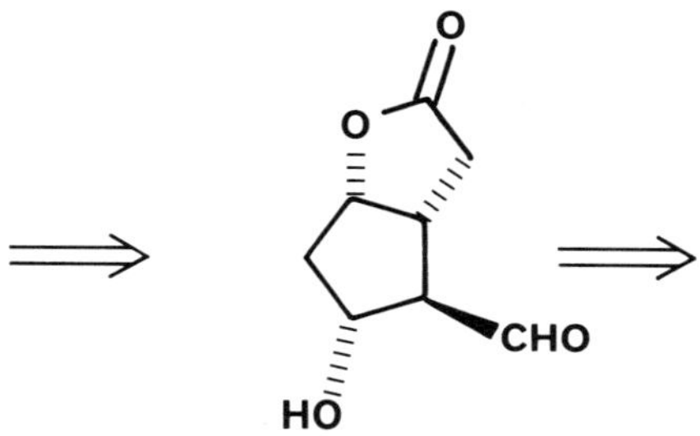

[3]
Corey Aldehyde

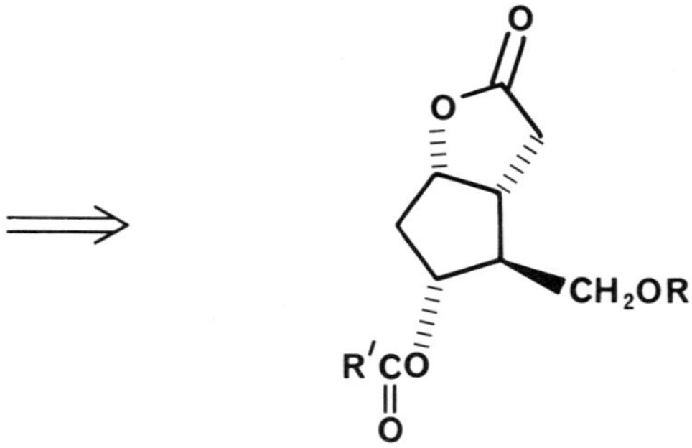

[4]
Corey lactone

To date the bicyclic lactone [4], commonly referred to as the Corey lactone, is the most widely used intermediate in the synthesis of naturally occurring prostaglandins and also in the synthesis of some of the analogs. The synthesis of the lactone [4] or the Corey aldehyde [3] by diverse synthetic methods has been accepted as constituting a formal synthesis of the prostaglandins.

Although the Corey lactone assures the stereochemistry of the substituents around the prostanoid nucleus, further elaboration into the prostaglandins necessitates the use of a remote functionality to induce the chirality at C_{15}.

The bicyclo[2.2.1]heptane route was designed within this context. Starting with a cyclopentane derivative sequential introduction of the appropriate substituents around the ring leads to Corey lactone. Thus Diels-Alder reaction of a 5-substituted cyclopentadiene with a ketene equivalent provides the C_6 and C_7 carbons and the formation of the *anti* adduct gives the required *trans* orientation of the α- and β- chain precursors at C_8 and C_{12}, respectively. Selective Baeyer-Villiger oxidation gives the δ-lactone, which is transformed to the γ-lactone via iodolactonization. Subsequent elaborations lead to $PGF_{2\alpha}$.

SYNTHETIC STRATEGY

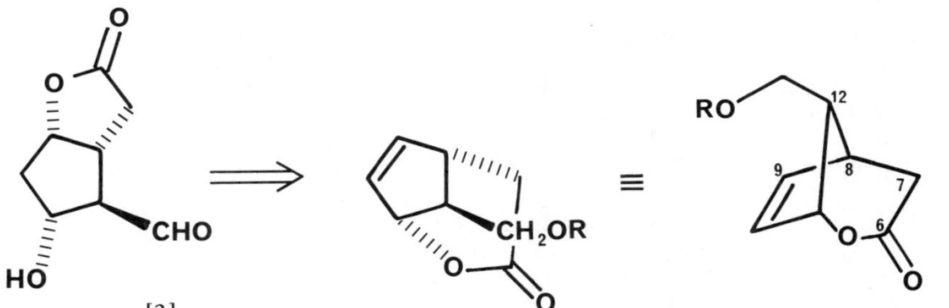

[3]

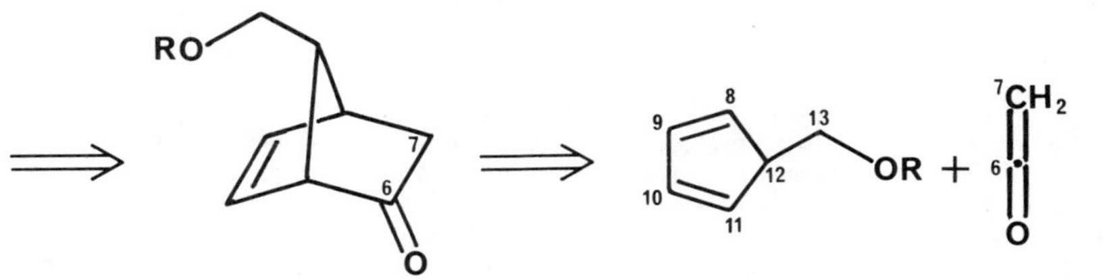

Ketene equivalent

SYNTHETIC PLAN[1]

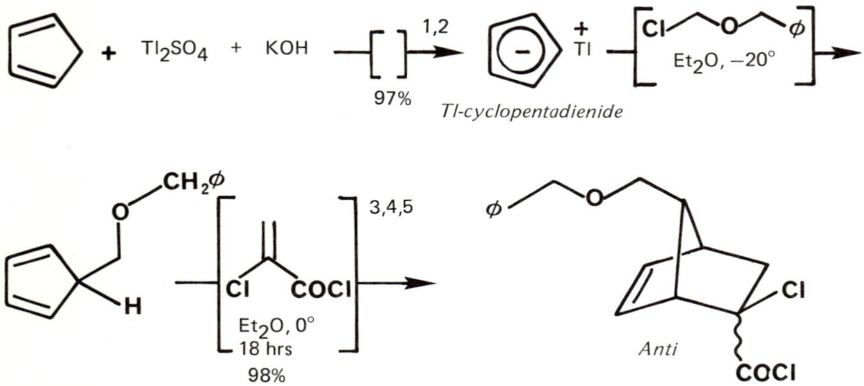

1. E. J. Corey, N. M. Weinshenker, T. K. Schaaf & W. Huber, *J. Am. Chem. Soc.*, **91**, 5675 (1969).
2. Similar modifications have been made by N. M. Weinshenker, *Prostaglandins*, **3**, 219 (1973). It is advantageous to use the less basic Tl-cyclopentadienide. The insoluble TlCl is removed by filtration (at –40° C), thereby avoiding aqueous work-up and minimizing any protropic rearrangements (0-3%). E. J. Corey, U. Koelliker & J. Neuffer, *J. Am. Chem. Soc.*, **93**, 1489 (1971).

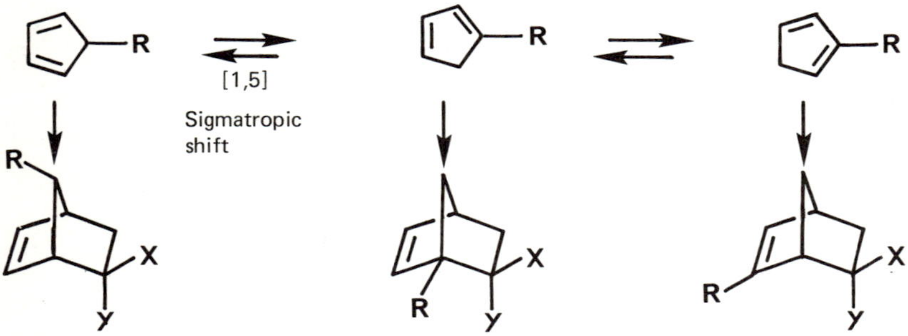

3. Owing to the fact ketenes react with 1,3-dienes to give cyclobutanones ($_{\pi}2_s + _{\pi}2_a$) rather than ($_{\pi}4_s + _{\pi}2_s$) adducts the use of suitable ketene equivalents was necessary. One early ketene equivalent, 2-acetoxyacrylonitrile, was first developed by Bartlett. P. D. Bartlett & B. E. Tate, *J. Am. Chem. Soc.*, **78**, 2473 (1956).
4. 2-Chloroacrylyl chloride is more reactive than 2-chloroacrylonitrile (D. A. Evans, W. L. Scott & L. K. Truesdale, *Tet. Lett.*, 121 (1972)) and exhibits a dienophilic reactivity comparable to maleic anhydride. On account of its geminal substitution, it reacts with 5-substituted cyclopentadienes to form Diels-Alder adducts with 7-*anti* configuration only.
E. J. Corey, T. Ravidranathan & S. Terashima, *J. Am. Chem. Soc.*, **93**, 4326 (1971).
The formation of the bicyclo[2.2.1]heptane derivative is based on the original observation of G. Kresze, *et al.*, *Ann. Chem.*, **666**, 45 (1963).

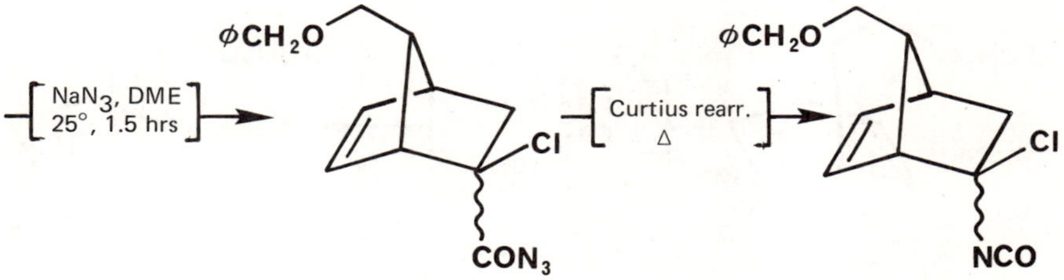

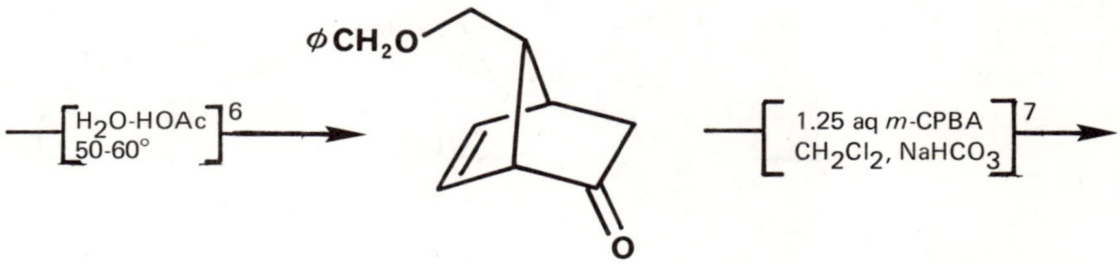

[5]

---

5. Dienophiles without geminal substitution give a mixture of *syn* and *anti* adducts.

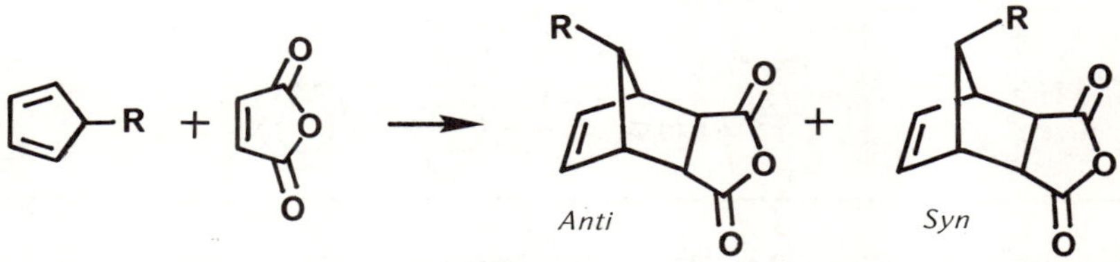

6. For another synthesis of this bicyclo[2.2.1]heptane ketone derivative [5] using acrylic acid as a ketene equivalent see:
B. M. Trost & Y. Tomaru, *J. Am. Chem. Soc.*, **97**, 3528 (1975).

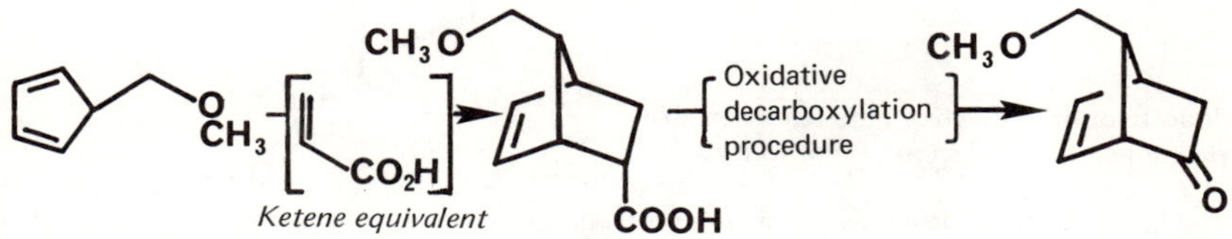

7. The norbornene double bond is not epoxidized.

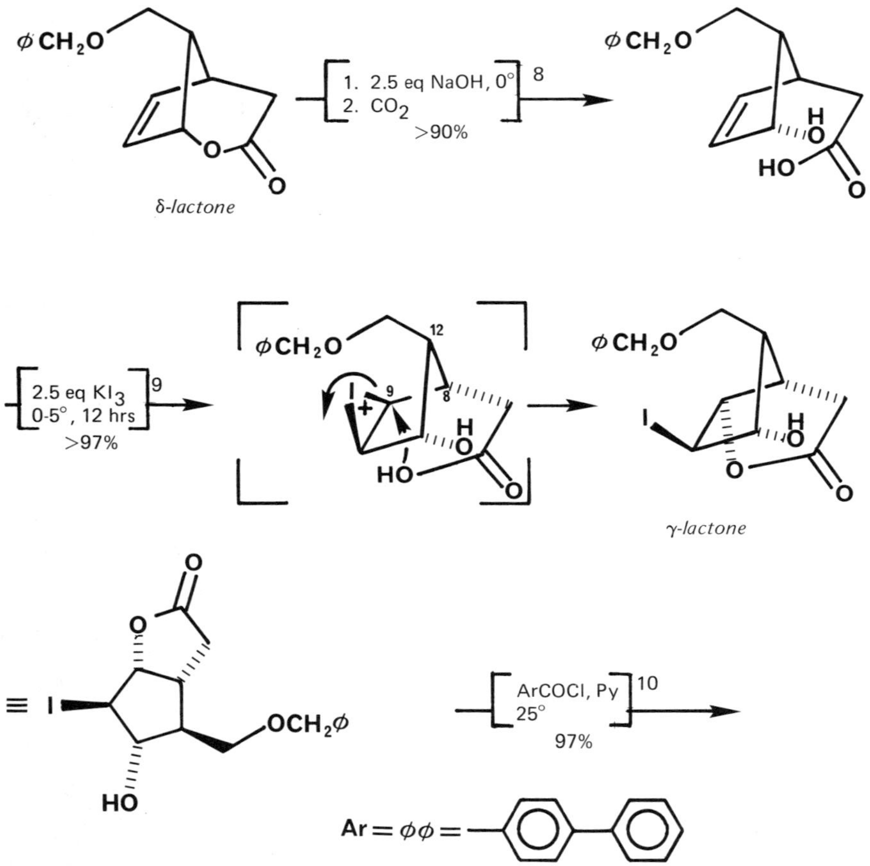

8. Use of alkaline hydrogen peroxide gives the hydroxy acid [6] directly in higher yields (99%). N. M. Weinshenker & R. Stephenson, *J. Org. Chem.*, 37, 3741 (1972).

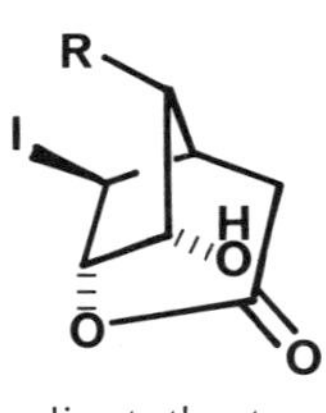

δ-lactone

9. Iodolactonization gives the more stable γ-lactone. The δ-lactone is not formed.

10. Unlike the acetate, the p-phenylbenzoate protecting group directs the stereochemical course of reduction of the C_{15} ketone. For further details see p. 107. Also, the *p*-phenylbenzoates are nice crystalline compounds.

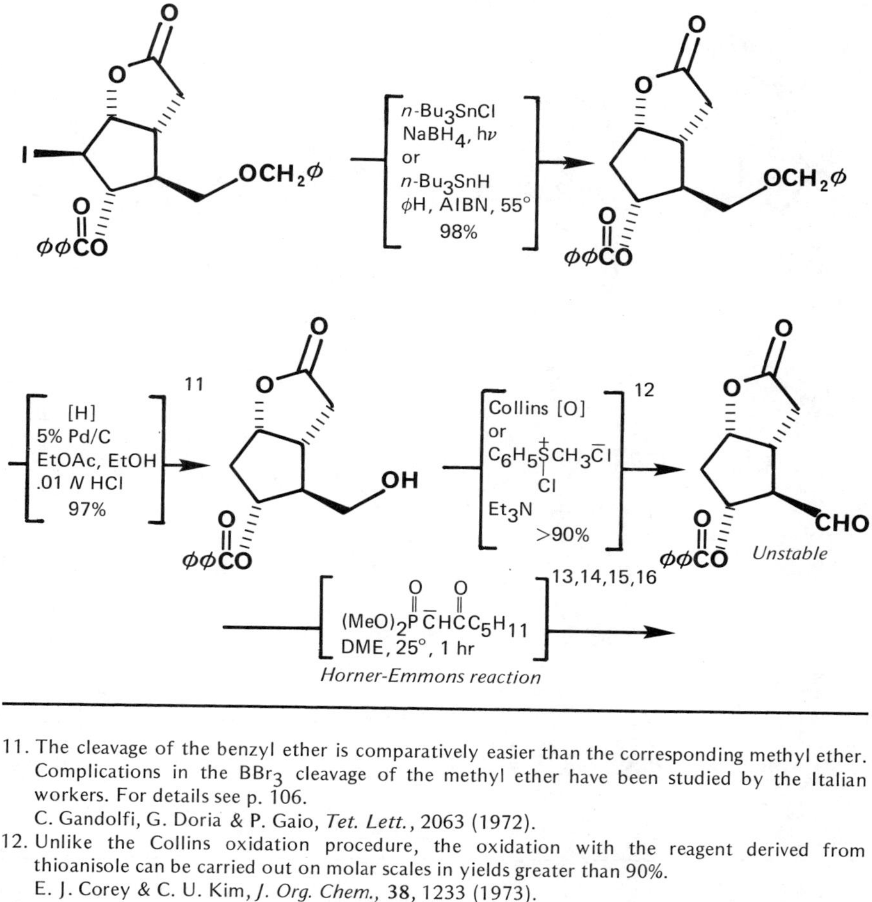

11. The cleavage of the benzyl ether is comparatively easier than the corresponding methyl ether. Complications in the BBr_3 cleavage of the methyl ether have been studied by the Italian workers. For details see p. 106.
    C. Gandolfi, G. Doria & P. Gaio, *Tet. Lett.*, 2063 (1972).
12. Unlike the Collins oxidation procedure, the oxidation with the reagent derived from thioanisole can be carried out on molar scales in yields greater than 90%.
    E. J. Corey & C. U. Kim, *J. Org. Chem.*, **38**, 1233 (1973).
13. W. S. Wadsworth & W. D. Emmons, *J. Am. Chem. Soc.*, **83**, 1733 (1961); L. Horner, H. Hoffmann, H. G. Wipper & G. Klahre, *Chem. Ber.*, **92**, 2499 (1959).
14. One of the side reactions in this Horner-Emmons reaction is the elimination of the ester to give the dienone [7].

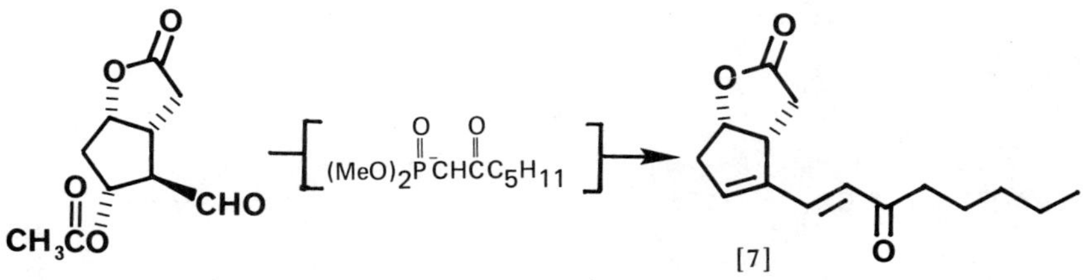

[7]

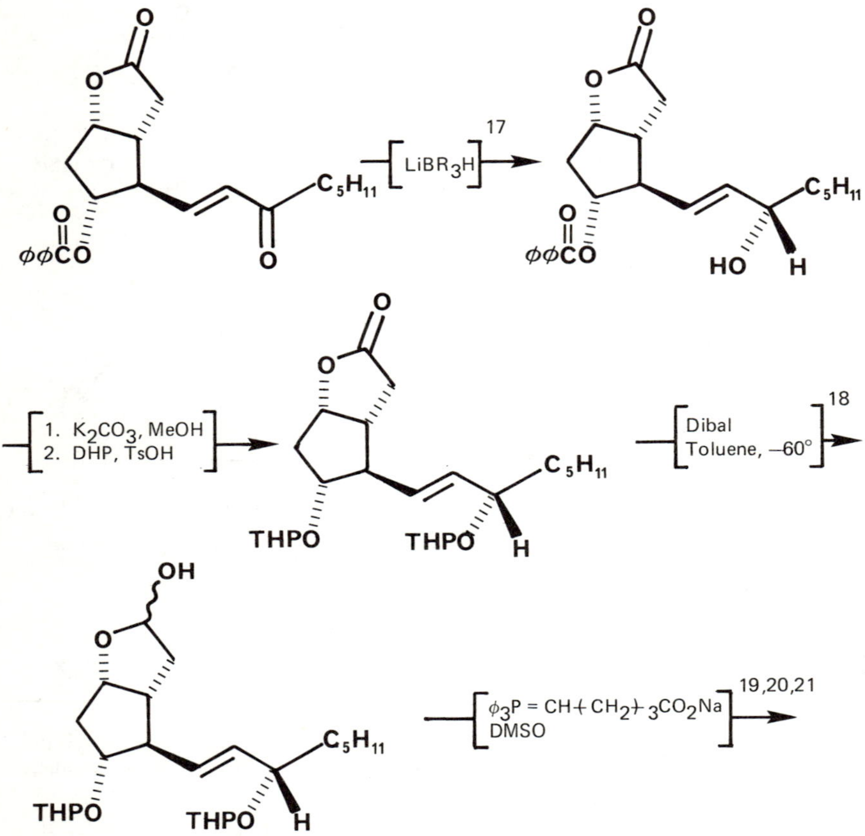

15. Similar eliminations in analogous cases have been observed also:
D. Taub, R. D. Hoffsommer, C. H. Kuo, H. L. Slates, Z. S. Zelawski & N. L. Wendler, *Tet.*, **30**, 819 (1974); D. Brewster, M. Myers, J. Ormerod, P. Otter, A. C. B. Smith, M. E. Spinner & S. Turner, *J. Chem. Soc., [Perkin I]*, 2796 (1973).
16. The phosphonate was prepared from ethyl-hexanoate and dimethyl-α-lithiomethane phosphonate. It has been made by a different method by P. A. Grieco & C. S. Pogonowski, *J. Am. Chem. Soc.*, **95**, 3071 (1973). See p. 357.

17. The stereoselective reduction of the C_{15} ketone by an exogeneous C_{11} substituent has been studied in detail.
E. J. Corey, S. M. Albonico, U. Koelliker, T. K. Schaaf & R. K. Varma, *J. Am. Chem. Soc.*, **93**, 1491 (1971); E. J. Corey, K. B. Becker & R. K. Varma, *J. Am. Chem. Soc.*, **94**, 8616 (1972). For the details of such studies see p. 107.
18. The reduction of lactones to hemiacetals was first shown by J. Schmidlin & A. Wettstein, *Helv. Chim. Acta.*, **46**, 2799 (1963).

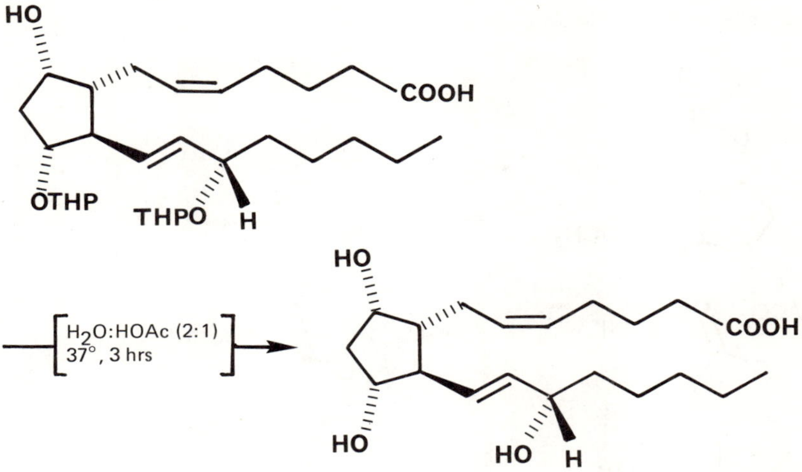

$PGF_{2\alpha}$

---

19. The ylid was generated from 5-triphenylphosphoniopentanoic acid and sodiomethylsulfinylcarbanide in DMSO. An excess of the ylid has to be used.
20. The use of methylsulfinylcarbanide in Wittig reaction was first shown by the Harvard group. R. Greenwald, M. Chaykovsky & E. J. Corey, *J. Org. Chem.*, **28**, 1128 (1963).
21. The formation of the *cis*-$\Delta^{5,6}$ olefin is in accord with the previous results obtained in the synthesis of humulene. E. J. Corey & E. Hamanaka, *J. Am. Chem. Soc.*, **89**, 2758 (1967).

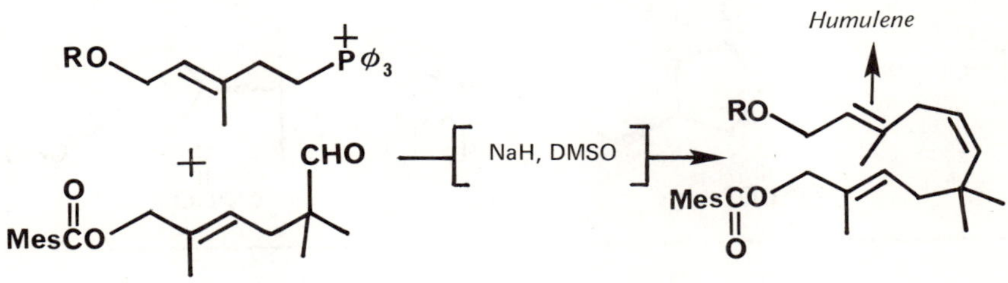

Complications in the BBr_3 Cleavage of the Methyl Ether [8][22]

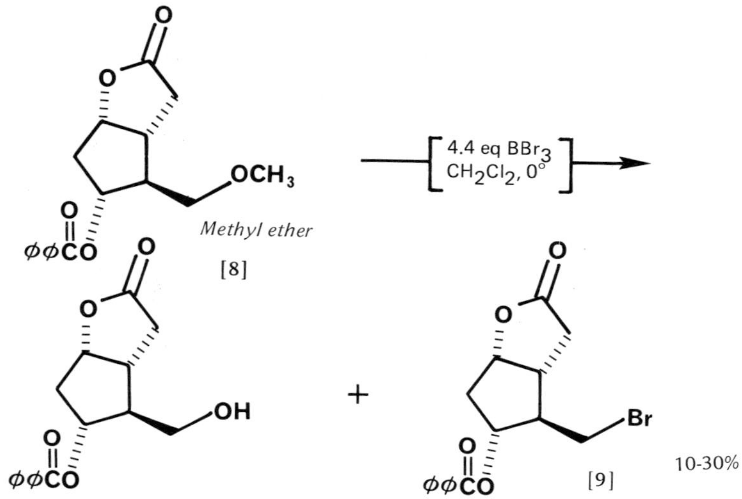

Conversion of the primary bromide [9] to the aldehyde [10] is carried out as follows:

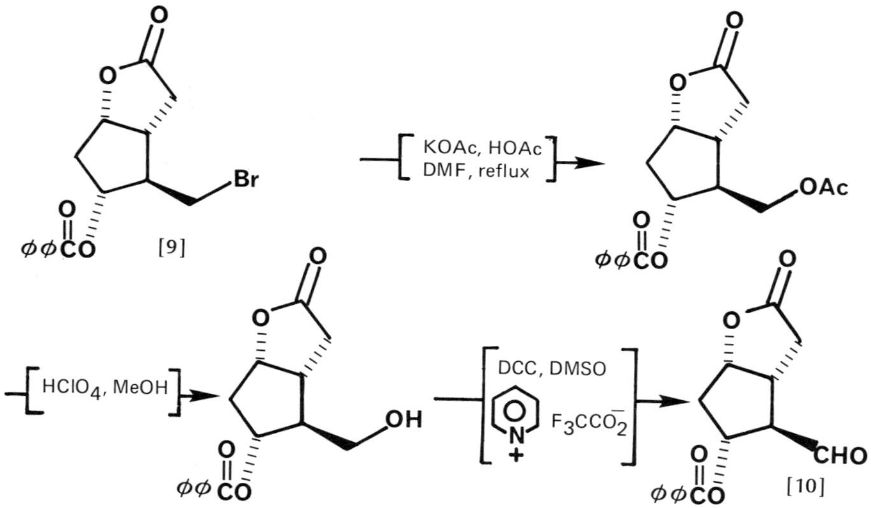

22. C. Gandolfi, G. Doria & P. Gaio, *Tet. Lett.*, 2063 (1972).

Stereospecific Reduction of the C_{15} Ketone[23,24]

A suitable alcohol protecting group was used to protect the C_{11} hydroxyl group such that this protecting group will stabilize the *S-cis*-enone conformer of transition state and block the approach of the hydride from the side b.

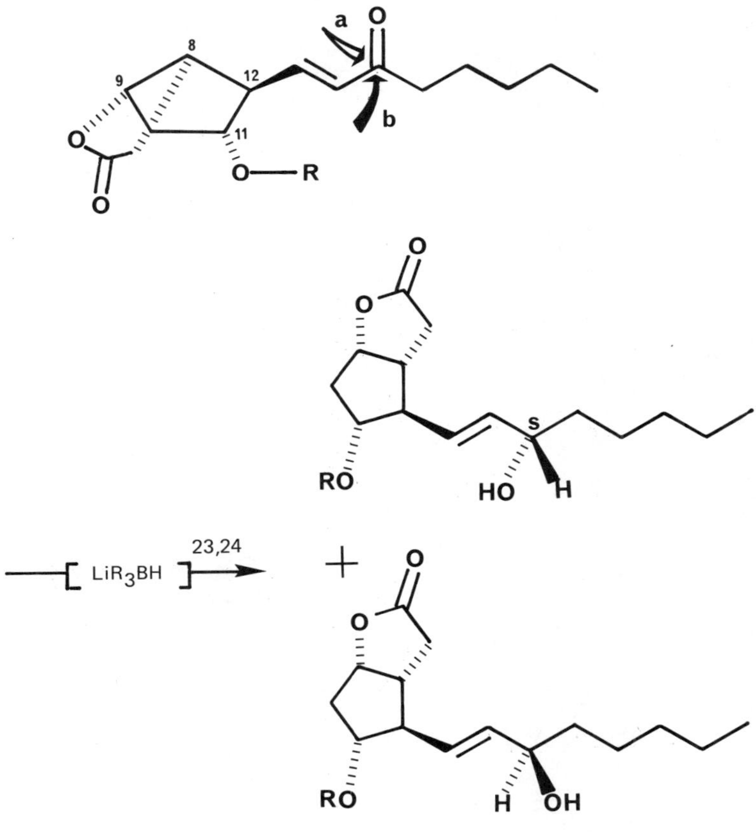

23. E. J. Corey, K. B. Becker & R. K. Varma, *J. Am. Chem. Soc.*, 94, 8616 (1972).
24. E. J. Corey in the Abstracts of 24th Organic Chemistry Symposium of the American Chemical Society held at Colorado State University, Fort Collins, June 22-26, 1975, p. 40-42.

Ratio of the C_{15} Epimeric Alcohols Obtained With Different Protecting Groups[24]

R =	15*S* : 15*R*
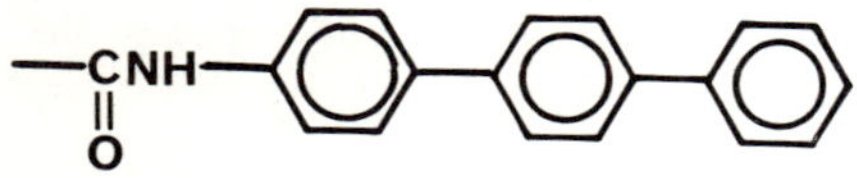	94 : 6
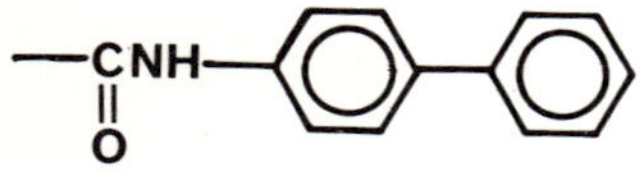	92 : 8
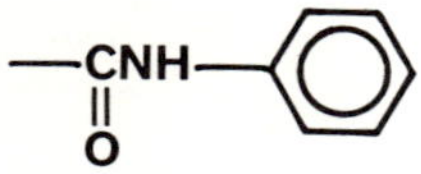	89 : 11
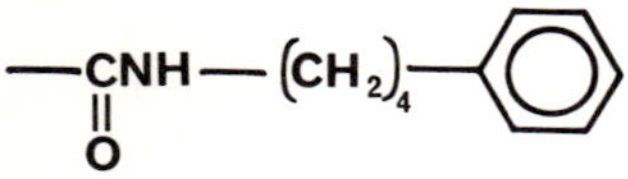	57 : 43
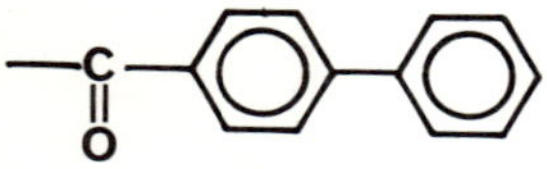	82 : 18
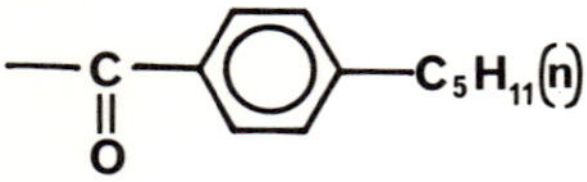	82 : 18
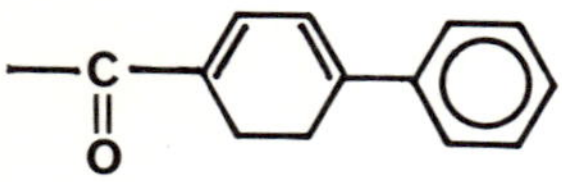	84 : 16
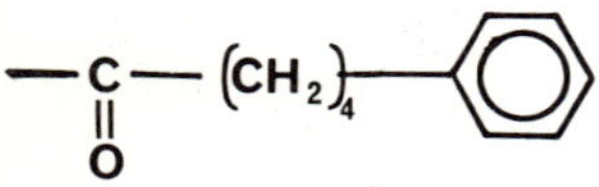	60 : 40
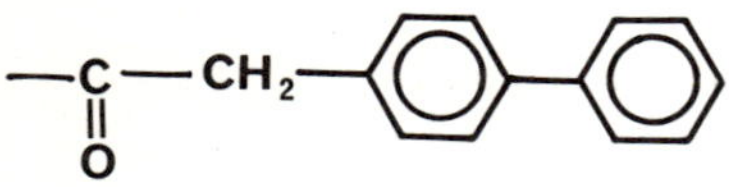	70 : 30
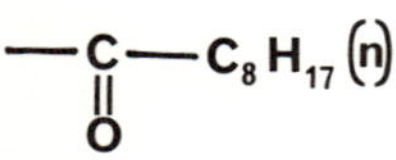	60 : 40

Synthesis of the Chiral Form of Corey Lactone[25]

The chiral form of the Corey lactone [11] has been synthesized via the Diels-Alder route using a chiral dienophile.[25]

SYNTHETIC PLAN[25]

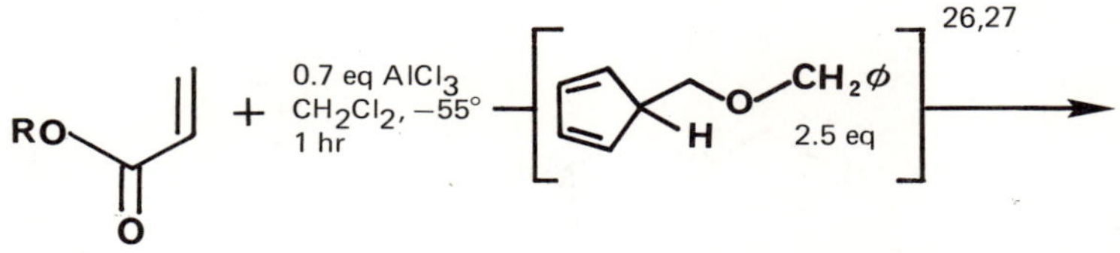

Chiral acrylate

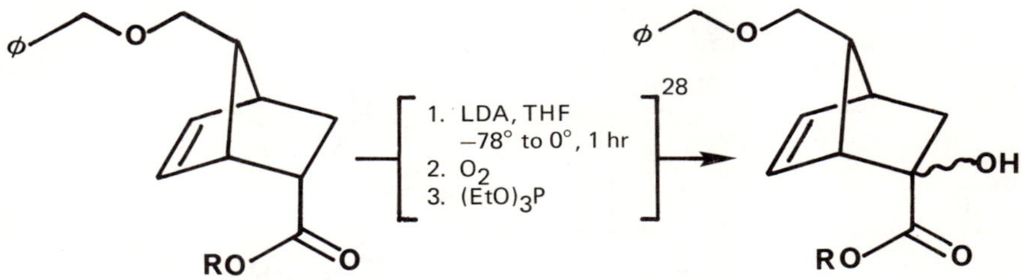

89% Endo adduct

$[\alpha]_D^{23} = -21.3°$

---

25. E. J. Corey & H. E. Ensley, *J. Am. Chem. Soc.*, **97**, 6908 (1976).
26. For a discussion of Diels-Alder reaction with various chiral dienes and dienophiles see J. D. Morrison & H. S. Mosher, *Asymmetric Organic Reactions*, Prentice-Hall, Englewood Cliffs, N.J., p. 252.
27. For examples of Diels-Alder Reaction of cyclopentadiene with various chiral acrylates see:
    J. Sauer, J. Kredel, *Angew. Chem. [Int. Edit.]*, **4**, 989 (1965).
    J. Sauer & J. Kredel, *Tet. Lett.*, 6359 (1966).
    R. F. Farmer & J. Hamer, *J. Org. Chem.*, **31**, 2418 (1966).
    O. Cervinka & O. Kriz, *Coll. Czech. Chem. Commun.*, **33**, 2342 (1968).

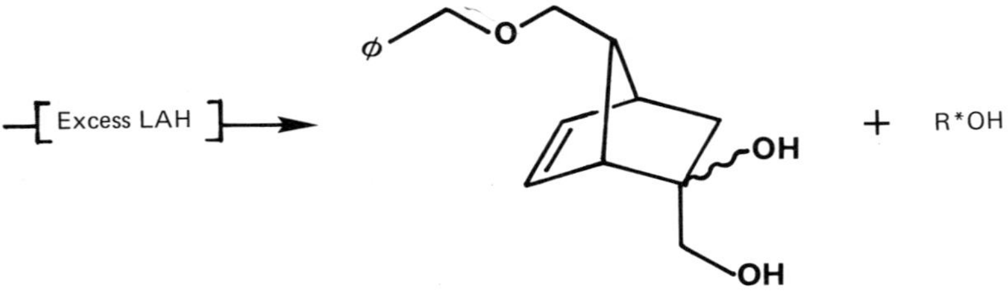

endo:exo(hydroxy) = 1:2

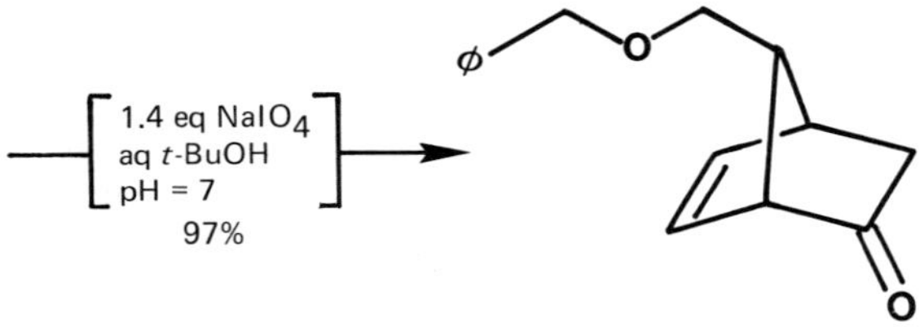

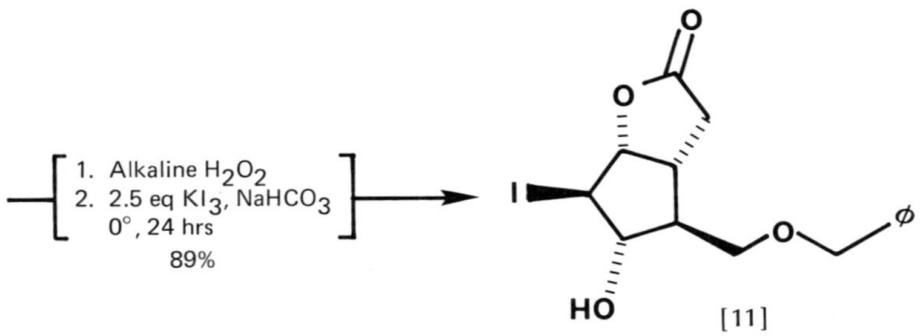

[11]

$[\alpha]_D^{23} = 33.3°$

28. This *in situ* formation and reduction of the α-hydroperoxy ester was found to be superior to other methods. See D. S. Watt & S. J. Selikson, *J. Org. Chem.*, **40**, 267 (1975); H. H. Wasserman & B. H. Lipshutz, *Tet. Lett.*, 1731 (1975).

Synthesis of the Chiral Acrylate[25]

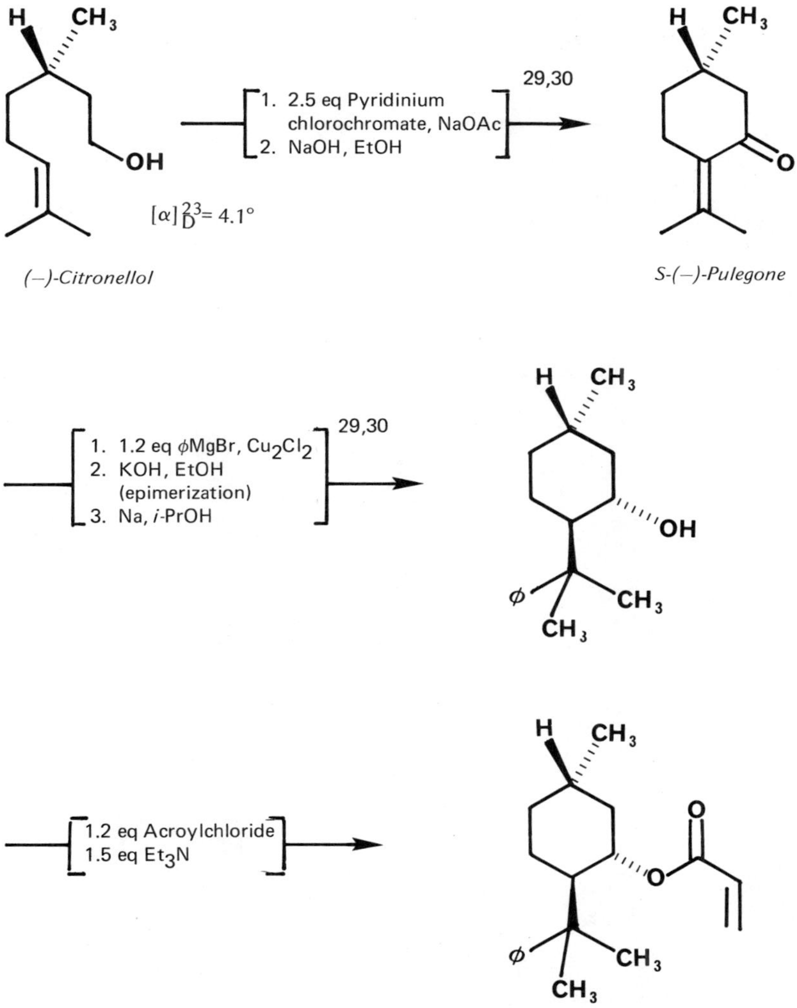

Chiral acrylate

---

29. E. J. Corey, H. E. Ensley & J. W. Suggs, *J. Org. Chem.*, **41**, 380 (1976).
30. E. J. Corey & J. W. Suggs, *Tet. Lett.*, 2647 (1975).

Synthesis of PGE_1 from Corey Lactone [12][31,32]

SYNTHETIC PLAN[31,32]

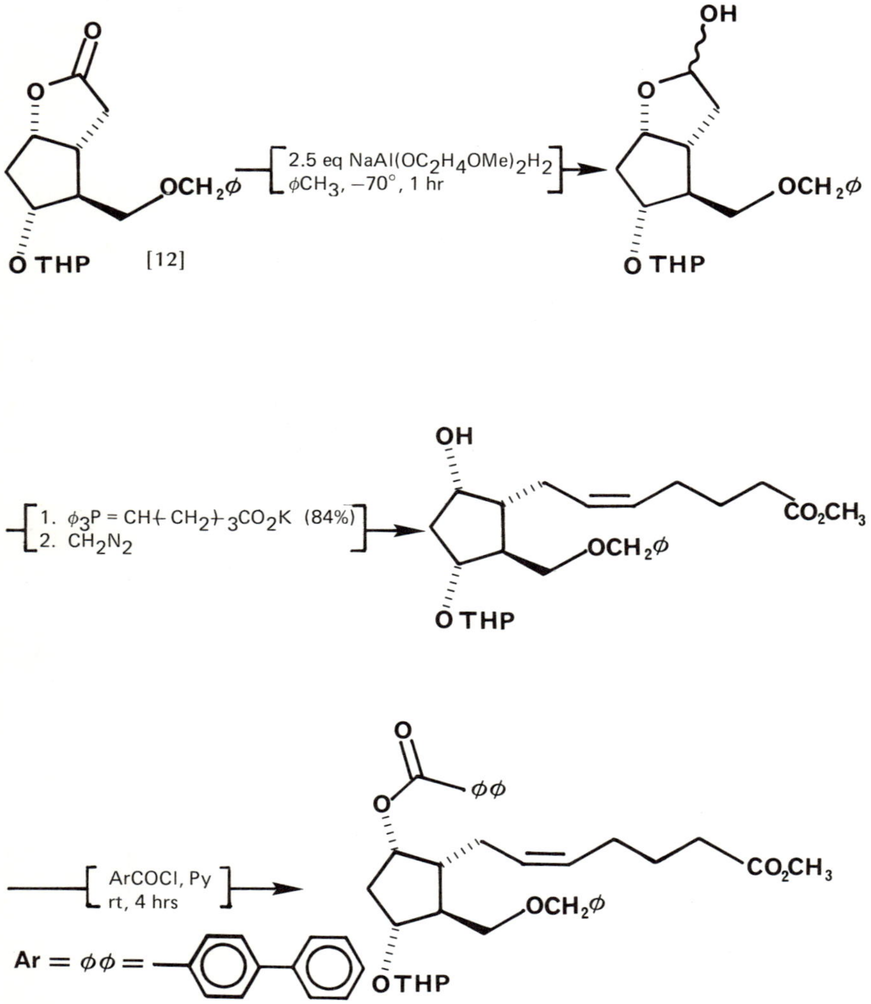

31. G. Doria, P. Gaio & C. Gandolfi, *Tet. Lett.*, 4307 (1972).
32. A similar approach to the synthesis of $PGF_{1\alpha}$ has also been reported. E. J. Corey & T. K. Schaaf, *J. Org. Chem.*, **37**, 2922 (1972).

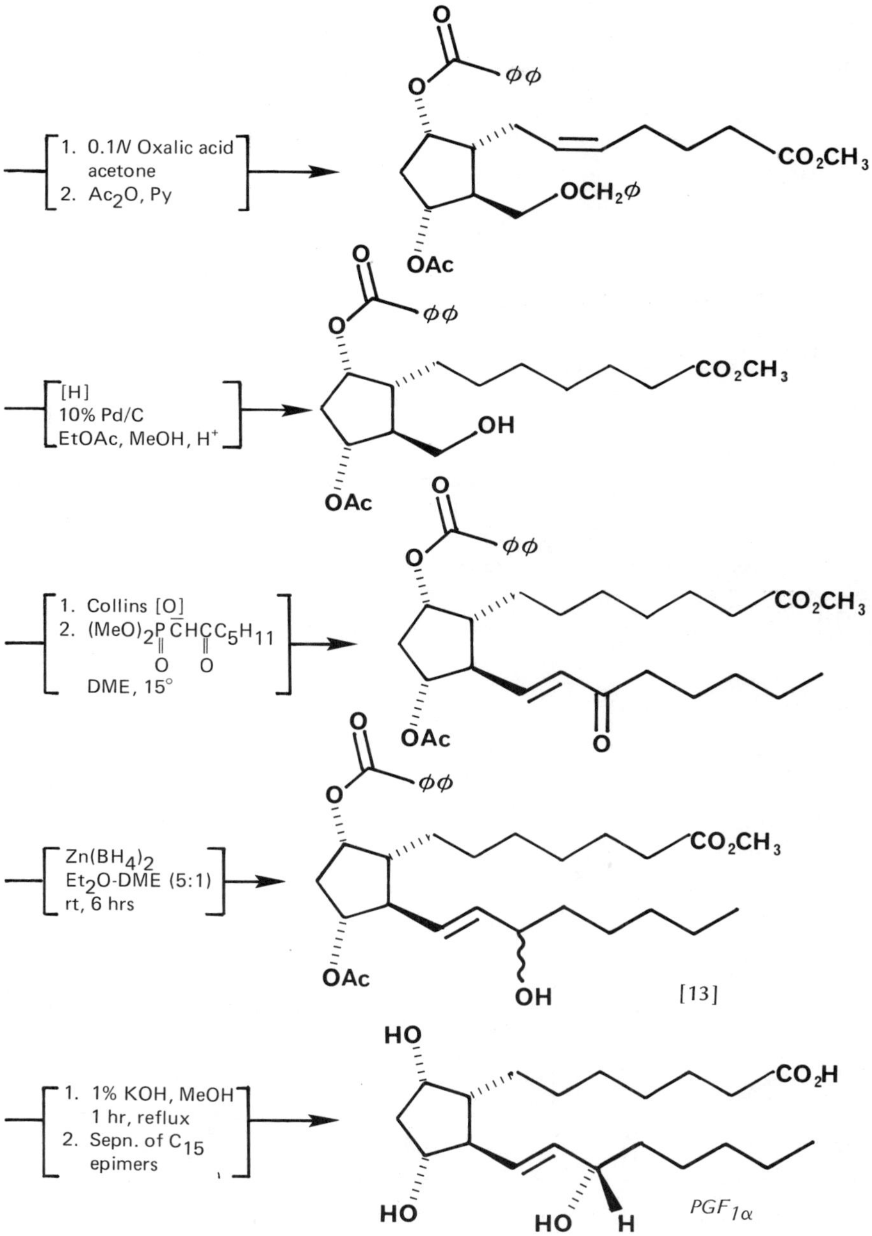
1. 0.1N Oxalic acid acetone
2. Ac2O, Py
OCH2ϕ
CO2CH3
ϕϕ
OAc
[H]
10% Pd/C
EtOAc, MeOH, H+
OH
1. Collins [O]
2. (MeO)2P(O)CHC(O)C5H11
DME, 15°
Zn(BH4)2
Et2O-DME (5:1)
rt, 6 hrs
[13]
1. 1% KOH, MeOH
1 hr, reflux
2. Sepn. of C15 epimers
HO
CO2H
H
PGF1α

Epimerization of C_{15}[31]

Hydrolysis of the C_{11}-acetate group of $PGF_{1\alpha}$ triester [13] by means of $HClO_4$/MeOH and with HCl/H_2O-dioxane was unsuccessful because of the partial isomerization of the hydroxyl group at C_{15}. Similar isomerization studies have also been done by the Upjohn group.[33]

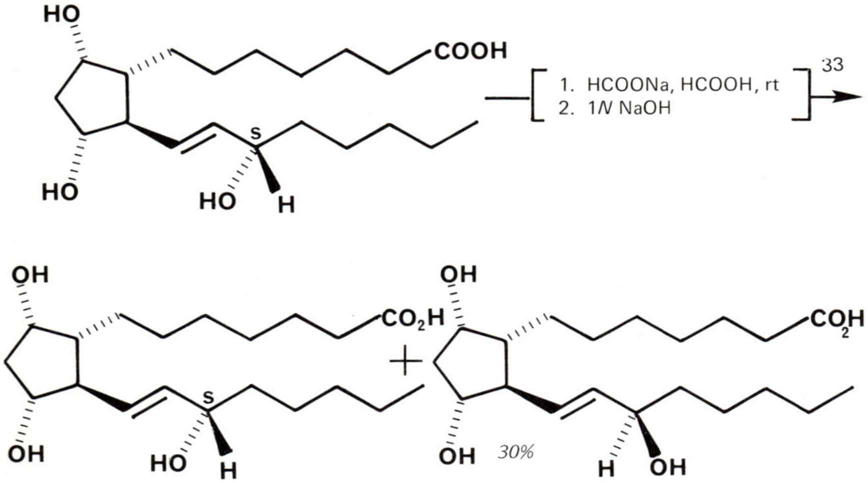

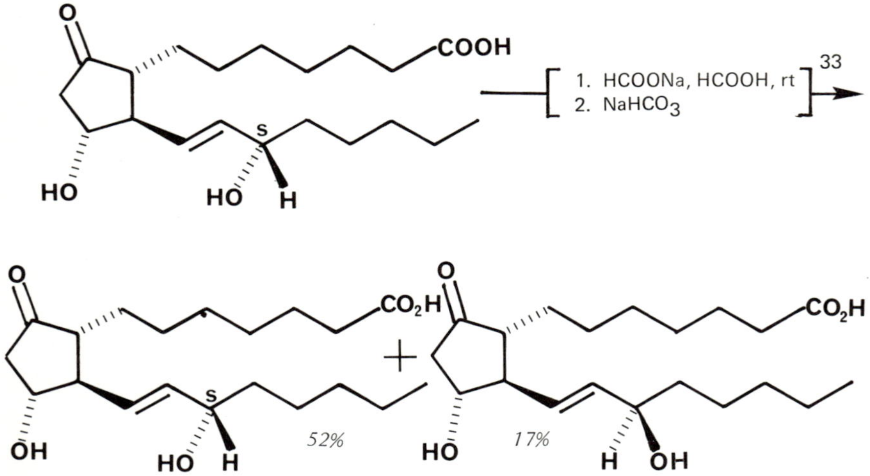

33. J. E. Pike, F. H. Lincoln & W. P. Schneider, *J. Org. Chem.*, **34**, 3552 (1969).

Synthesis of PGE_2 from the Protected Triol [14][34]

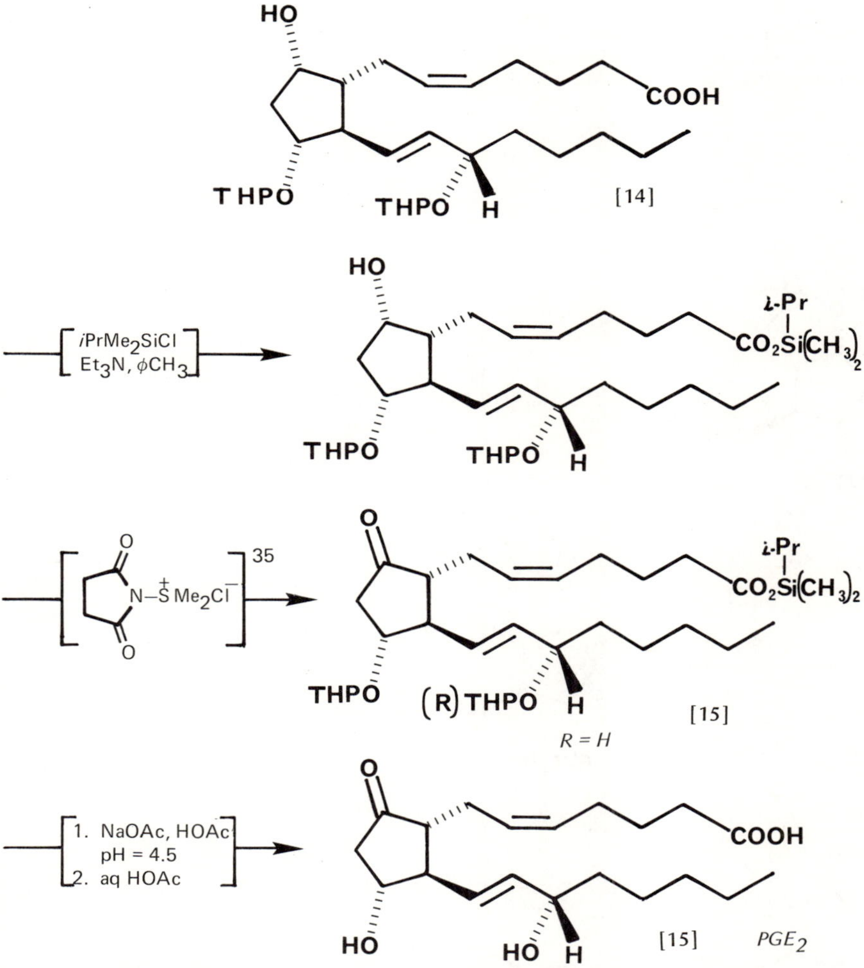

---

34. E. J. Corey & C. U. Kim, *J. Org. Chem.*, **38**, 1233 (1973).
35. Oxidation of the acid-sensitive keto-alcohol with Jones reagent at −20° C gave only 70% yield of the keto acid (**15**, R=H). Previously known non-acidic oxidizing agents (e.g. Collins reagent)[36] were ineffective. This problem led to the development of a new neutral oxidizing agent. E. J. Corey, T. K. Schaaf, W. Huber, U. Koelliker & N. M. Weinshenker, *J. Am. Chem. Soc.*, **92**, 397 (1970).
36. J. C. Collins, W. W. Hess & F. J. Foank, *Tet. Lett.*, 3363 (1968).

Synthesis of $PGF_{3\alpha}$ [18][37]

A desire to introduce the β-chain with the 15*S* alcohol[37] without having to use bulky directing groups for stereocontrolled reduction of C_{15} ketone[38] motivated the development of the chiral β-oxido ylid [16] for the synthesis of $PGF_{3\alpha}$

SYNTHETIC PLAN[37]

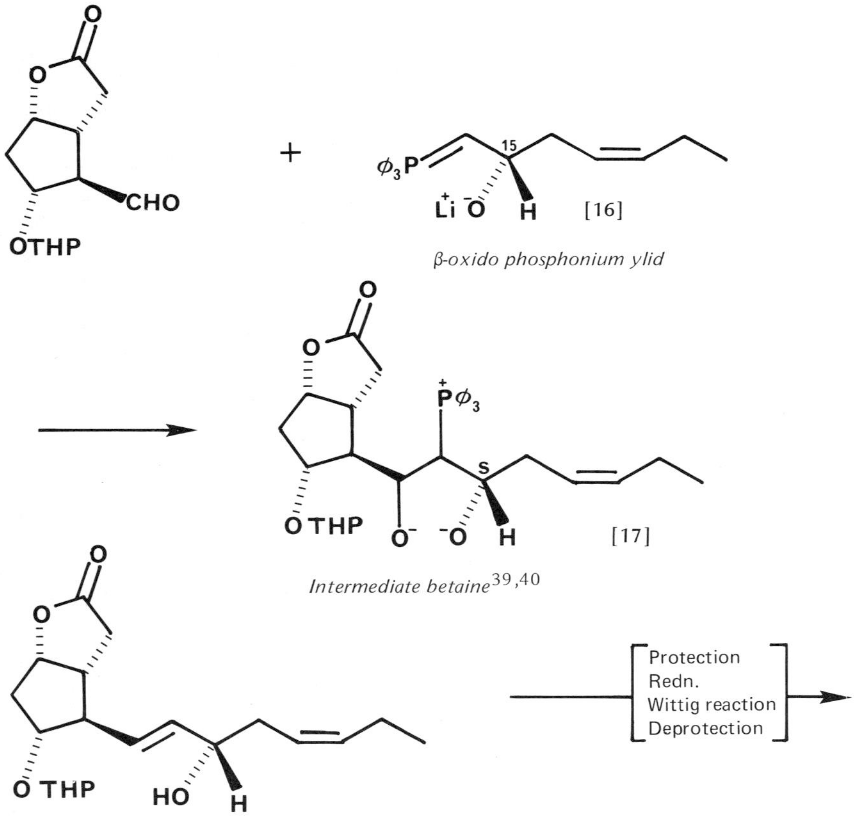

[16]

β-oxido phosphonium ylid

[17]

Intermediate betaine[39,40]

---

37. E. J. Corey, H. Shirahama, H. Yamamoto, S. Terashima, A. Venkateswarlu & T. K. Schaaf, *J. Am. Chem. Soc.*, 93, 1490 (1971).
38. E. J. Corey, K. B. Becker & R. K. Varma, *J. Am. Chem. Soc.*, 94, 8616 (1972).

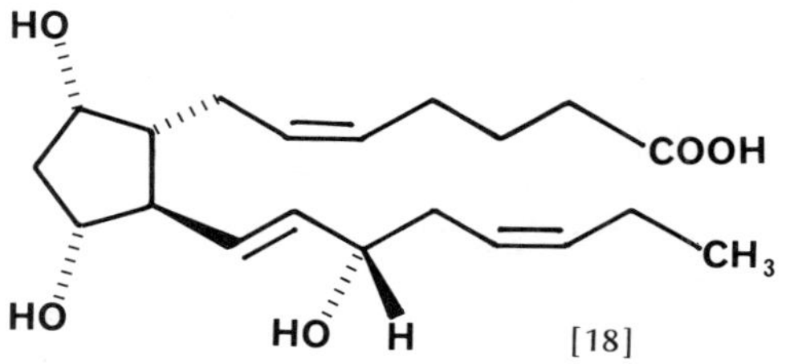

[18]

PGF$_{3\alpha}$[41]

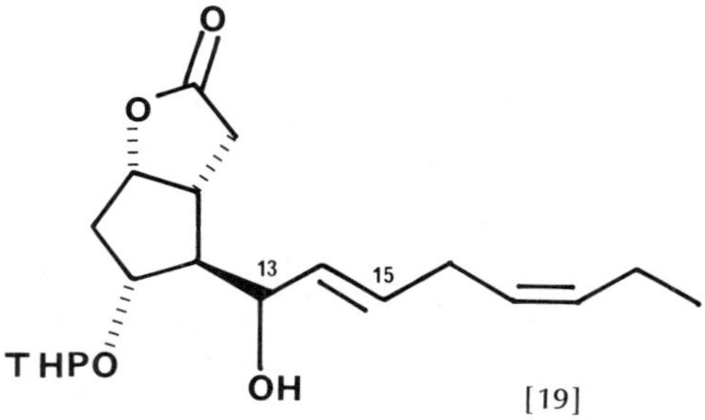

[19]

39. It is not obvious why the intermediate betaine [17] decomposes to give the desired allylic alcohol. The other allylic alcohol [19] is not formed. Exploratory studies show that the betaine undergoes elimination in the direction of that carbonyl moiety which was added last except in the case of formaldehyde. E. J. Corey & H. Yamamoto, *J. Am. Chem. Soc.*, **92**, 226 (1970).
40. Dialkoxyphosphonium betaines have been similarly applied to the syntheses of juvenile hormones. E. J. Corey & H. Yamamoto, *J. Am. Chem. Soc.*, **92**, 6636 (1970); and farnesol, E. J. Corey & H. Yamamoto, *J. Am. Chem. Soc.*, **92**, 6637 (1970).
41. For an alternate synthesis of *racemic* PGE$_3$ methyl ester via the bicyclo[3.1.0]hexane route see: U. Axen, J. L. Thompson & J. E. Pike, *Chem. Commun.*, 602 (1970).

Synthesis of the Chiral Ylid [20][37]

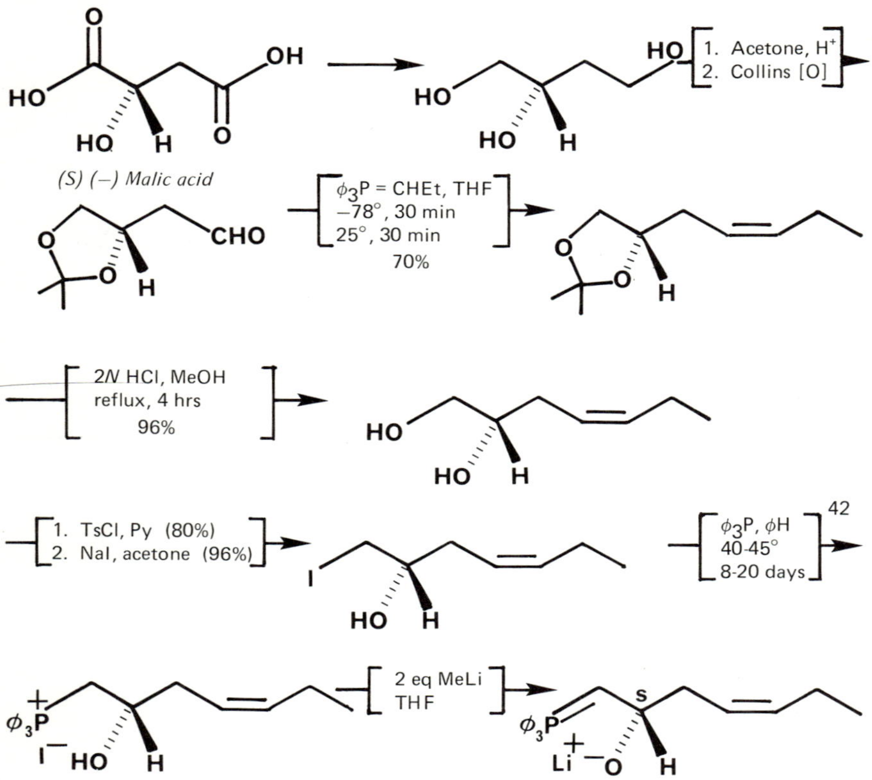

[20]

42. Only those phosphonates in which R_1 can further stabilize the carbanion by resonance can be employed successfully in olefin synthesis (R_1 = COR_1, CN, ϕ, etc.). J. Boutagy & R. Thomas, *Chem. Rev.*, 74, 87 (1974).

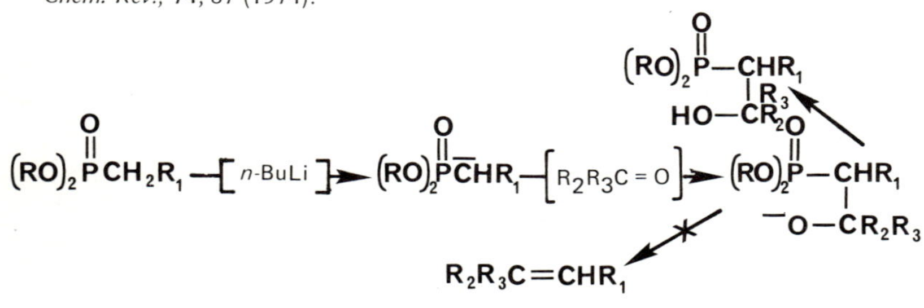

Synthesis of Optically Active β-Chain [21][43]

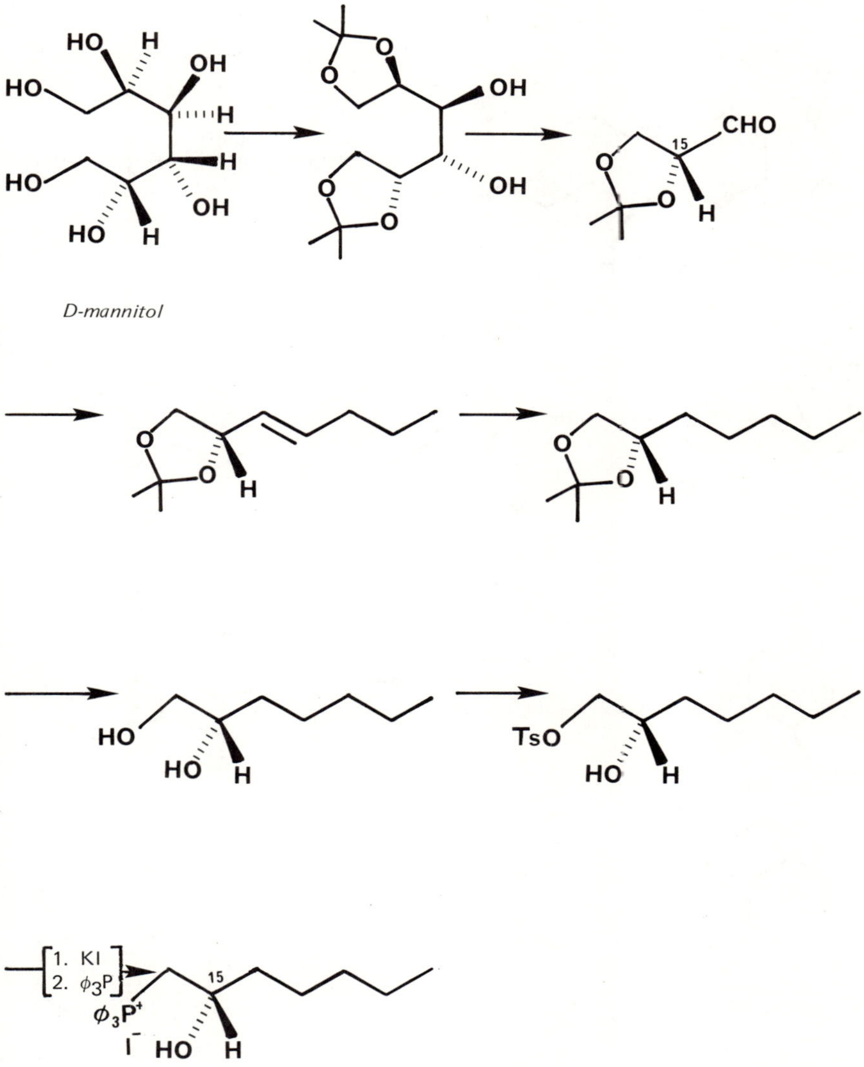

[21]

---

43. F. Johnson *et al.*, personal communication.

Stereospecific Reduction of PGE_2 to $PGF_{2\alpha}$[44]

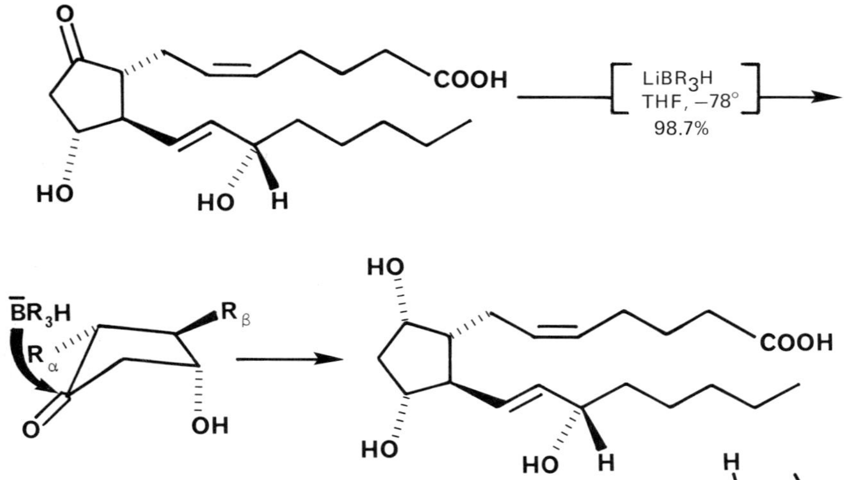

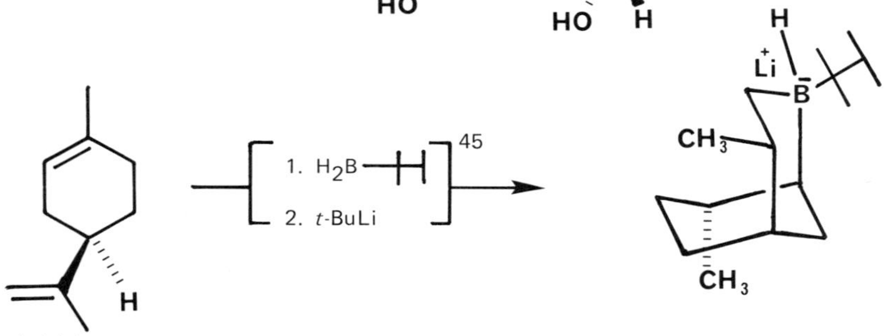

(D) (+) Limonene

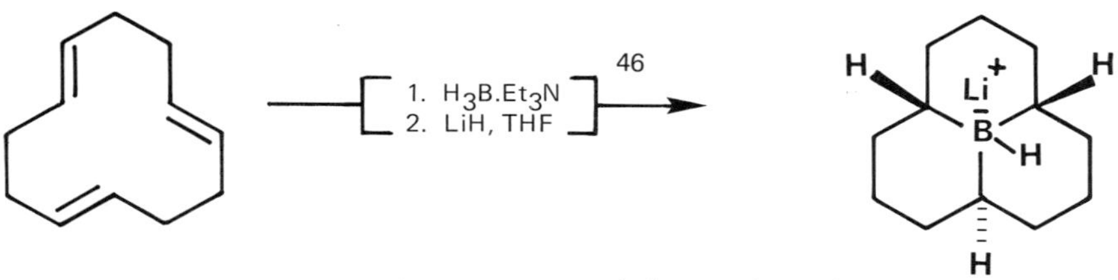

Lithium perhydro-9b-boraphenalyl hydride

---

44. E. J. Corey & R. K. Varma, *J. Am. Chem. Soc.*, **93**, 7319 (1971).
45. H. C. Brown & C. D. Pfaffenberger, *J. Am. Chem. Soc.*, **89**, 5475 (1967).
46. H. C. Brown & W. C. Dickason, *J. Am. Chem. Soc.*, **92**, 709 (1970).

Reduction of PGE_2 to PGE_1[47]

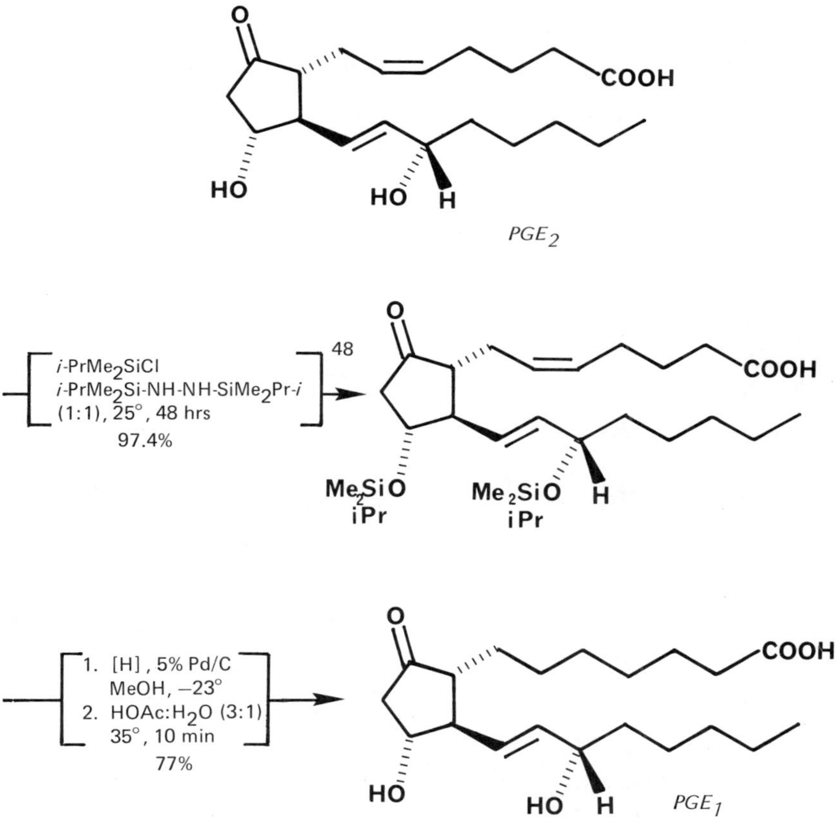

---

47. E. J. Corey & R. K. Varma, *J. Am. Chem. Soc.*, 93, 7319 (1971).
48. The use of dimethylisopropylsilyl (DMIS) ethers protecting group offers several advantages:
    i. Cleavage of the DMIS-ethers require comparatively milder conditions than the corresponding THP-ethers.
    ii. DMIS-ethers are frequently crystalline substances whereas the THP-ethers are usually oils.
    iii. Unlike the THP-ethers, DMIS-ethers have no additional chiral centers.
    iv. Better screening of the C_{13}-C_{14} double bond by the DMIS ether than the THP-ether increases the selectivity of the hydrogenation.[49]
49. E. J. Corey, R. Noyori & T. K. Schaaf, *J. Am. Chem. Soc.*, 92, 2586 (1970).

Alternate Synthesis of the Corey Lactone [22][50]

This novel and practical approach[50] involves the one-step transformation of the bicyclo[2.2.1]heptane skeleton arising from the cycloaddition of nitroethylene to 5-substituted cyclopentadienes to the oxabicyclo[3.3.0]octane [23] framework directly related to PGA_2. This intermediate has also been converted to the Corey aldehyde by a regiospecific addition of the elements of BrOH.[51]

SYNTHETIC STRATEGY

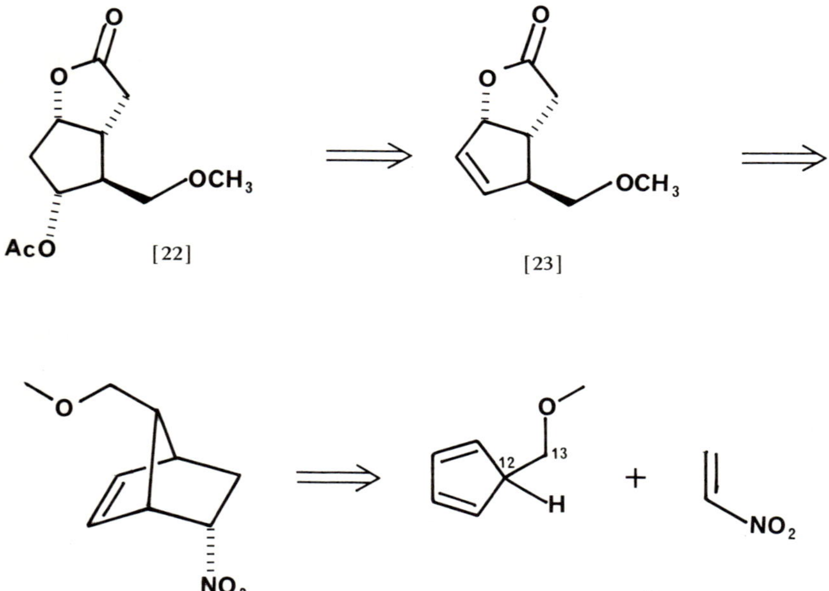

Ketene equivalent

---

50. S. Ranganathan, D. Ranganathan & A. K. Mehrotra, *J. Am. Chem. Soc.*, **96**, 5261 (1974).
51. S. Ranganathan, D. Ranganathan & A. K. Mehrotra, *Tet. Lett.*, 1215 (1975).
52. S. Ranganathan, D. Ranganathan & R. Iyengar, *Tet.*, **32**, 961 (1976).

SYNTHETIC PLAN[50]

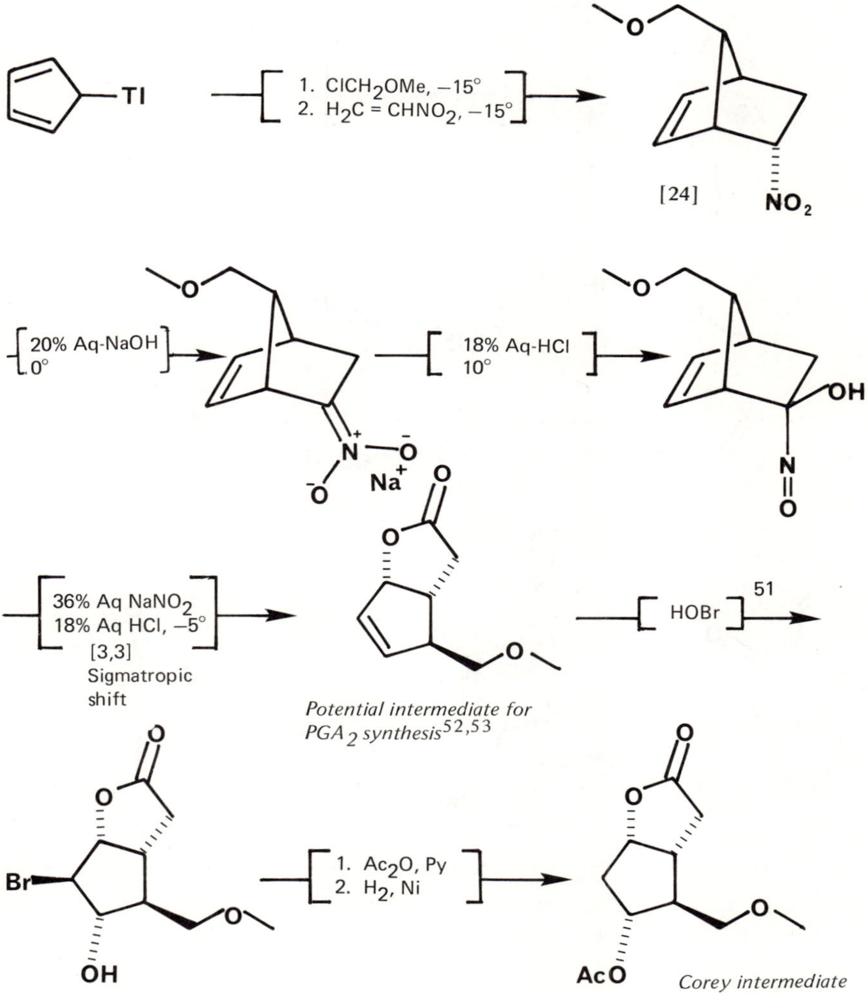

Potential intermediate for PGA 2 synthesis[52,53]

Corey intermediate

Proposed Mechanism for the Transformation of the Adduct [24] to [25]

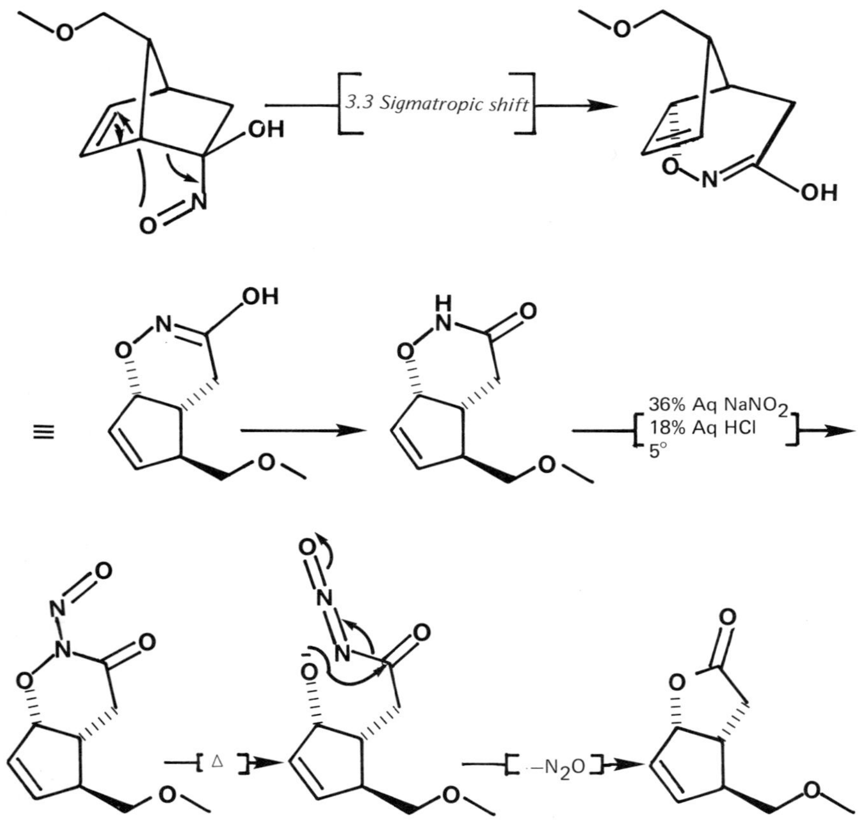

[25]

53. Catalytic hydrogenation of [25] leads to the dihydro-compound [26] from which the 11-deoxyprostaglandins can be synthesized.

[26] 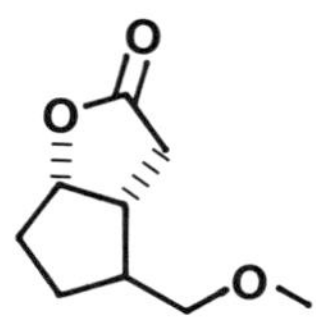

Another synthesis of the intermediate [**25**] has been reported by Fleming.[54] This approach is based on the reaction of allylsilanes as shown in the following:[55,56,57,58]

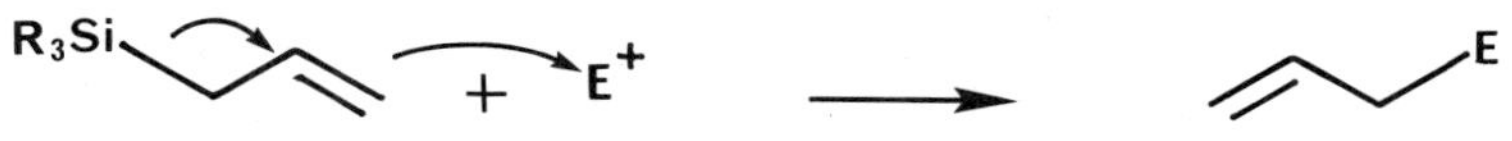

Such an approach has also been used by Fleming in the synthesis of loganin.[59]

SYNTHETIC STRATEGY

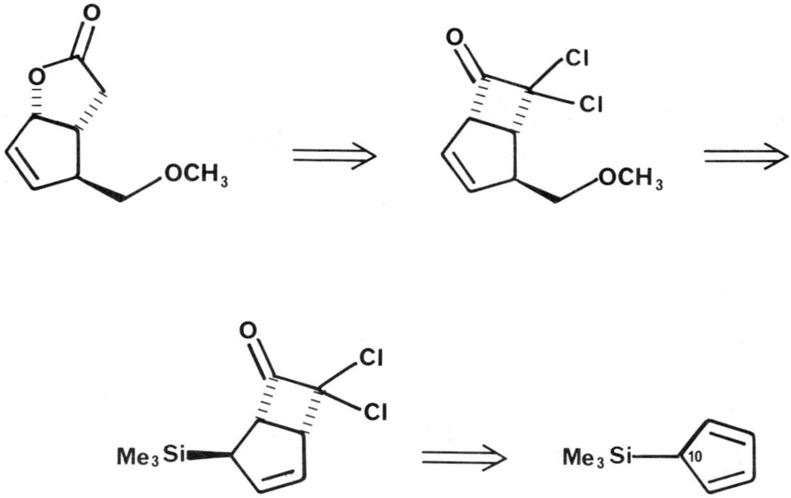

54. B. A. Yeung & I. Fleming, *Chem. Commun.*, 79 (1977).
55. R. Callas, J. Dunogues, J. P. Pillot, C. Biran, F. Pisciotti & B. Arreguy, *J. Orgmet. Chem.*, **85**, 149 (1975); G. Deleris, J. Dunogues & R. Callas, *J. Orgmet. Chem.*, **93**, 43 (1975).
56. A. Hosomi & H. Sakurai, *Tet. Lett.*, 1295 (1976).
57. G. D. Hartman & T. G. Traylor, *Tet. Lett.*, 939 (1975).
58. M. J. Carter & I. Fleming, *Chem. Commun.*, 679 (1976).
59. B. A. Yeung & I. Fleming, *Chem. Commun.*, 81 (1977).

SYNTHETIC PLAN[54]

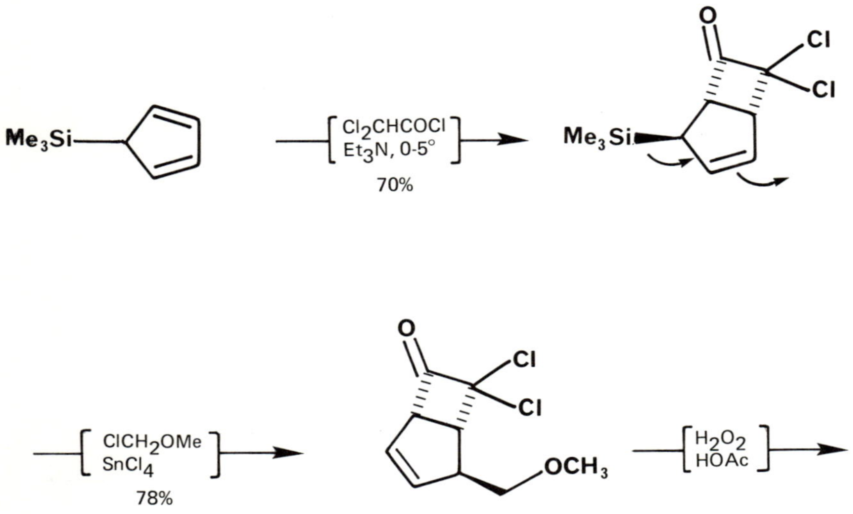

[27]

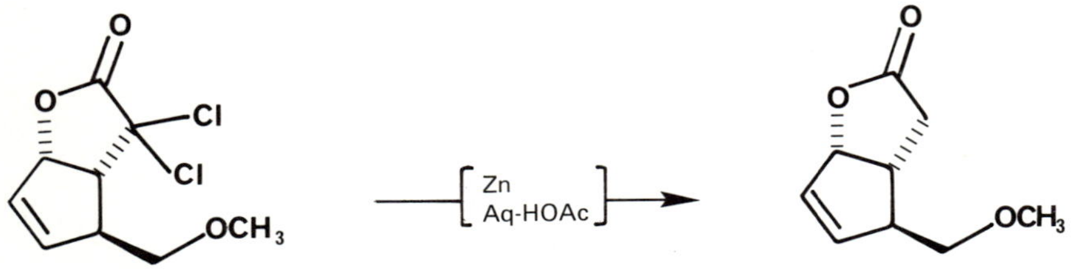

62% from [27]

Conversion of $PGF_{2\alpha}$ into PGX (Prostacyclin)

The proposed structure of PGX has been unambiguously proved by its synthesis from $PGF_{2\alpha}$.[60]

SYNTHETIC PLAN[60]

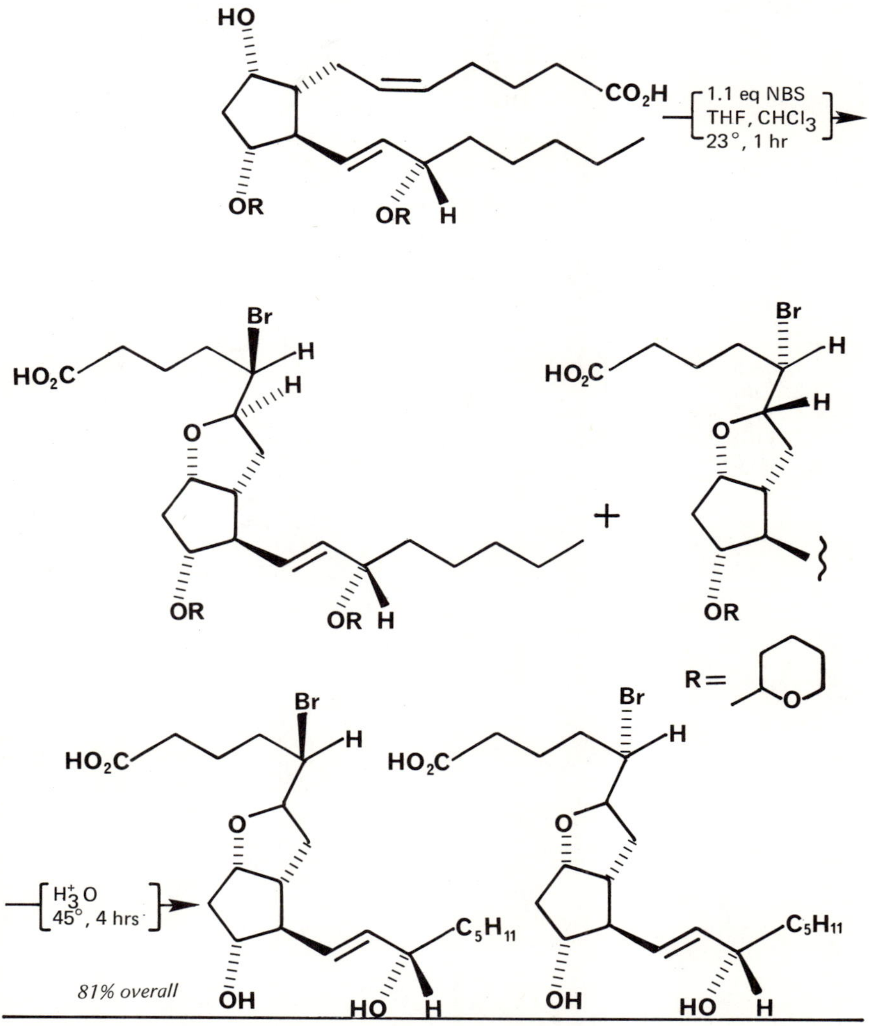

60. E. J. Corey, G. E. Keck & I. Szekely, *J. Am. Chem. Soc.*, 99, 2006 (1977).

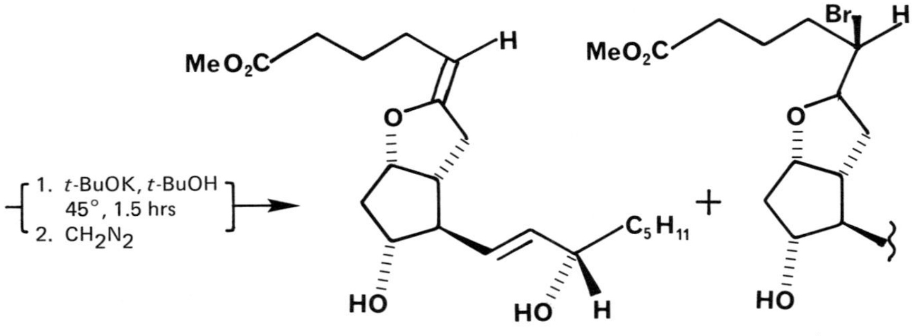

Recovered unchanged

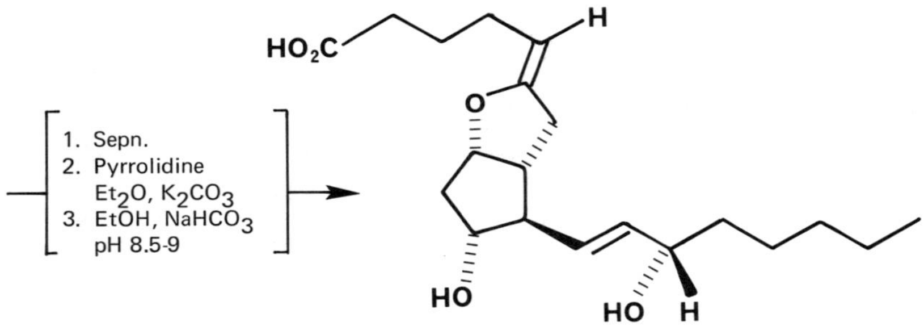

Prostacyclin

Analogues of Prostacylin

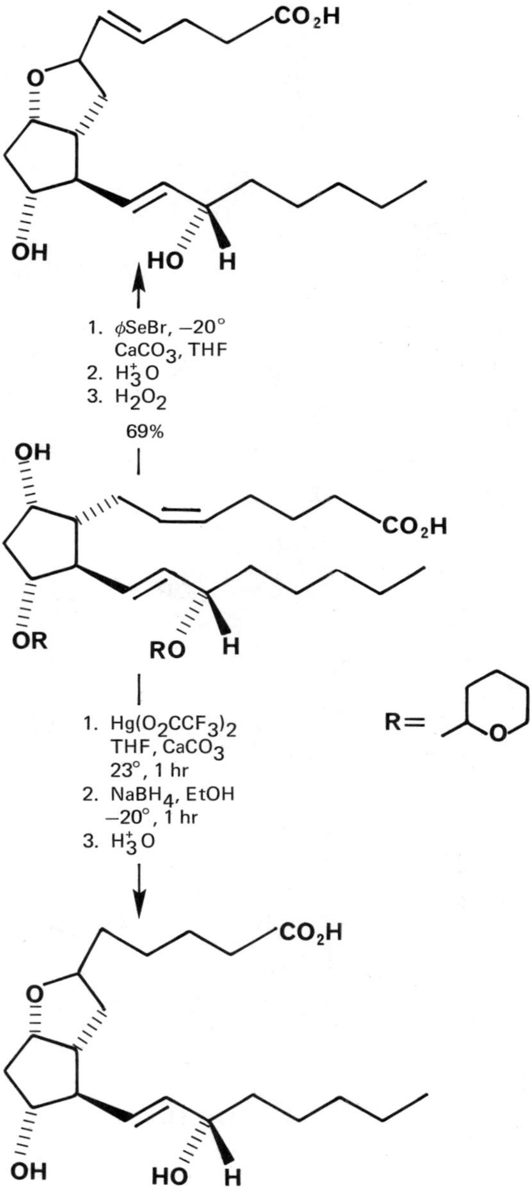

APPROACHES TO COREY LACTONE

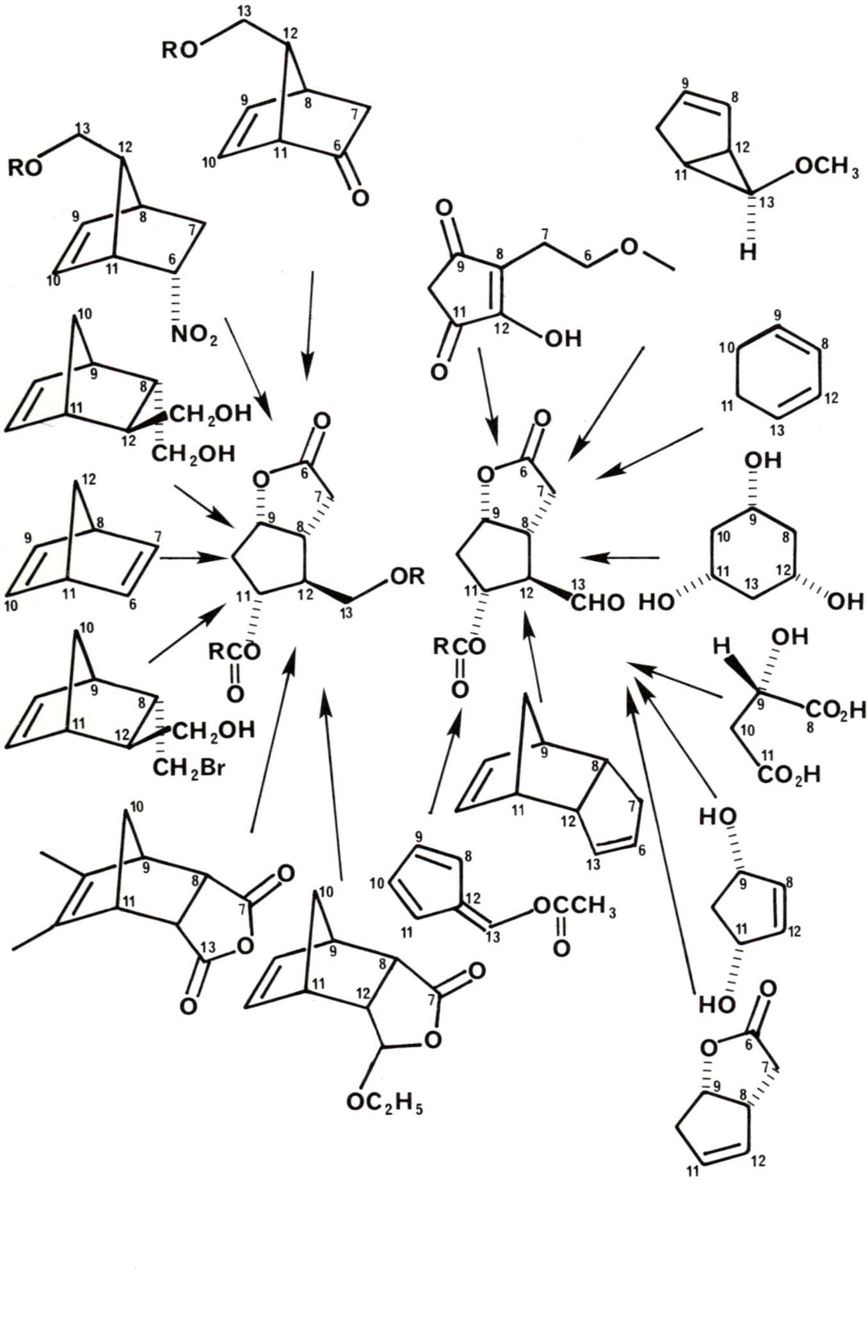

6

Bicyclo[3.2.0]heptene Approach

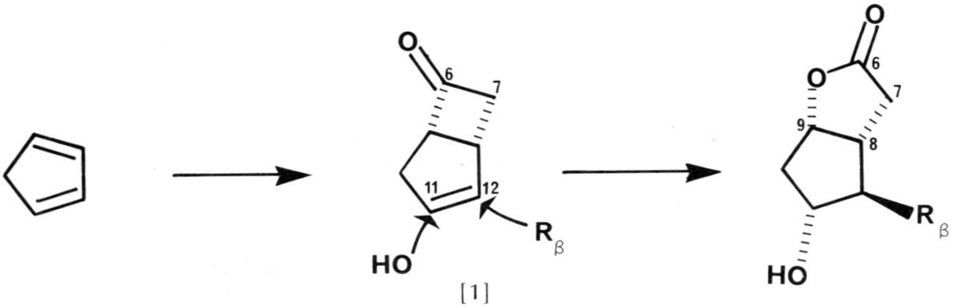

[1]

After the successful synthesis of prostaglandins via the bicyclo[2.2.1]heptane approach a different route was sought to the bicyclic lactone. Thus in the bicyclo[3.2.0]heptene route, developed subsequently, the potential two carbon aldehyde unit (C_6-C_7) was introduced by a ($_{\pi}2_s + {}_{\pi}2_a$) cycloaddition rather than a ($_{\pi}4_s + {}_{\pi}2_s$) cycloaddition sequence. The problem was how to introduce the β-chain and the C_{11} hydroxyl function by a suitable functionalization sequence of the cyclopentene double bond [1].

In the first such synthetic route the functionalization of the cyclopentene double bond was done by the prior formation of a cyclopropyl ether [2]. Subsequent oxidative cleavage of the cyclopropanol [4] gives hydroxyaldehyde [5] required for further elaboration into prostaglandin.

1. E. J. Corey, Z. Arnold & J. Hutton, *Tet. Lett.*, 307 (1970).

SYNTHETIC STRATEGY

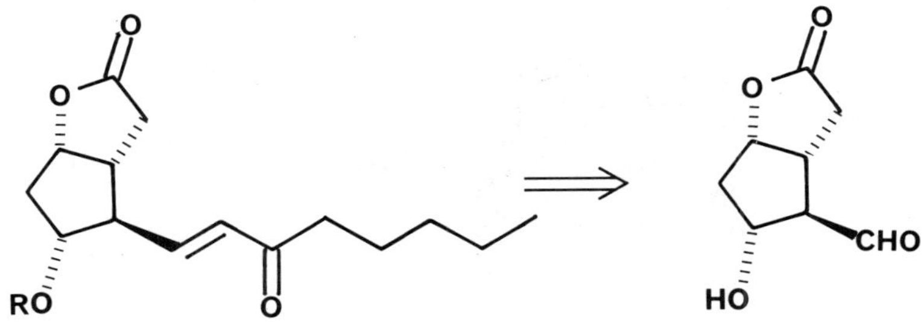

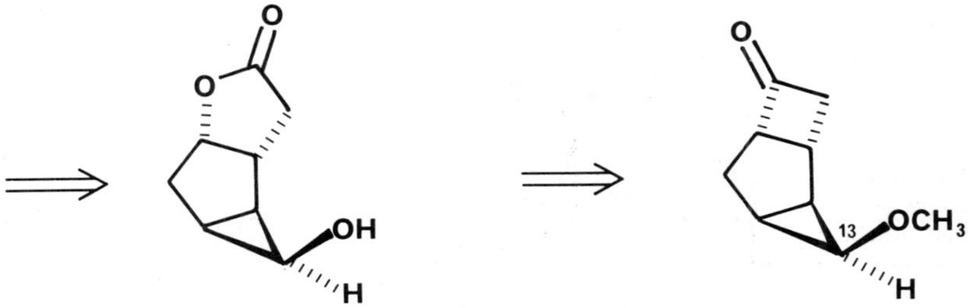

[4]

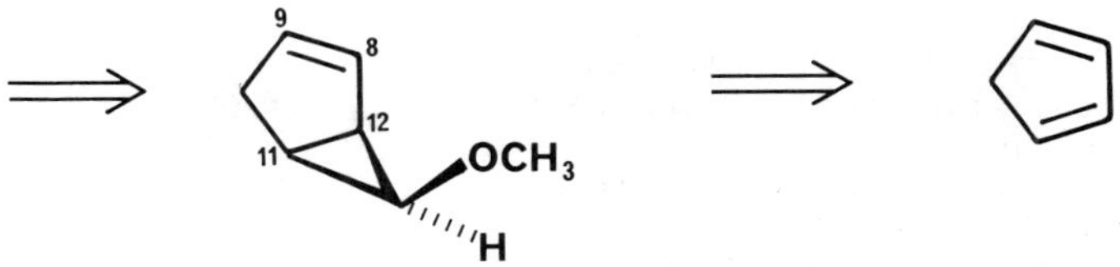

SYNTHETIC PLAN[1]

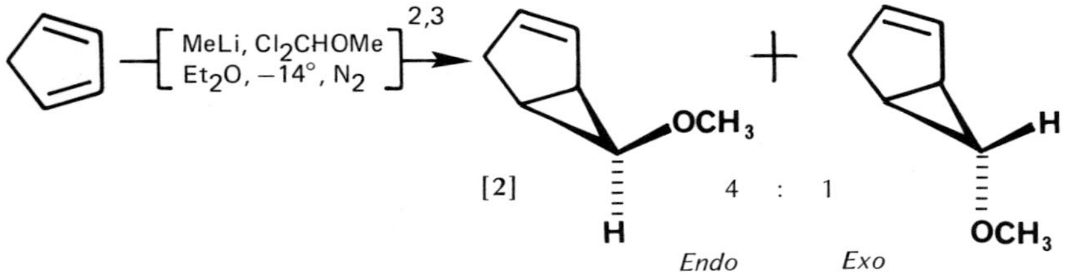

[2]

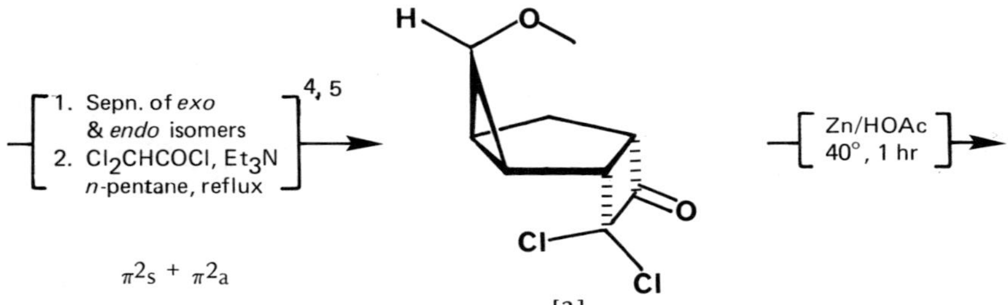

[3]

2. U. Schollkopf, *Angew. Chem. [Int. Edit.]*, 7, 588 (1968).
3. Cu catalyzed addition of diazoacetate by contrast gives the *exo* isomer as the major product. For details see ref. 5, p. 16.
4. The *anti* relationship of the three and the four membered rings about the cyclopentane ring in [3] can be easily explained on steric grounds.
5. The regiospecificity of the cycloaddition process is explained by assuming that the electrophilic carbonyl carbon of the dichloroketene initiates the addition by attaching itself to C_3 rather than C_2 which leads to the stabilization of the transition state either by the electron supplying cyclopropyl- or the *endo*-methoxy group as shown in the following:

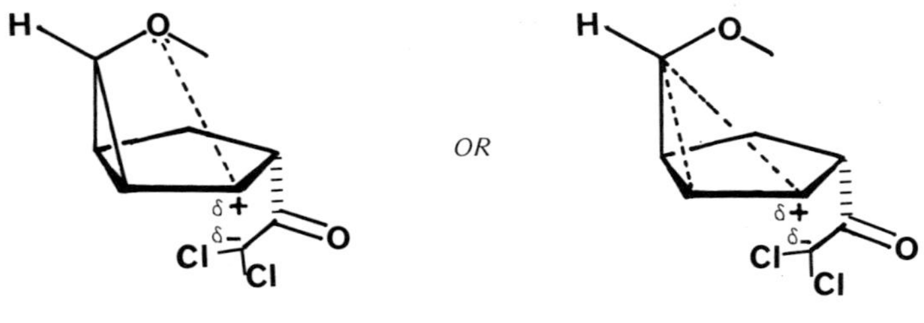

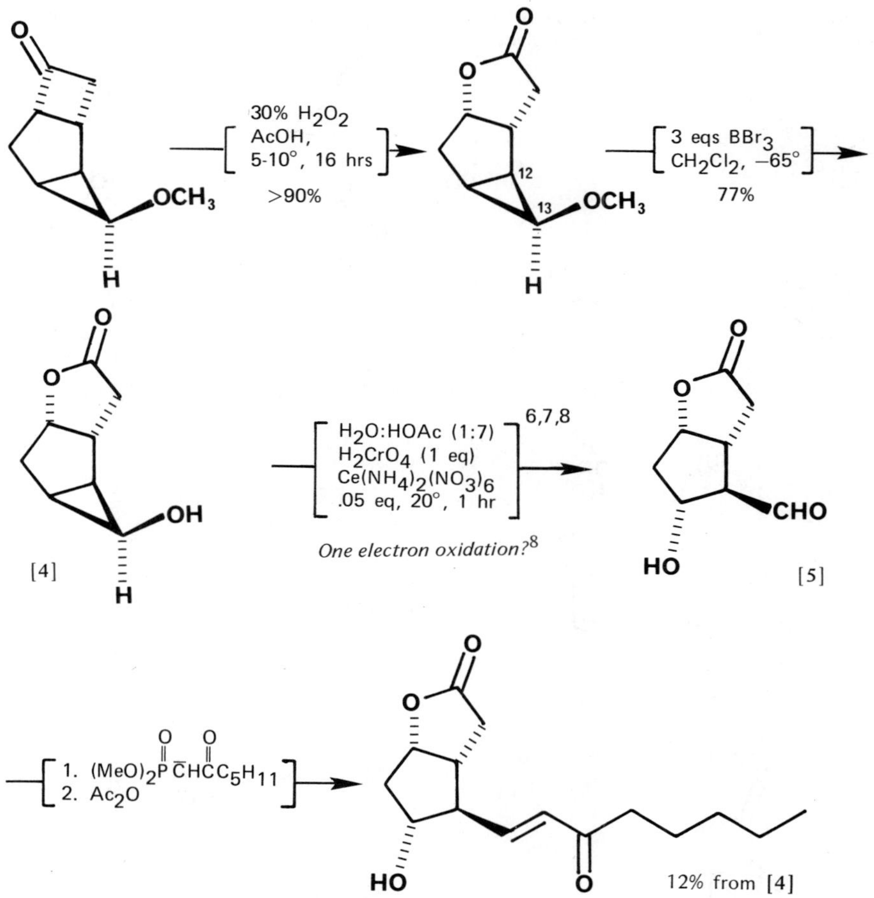

---

6. This is unfortunately a low yield step.
7. Other oxidizing agents, for example, $Hg(OAc)_2$, $Tl(OAc)_2$ & $Pb(OAc)_4$, were also tried. R. J. Ouellette, A. South, Jr., D. L. Shaw, *J. Am. Chem. Soc.*, **87**, 2602 (1965).
8. It is known that one electron oxidants such as Cr(IV), Ce(IV), V(V), and Mn(III) oxidize cyclobutanol and some other alcohols to afford cleavage products. Thus, cyclobutanol gives 4-hydroxybutyraldehyde.
   J. Rocek & A. E. Radkowsky, *J. Am. Chem. Soc.*, **90**, 2986 (1968).
   It is not clear why Ce(IV) was added to the chromic acid in this particular case because recently Rocek has shown that chromic acid itself oxidizes cyclopropanol to give 3-hydroxypropionaldehyde (30% yield).
   J. Rocek, A. M. Martinez & G. E. Cushmac, *J. Am. Chem. Soc.*, **95**, 5425 (1973).

The key *cis-anti-cis* tricyclic lactone [6] can also be prepared by a reverse cycloaddition sequence, namely (2+2) & (2+1) to cyclopentadiene.

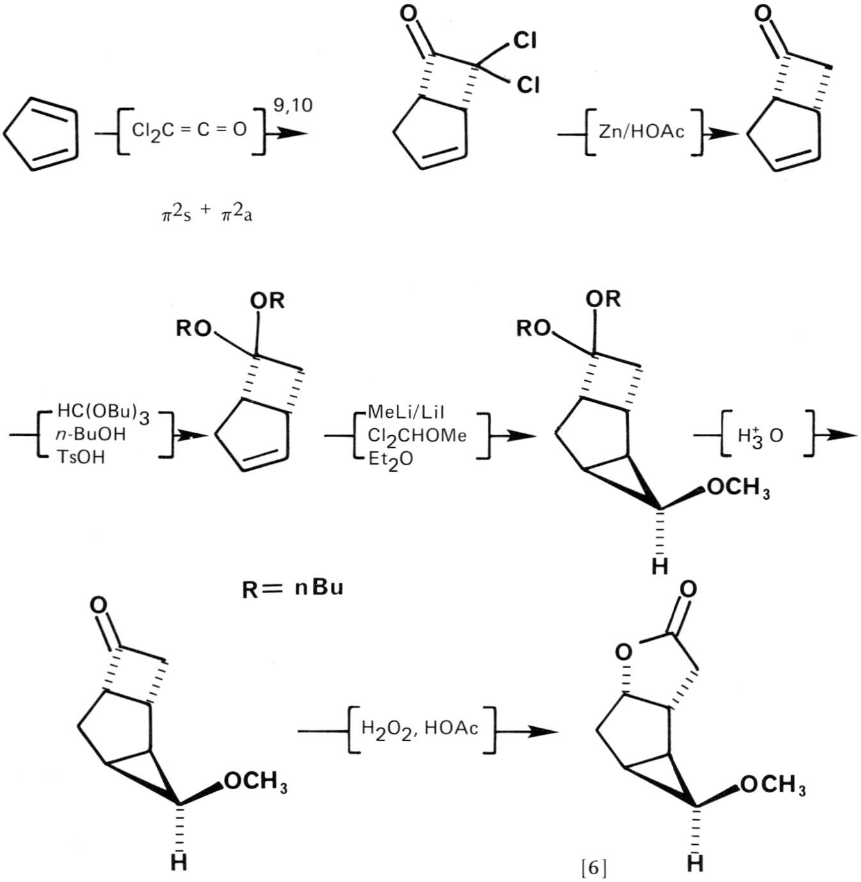

[6]
cis-anti-cis
Tricyclic lactone

9. "Halogenated ketenes: Valuable intermediates in organic synthesis," W. T. Brady, *Synthesis*, 415 (1971).
10. "Cycloadditions of dichloroketene to olefins and dienes," L. Ghosez, R. Montaigne, A. Roussel, H. Vanlierde & P. Mollet, *Tet.*, **27**, 615 (1971).

A better functionalization sequence was devised in order to circumvent the oxidative cleavage of the cyclopropanol [4] which is a low yield step. Epoxidation was followed by regioselective opening of the *cis-syn-cis* bicyclic epoxide [7] by the lithio-derivative of the vinylsulfide MeS-CH_2-CH=CH-SMe (a β-nucleophilic acrolein unit $^{-}$CH=CH-CHO) which already contains a latent C_{13}-C_{14} *trans* double bond. Another interesting feature is the introduction, albeit nonstereoselective, of the C_5H_{11} alkyl chain by the addition of n-C_5H_{11}Li to the C_{15} aldehyde [8].[11]

SYNTHETIC STRATEGY

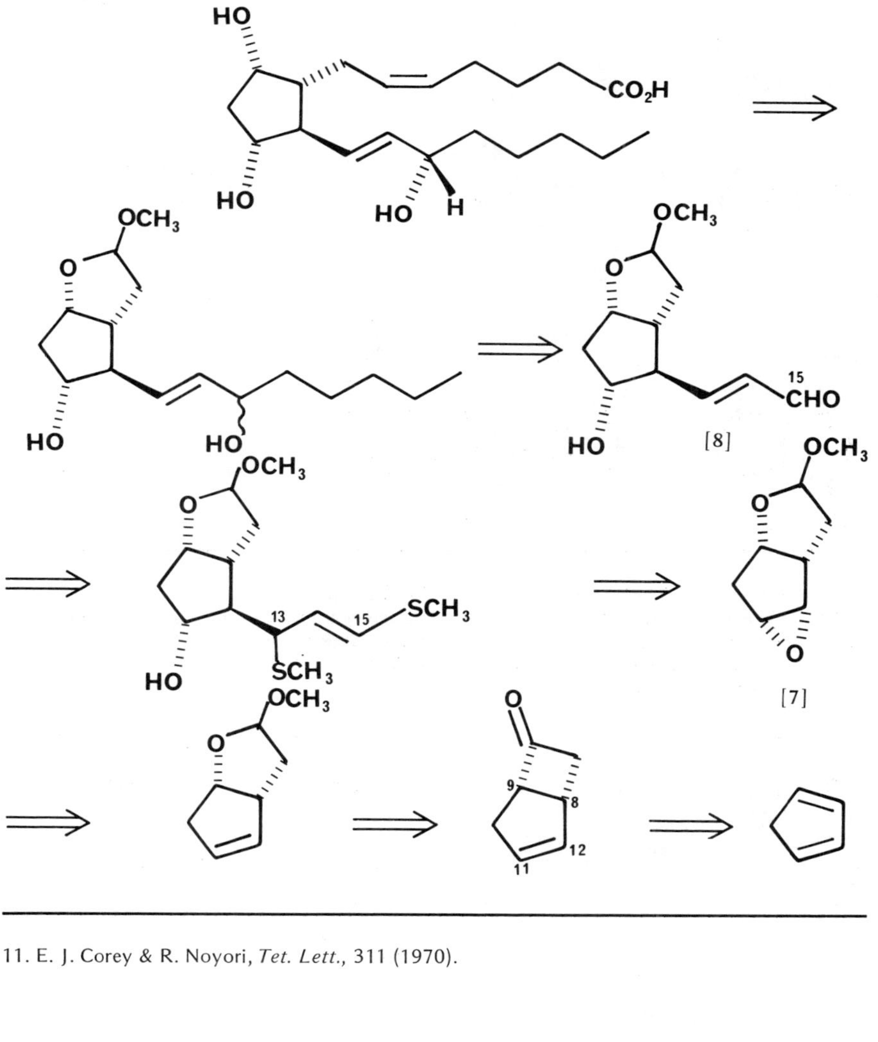

11. E. J. Corey & R. Noyori, *Tet. Lett.*, 311 (1970).

SYNTHETIC PLAN[11]

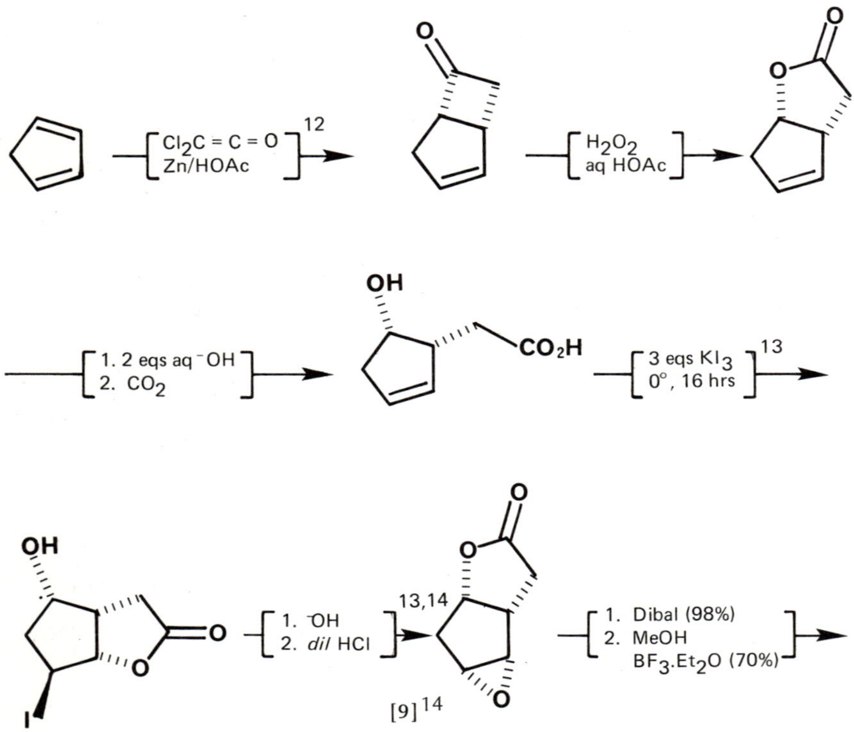

---

12. E. J. Corey, Z. Arnold & J. Hutton, *Tet. Lett.*, 307 (1970).
13. These sequence of reactions insures the *cis-syn-cis* stereochemistry of the oxido-lactone [9].
14. The same lactone [9] can be made by direct epoxidation. The desired stereoselectivity is observed only in acetic acid medium. The epoxidation takes place from the hindered side which may be due to solvation effects.

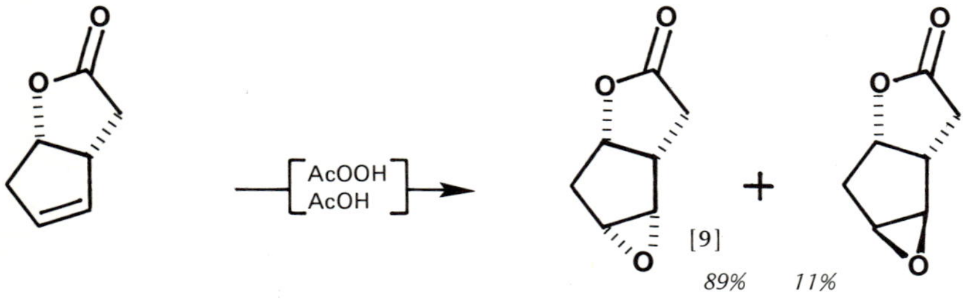

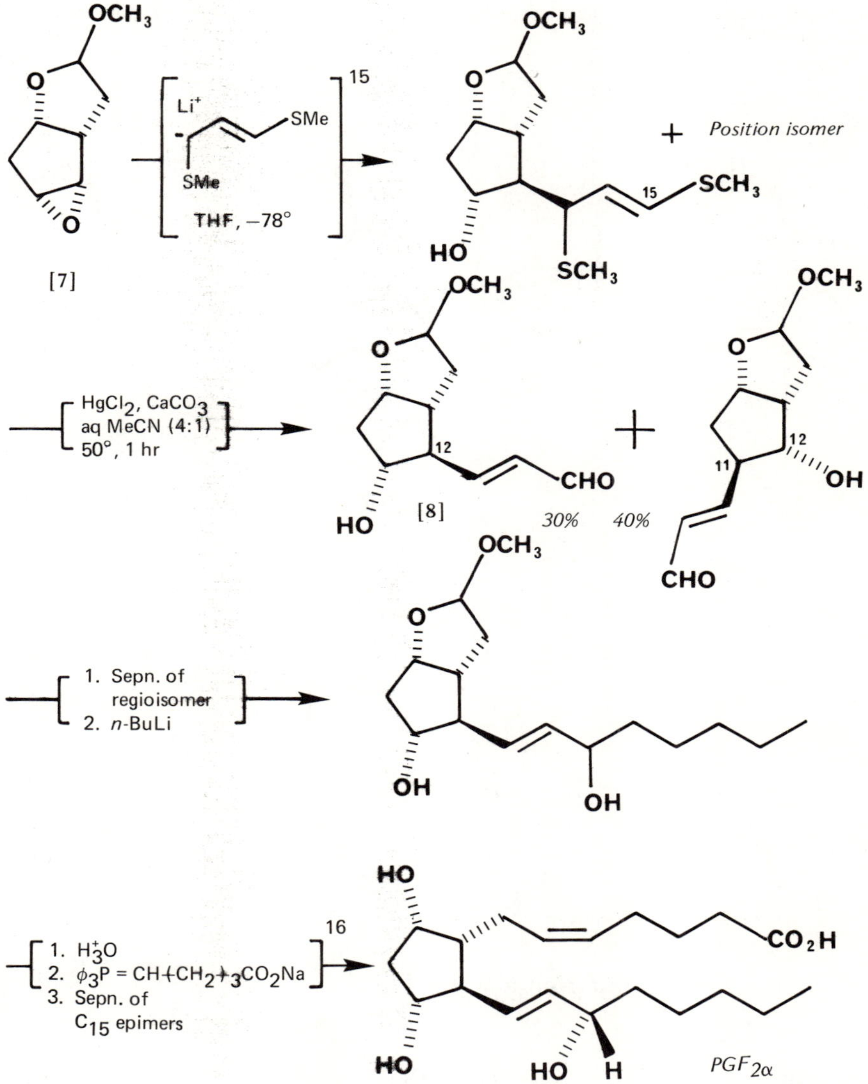

15. For the application of this reagent to a new synthesis of α,β-unsaturated aldehydes see: E. J. Corey, B. W. Erickson & R. Noyori, *J. Am. Chem. Soc.*, 91, 1724 (1971).
16. E. J. Corey, N. M. Weinshenker, T. K. Schaaf & W. Huber, *J. Am. Chem. Soc.*, 91, 5675 (1969).

In a later modification the same tricyclic epoxide [7] was opened with higher regioselectivity by divinylcuprate.

SYNTHETIC PLAN[17]

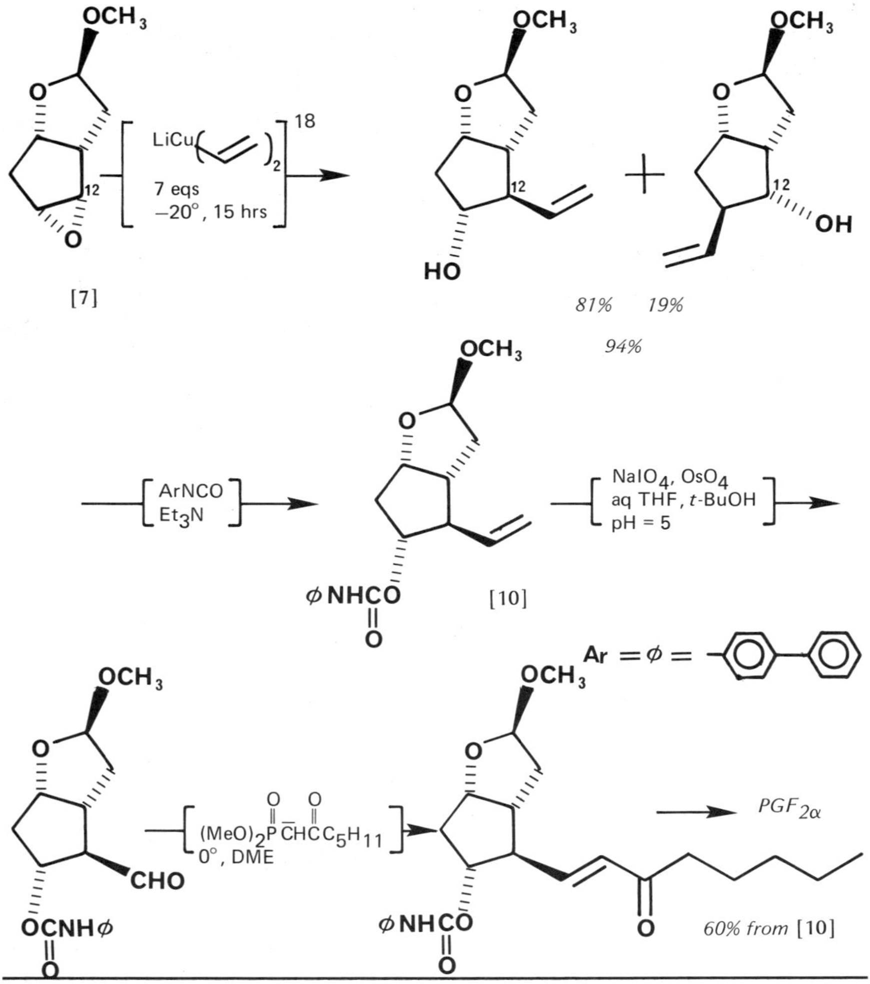

17. E. J. Corey, K. C. Nicolaou & D. J. Beames, *Tet. Lett.*, 2439 (1974).
18. The opening of the epoxides [7] where R = *t*-butyldimethylsilyl-, tribenzylsilyl- and methyl with divinyl cuprate gave almost identical results in all three cases.

Kelly's route to $PGF_{2\alpha}$[19] utilizes the Corey method of constructing the α-side chain[20] but adopts the Just-Upjohn method for the generation of the β-chain by solvolysis of cyclopropylcarbinol derivative.[21]

SYNTHETIC STRATEGY

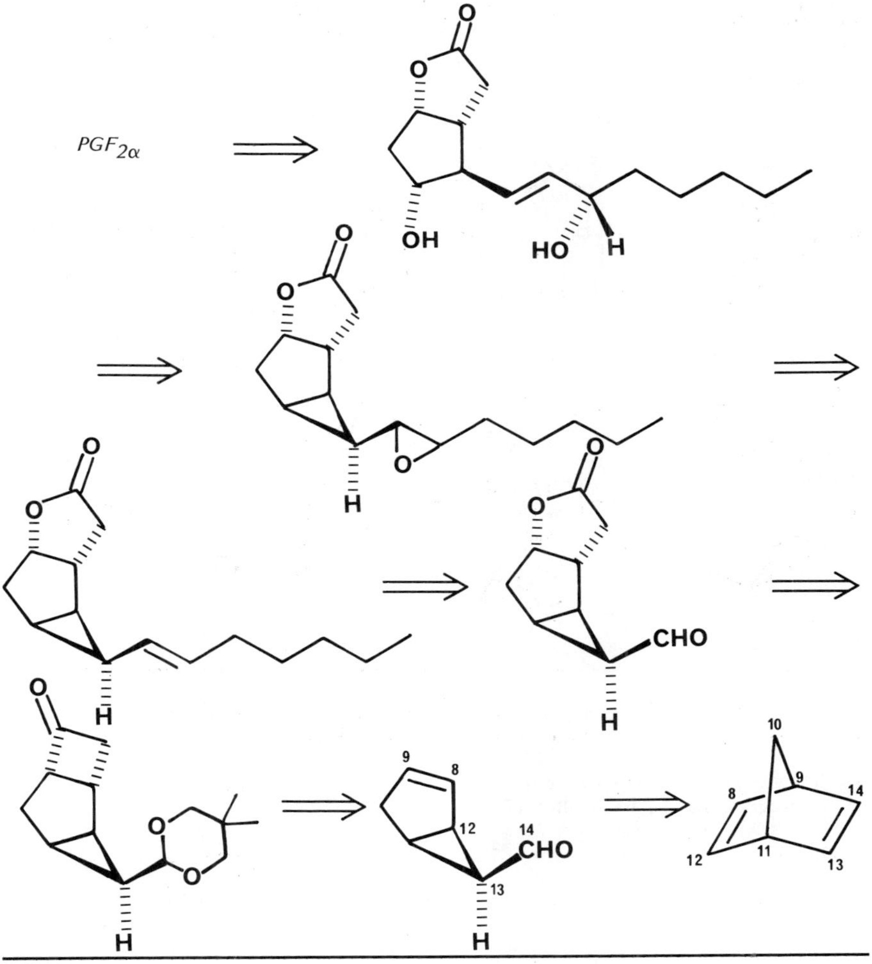

19. R. C. Kelly, V. Van Rheenen, I. Schletter & M. D. Pillai, *J. Am. Chem. Soc.*, **95**, 2746 (1973).
20. E. J. Corey, Z. Arnold & J. Hutton, *Tet. Lett.*, 307 (1970).
21. U. Axen, F. H. Lincoln & J. L. Thompson, *Chem. Commun.*, 303 (1969).
22. J. Meinwald, S. S. Cabana & M. S. Chadha, *J. Am. Chem. Soc.*, **85** 582 (1963).

SYNTHETIC PLAN[19]

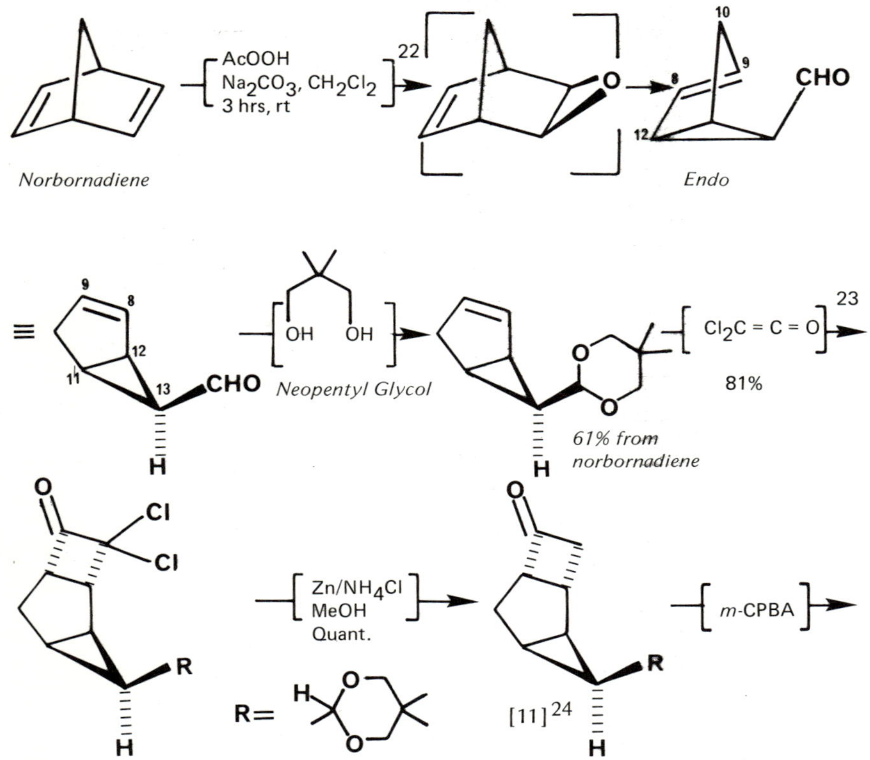

23. The regio- and stereo- chemistry of the dichloroketene addition may be explained by the same argument as put forward by Corey. For details see ref. 4&5, p. 134.

24. The cyclobutanone [11] was resolved with *l*-ephedrine via the oxazolidine [12]. R. Kelly & V. Van Rheenen, *Tet. Lett.*, 1709 (1973).

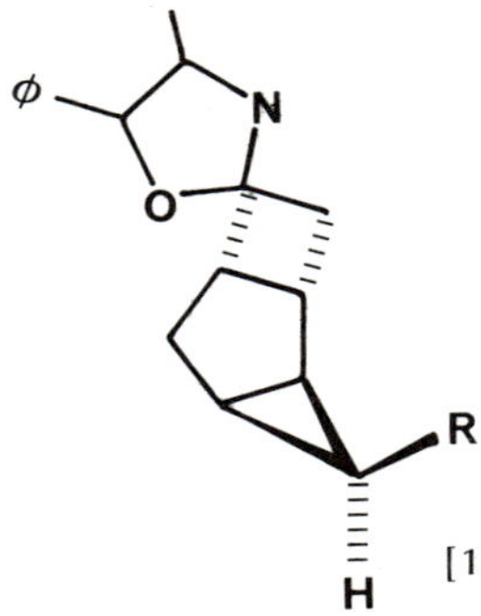

[12]

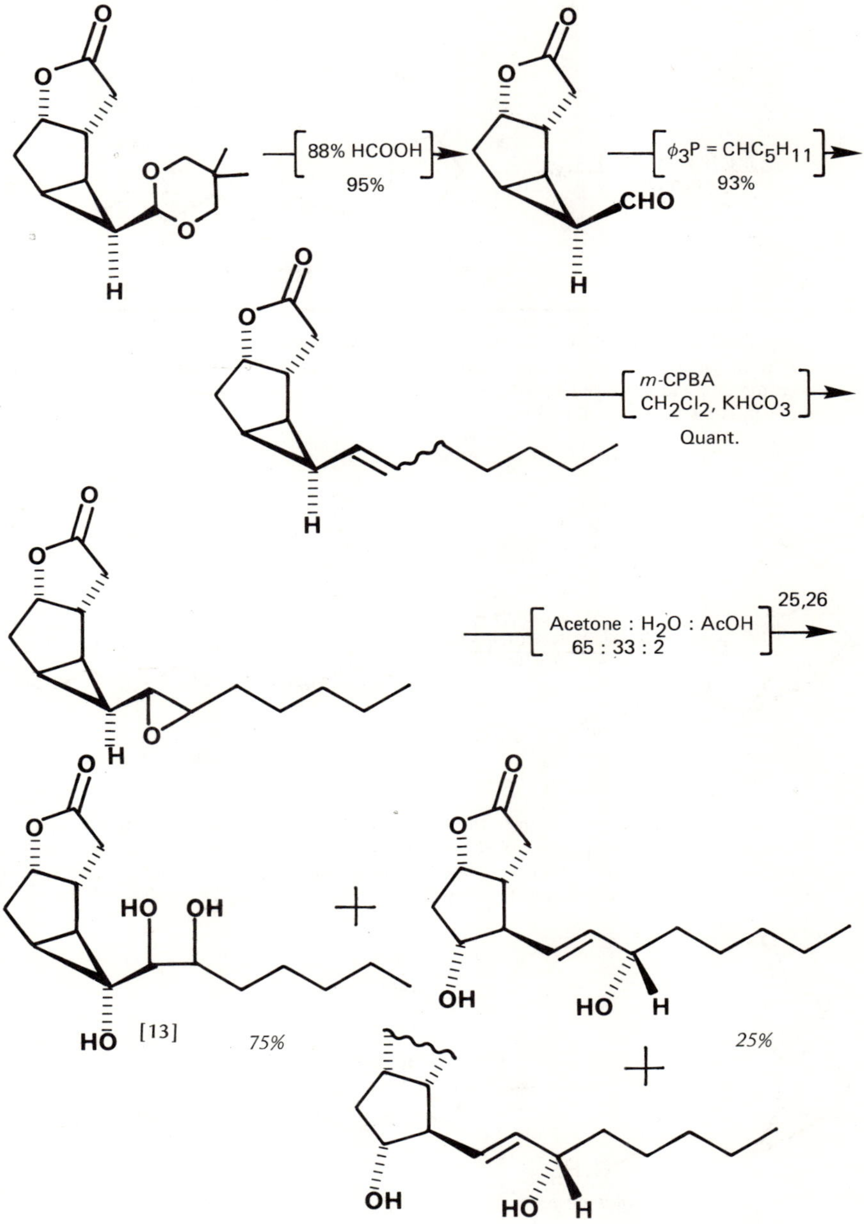

O
O
O
O
H
88% HCOOH
95%
CHO
ϕ3P = CHC5H11
93%
m-CPBA
CH2Cl2, KHCO3
Quant.
Acetone : H2O : AcOH
65 : 33 : 2
25,26
HO
OH
[13]
75%
OH
HO
25%

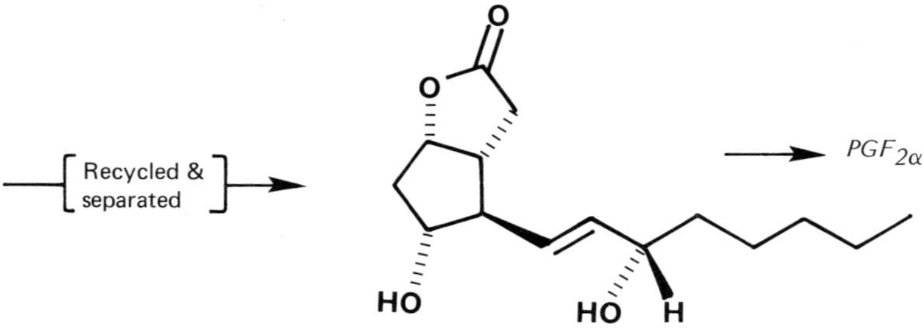

25. The possibility of an orthoformate intermediate [14] in the solvolysis of the diol [13] with dry formic acid has been proposed. To test this hypothesis the orthoformate was prepared from the diol and subjected to solvolytic conditions. The solvolysis was much faster and over in five minutes as compared to 3 hrs.

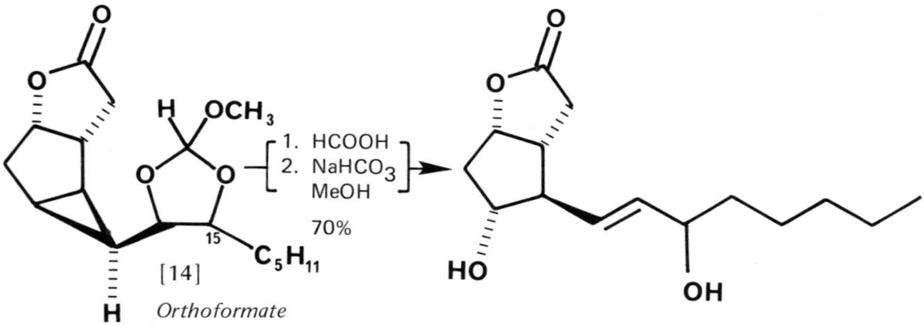

26. It has also been proposed that since the C_{15}-O bond is not broken during the solvolysis the stereochemistry of the C_{15} alcohol should be maintained. Partial success has been achieved along these lines. Only the orthopropionate [15] on solvolysis gives the product with complete retention of C_{15} configuration. R. C. Kelly & V. Van Rheenen, *Tet. Lett.*, 1067 (1976).

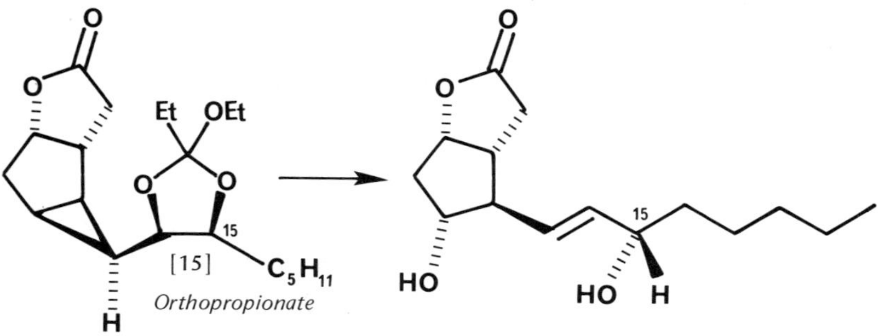

In a subsequent modification the elaboration of the β-chain is carried out by using a masked acylcarbanion (ACE) equivalent to give the epoxynitrile [16] which on solvolysis and base treatment gives the enone.[27,28]

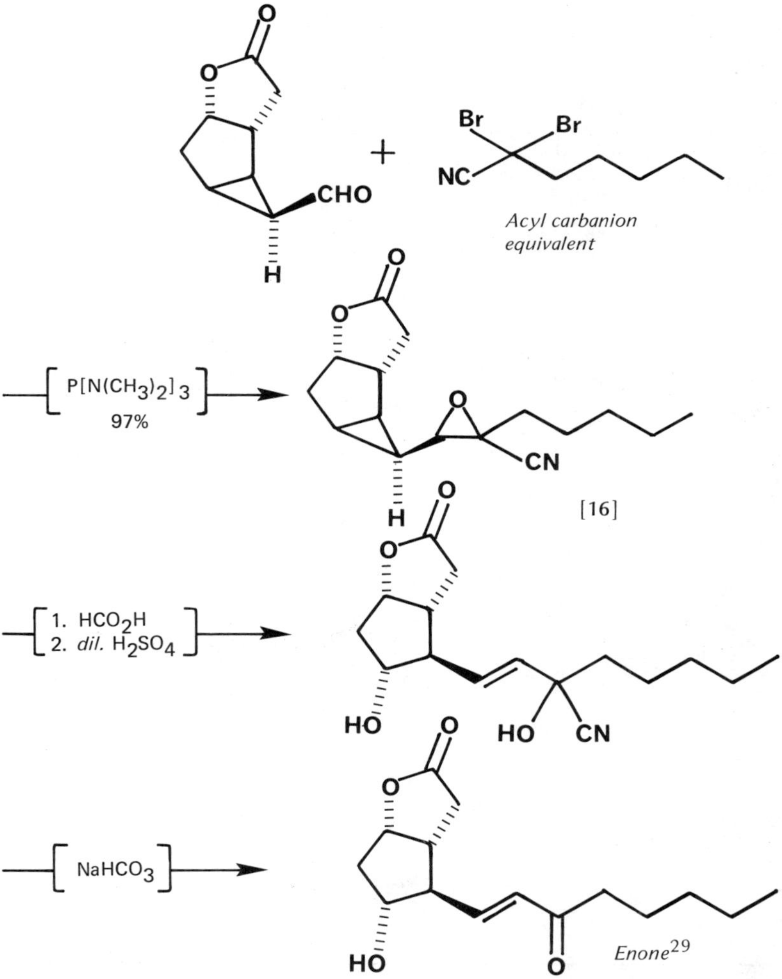

---

27. D. R. White, *Tet. Lett.*, 1753 (1976).
28. For references to acylcarbanions see: J. E. Baldwin, G. A. Hofle & W. Lever Jr., *J. Am. Chem. Soc.*, **96**, 7125 (1974).
29. E. J. Corey, K. B. Becker & R. K. Varma, *J. Am. Chem. Soc.*, **94**, 8616 (1972).

In this last approach a regio- as well as stereo- specific Prins reaction has been used to functionalize the $C_{11}-C_{12}$ double bond.[30]

SYNTHETIC PLAN[30]

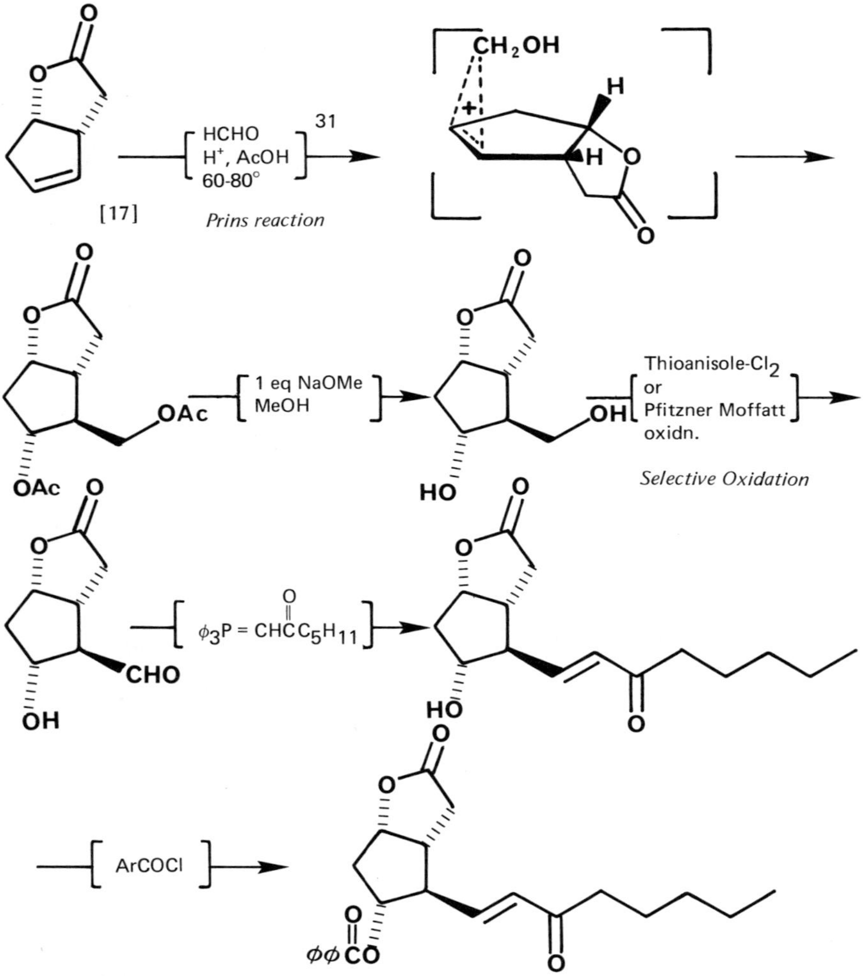

30. G. Kovacs, I. Szekely, V. Simonidesz, I. Tomoskozi & L. Gruber, *Tet. Lett.*, 4639 (1976).
31. The regio- and stereo- specificity of the reaction seems to be characteristic of the lactone [17] or analogous bicyclic olefins in electrophilic addition reactions. J. C. Gilbert, T. Luo & R. E. Davis, *Tet. Lett.*, 2545 (1975), and Z. Grudzinski & S. M. R. Roberts, *J. Chem. Soc., [Perkin I]*, 1767 (1975).

7

Syntheses from 2-Alkylcyclopentane 1,3,4-trione

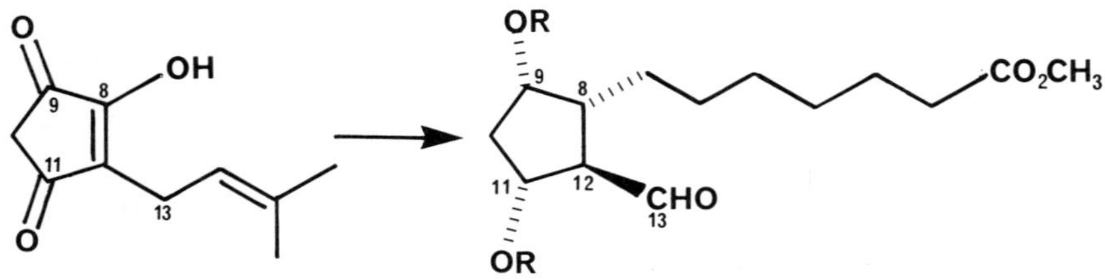

In all the approaches going through the 3-alkyl-1,2,4-cyclopentatrione [1] the three carbonyl groups are distinguished. The differentiation became possible because one would expect the formation of the more substituted vinylogous ester and because of the important observation that the diethyl ketal that is formed, under thermodynamically equilibrating conditions, is alpha to the carbonyl to give the useful vinylogous ester [2].

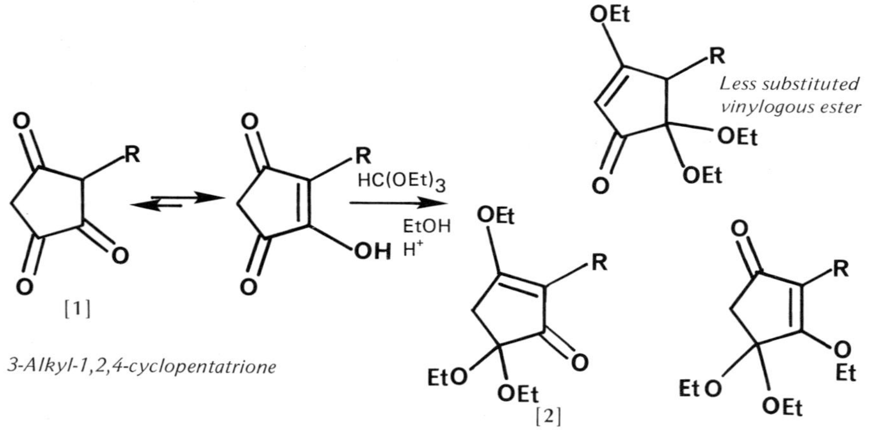

[1]

3-Alkyl-1,2,4-cyclopentatrione

[2]

More substituted vinylogous ester

Not formed

The sequence then proceeds[1] through a 2,3-disubstituted 2-cyclopentene-1,4-dione [3]. Although this can be further manipulated, the number of steps is quite large and some of the reactions lack selectivity.

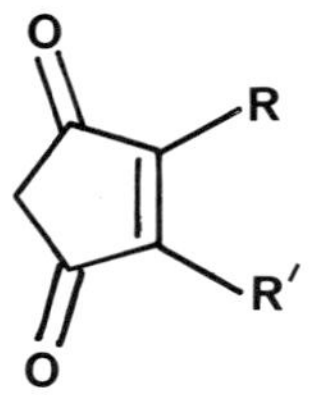

[3]

1. P. De Clercq & M. Vandewalle, *Bull. Soc. Chim. Belg.*, 83, 305 (1974).

SYNTHETIC STRATEGY

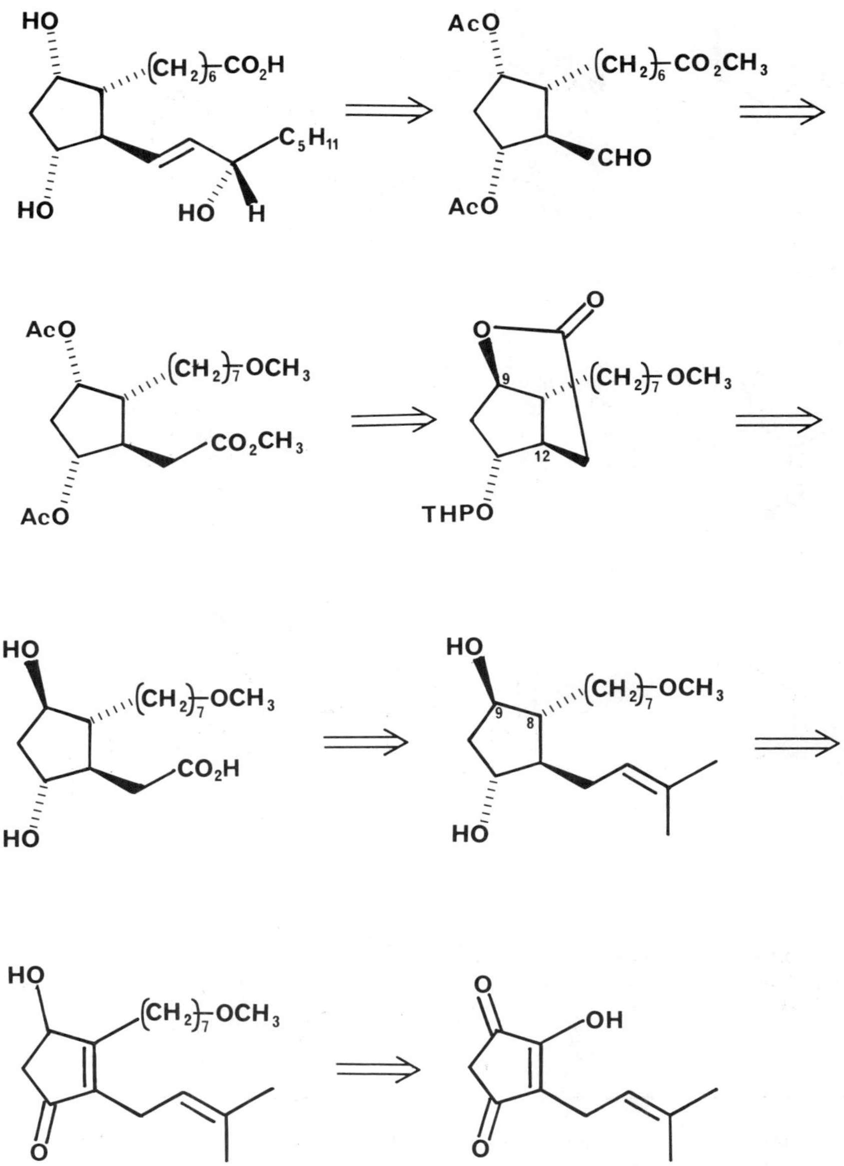

SYNTHETIC PLAN[1]

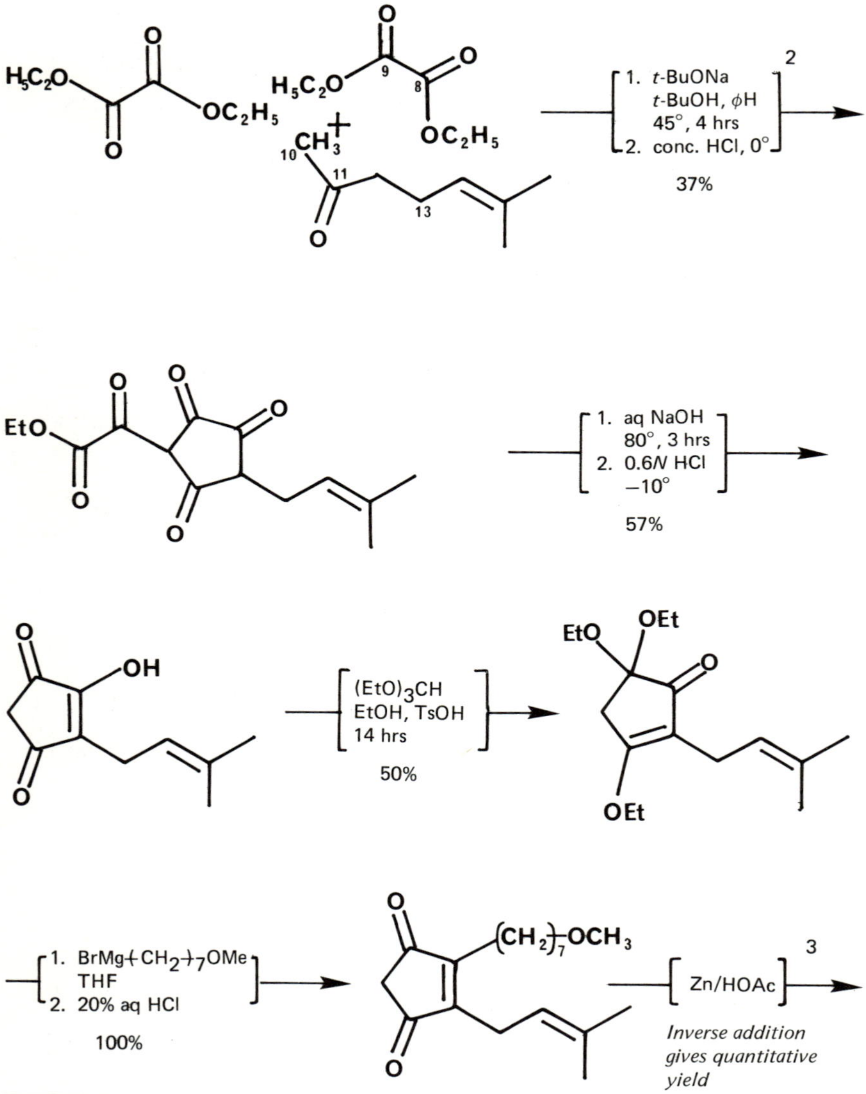

2. The use of 6-methyl-5-heptene-2-one necessitates a subsequent one carbon degradation sequence.

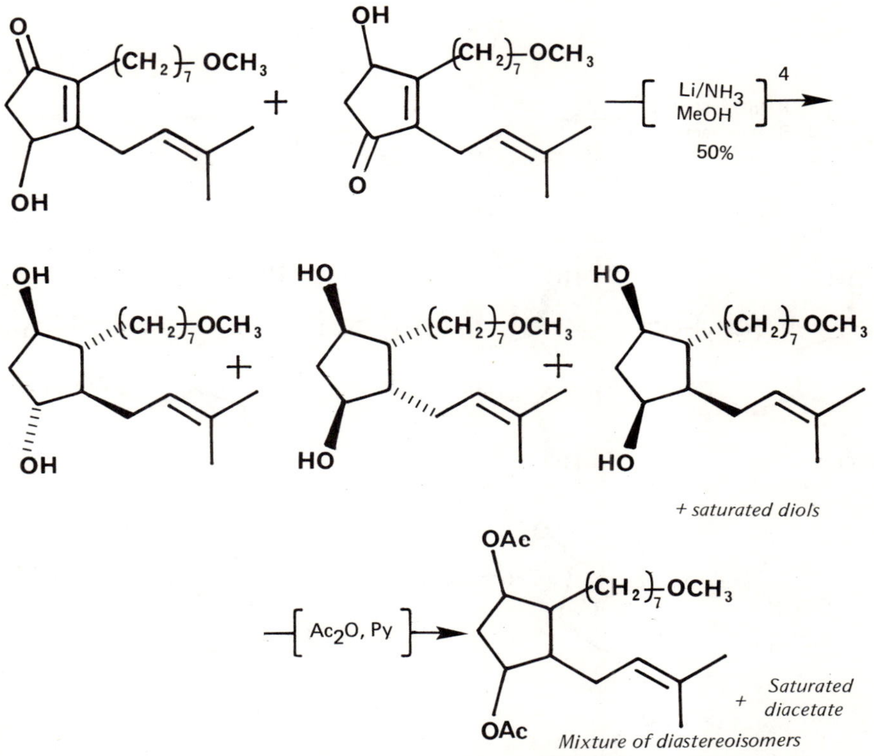

3. Zn/H⁺ reduction of the dimethyl ether [4] gave the cyclopentane-1,3-dione [5]:

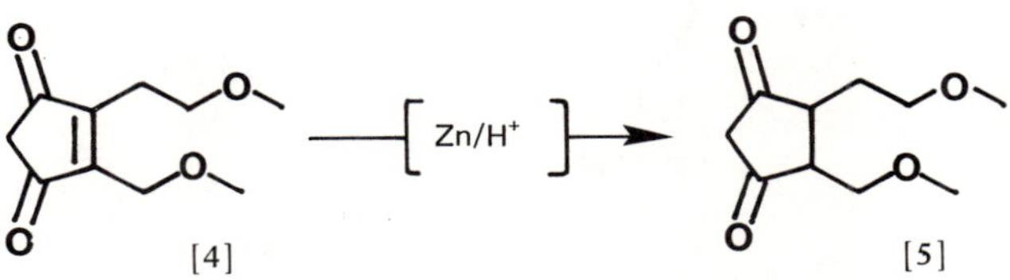

[4] [5]

It is difficult to rationalize the effect of the oxygen lone pair electrons of the extra methyl ether on the course of reduction. This problem required devising more complex latent functionalities lacking this second oxygen function.

4. The stereoselectivity of the reduction was increased subsequently by using a proton donor of lower pK_a value. For details see footnote 8, p. 156.

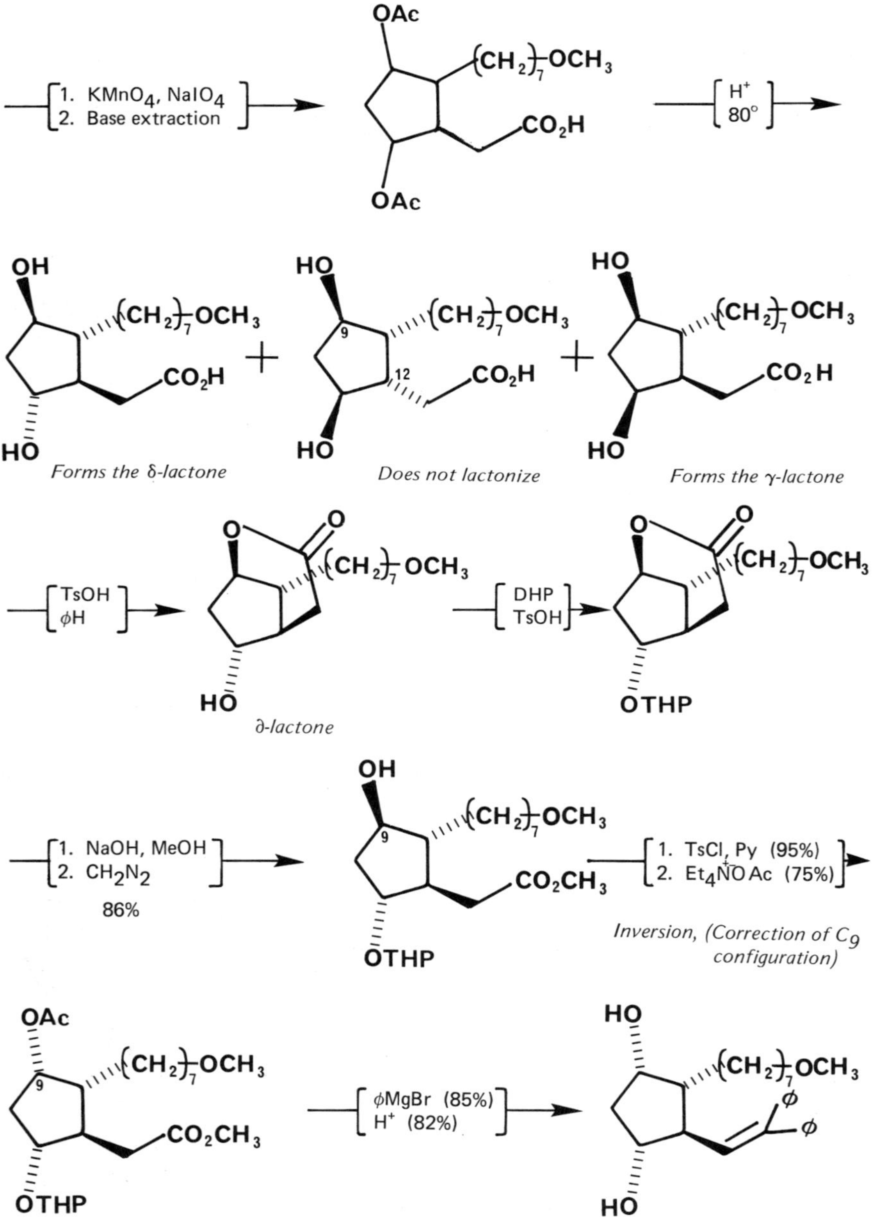
1. KMnO4, NaIO4
2. Base extraction
OAc
(CH2)7OCH3
CO2H
OAc
H+
80°
OH
HO
Forms the δ-lactone
Does not lactonize
Forms the γ-lactone
TsOH
φH
∂-lactone
DHP
TsOH
OTHP
1. NaOH, MeOH
2. CH2N2
86%
CO2CH3
1. TsCl, Py (95%)
2. Et4NOAc (75%)
Inversion, (Correction of C9 configuration)
φMgBr (85%)
H+ (82%)

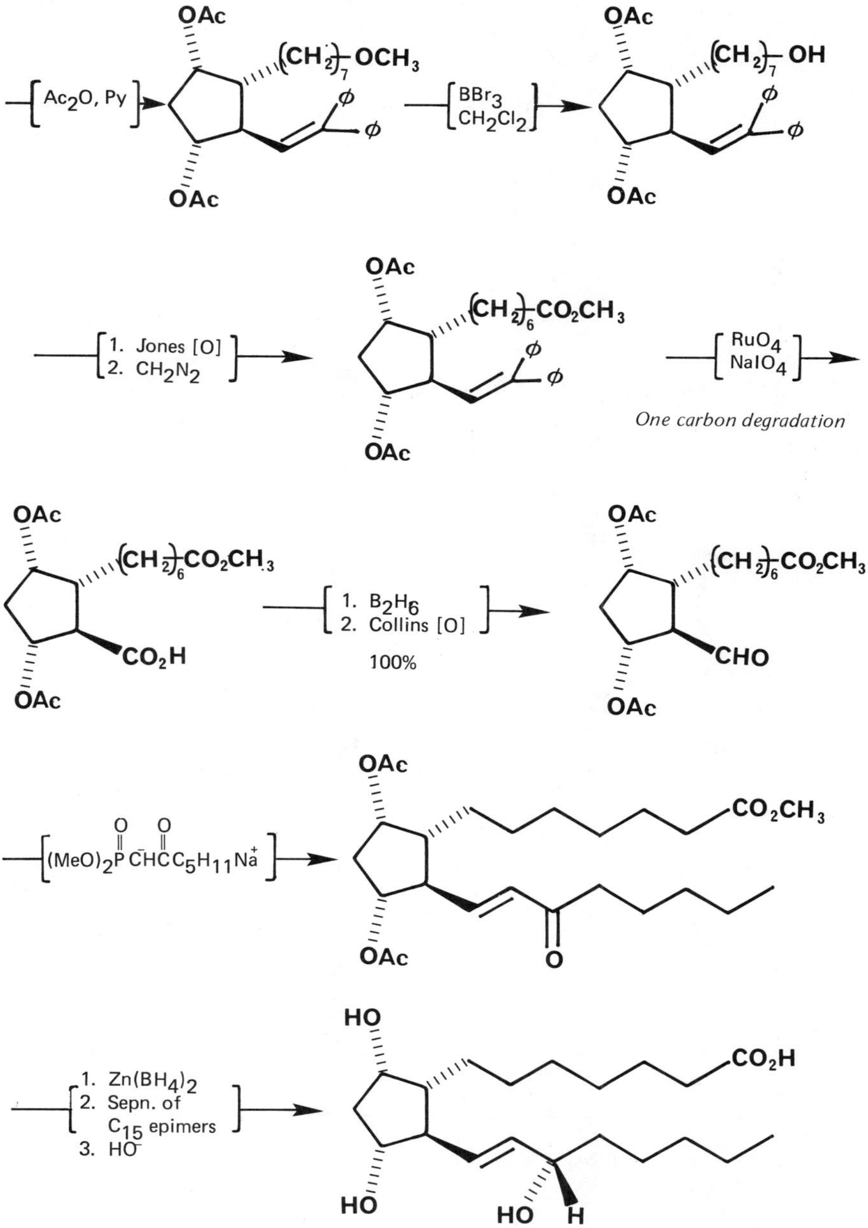

Ac2O, Py
OAc
(CH2)7 OCH3
ϕ
ϕ
OAc
BBr3
CH2Cl2
OAc
(CH2)7 OH
ϕ
ϕ
OAc
1. Jones [O]
2. CH2N2
OAc
(CH2)6 CO2CH3
ϕ
ϕ
OAc
RuO4
NaIO4
One carbon degradation
OAc
(CH2)6 CO2CH3
CO2H
OAc
1. B2H6
2. Collins [O]
100%
OAc
(CH2)6 CO2CH3
CHO
OAc
(MeO)2P CHC C5H11 Na+
OAc
CO2CH3
OAc
O
1. Zn(BH4)2
2. Sepn. of C15 epimers
3. HO−
HO
CO2H
HO
HO
H

In this modified approach,[5,6] the one carbon degradation sequence to get the aldehyde [6] was avoided by the migration of the double bond and its subsequent oxidative cleavage. The C_9 stereochemistry had to be corrected again.

SYNTHETIC STRATEGY

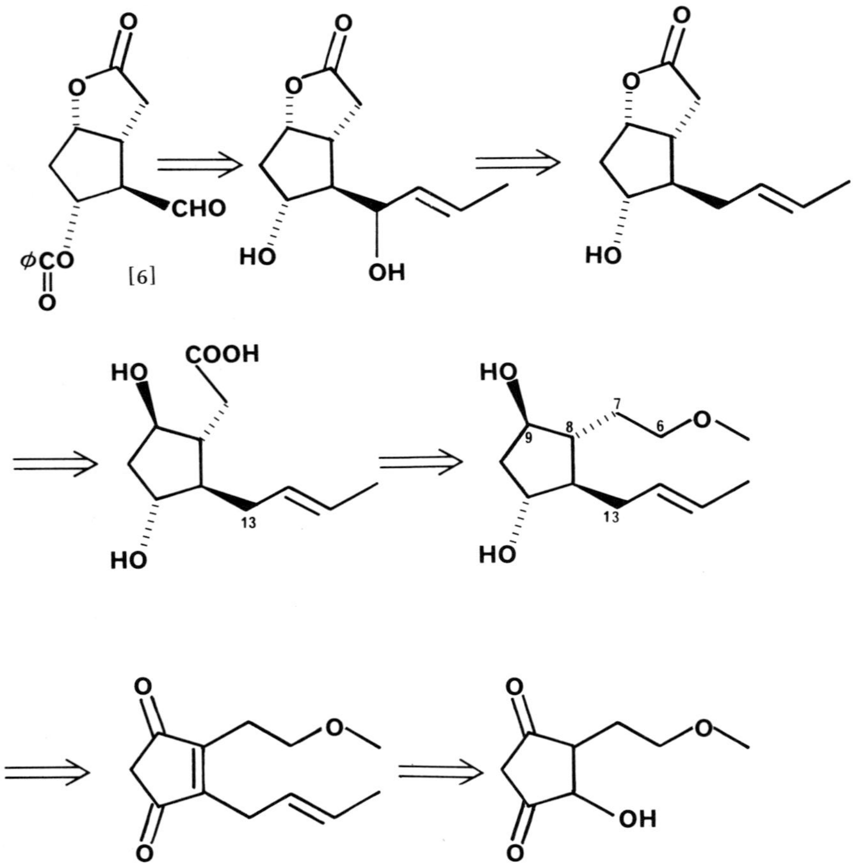

5. J. Van Hooland, P. De Clercq & M. Vandewalle, *Tet. Lett.*, 4343 (1974).
6. W. Van Brussel, J. Van Hooland, P. De Clercq & M. Vandewalle, *Bull. Soc. Chim. Belg.*, **84**, 813 (1975).

SYNTHETIC PLAN[5,6]

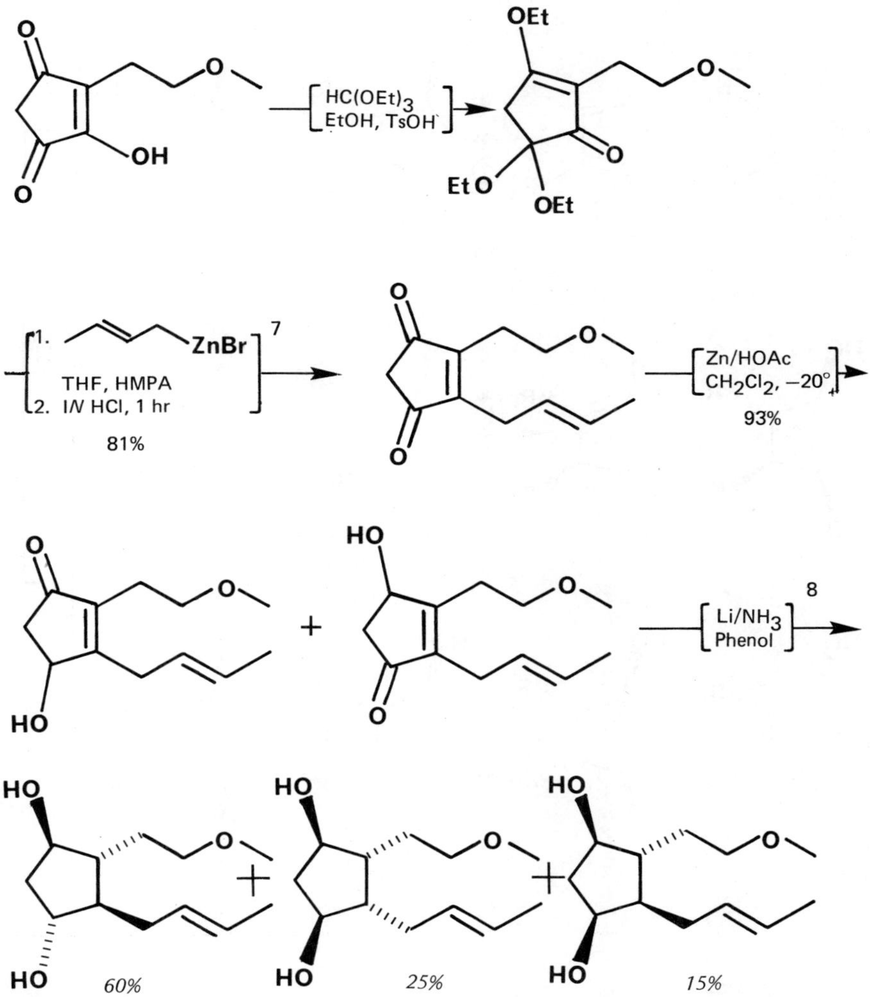

7. Unlike crotylmagnesium bromide, the addition of the crotylzinc bromide takes place without rearrangement.
Ph. Migniac,. *Bull. Chim. Soc. Fr.*, 1077 (1970) and references cited therein.
It has also been shown that diallyl zinc reagents react exclusively via rearrangement. D. Abenhaim, *J. Orgmet. Chem.*, 92, 275 (1975).

Proposed Mechanism for the Reduction[8]

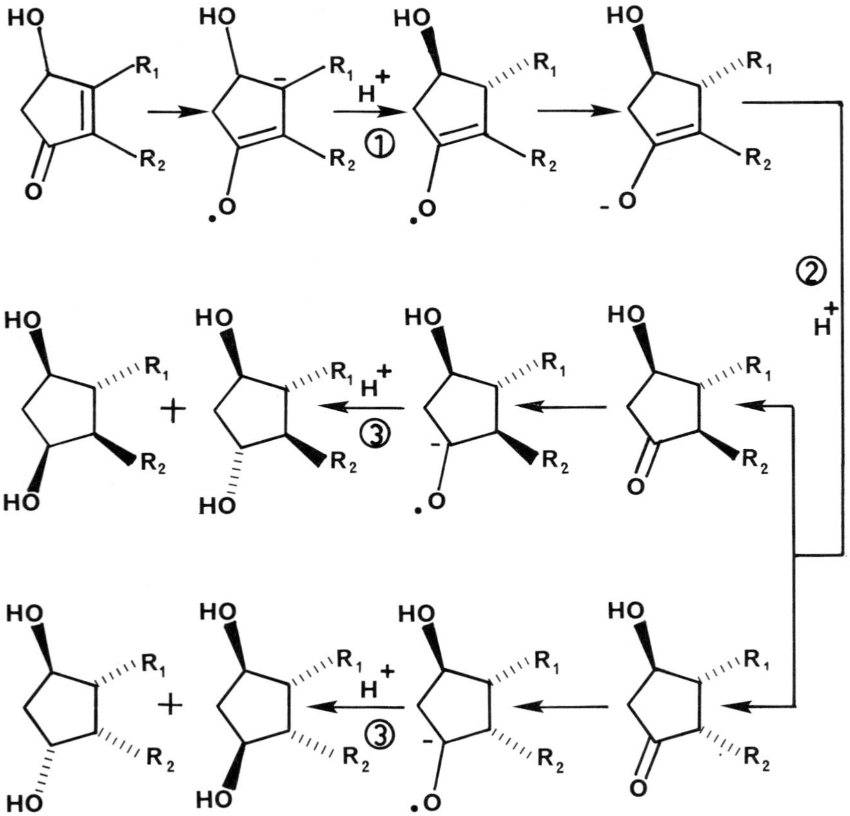

8. There are three protonation steps in the reduction. The first and the third protonations are highly stereoselective. It is the second protonation that determines the relative amounts of the diastereoisomers formed. The stereochemistry of the second protonation depends on the pK_a value of the proton source used (see Table 1).
P. De Clercq, D. Van Haver, D. Tavernier & M. Vandewalle, *Tet.*, 30, 55 (1974).
M. Samson, P. De Clercq & M. Vandewalle, *Tet.*, 31, 1233 (1975).

Table 1. Effect of Acidity of the Proton Source on the Stereochemistry of Reduction

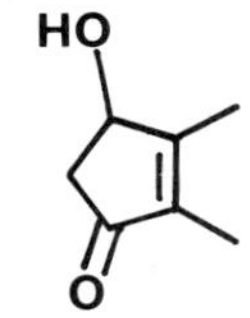	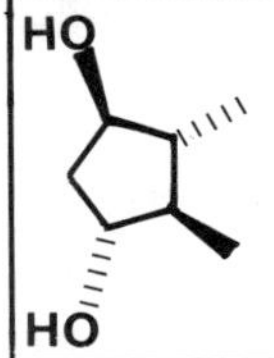	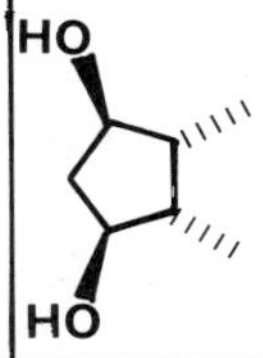	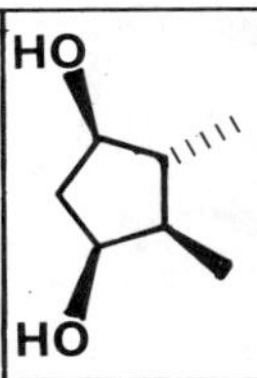	Total diol *trans*-alkyl	Total diol *cis*-alkyl
Phenol	67%	26%	7%	74%	26%
Methanol	62%	28%	10%	72%	28%
Ethanol	52%	43%	5%	57%	43%
i-Propanol	33%	60%	7%	40%	60%
t-Butanol	21%	74%	5%	26%	74%

(← Increasing Acidity: from *t*-Butanol up to Phenol)

Competition between intra- and intermolecular protonation determines the stereochemical outcome of the reduction. With the more acidic proton donors intermolecular reaction occurs whereas with less acidic external proton sources the competing intramolecular protonation becomes more effective.[8]

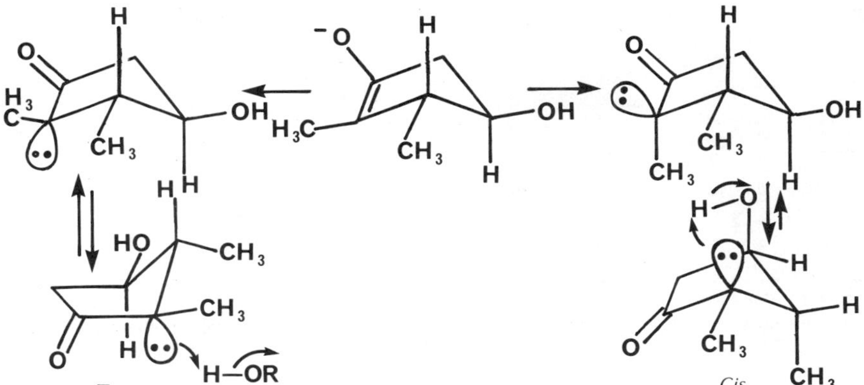

Trans — *Intermolecular protonation*

Cis — *Intramolecular protonation*

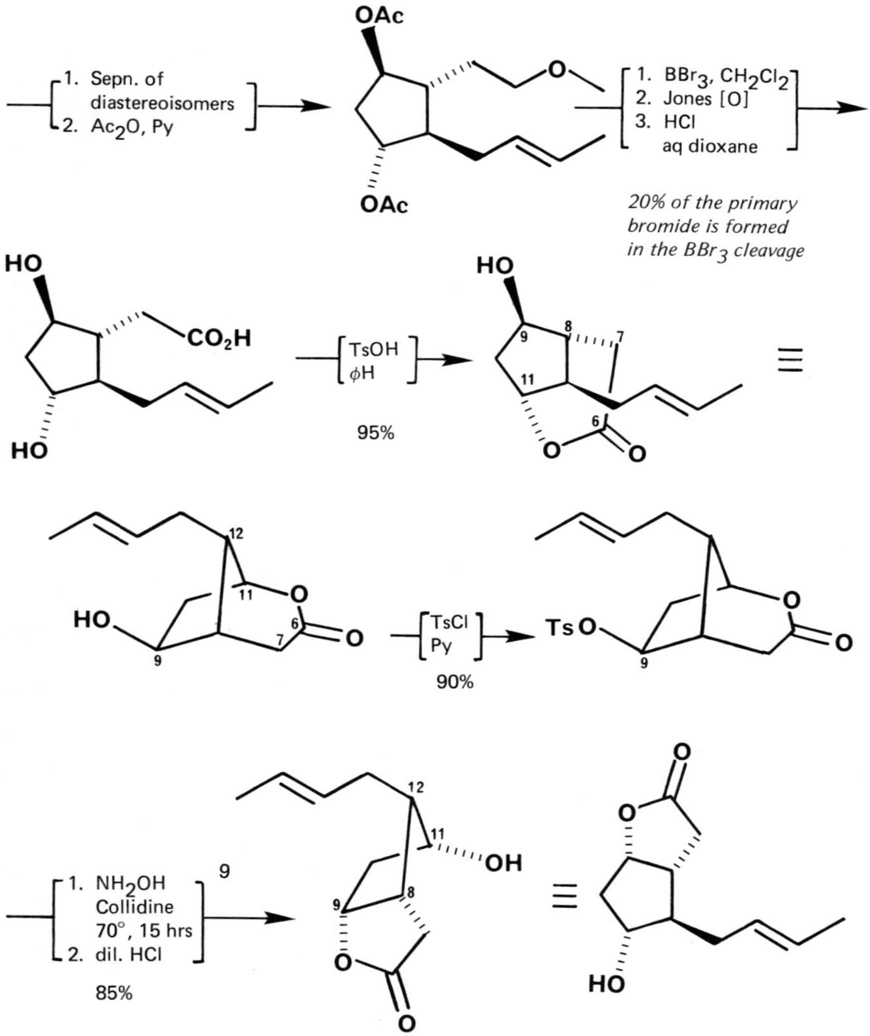

9. This nucleophile (hydroxylamine) is chosen to give the best ratio of carbonyl attack to proton removal (which gives a cyclopropane ring). The hydroxamic acid then goes to the lactone via participation of the amide carbonyl in the tosylate displacement.
A similar problem was also faced by the English group. R. Peel & J. K. Sutherland, *Chem. Commun.*, 151 (1974). For details see footnote 7, p. 220.

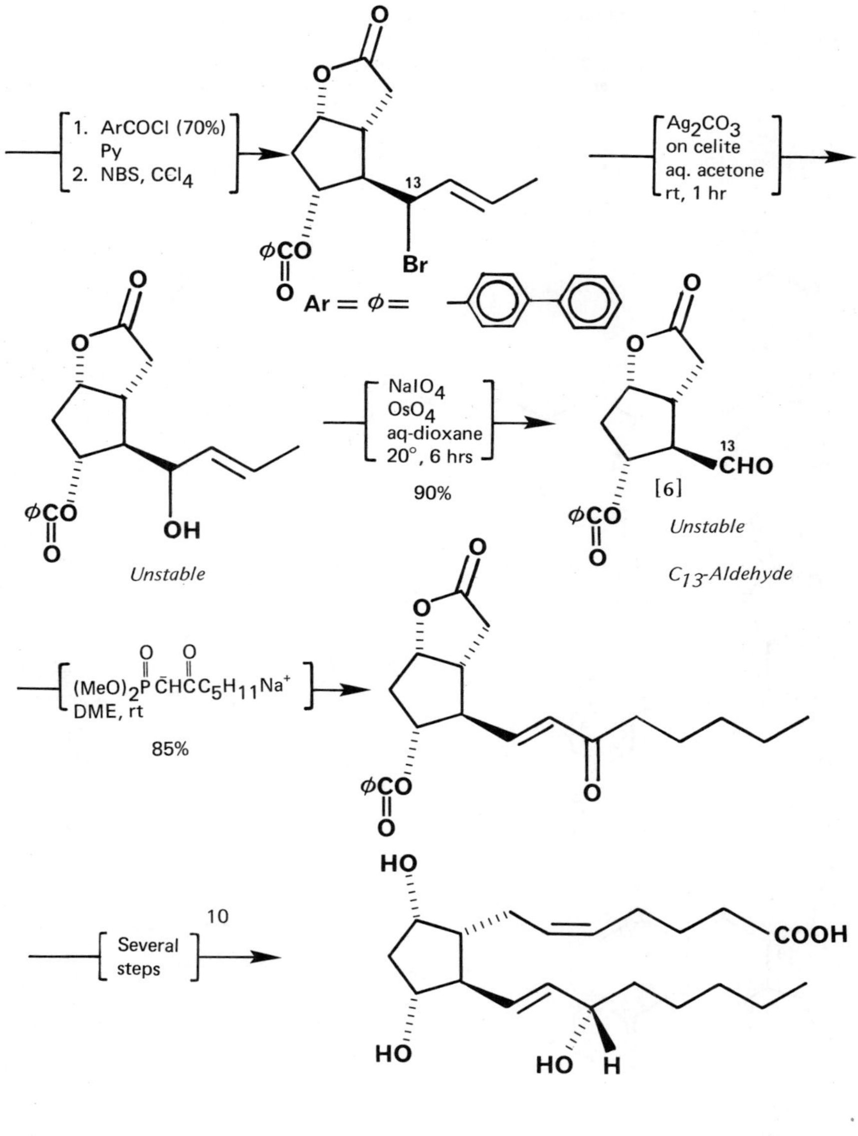

---

10. E. J. Corey, N. M. Weinshenker, T. K. Schaaf & W. Huber, *J. Am. Chem. Soc.*, 91, 5675 (1969).

In this approach[11,12] the problem of obtaining the C_{13}-aldehyde is simplified by using the (2'-phenyl)-ethyl substituent at C_{12}. This, also, avoids the problem of getting some saturated side chain during the reduction of the hydroxycyclopentenone [7]. Catalytic hydrogenation of [7] produces the wrong C_{12} stereochemistry which partially epimerizes during the Horner-Emmons reaction.

SYNTHETIC STRATEGY

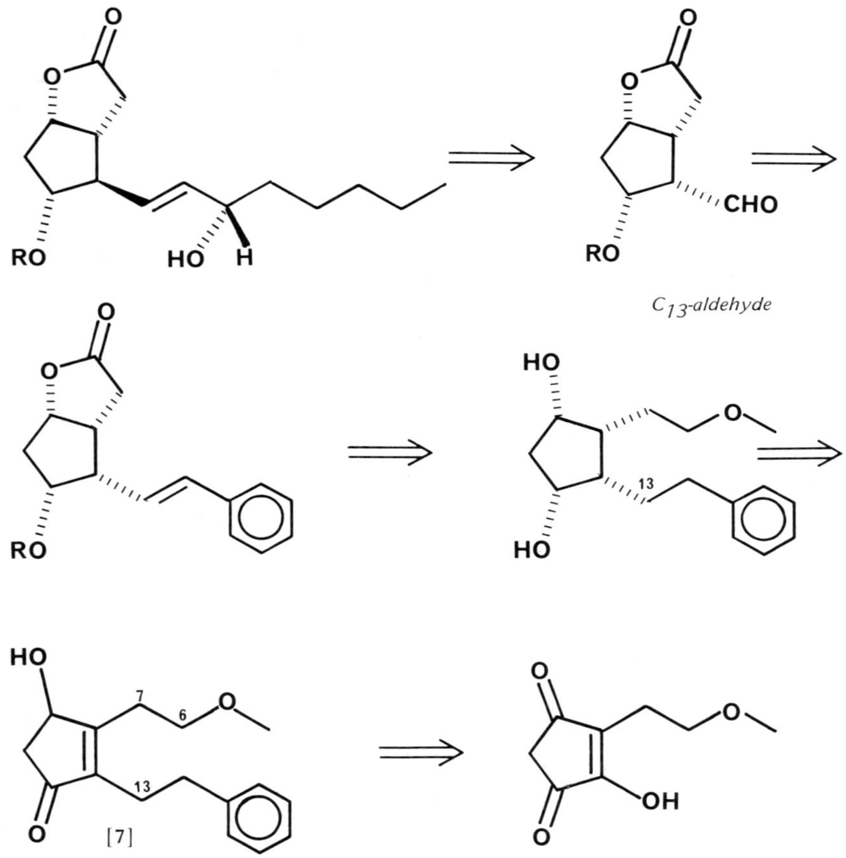

11. P. De Clercq, R. Coen, E. Van Hoof & M. Vandewalle, *Tet.*, 32, 2747 (1976).
12. R. Coen, P. De Clercq, D. Van Haver & M. Vandewalle, *Bull. Soc. Chim. Belg.*, 84, 203 (1975).

SYNTHETIC PLAN[11,12]

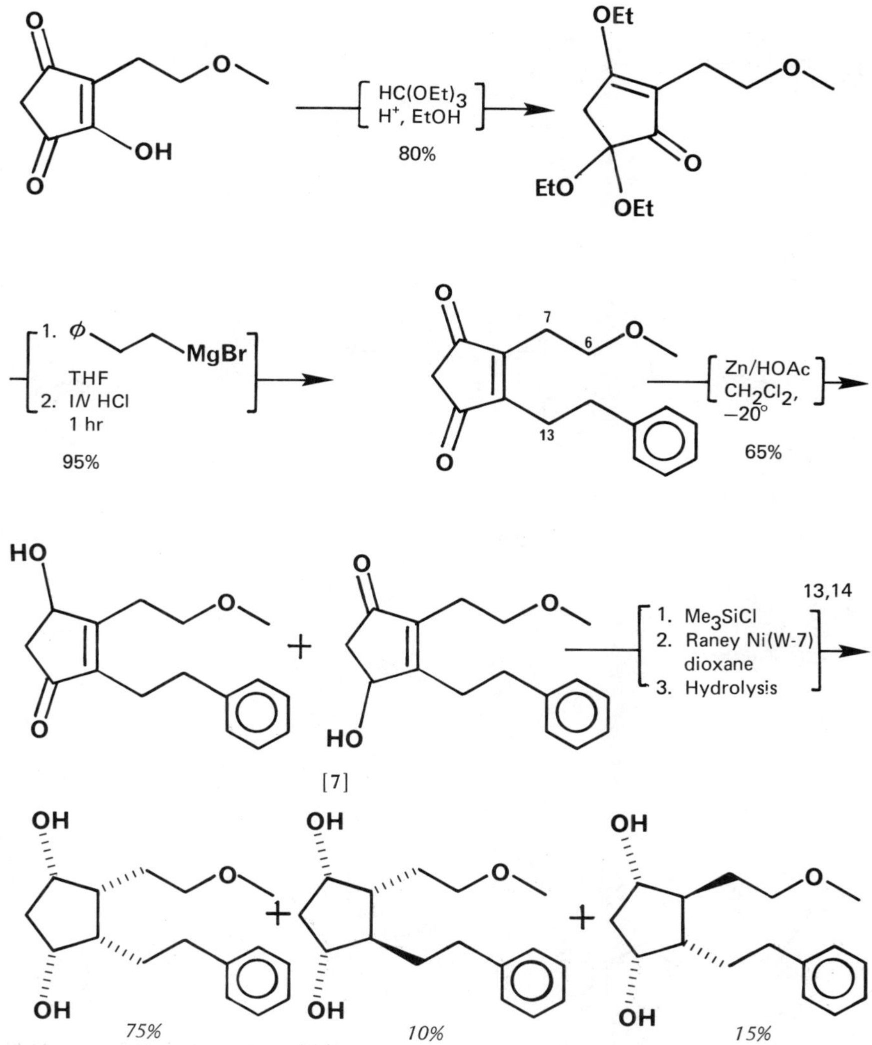

13. The protection of the alcohol as the trimethylsilyl ether was necessary to avoid hydrogenolysis during the catalytic hydrogenation.
D. Van Haver, D. Tavernier, M. Ateunis & M. Vandewalle, *Tet.*, **30**, 105 (1974).

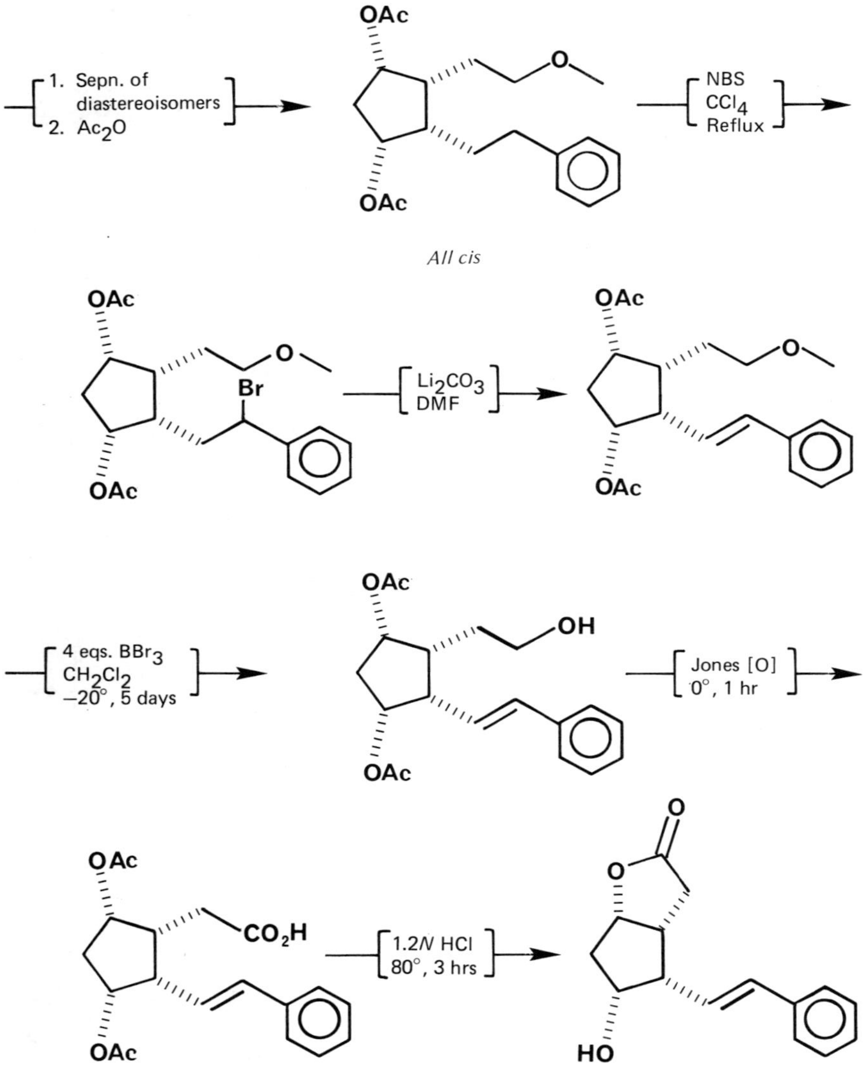

14. The size of the trimethylsilyl group probably enhances the stereoselectivity of the hydrogenation. N. Finch, L. Della Vecchia, J. J. Fitt, R. Stephani & I. Vlattas, *J. Org. Chem.*, **38**, 4412 (1973).

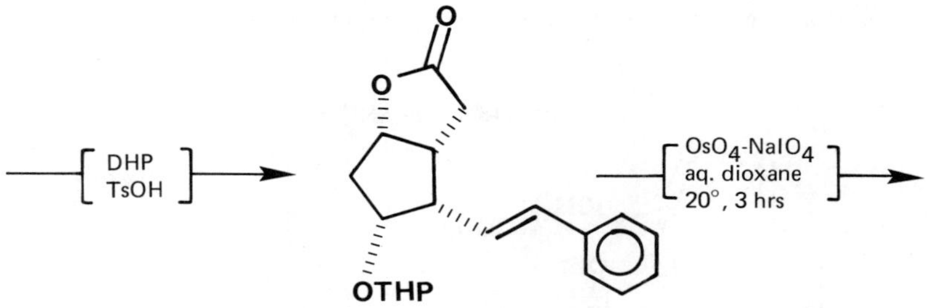

[8]

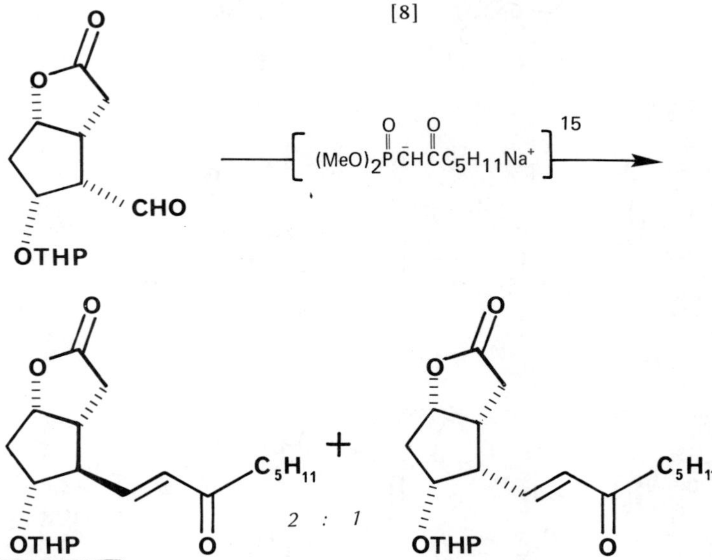

55% from [8]

Epimerization

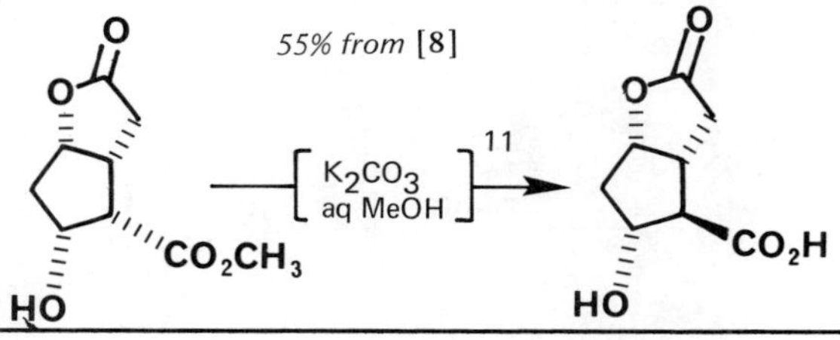

15. The desired equilibration during the Horner-Emmons reaction is to be contrasted with unsuccessful attempts to epimerize the C_{12} formyl group to the more stable *trans* configuration before the condensation.

D. Brewster, M. Myers, J. Ormerod, P. Otter, A. C. B. Smith, M. E. Spinner & S. Turner, *J. Chem. Soc. (Perkin I)*, 2796 (1973). For details see p. 204.

Another synthesis going through the cyclopentane-1,3,4-trione has been reported.[16]

SYNTHETIC PLAN[16]

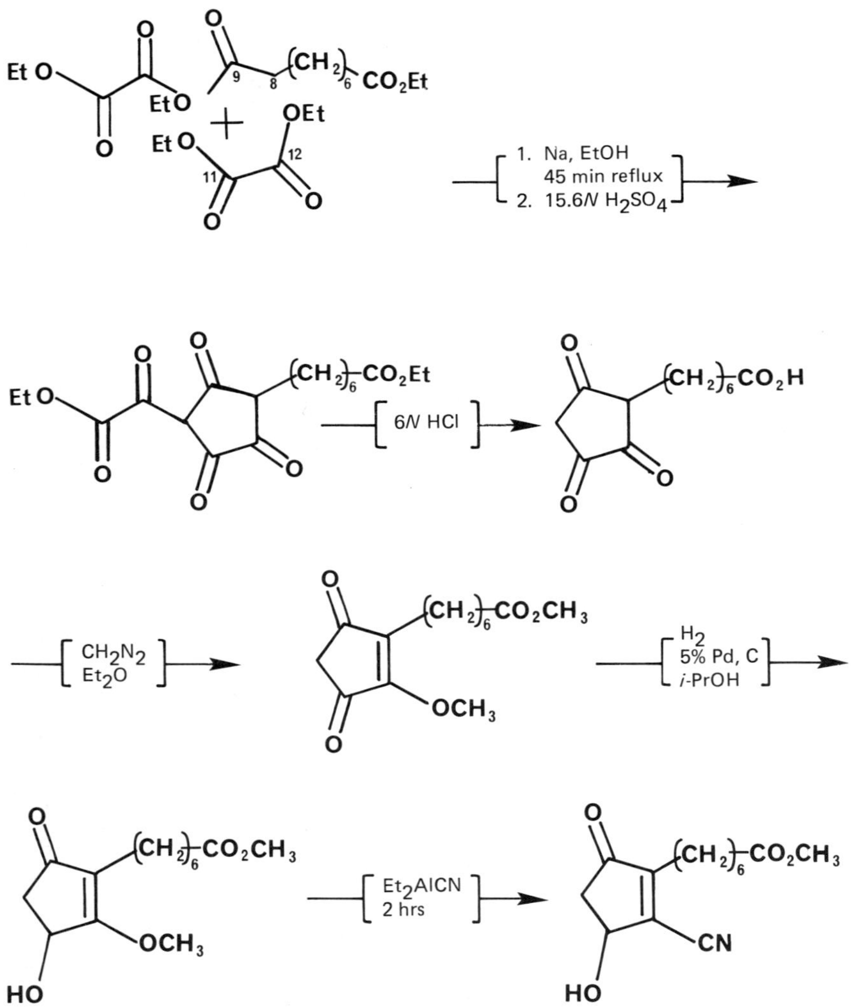

16. J. Katsube, H. Shimomura, E. Murayama, K. Toki & M. Matsui, *Agr. Biol. Chem.*, 35, 1768 (1971).

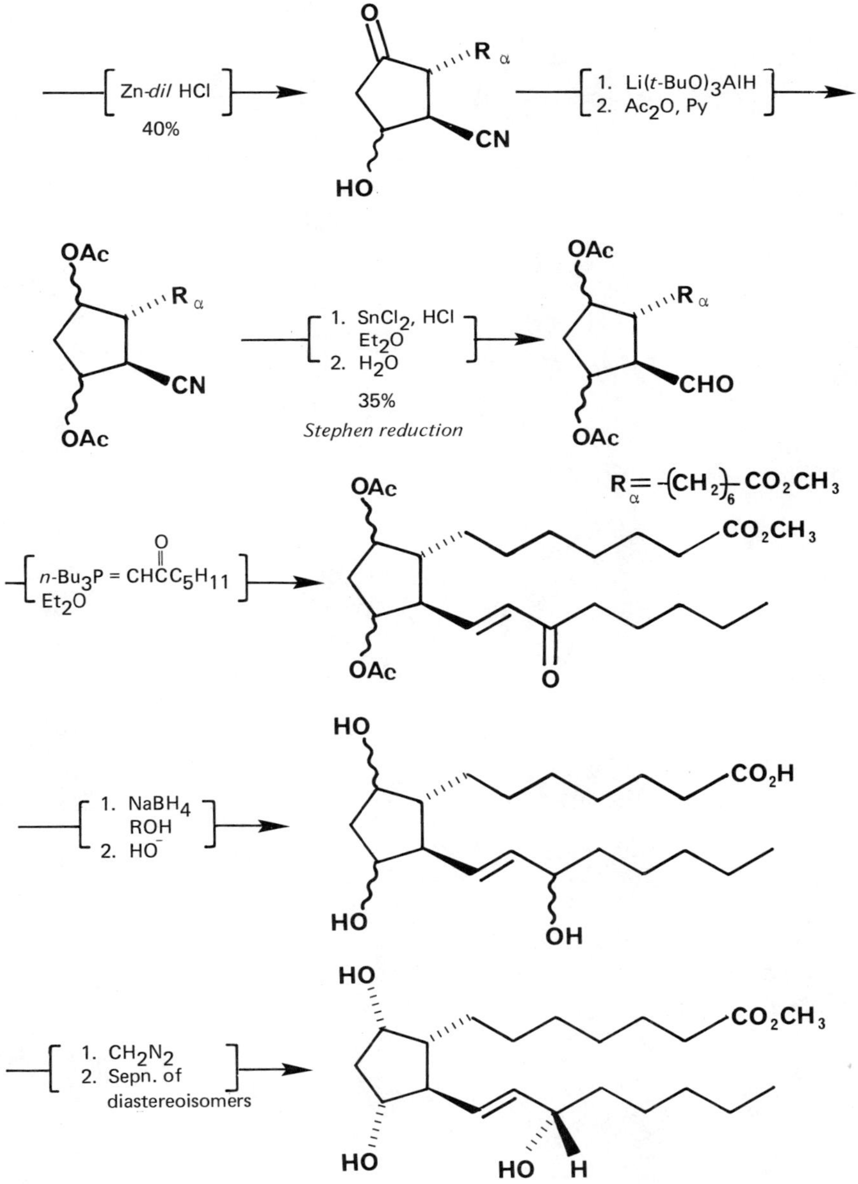

Zn-dil HCl
40%
1. Li(t-BuO)3AlH
2. Ac2O, Py
1. SnCl2, HCl
Et2O
2. H2O
35%
Stephen reduction
R = (CH2)6 CO2CH3
n-Bu3P = CHCC5H11
Et2O
1. NaBH4
ROH
2. HO
1. CH2N2
2. Sepn. of diastereoisomers

8

Cyclohexane Ring Contraction Approach

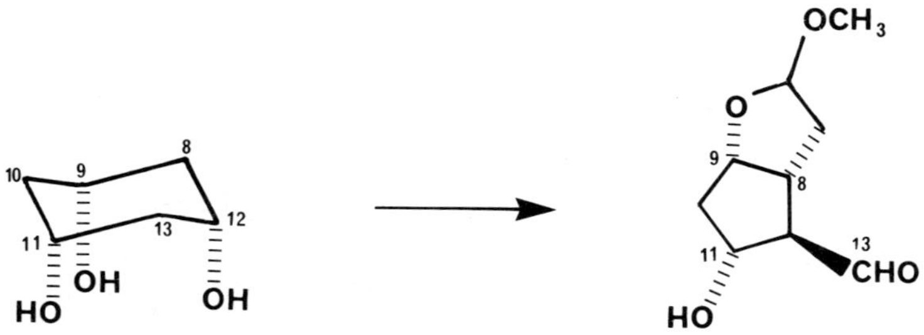

In this ingenious approach[1] to the synthesis of prostaglandins, the adequately developed chemistry of the cyclohexanes has been exploited to create the four contiguous asymmetric centers of the prostaglandin nucleus; the extra ring carbon then becomes the aldehyde attached to the cyclopentane ring in a fascinating ring contraction. A noteworthy feature of this synthesis is that it largely succeeds in avoiding the use of extrinsic protecting groups.[2]

---

1. R. B. Woodward, J. Gosteli, I. Ernest, R. J. Friary, G. Nestler, H. Raman, R. Sitrin, Ch. Suter & J. K. Whitesell, *J. Am. Chem. Soc.*, **95**, 6853 (1973).
2. For an interesting review of the synthetic strategy see: I. Ernest, *Angew. Chem. [Int. Edit.]*, **15**, 207 (1976).

SYNTHETIC STRATEGY

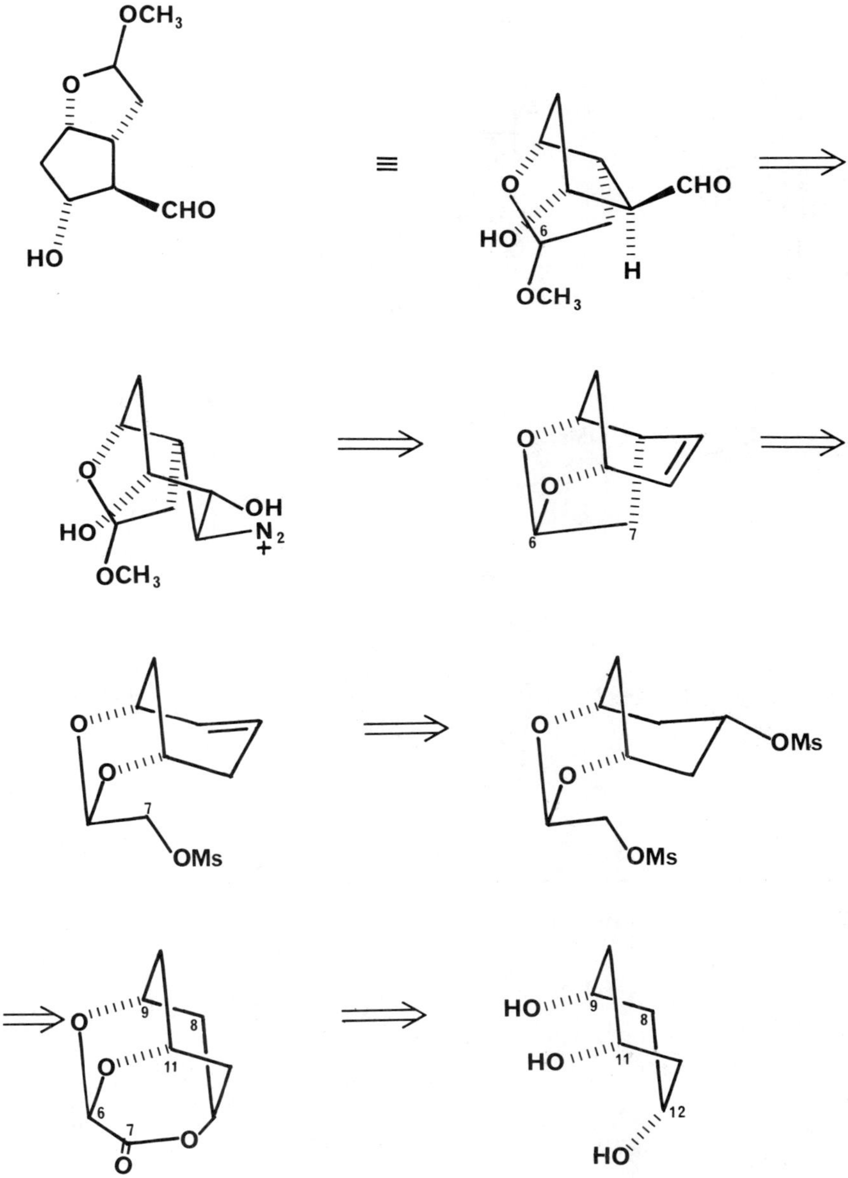

SYNTHETIC PLAN[1]

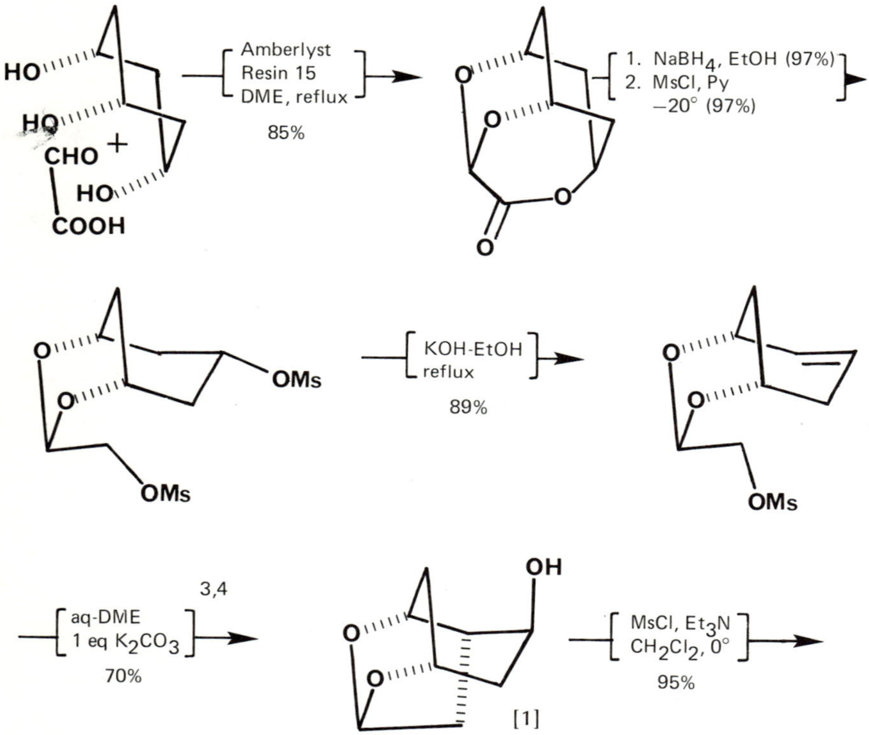

Resolved as the ketopinic ester

---

3. Examples of similar cyclizations through π-bond participation are known in the literature. D. J. Raber, G. J. Kane & P. von R. Schleyer, *Tet. Lett.*, 4117 (1970).

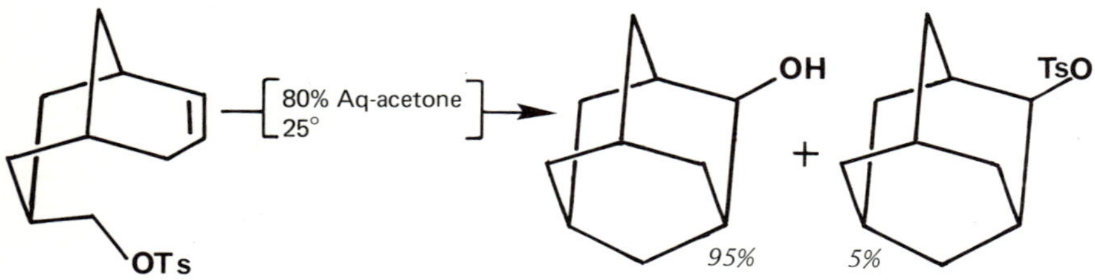

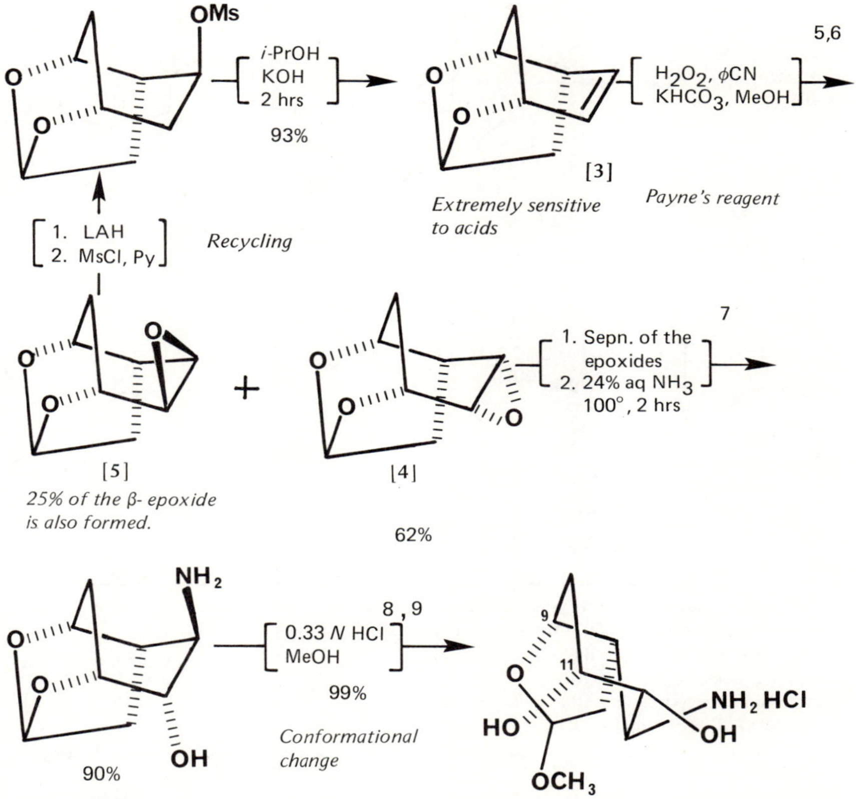

4. The three centered electron deficient intermediate accepts elements of water at the most favorable location to give exclusively this isomer [1]. 5-8% of the undesirable isomeric dioxaadamantanol is [2] also formed.

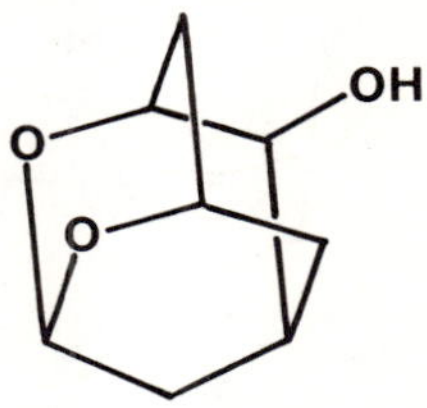

[2]

5. The highly acid sensitive olefin [3] is epoxidized under basic conditions with Payne's reagent. G. B. Payne, **18**, 763 (1962). It is not clear why the desired epoxide is formed.
6. The undesired epoxide [5], which is formed as the main product when *m*-CPBA -$NaHCO_3$ is used as the reagent, can be recycled as shown.
7. The regiospecific opening of the epoxide is a consequence of the rigid conformation of [4].

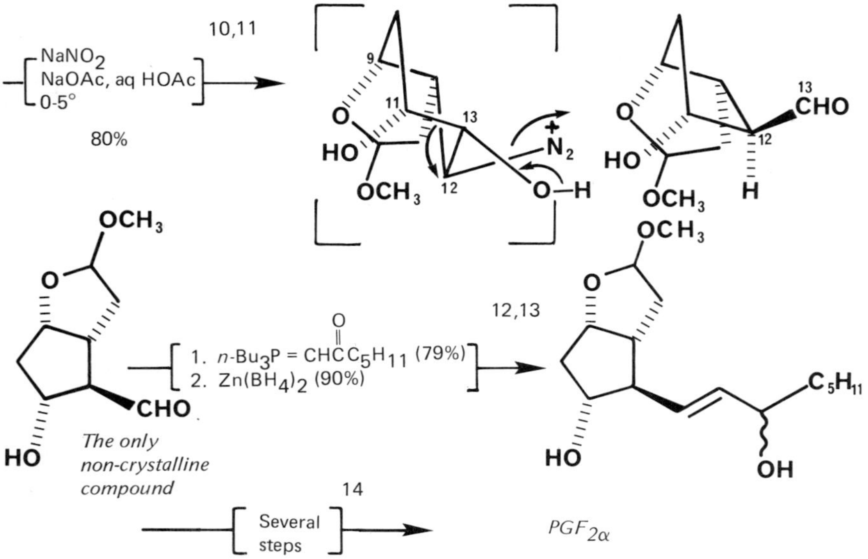

8. The ring contraction of a 1,2-disubstituted cyclohexane can take place only when the leaving substituent is equatorial and thus *anti* periplanar to migrating C—C bond.

9. The other possible seven membered [3.2.2] bicyclic ketal [6] is not formed. Only the more stable five membered ketal is formed. The formation of this [4.3.0] bicyclic ketal fixes the stereochemistry for the subsequent rearrangement.

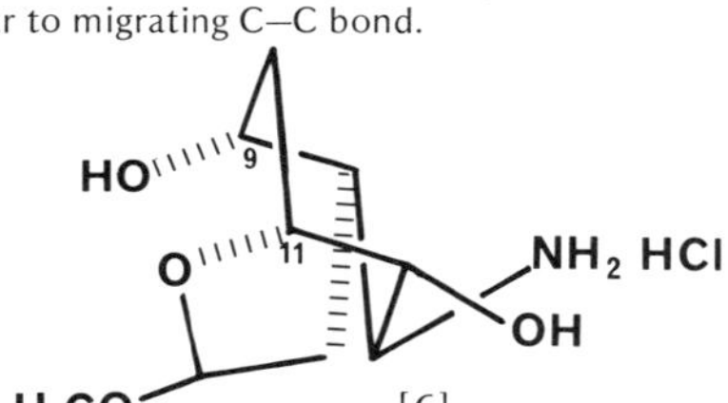

[6]

10. Direct ring contraction of the tricyclic olefin [3] with thallium salts failed under various conditions.

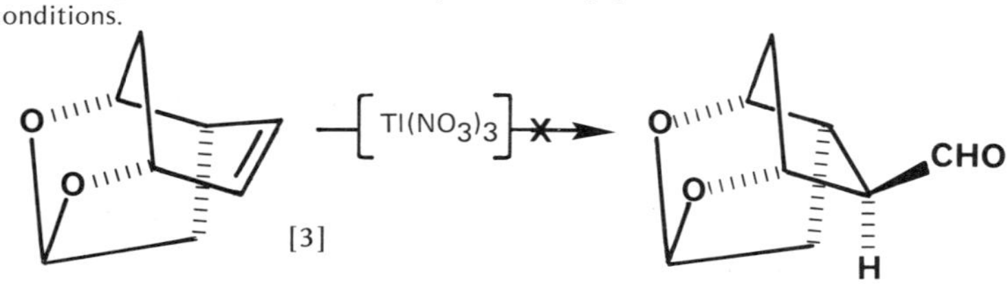

11. Tiffeneau-Demjanov rearrangement: see D. Redmore & C. D. Gutsche, *Adv. Alicyclic Chem.*, 3, 2 (1971).
12. N. Finch & J. J. Fitt, *Tet. Lett.*, 4639 (1969).
13. The triphenyl phosphorane has also been used. M. Miyano & C. R. Dorn . *J. Org. Chem.*, **37**, 1818 (1972).
14. E. J. Corey & R. Noyori, *Tet. Lett.*, 311 (1970).

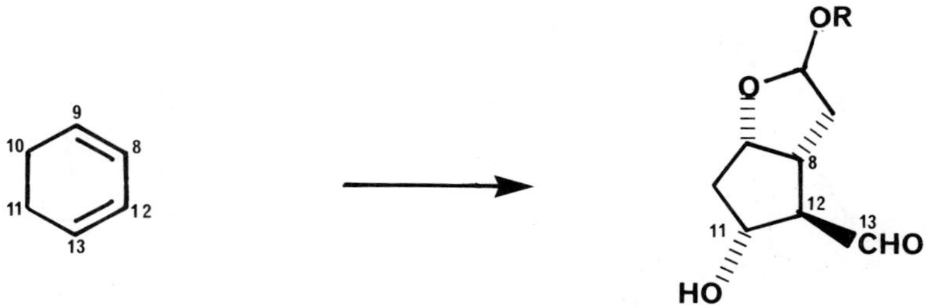

In the Corey[15] ring contraction route the Woodward intermediate (I, R=Me) is made from cyclohexa-1,3-diene by allylic functionalization via the ene reaction followed by the cleavage of the N-phenyltriazolindione (enophile).[16]

15. E. J. Corey & B. B. Snider, *Tet. Lett.,* 3091 (1973).
16. B. B. Snider, Ph.D. Dissertation, Harvard University (1973).

SYNTHETIC STRATEGY

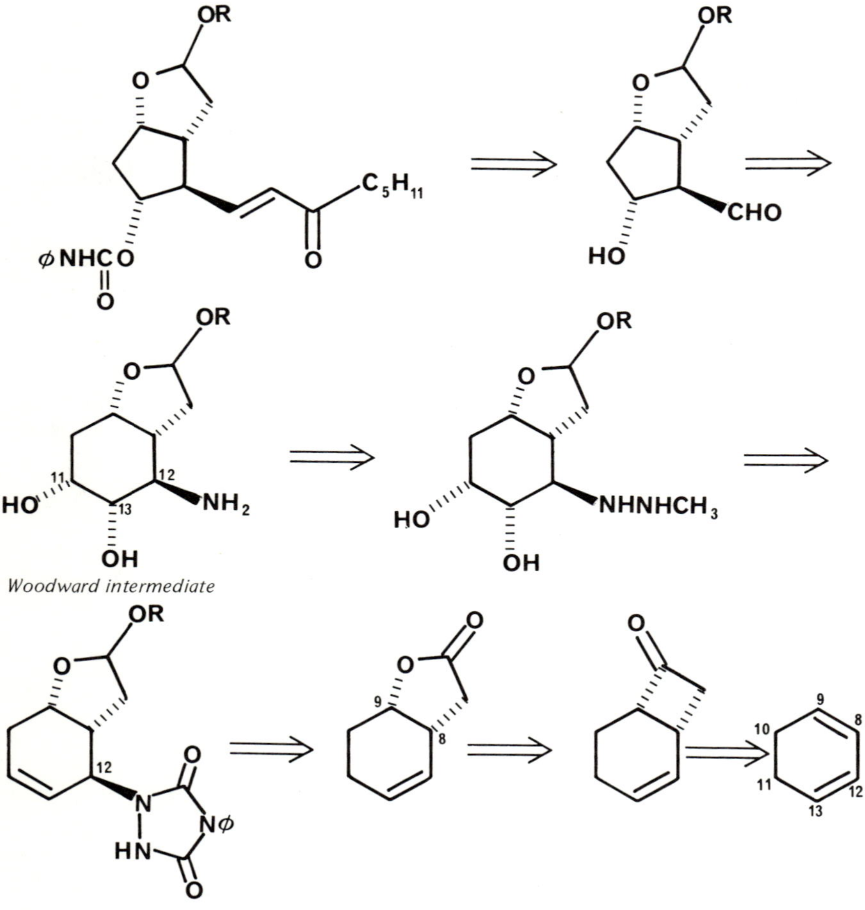

SYNTHETIC PLAN[15,16]

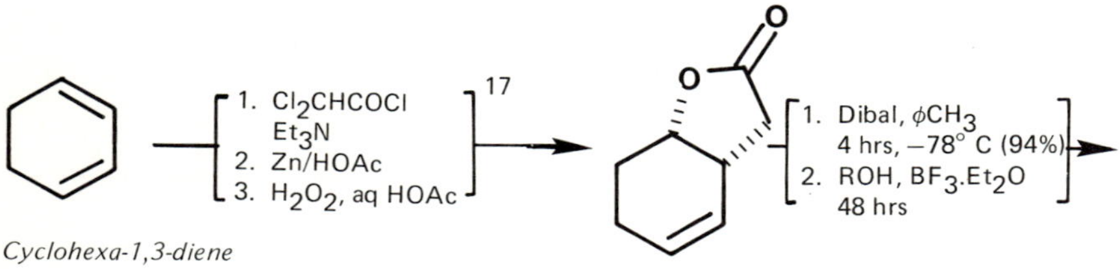

Cyclohexa-1,3-diene

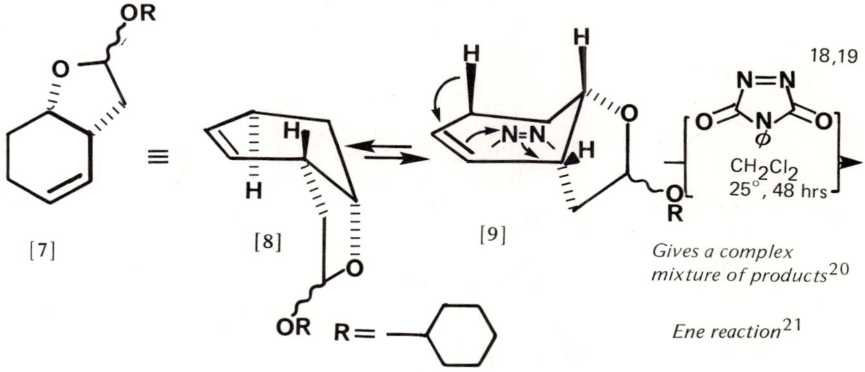

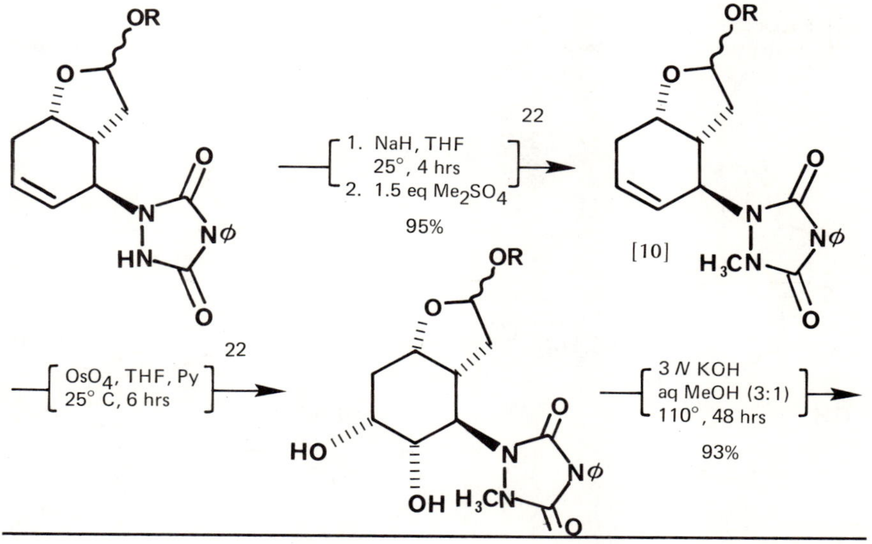

17. E. J. Corey & T. Ravindranathan, *Tet. Lett.*, 4753 (1971).
18. N-Phenyltriazolinedione is one of the most reactive enophile (or dienophile) known. It was first used by Cookson.
    R. S. Cookson, S. S. H. Gilani & I. D. R. Stevens, *J. Chem. Soc.C.*, 1905 (1967); R. S. Cookson *et al.*, *Org. Syn.*, **51**, 121 (1971).
19. The cyclohexene [7] does not undergo the ene reaction with azodicarboxylate.
20. The cyclohexene [7] exists in two conformations [8] and [9]. Abstraction of the allylic hydrogen from [9] by N-phenyltriazolinedione gives the desired product (30-45% yield) along with other products.
21. For other examples of ene reactions with triazolinediones see:
    W. H. Pirkle & J. C. Stickler, *Chem. Commun.*, 760 (1967) and D. J. Pasto & A. F. Chan, *Tet. Lett.*, 713 (1973).

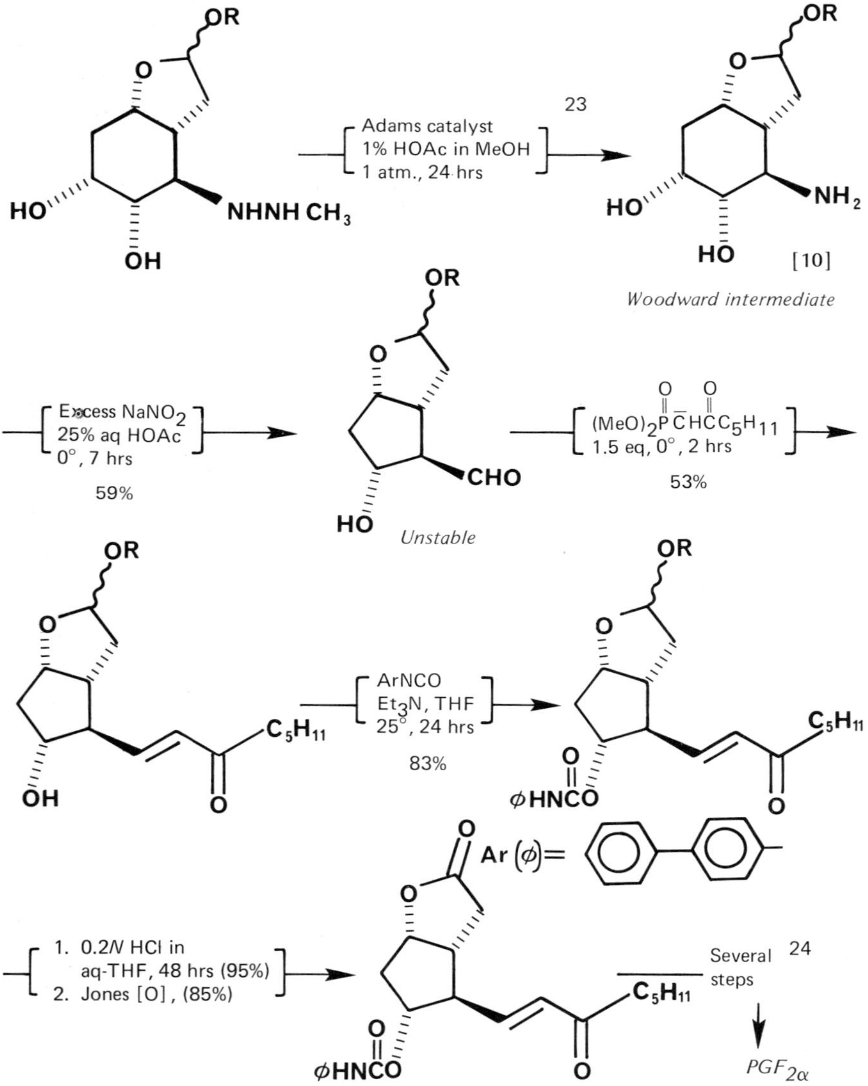

22. The OsO_4 hydroxylation reaction on the -NH- compound gave an intractable black solid.
23. For other examples of hydrogenolysis of hydrazines see P. N. Rylander, *Catalytic Hydrogenation Over Platinum Metals*, Academic, New York, 1967, p. 491.
24. E. J. Corey, K. B. Becker & R. V. Varma, *J. Am. Chem. Soc.*, 94, 8616 (1972).

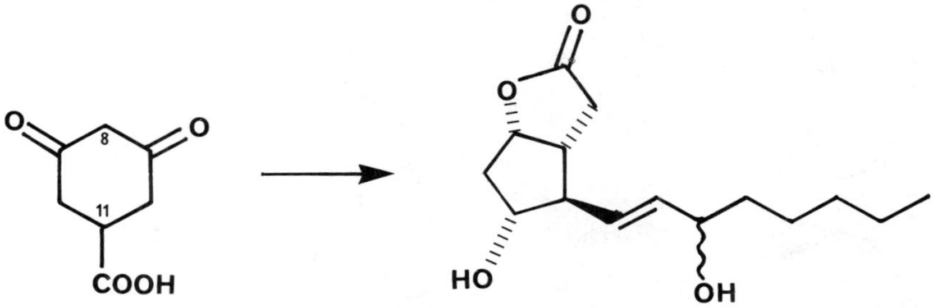

In this approach[25] the prostanoid nucleus is constructed from cyclohexadione carboxylate by a sequence involving a Favorski-type ring contraction[26] and a carboxy inversion step.[32] This procedure allows the preparation of the C_{11} ring analogs by using appropriate substituents at that position.

---

25. F. Kienzle, G. W. Holland, J. L. Jernow, S. Kwoh & Perry Rosen, *J. Org. Chem.*, 38, 3440 (1973).

SYNTHETIC STRATEGY

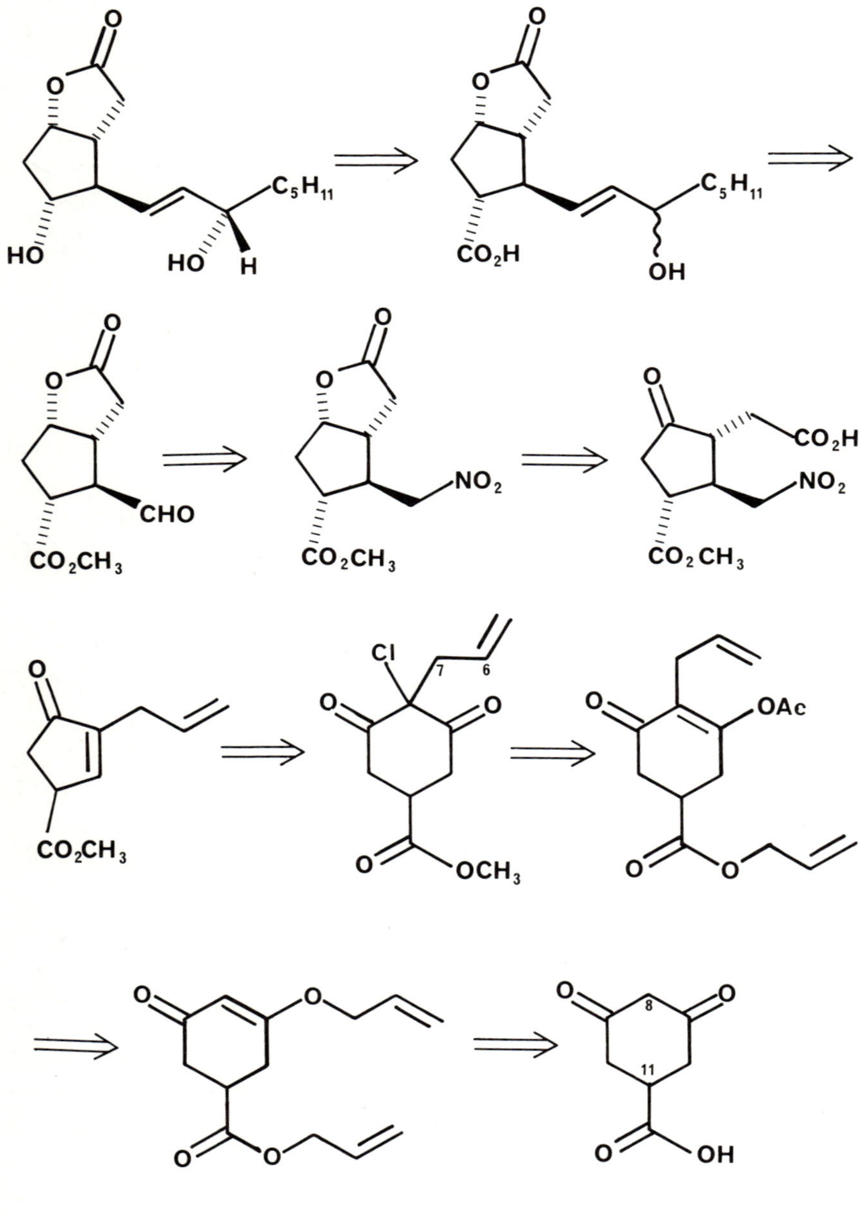

SYNTHETIC PLAN[25]

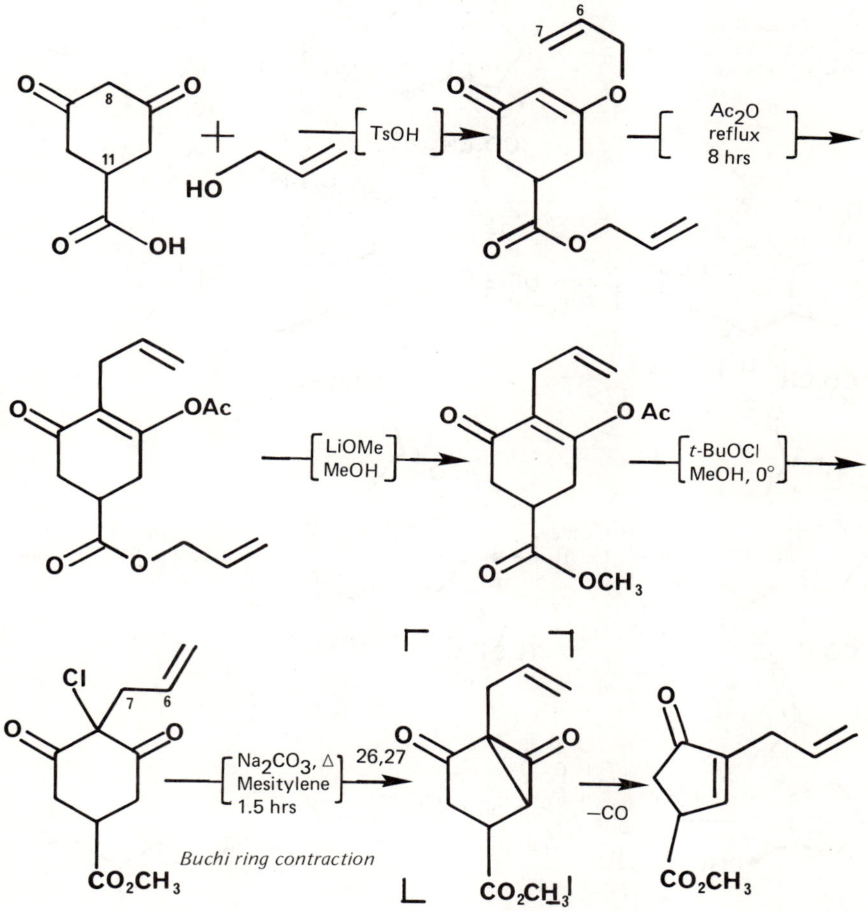

26. G. Buchi & B. Egger, *J. Org. Chem.*, 36, 2021 (1971).
27. This ring contraction method was first applied to the synthesis of a prostaglandin by Dr. J. Bagli.
    J. Bagli & T. Bogri , *Tet. Lett.*, 3815 (1972).
28. The dihydrofuran [11] is formed in substantial quantity when the rearrangement is carried out in solvents other than acetic anhydride.

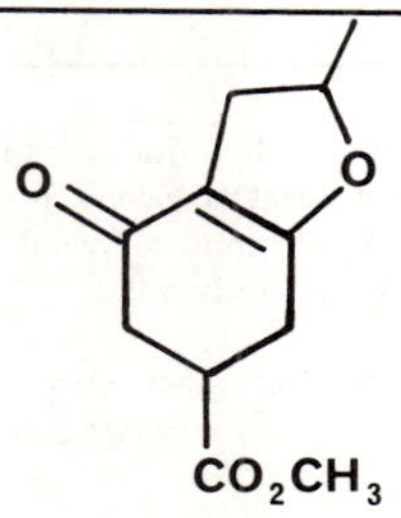

[11]

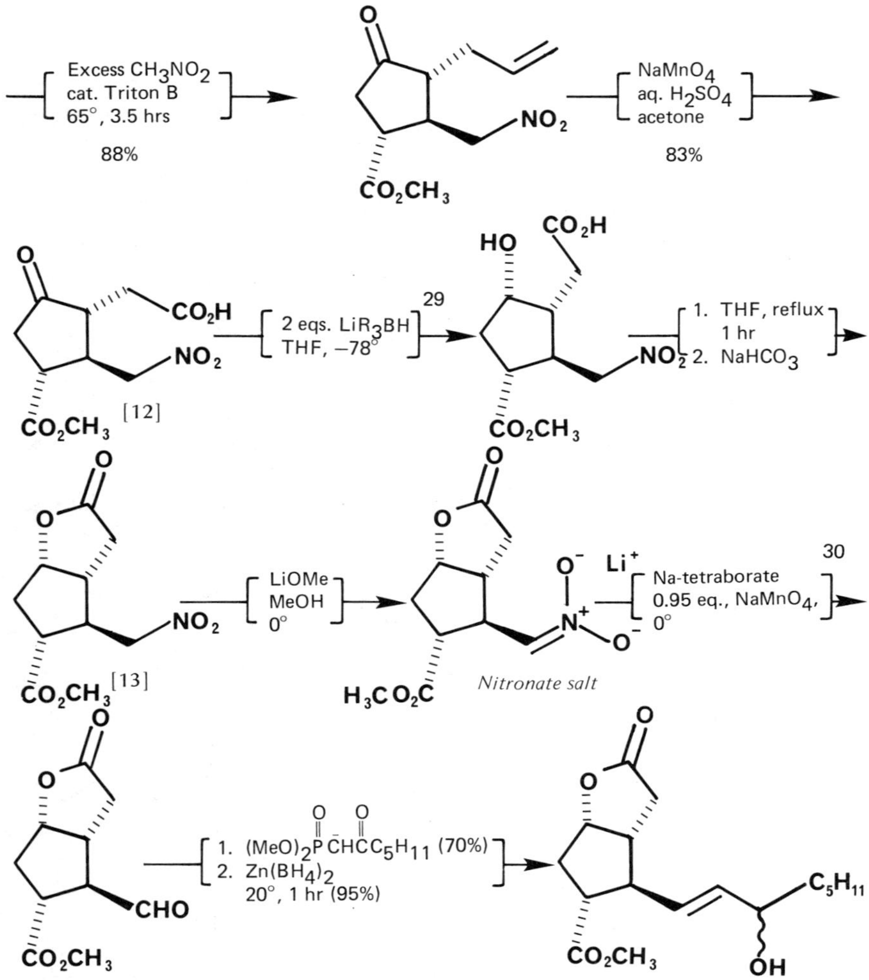

29. Reduction of the cyclopentanone [12] with $NaBH_4$/LiOMe in MeOH gave a mixture of epimeric C_9-alcohols and the overall yield of the lactone [13] was only 54%.

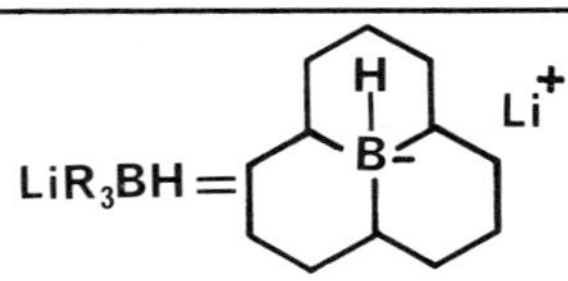

30. For a review on Nef reaction see "Nitronic acids and esters" by A. T. Nielsen, in *The Chemistry of the Nitro and Nitroso Groups*, H. Feuer (Ed.), Wiley, New York, 1969, Ch. 7, p. 349.

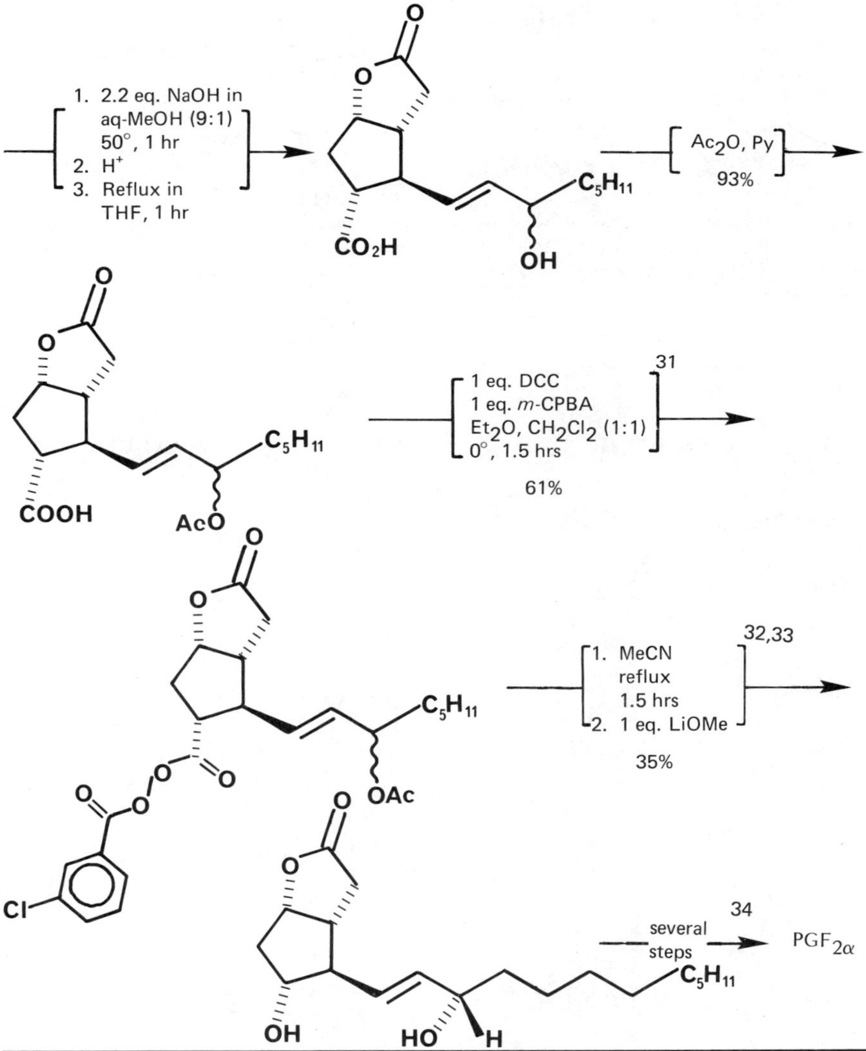

31. F. D. Greene & J. Kazan, *J. Org. Chem.*, **28**, 2168 (1963).
32. D. B. Denney & N. Sherman, *J. Org. Chem.*, **30**, 3760 (1965).
33. The carboxy inversion takes place with retention of configuration. T. Kashiwagi, S. Kozuka & S. Oae, *Tet.*, **26**, 3619 (1970).
34. E. J. Corey, N. M. Weinshenker, T. K. Schaff & W. Huber, *J. Am. Chem. Soc.*, **91**, 5675 (1969).

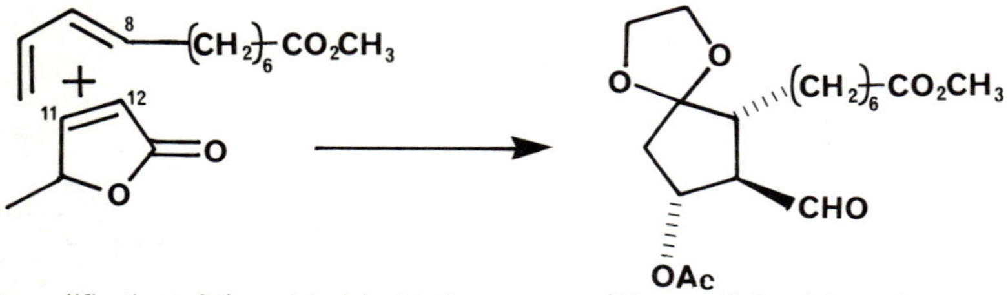

This modification of the original hydrindenone route (Chapter 4), involving a ring contraction, leads directly to the aldehyde [14] without having to resort to a four-carbon degradation sequence.[35] One of the limitations of this route is its inapplicability to the synthesis of PG_2 compounds.

SYNTHETIC STRATEGY

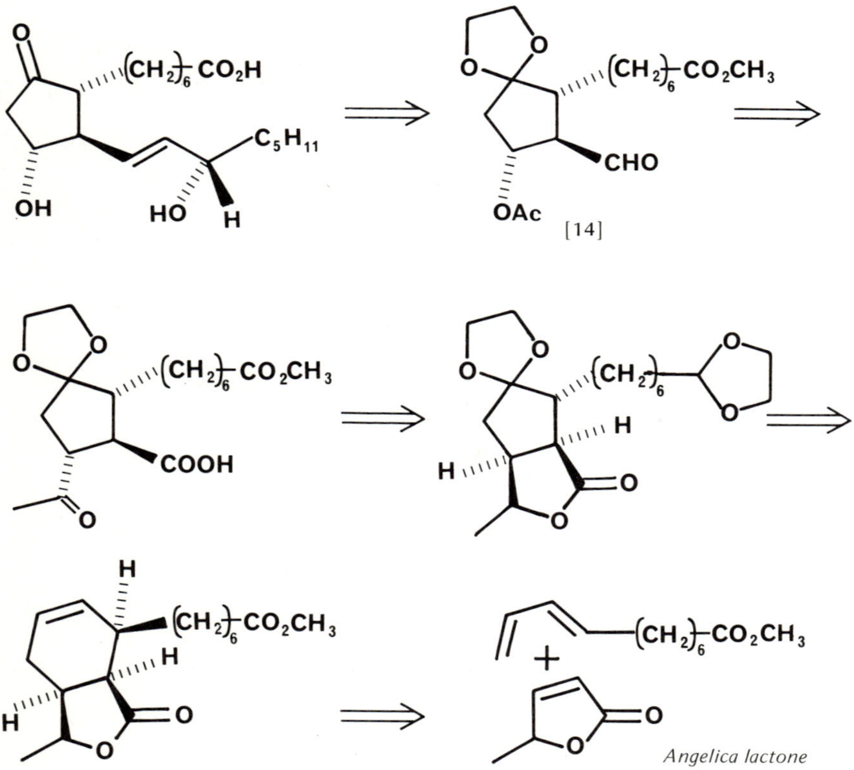

35. C. H. Kuo, D. Taub & N. L. Wendler, *Tet. Lett.*, 5317 (1972).

SYNTHETIC PLAN[35]

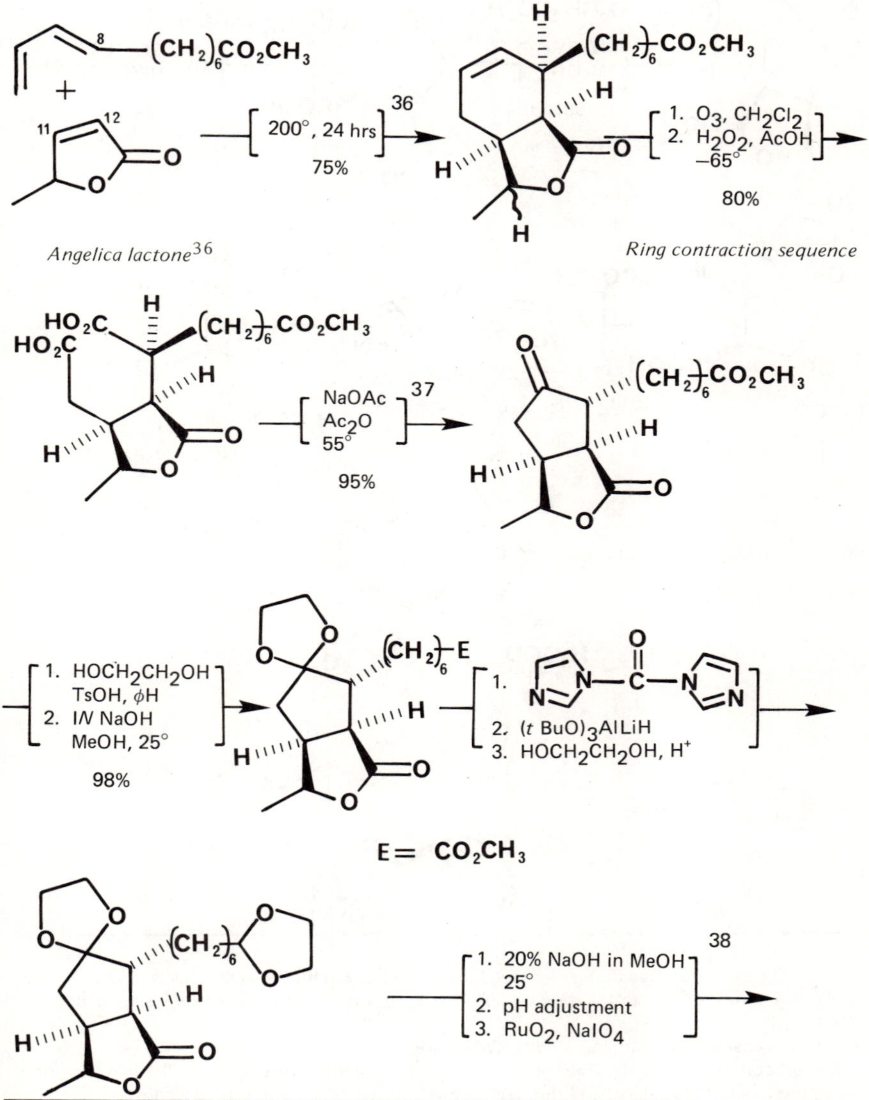

36. This may be the first example of Diels-Alder reaction with angelica lactone.
37. Dieckmann cyclization and subsequent decarboxylation.

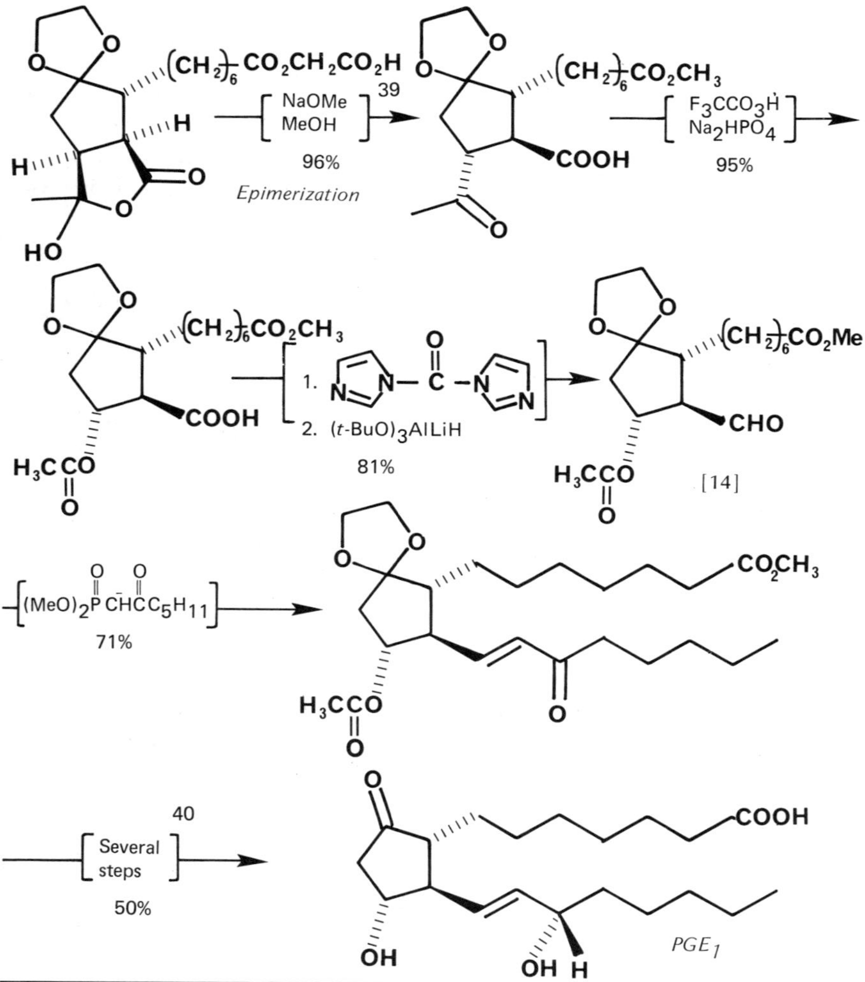

38. The RuO_4 oxidation transforms the acetal into the ester of glycolic acid. This is, probably, the only oxidation of an acetal directly into an ester other than the ozonolysis method of Deslongchamps.
P. Deslongchamps & C. Moreau, *Can. J. Chem.*, **49**, 2465 (1971).

39. This process allows distinction of the two acid functions because the hydroxy-lactone tautomerizes to the acid salt and the ester of glycolic acid undergoes ester exchange.

40. For another synthesis of PGE_1 see E. J. Corey, N. H. Anderson, R. M. Carlson, J. Paust, E. Vedejs, I. Vlattas & R. E. K. Winter, *J. Am. Chem. Soc.*, **90**, 3245 (1968).

In this modification, 1,3-butadiene was used as the diene in the Diels-Alder reaction to obtain compounds of the PG_2 series.[41] Subsequent ring contraction sequence leads to the carbomethoxycyclopentanone [15] derivative which is alkylated with allyl bromide (an acetaldehyde synthon) for further elaboration of the C_5-C_6 *cis* double bond of the PG_2 compounds.

SYNTHETIC PLAN[41]

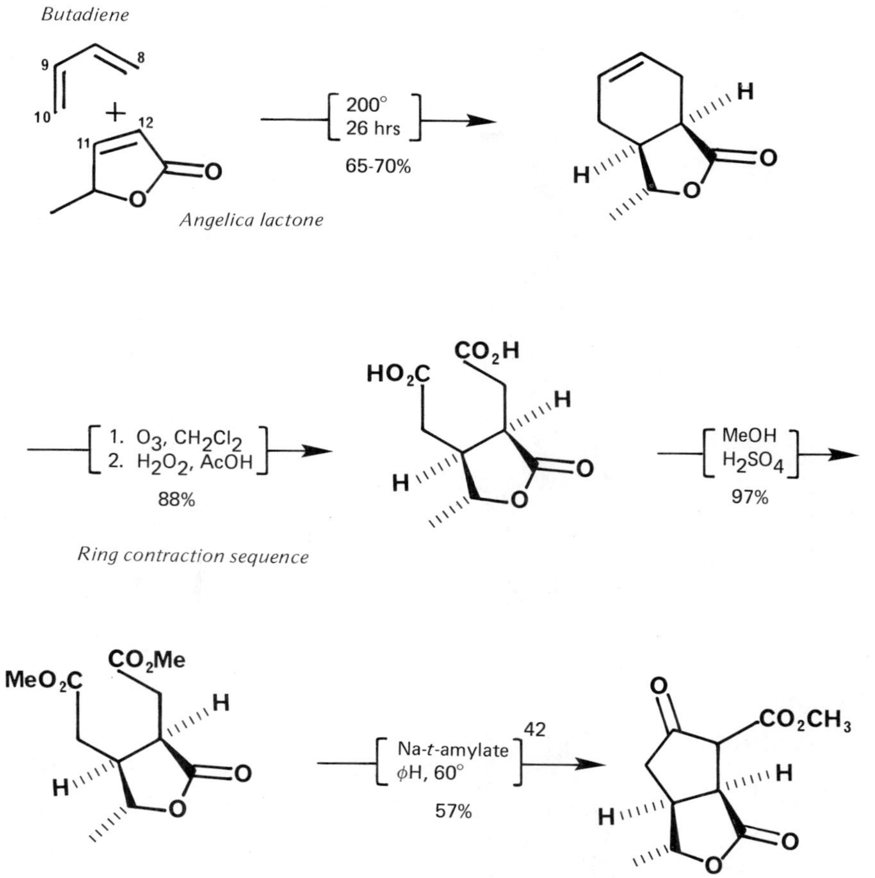

[15]

---

41. D. Taub, Z. Zelawski & N. L. Wendler, *Tet. Lett.*, 3667 (1970).
42. Steric considerations direct the Dieckmann cyclization to the desired carbomethoxycyclopentanone [15] which controls the regioselectivity of the subsequent alkylation to introduce the truncated α-chain.

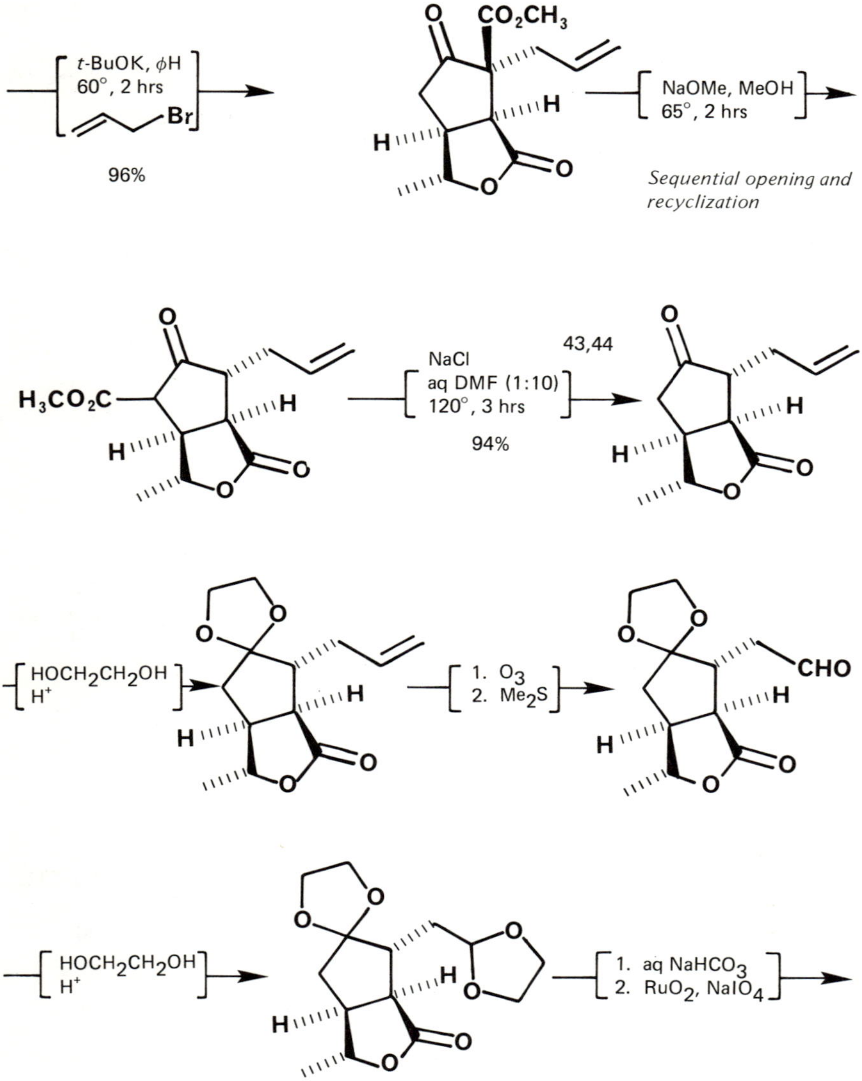

---

43. A. P. Krapcho & A. J. Lowey, *Tet. Lett.*, 957 (1973).
44. Compare this with the direct decarboxylation of a similar intermediate. For further details see footnote 37, p. 183.

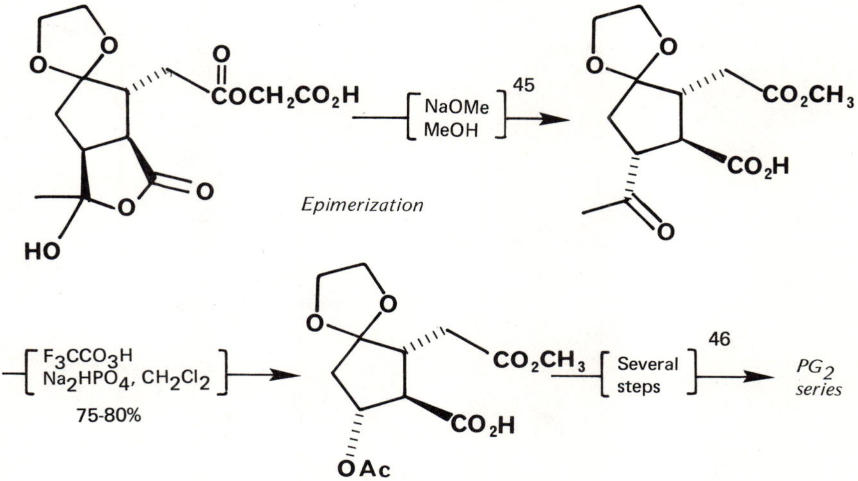

45. This process allows the distinction of the two acid functions. For further details see footnote 39, p. 184.

46. Personal communication.

9

Bicyclo[2.2.1]heptene Approach

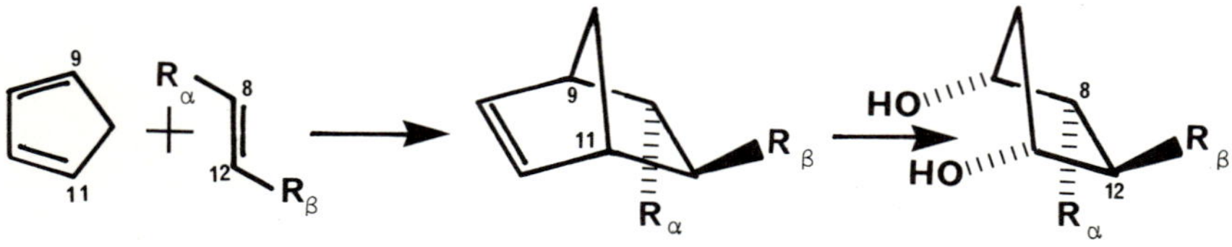

[1]

The 5,6-disubstituted bicyclo[2.2.1]hept-2-ene can be a convenient precursor for the prostanoid nucleus if the C_2 and C_3 carbon atoms can be replaced by two oxygen atoms. The substituents at C_6 and C_5 become the α- and β- chains, respectively.

This type of synthetic strategy was first developed, and subsequently modified, by Katsube.[1,2,3] Later variations along these lines were made by Raphael and Jones.[4,5] The disubstituted bicyclo[2.2.1]heptene [1] is made via the Diels-Alder reaction and the dienophile provides the C_8 and C_{12} carbons of the prostanoid nucleus. The dienophile is differentially substituted so as to enable further elaboration of the substituents to the appropriate side chains. Oxidative cleavage of the norbornene double bond leads to the Corey lactone which has been converted to the prostaglandins.

1. J. Katsube, H. Shimomura & M. Matsui, *Agr. Biol. Chem.*, **35**, 1828 (1971).
2. J. Katsube, H. Shimomura & M. Matsui, *Agr. Biol. Chem.*, **36**, 1997 (1972).
3. H. Shimomura, J. Katsube & M. Matsui, *Agr. Biol. Chem.*, **39**, 657 (1975).
4. G. Jones, R. A. Raphael & S. Wright, *Chem. Commun.*, 609 (1972).
5. G. Jones, R. A. Raphael & S. Wright, *J. Chem. Soc.*, [Perkin I], 1676 (1974).

SYNTHETIC STRATEGY

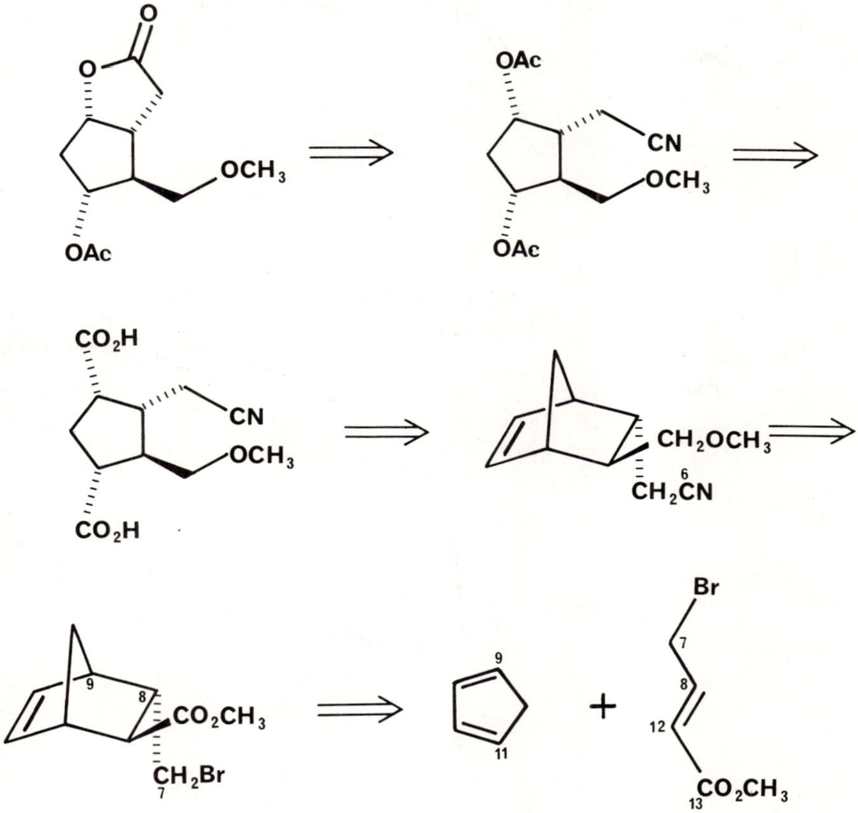

SYNTHETIC PLAN[1,2,3]

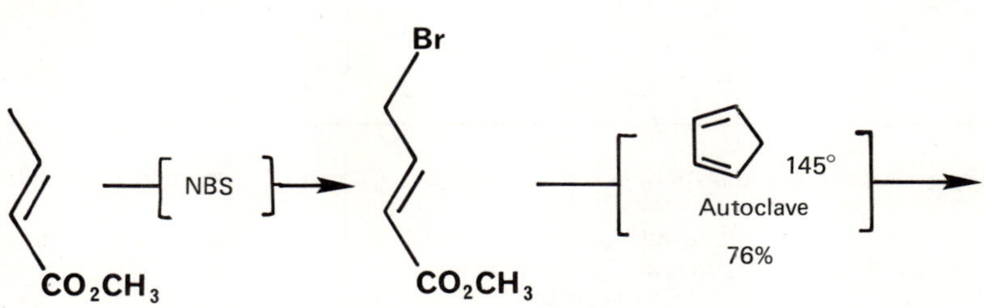

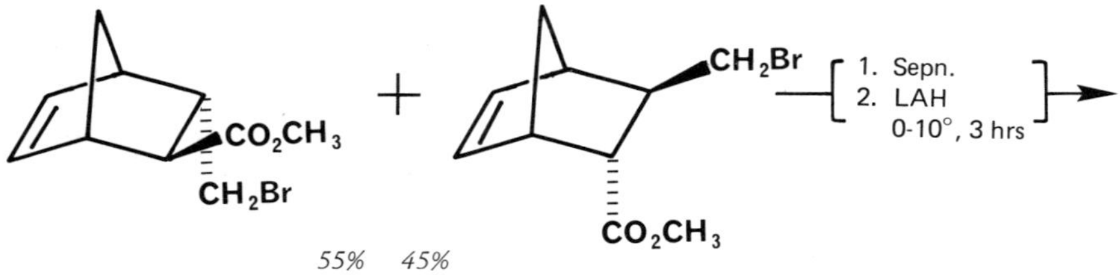

55% *45%*

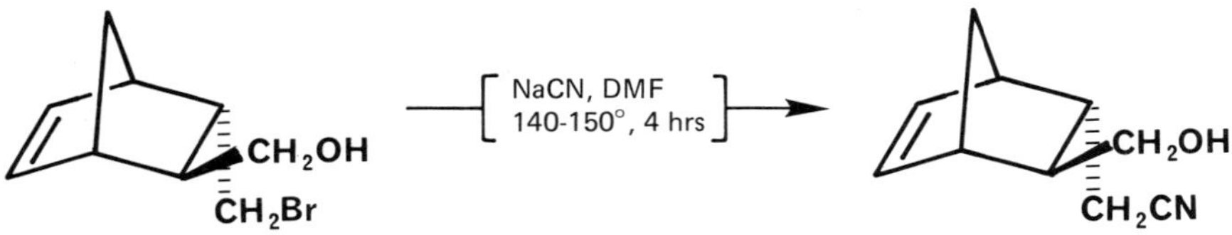

Homologation [6]

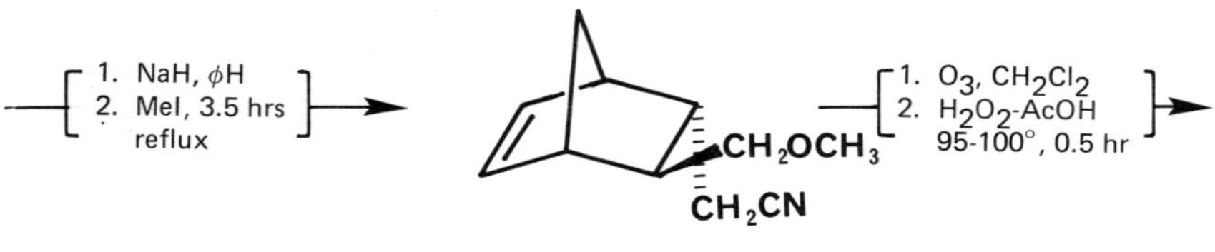

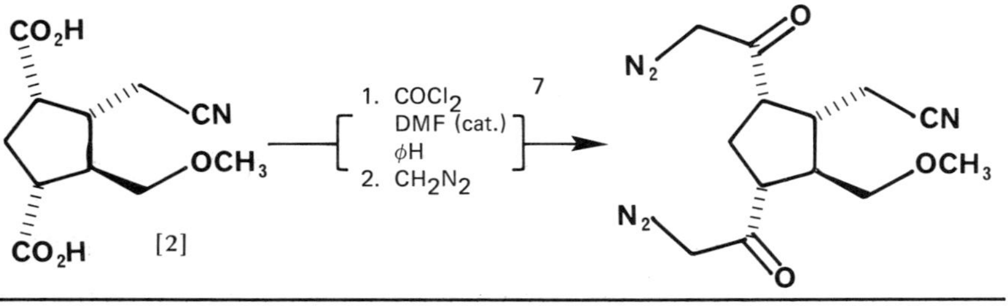

6. In this case the homologation is done prior to the oxidative cleavage of the norbornene double bond.
7. Any compound which has the function -X-Y=Z- can catalyze the reaction of phosgene with a carboxylic acid to give an acid chloride.
   C. F. Hauser & L. F. Theiling, *J. Org. Chem.*, 39, 1134 (1974).

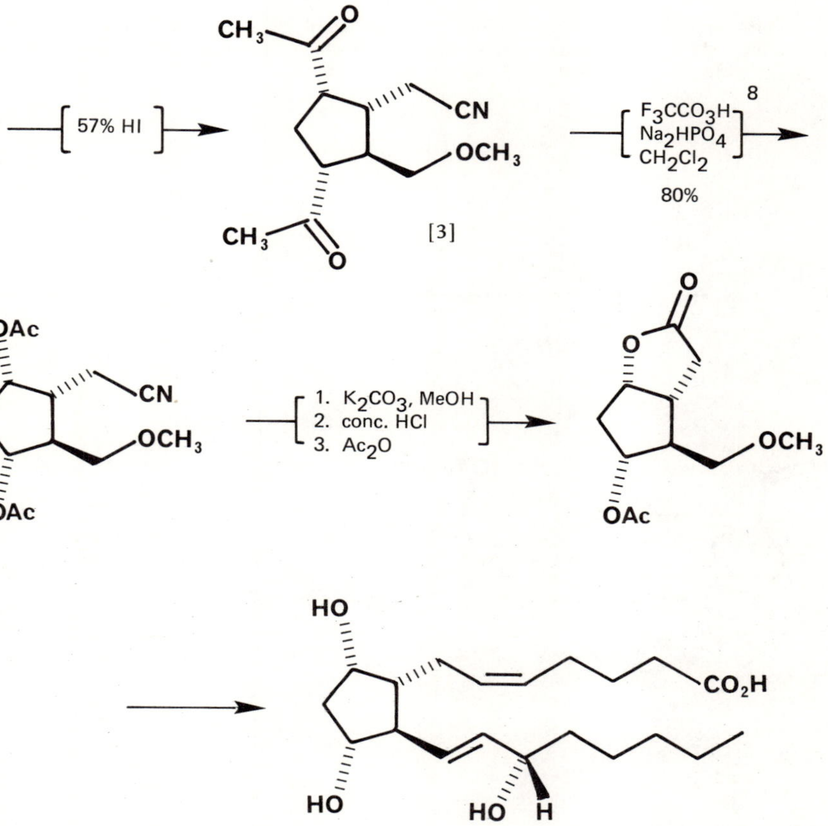

[3]

---

8. Baeyer-Villiger oxidation of aliphatic aldehydes in general gives formic acids and not formates. J. B. Lee & B. C. Uff, *Quart. Rev.*, 21, 429 (1967).

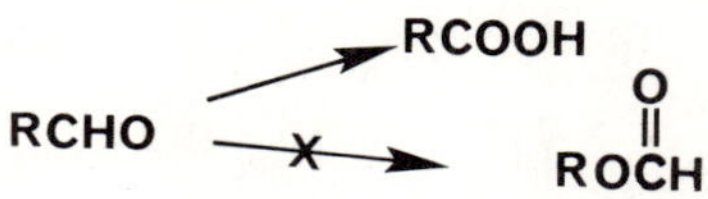

This necessitated the conversion of the intermediate aldehyde to the methyl ketone [3] via the acid [2].

In a similar approach,[9] previously published, an enone [4] was obtained which could not be converted to $PGF_{1\alpha}$. This enone was in fact the epimer which was obtained by the Baeyer-Villiger oxidation of the all *trans* methyl ketone with *m*-CPBA.

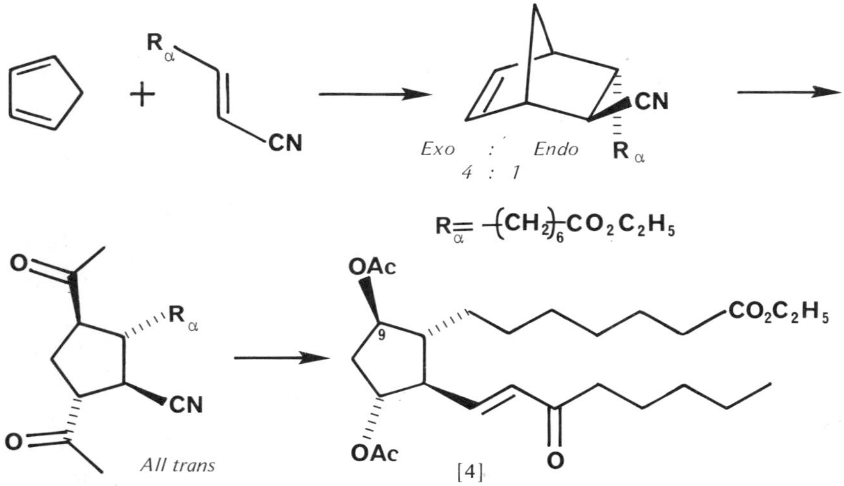

Synthesis of the Dienophile

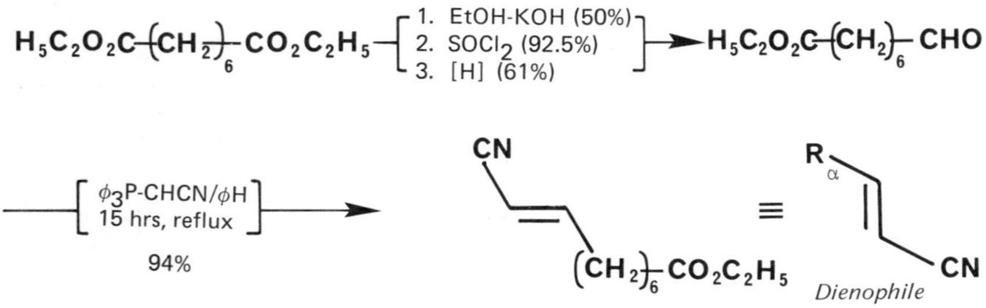

9. J. Katsube, H. Shimomura & M. Matsui, *Agr. Biol. Chem.*, 35, 1828 (1971).

Anomalous Behavior of the *Cis* and *Trans* Methyl Ketones
(In the case of Baeyer-Villiger oxidation with *M*CPBA)

Some epimeric ($C_9\beta$) dicarboxylic acid [5] is formed. It is not known at which stage this occurs. The corresponding all *trans* methyl ketone [6] undergoes Baeyer-Villiger oxidation (with *m*CPBA) to the diacetoxy compound [7].

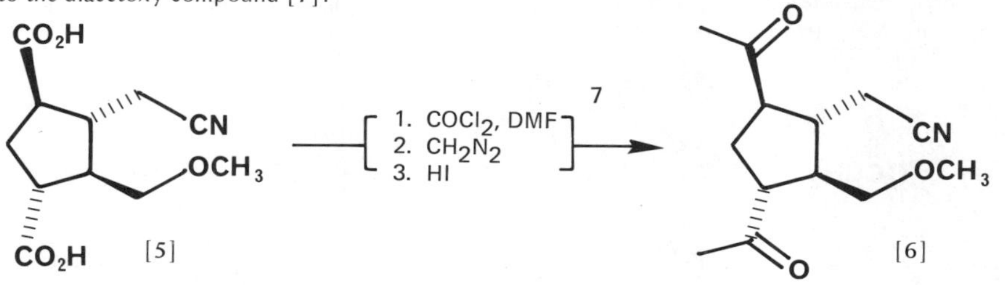

[5] [6]

Trans methyl ketone

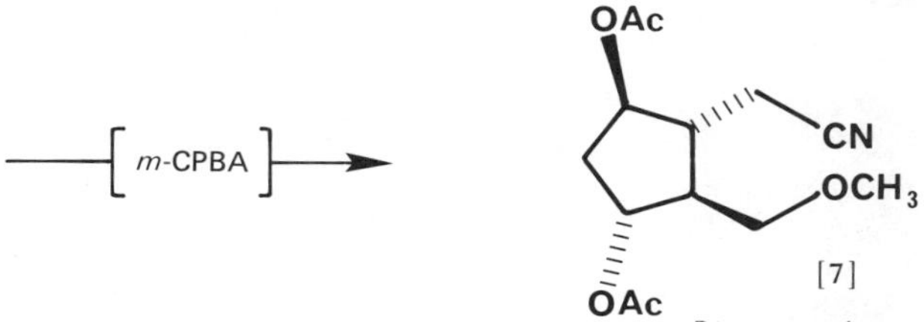

[7]
Diacetoxy derivative

However, the *cis* methyl ketone [8] undergoes Baeyer-Villiger oxidation solely to the monoacetoxy compound [9].

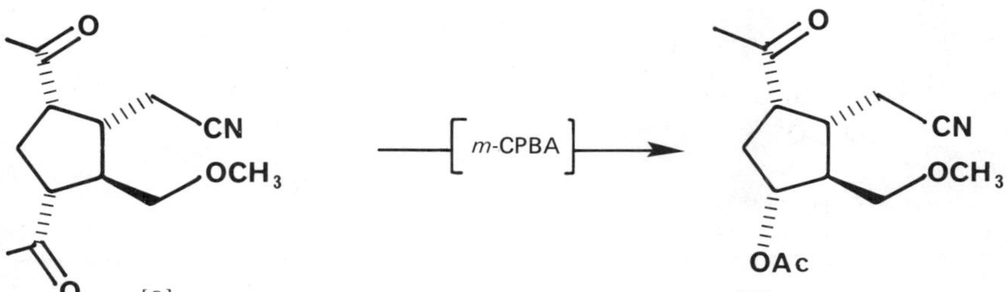

[8]
Cis methyl ketone

[9]
Monoacetoxy derivative

The approach of Katsube,[1,2,3] as shown previously, starts with a Diels-Alder reaction between cyclopentadiene and an appropriately substituted *trans* olefin. This gives a mixture of *exo* and *endo* adducts. The formation of these diastereoisomers and their separation creates an additional problem which was circumvented[10,11] by using a dienophile [10] (pseudo ester of β-formylacrylic ester) which gave exclusively the *endo* isomer, followed by an equilibration at C_{12} to give the requisite *trans* stereochemistry.

SYNTHETIC STRATEGY

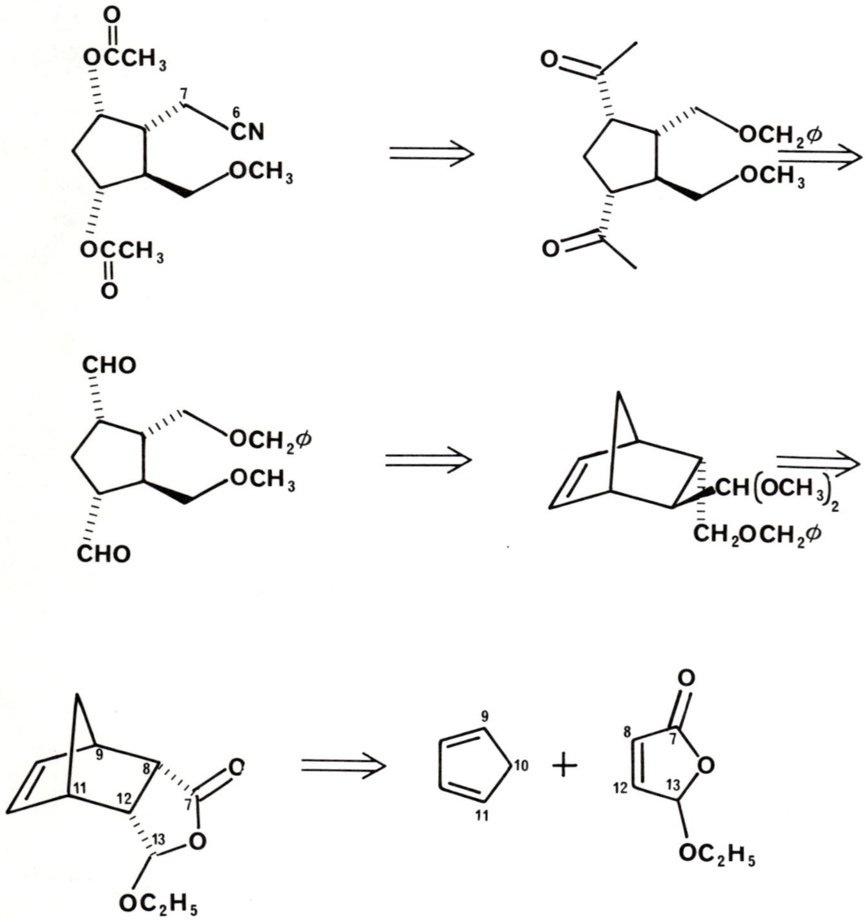

10. G. Jones, R. A. Raphael & S. Wright, *Chem. Commun.*, 609 (1972).
11. G. Jones, R. A. Raphael & S. Wright, *J. Chem. Soc., [Perkin I]*, 1676 (1974).

SYNTHETIC PLAN[10,11]

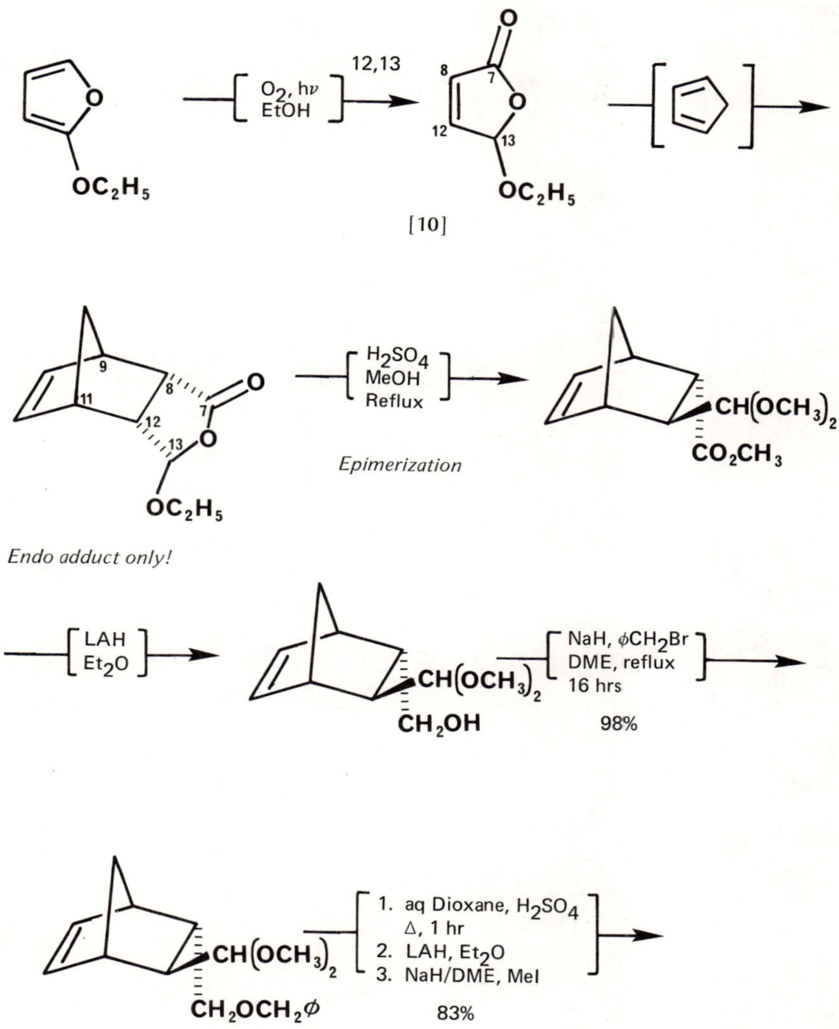

12. G. O. Schenk, *Annalen,* **584**, 156 (1953).
13. G. O. Schenk, *Annalen,* **697**, 42 (1966).

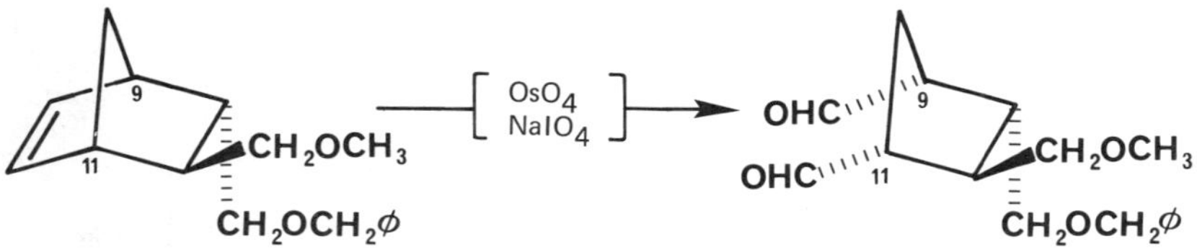

[11]

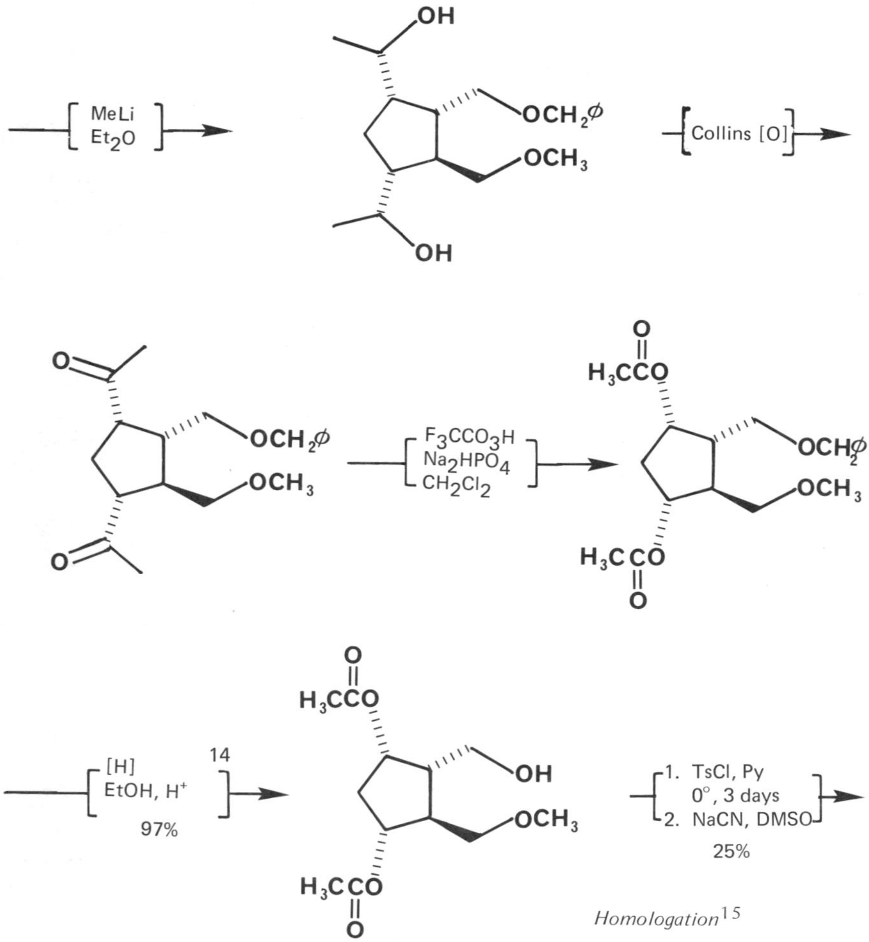

Homologation[15]

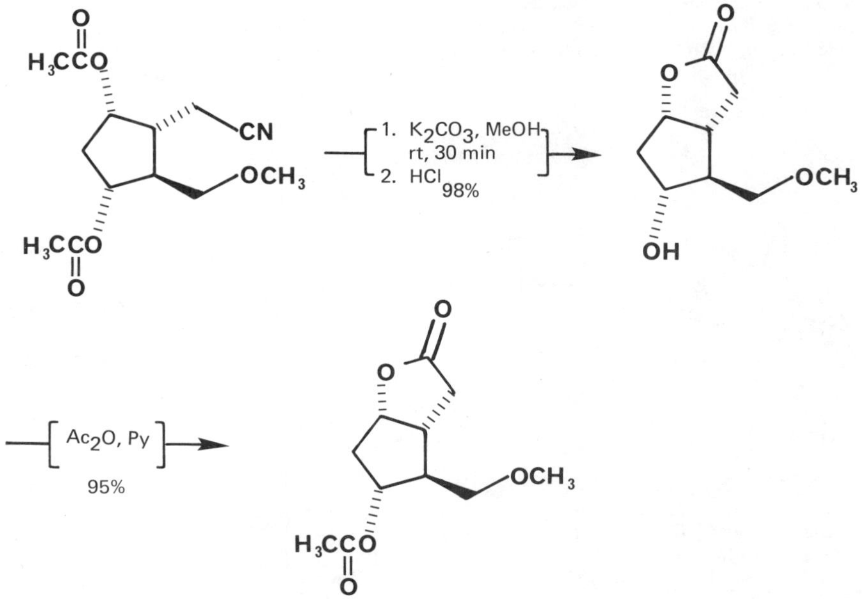

14. 1,3-Acetate shift takes place during hydrogenolysis.

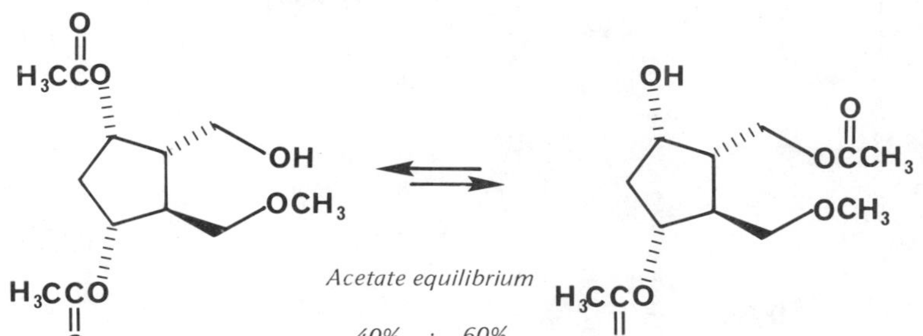

15. In contrast to Katsube's approach, the homologation is done after the oxidative cleavage of the norbornene double bond. For further details see footnote 6, p. 192.

In order to circumvent the unwieldy route to the *trans* norbornene diether[16] [11] an alternate route was devised starting from a symmetrically substituted norbornene diether [12]. In this modified approach the differentiation of the diol functions is postponed until after the olefin cleavage. This differentiation is achieved by means of the erstwhile undesirable acetate equilibrium.[10,11]

SYNTHETIC PLAN[10,11]

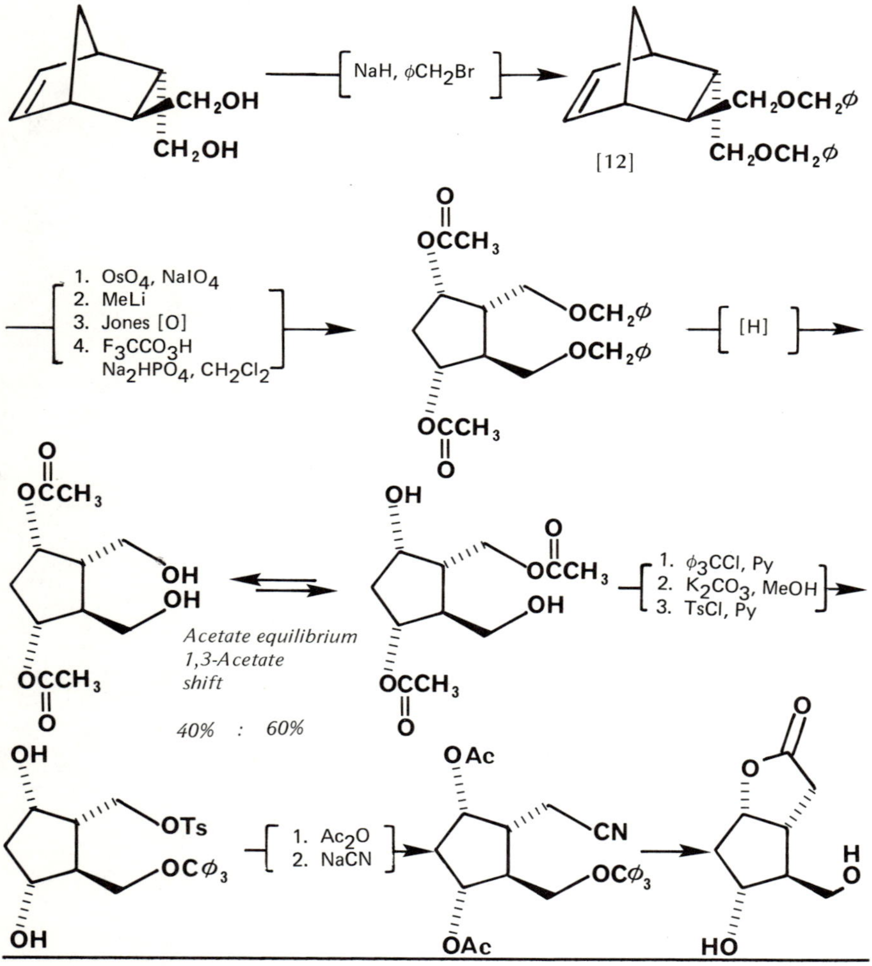

16. See p. 198.

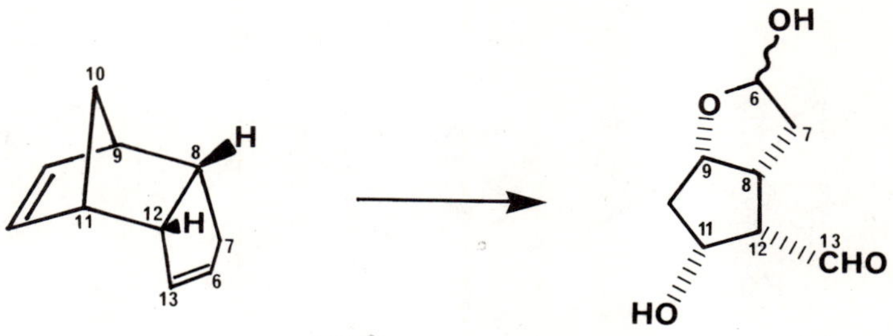

Turner intermediate

The Turner modification of these bicyclo[2.2.1]heptene approaches starts with the readily available *endo*-dicyclopentadiene. This avoids the Diels-Alder reaction with a symmetrically substituted dienophile. The cyclopentene ring of dicyclopentadiene serves as the latent one- and two- carbon aldehyde units necessary for the further elaboration of the β- and α- chains respectively. Again, epimerization of C_{12} is necessary to achieve the requisite *trans* orientation of the alkyl chains at C_8 and C_{12}.[17,18,19]

---

17. D. Brewster, M. Myers, J. Ormerod, P. Otter, A. C. B. Smith, M. E. Spinner & S. Turner, *J. Chem. Soc. [Perkin I]*, 2796 (1973).
18. D. Brewster, M. Myers, J. Ormerod, M. E. Spinner, S. Turner & A. C. B. Smith, *Chem. Commun.*, 1235 (1972).
19. S. Turner, *Prostaglandin Synthesis: Design*, Third International Symposium On Organic Synthesis, Oxford, 1973.

SYNTHETIC STRATEGY

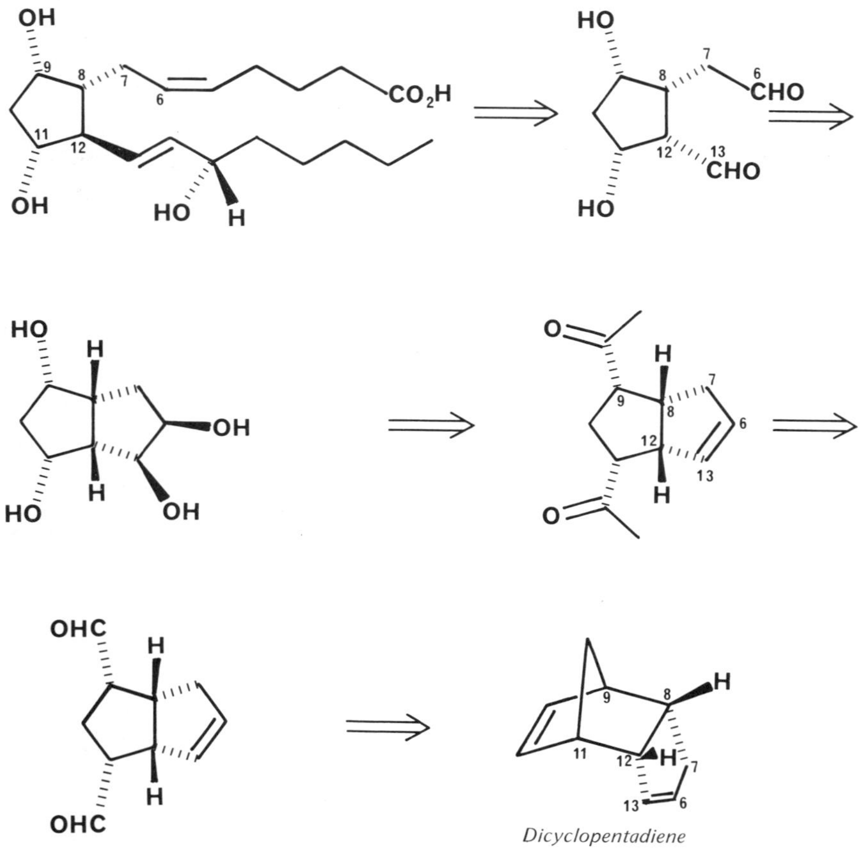

SYNTHETIC PLAN[17,18,19]

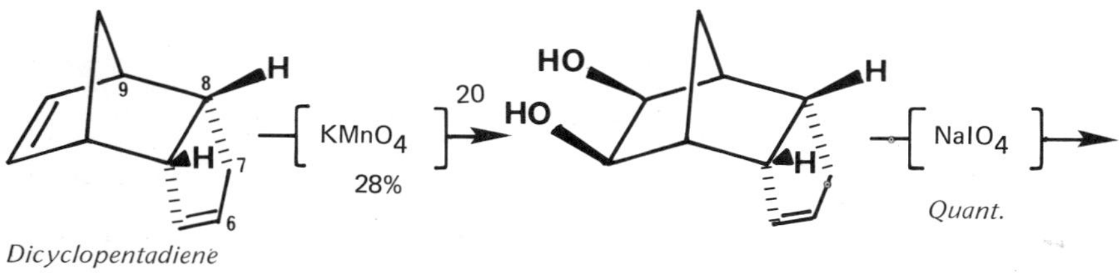

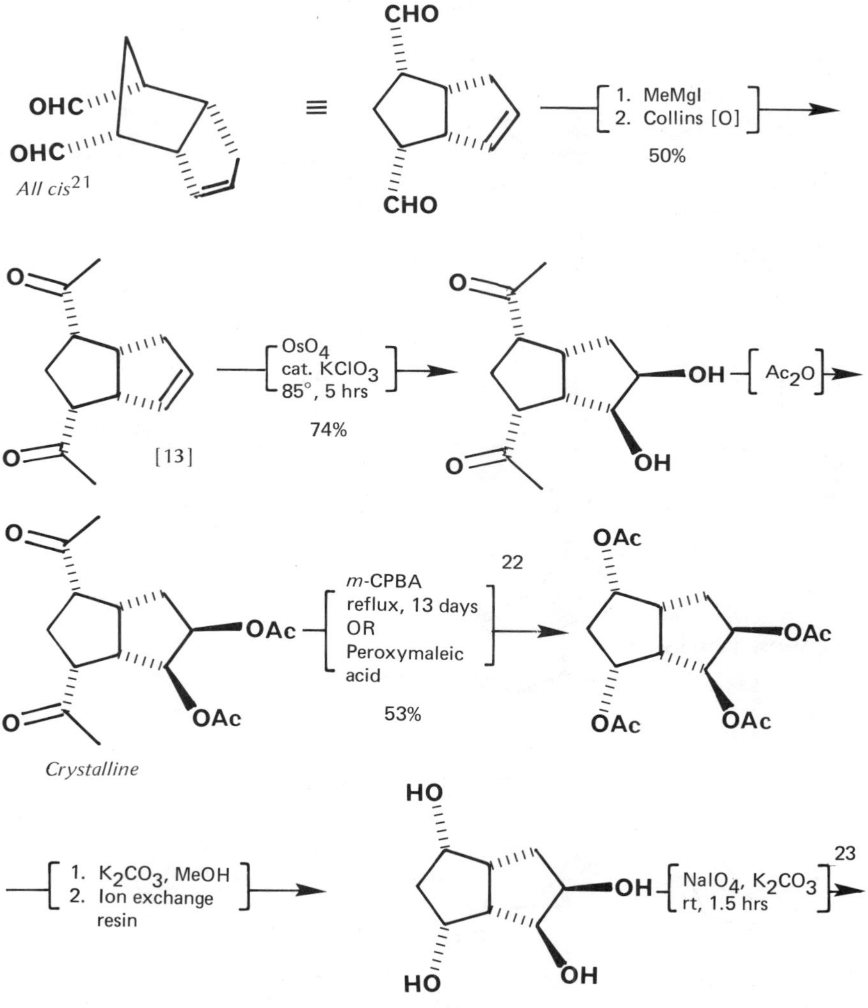

---

20. The norbornene double bond is distinguished by its greater reactivity.
21. The all-*cis* diketone is the least stable of the four possible diastereoisomers. A. C. Cope & M. Brown, *J. Am. Chem. Soc.*, **80**, 2859 (1958).
22. Baeyer-Villiger oxidation of the unsaturated methylketone [13] gave a complex mixture of products. This may be due to the epoxidation of the olefin followed by the opening of the epoxide [14] to give the hemiketal [15]. Therefore the double bond had to be converted to the diacetate prior to the Baeyer-Villiger oxidation step.

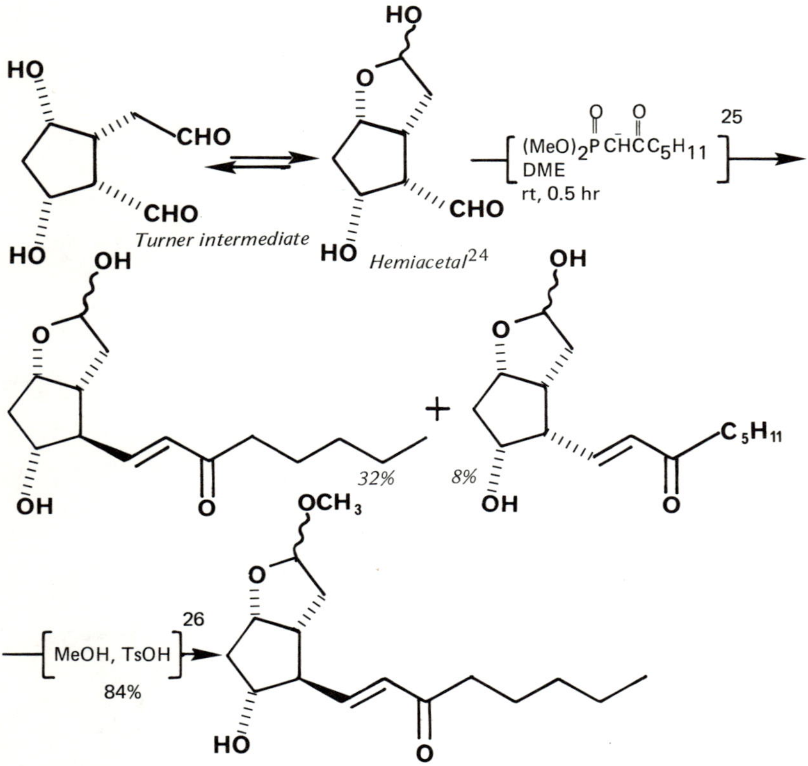

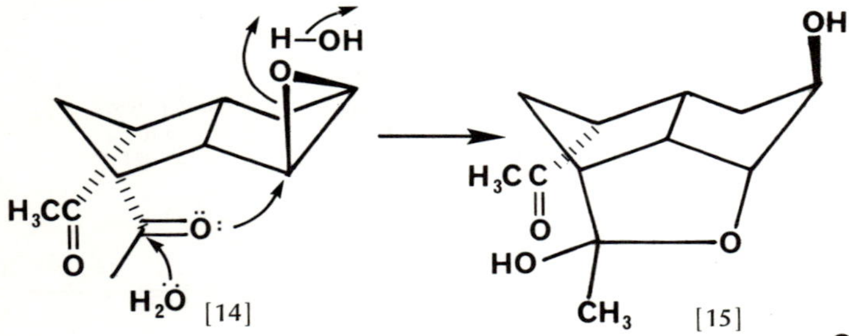

[14] [15]

23. When the periodate cleavage was carried out without K_2CO_3 the unsaturated aldehyde [16] was formed in 10%-20% yield.

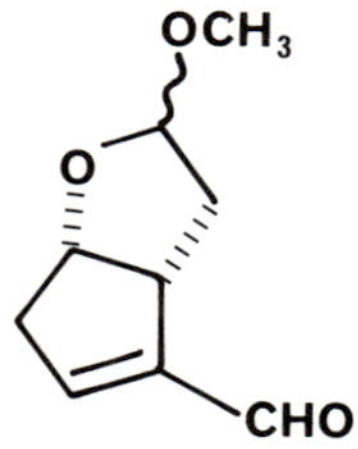

[16]

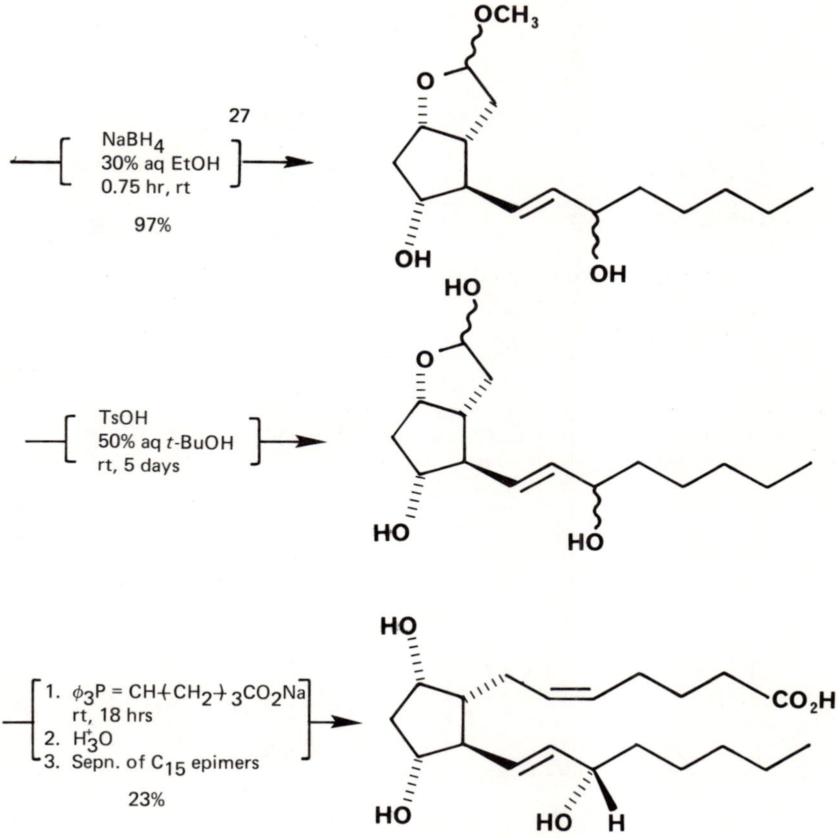

PGF$_{2\alpha}$

---

24. The formation of the hemiacetal differentiates the two aldehyde units.
25. The epimerization of the aldehyde probably takes place at the early stages of the Wittig reaction.
    P. Crabbe, A. Cervantes & M. Carmen Meana, *Chem. Commun.*, 119 (1973).
    For a similar epimerization during Wittig reaction see p. 163.
26. Although the subsequent steps could be carried out without protecting the hemiacetal, its protection as the methyl ether led to improved yields.
27. It has been previously observed that $NaBH_4$ leads to 1,4-reduction and consequently $Zn(BH_4)_2$ has been used routinely.

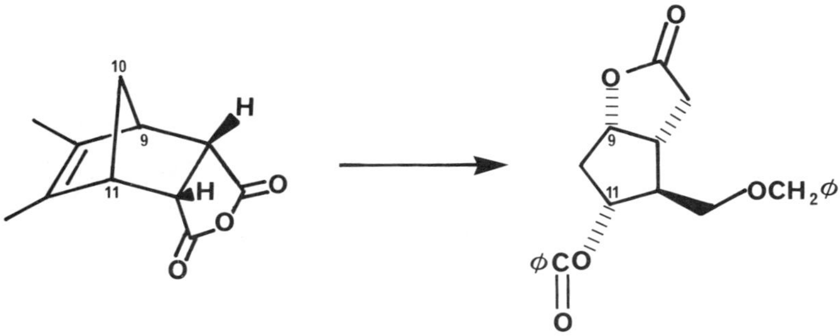

The bicyclo[2.2.1]heptene approaches culminated in this elegant approach developed by the Hoffmann-La Roche group (Basel).[28] A symmetric intermediate [17] is dissymmetrized with a chiral reagent to give two enantiomers. The one with the desired chirality at C_8 and C_9 was converted to the natural $PGF_{2\alpha}$ via the Corey lactone.

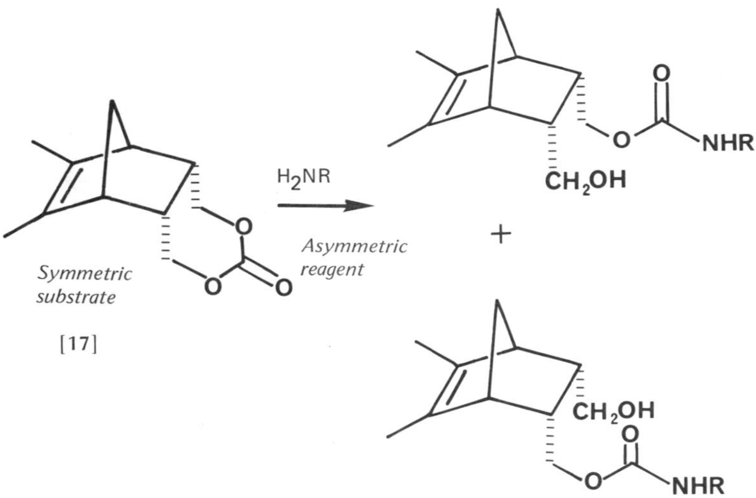

The Diels-Alder reaction is carried out with 2,3-dimethylcyclopenta-1,3-diene to give the 2,3-dimethylbicyclo[2.2.1]heptene derivative [20]. Oxidative cleavage gives the *bis*-methyl ketone which can undergo the Baeyer-Villiger oxidation directly to the *bis*-acetoxy compound [23]. This avoids the aldehyde to methyl ketone transformation.

---

28. A. Fischli, M. Klaus, H. Mayer, P. Schonholzer & R. Ruegg, *Helv. Chim. Acta,* **58**, 564 (1975).

SYNTHETIC STRATEGY

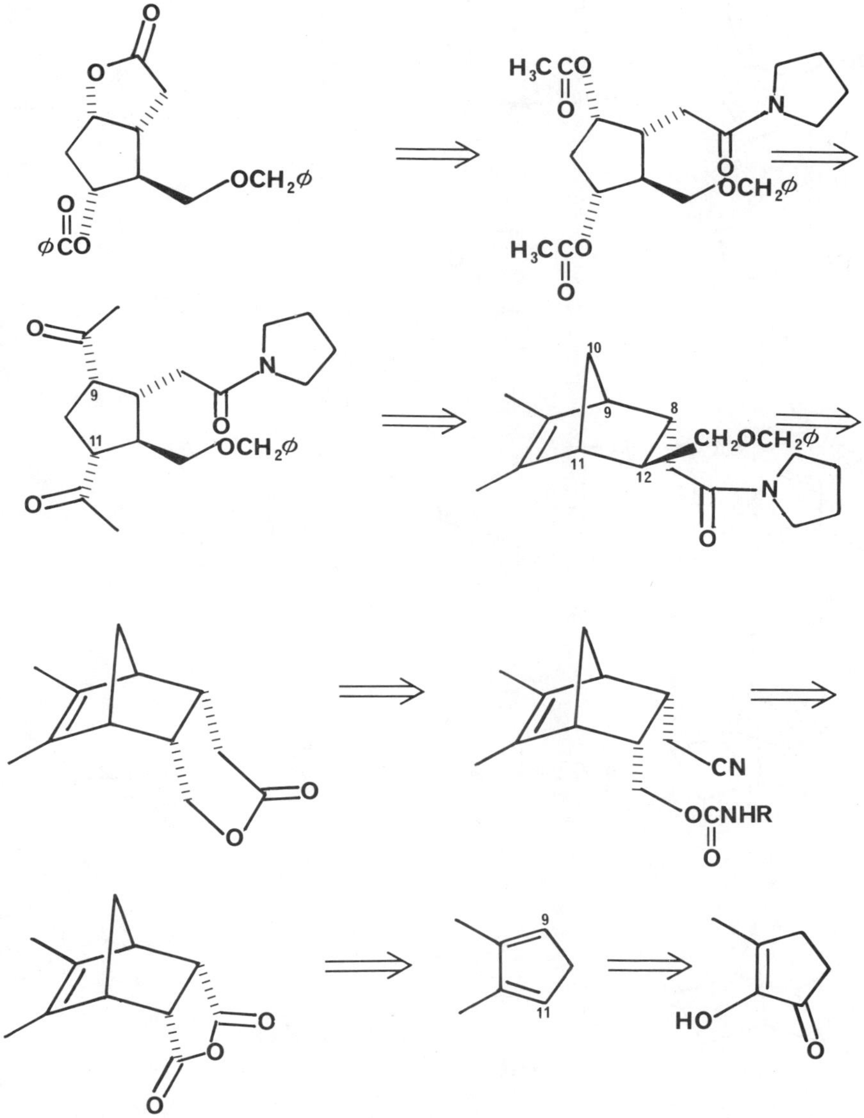

SYNTHETIC PLAN[28]

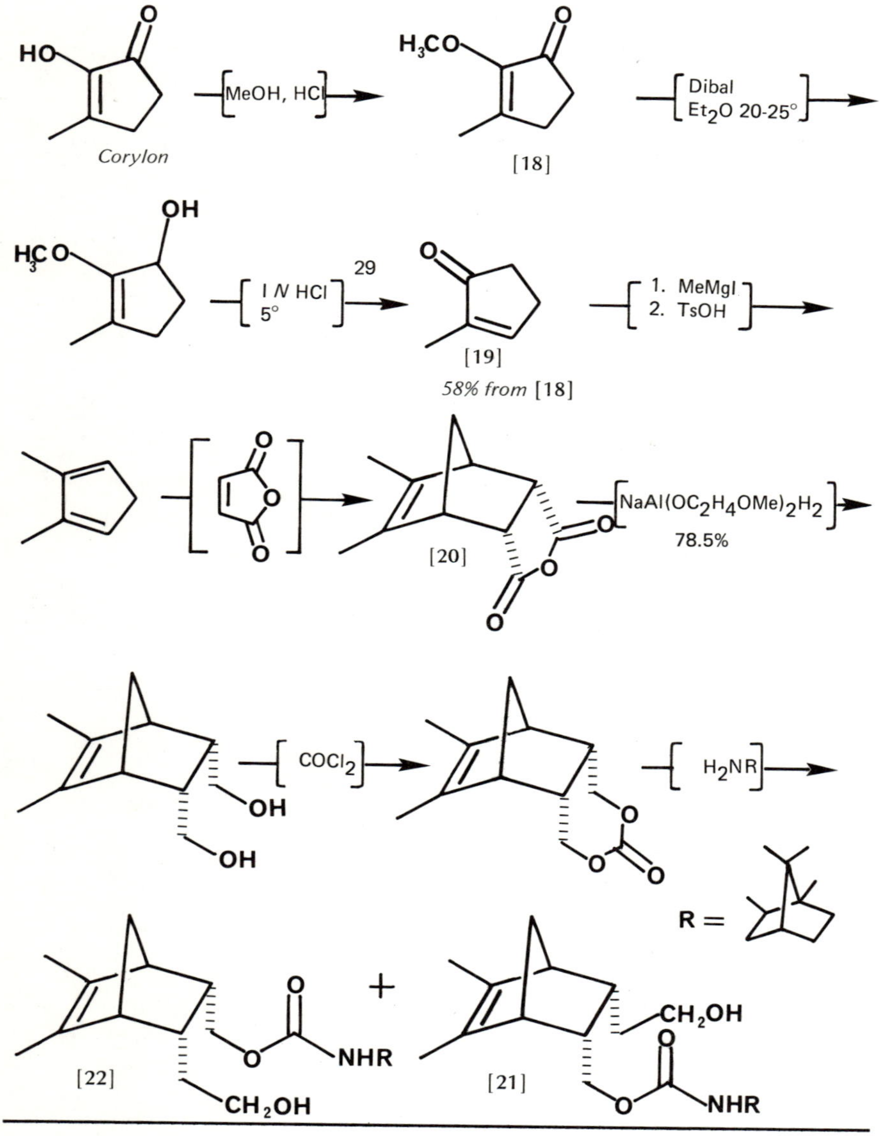

29. The mechanism of dehydration!

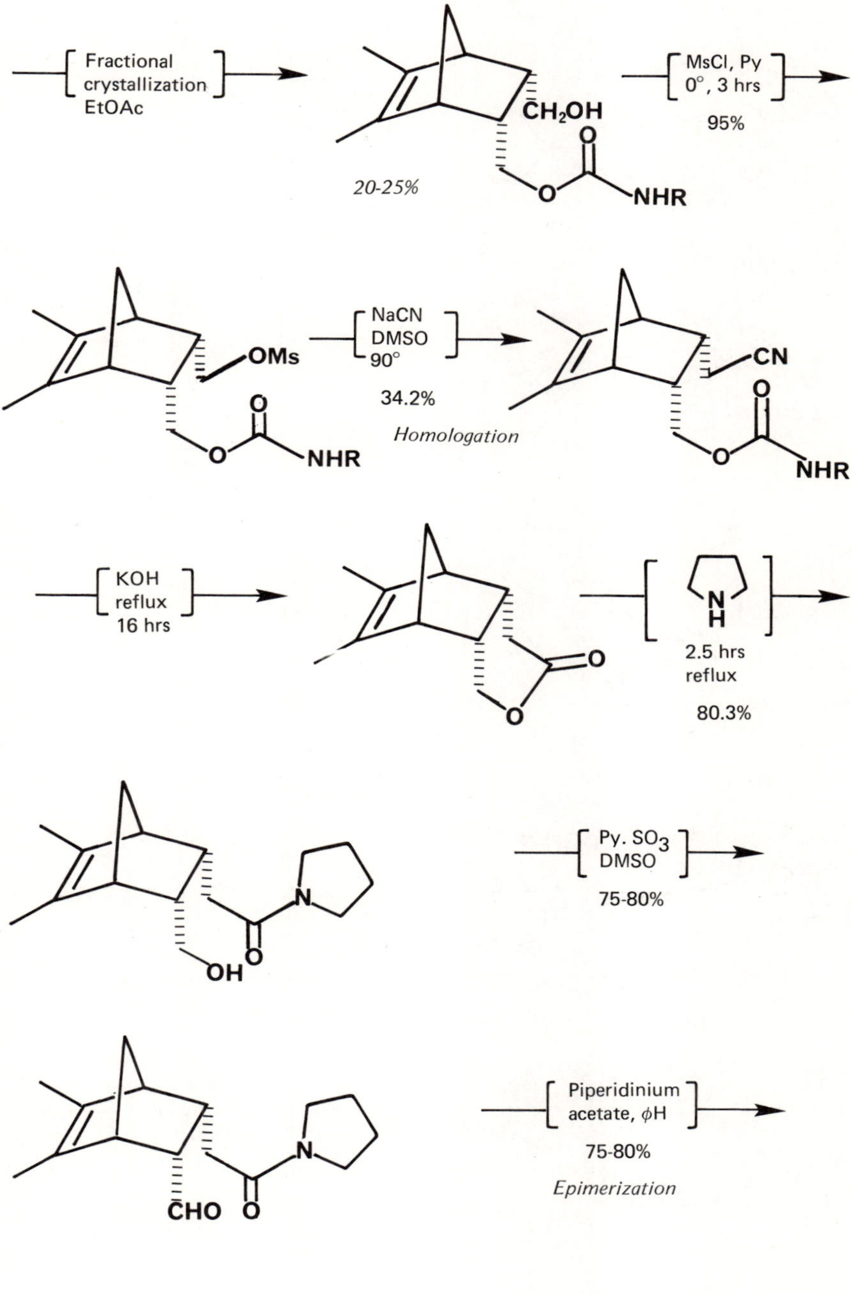
Fractional
crystallization
EtOAc
CH2OH
O
NHR
20-25%
MsCl, Py
0°, 3 hrs
95%
OMs
O
NHR
NaCN
DMSO
90°
34.2%
Homologation
CN
O
NHR
KOH
reflux
16 hrs
O
O
N
H
2.5 hrs
reflux
80.3%
N
O
OH
Py. SO3
DMSO
75-80%
N
CHO
O
Piperidinium
acetate, φH
75-80%
Epimerization

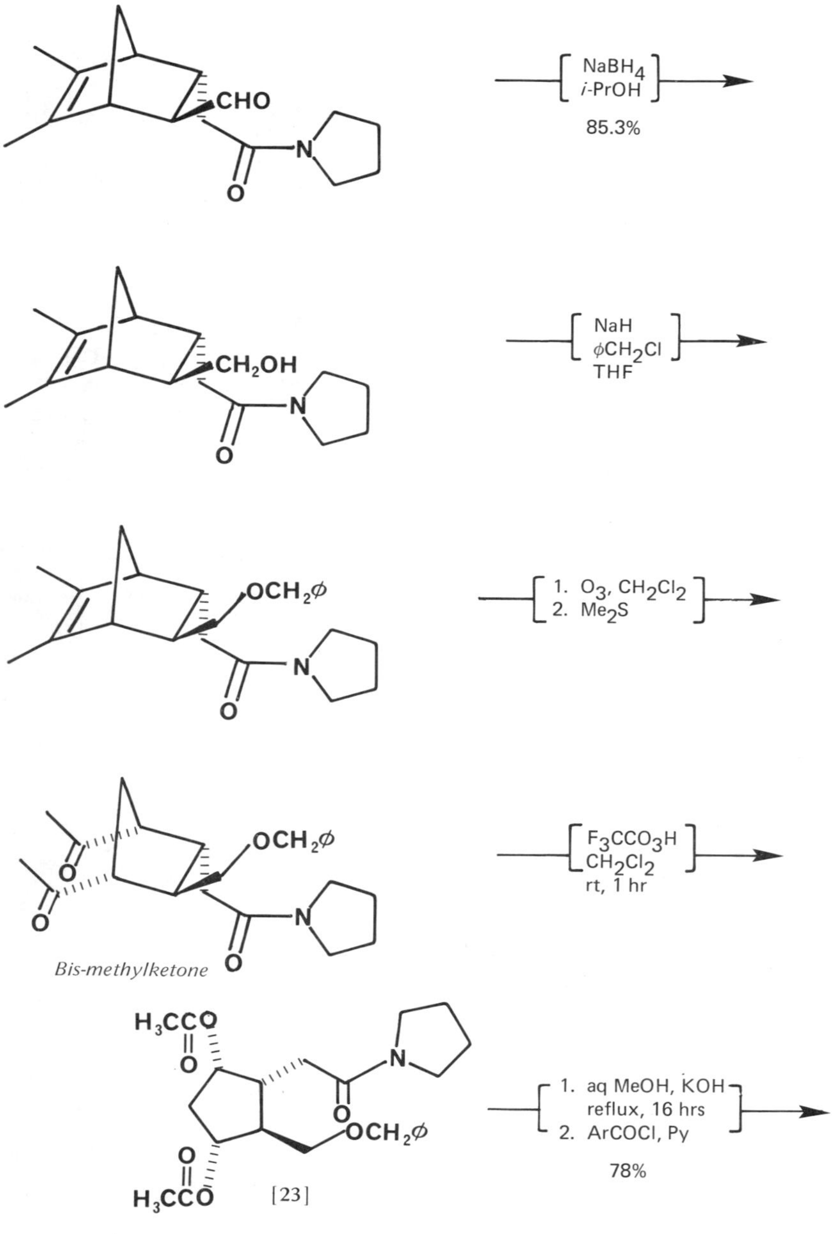

Bis-methylketone

[23]

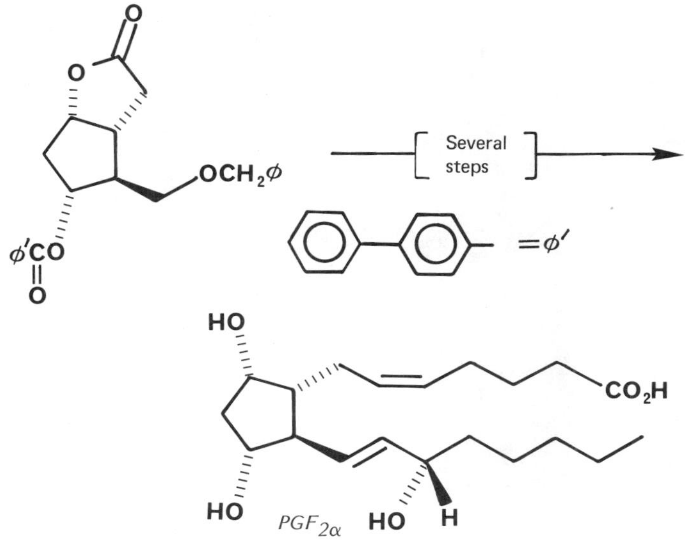

The enantiomer [21] used for the synthesis of natural PGF$_{2\alpha}$, and not the other one [22] was converted to the enantiomeric PGF$_{2\alpha}$. This was done because only the enantiomer [21] crystallized out during fraction crystallization.

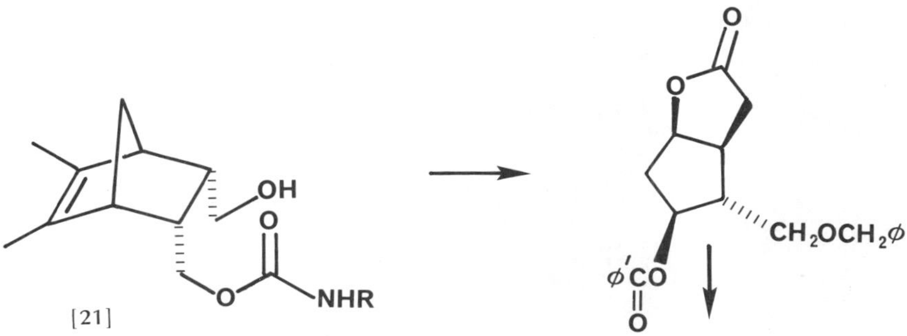

[21]

Enantiomeric PGF$_{2\alpha}$

10

Bicyclo[2.2.1]heptadiene Approach

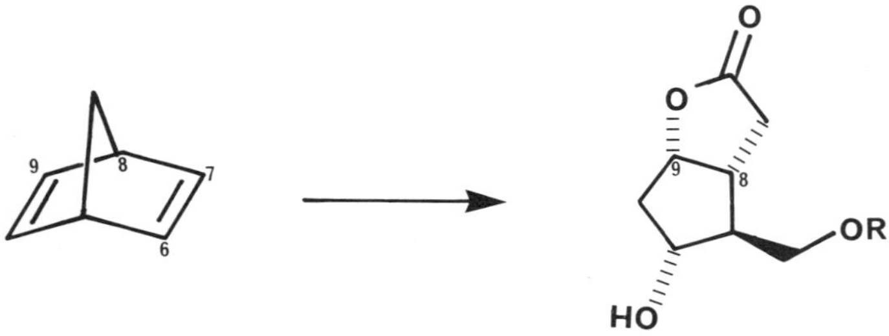

The bicyclo[2.2.1]hepta-2,5-diene approach developed independently by Corey[1] and Sutherland,[2] provides an alternate use of the bicyclo[2.2.1]heptane[3] system. The tricyclic intermediate [1], derived from norbornadiene via the Prins reaction with formaldehyde and formic acid is elaborated through an imaginative sequence to the Corey intermediate by transforming the δ-lactone to the γ-lactone.

There is a fundamental strategic difference between the bicyclo[2.2.1]heptene and the bicyclo[2.2.1]heptadiene routes. In the latter approach the carbons that eventually become the prostanoid nucleus include the double bond and the bridgehead carbons. In the bicyclo[2.2.1]heptene approaches the olefinic carbons are in fact precursors to the *cis*-hydroxyl groups at C_9 and C_{11}.

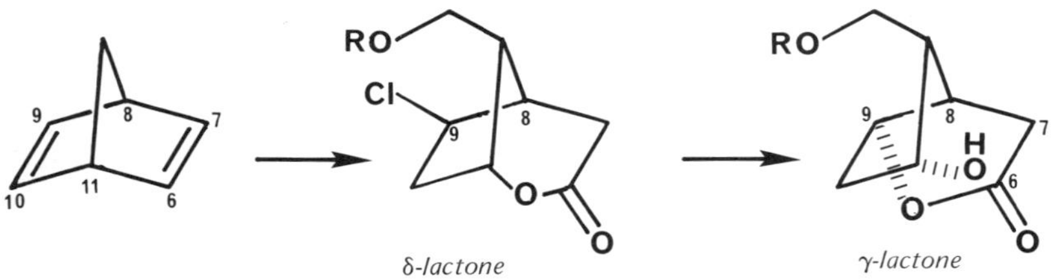

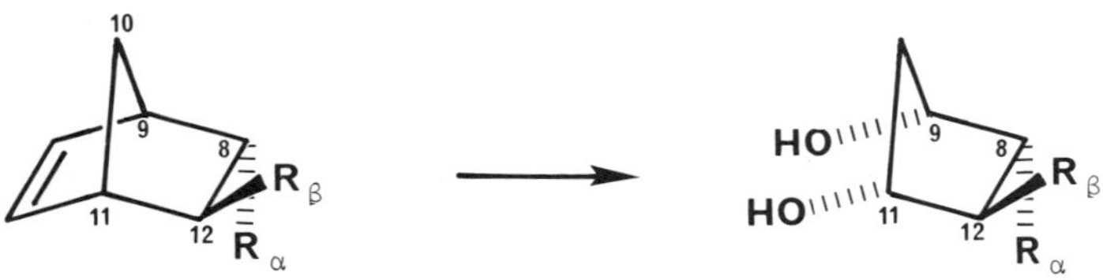

1. J. S. Bindra, A, Grodski, T. K. Schaaf & E. J. Corey, *J. Am. Chem. Soc.*, **95**, 7522 (1973).
2. R. Peel & J. K. Sutherland, *Chem. Commun.*, 151 (1974).
3. E. J. Corey, N. M. Weinshenker, T. K. Schaaf & W. Huber, *J. Am. Chem. Soc.*, **91**, 5675 (1969).

SYNTHETIC STRATEGY

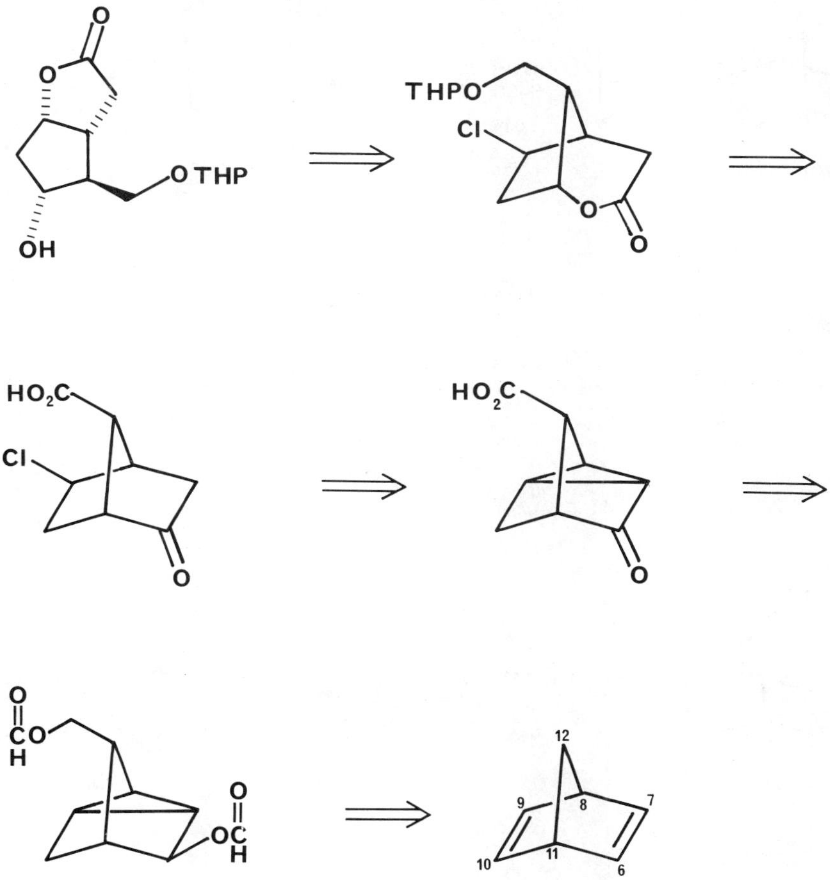

Norbornadiene

SYNTHETIC PLAN[1]

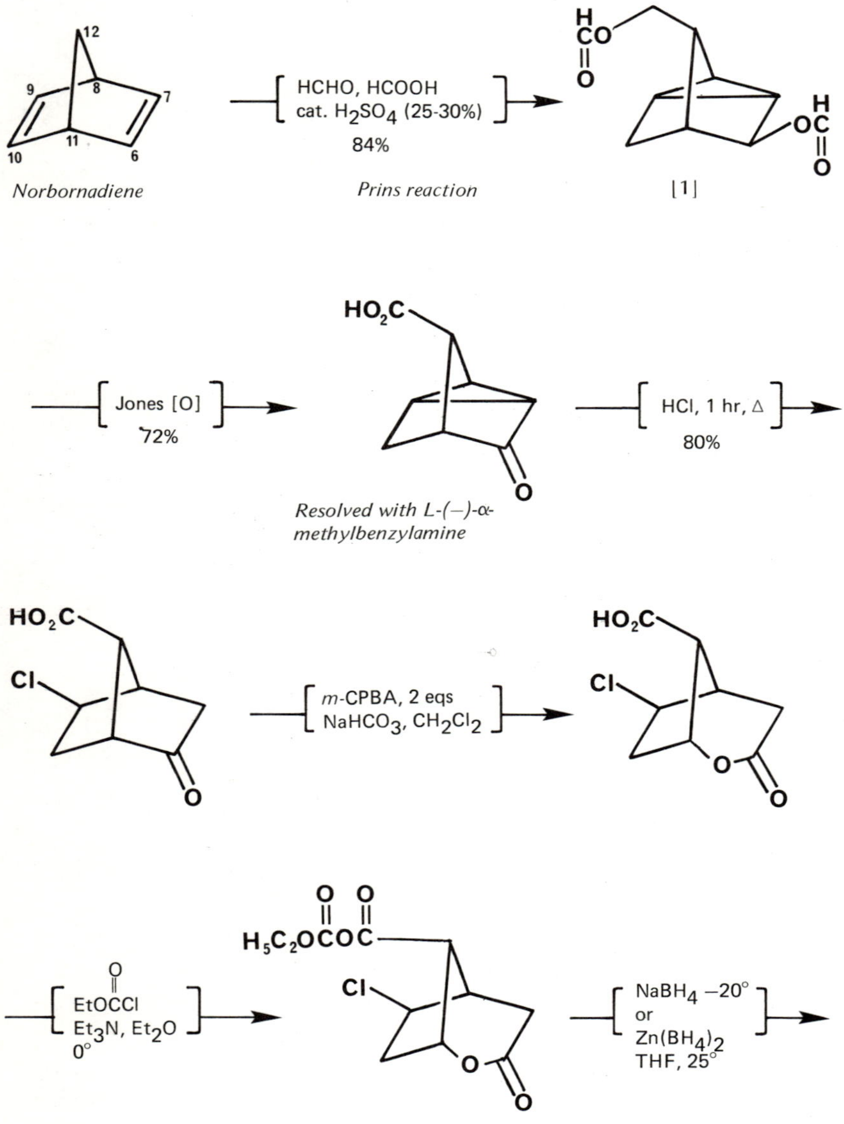

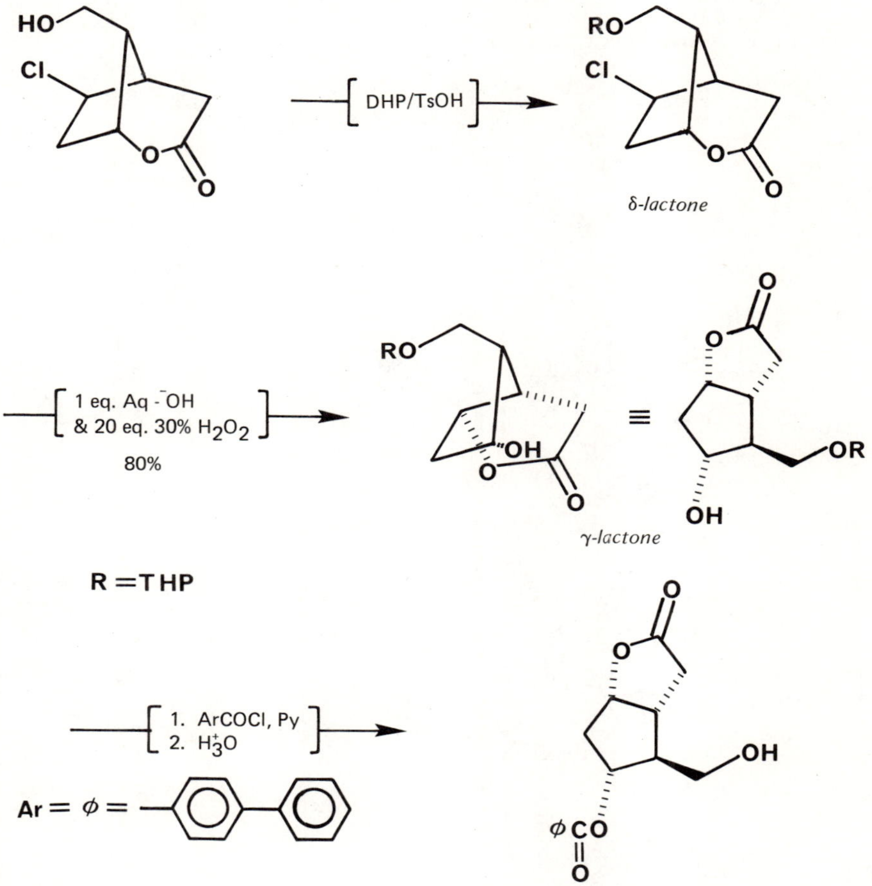
HO
Cl
DHP/TsOH
RO
Cl
O
O
δ-lactone
1 eq. Aq - ¯OH
& 20 eq. 30% H2O2
80%
RO
OH
O
O
≡
O
O
OR
OH
γ-lactone
R = THP
1. ArCOCl, Py
2. H3+O
Ar = φ =
O
O
OH
φCO
O

One of the advantages of this bicyclo[2.2.1]heptadiene approach is that it can also lead to the all *trans* stereochemistry of the four contiguous asymmetric centers of the prostanoid nucleus. Thus it leads to a direct synthesis of PGF_{β} compounds.[1]

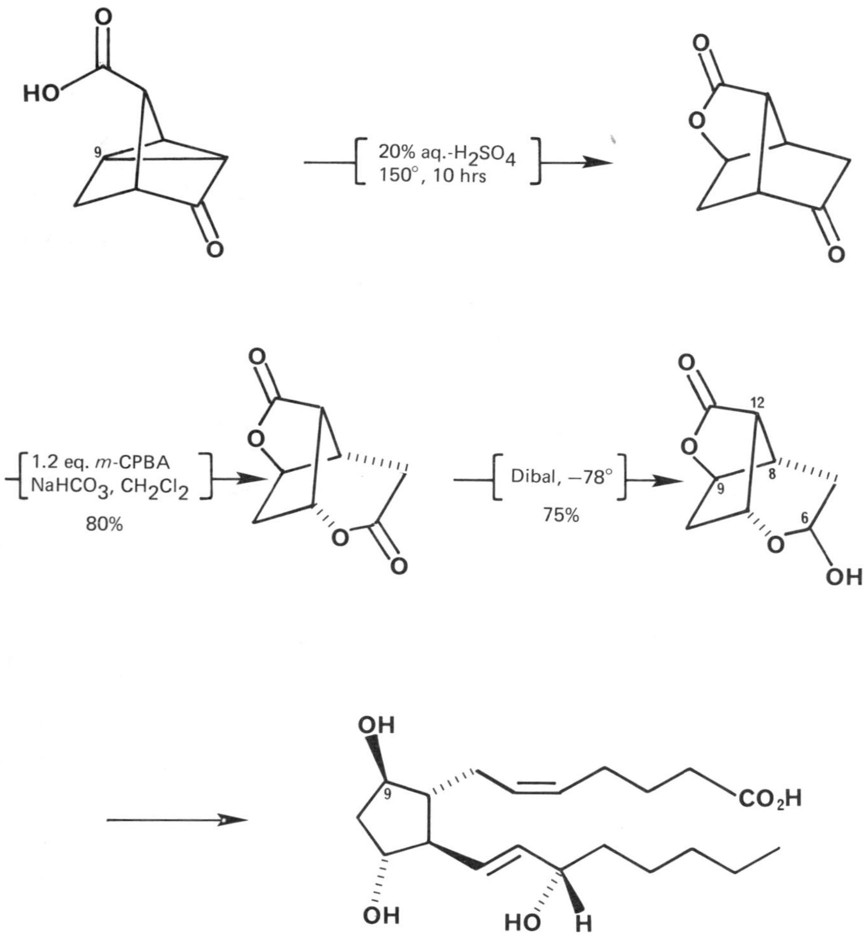

PGF_{β}

A similar route was developed independently by J. K. Sutherland at the University of Manchester.[4]

SYNTHETIC PLAN[4]

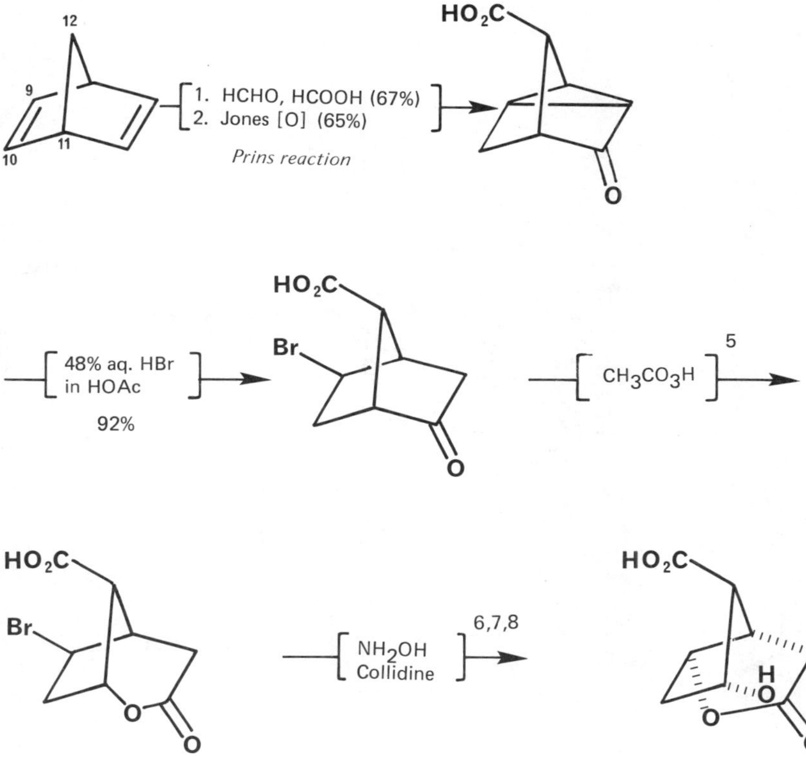

4. R. Peel & J. K. Sutherland, *Chem. Commun.*, 151 (1974).
5. Some of the other lactone [2] is also formed.

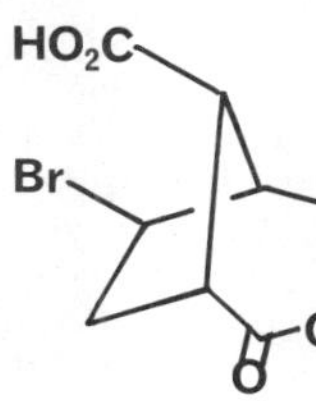

[2]

20%

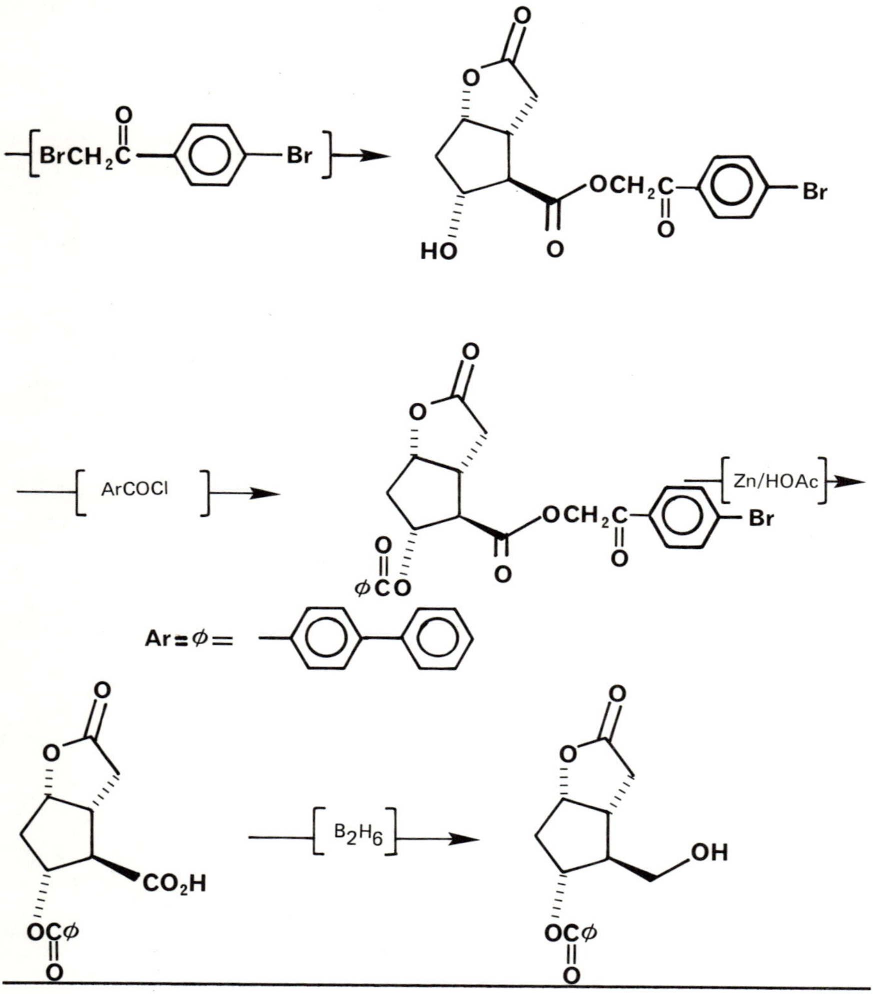

6. Use of aqueous alkali led to the predominant formation of the cyclopropane derivative [3] by 1,3 elimination.
7. The enhanced nucleophilicity of those nucleophiles bearing a lone pair of electrons on adjacent atom is known as the α-effect. Bunnett, *Ann. Rev. Phys. Chem.*, 14, 271 (1963) and Edwards & Pearson, *J. Am. Chem. Soc.*, 84 26 (1963).

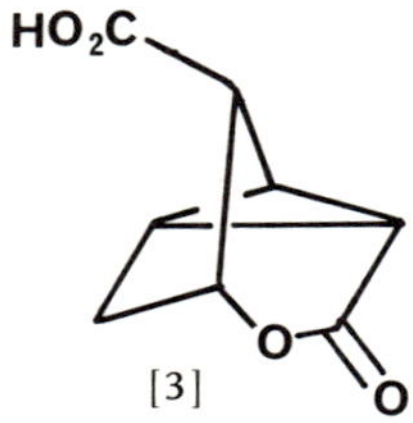

[3]

In an alternative pathway, the β-chain is introduced before the conversion of the δ-lactone to the γ-lactone.

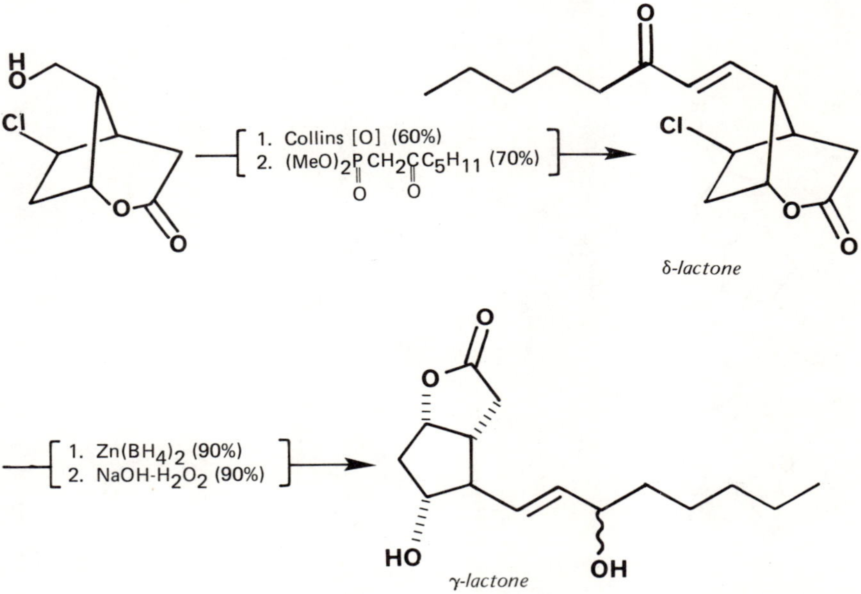

8. Other methods of lactonization were also used to avoid the cyclopropane formation (by 1,3 elimination). One example is shown in the following:

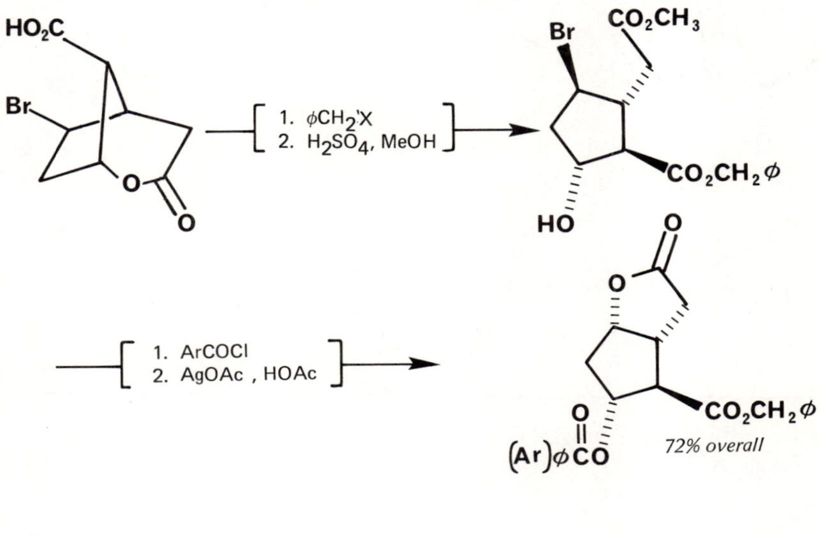

An acid catalyzed addition of chloral (the methyl group of chloral becomes the C_{13} of the prostanoid) to norbornadiene[9] has been by Ogasawara in another synthesis of the Corey lactone.[10]

SYNTHETIC STRATEGY

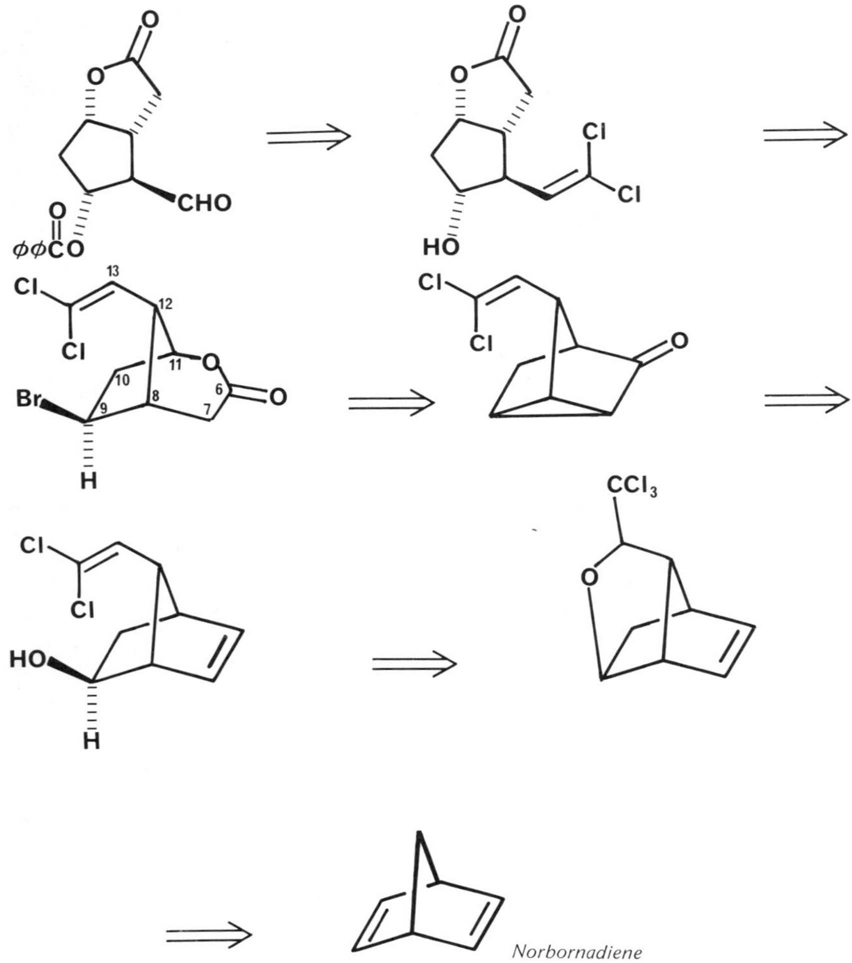

Norbornadiene

---

9. H. Fritz, C. D. Weis & T. Winkler, *Helv. Chim. Acta.*, **58**, 1345 (1975).
10. S. Takano, N. Kubodera & K. Ogasawara, *J. Org. Chem.*, **42**, 786 (1977).

SYNTHETIC PLAN[10]

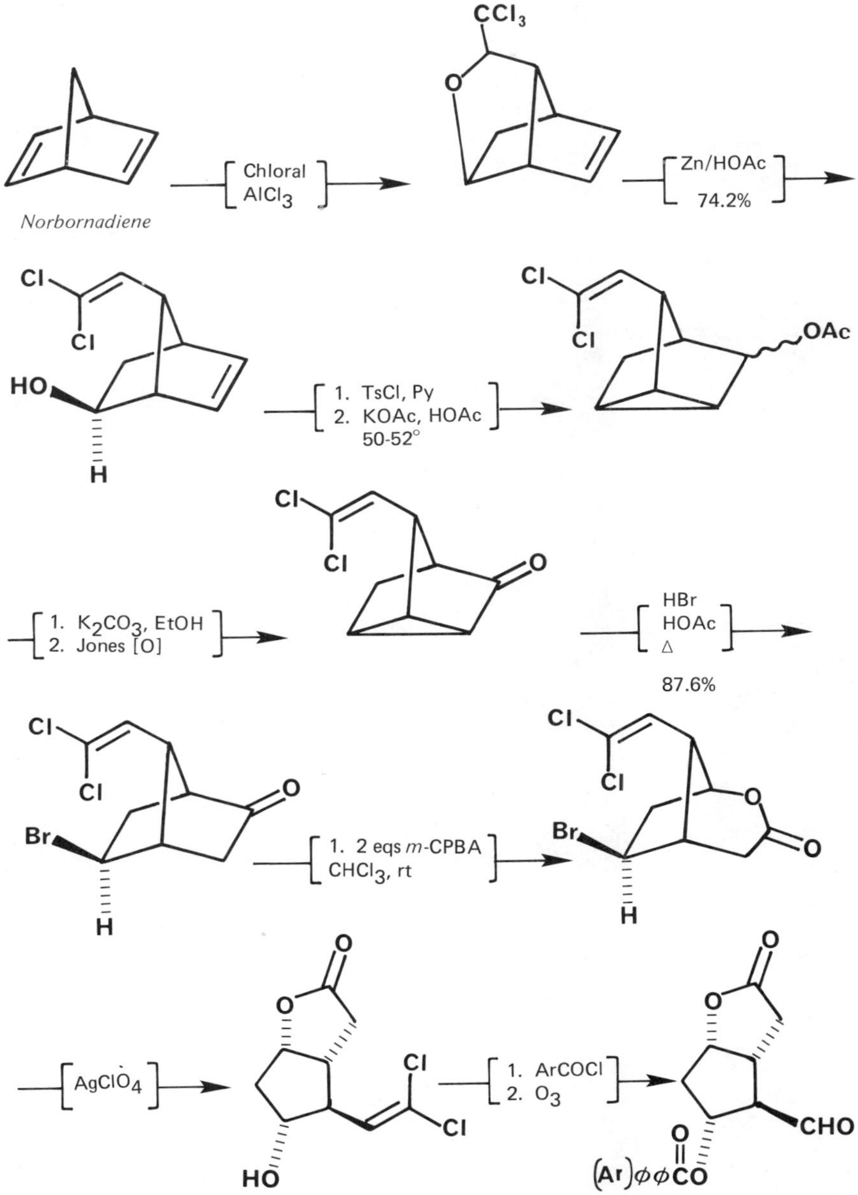

11

Acetoxyfulvene Approach

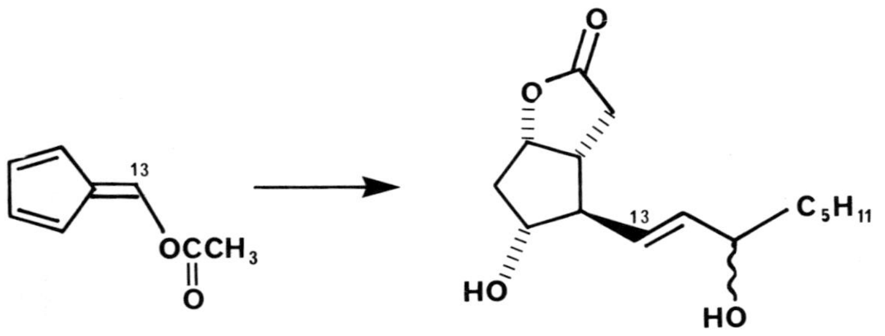

Acetoxyfulvene

This alternative synthesis of $PGF_{2\alpha}$ from acetoxyfulvene circumvents the use of sensitive 5-alkylated cyclopentadienes made from the toxic thallium cyclopentadienide. Also, the formyl group on C_{12} is introduced in the right oxidation state.[1]

---

1. E. D. Brown & T. L. Lilley, *Chem. Commun.* 39 (1975).

SYNTHETIC STRATEGY

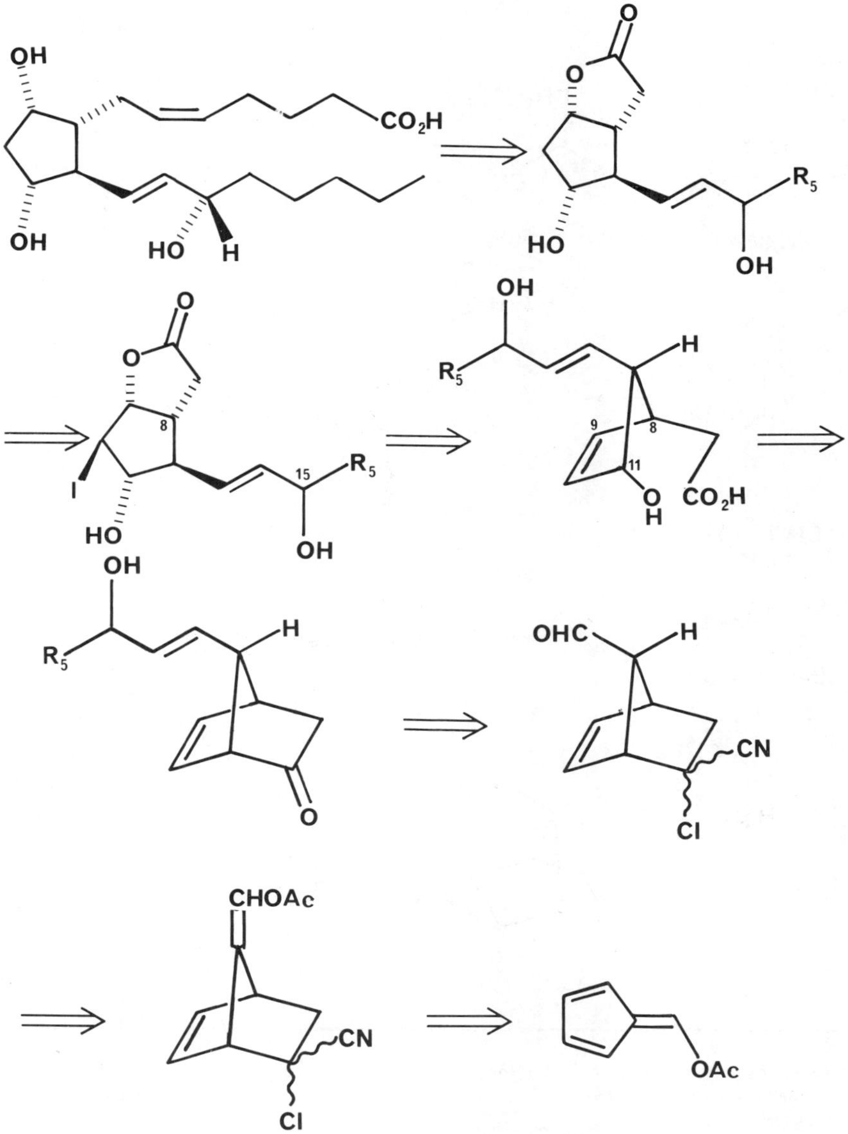

R= C_5H_{11}

SYNTHETIC PLAN[1]

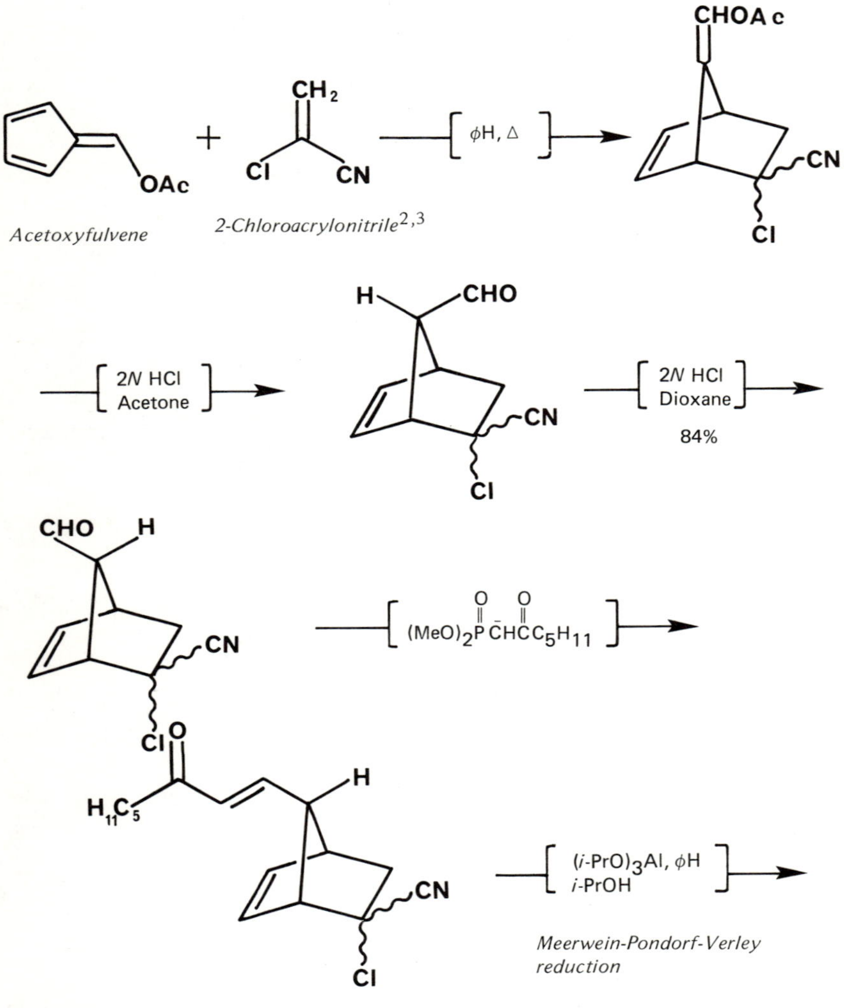

2. Comparison between 2-chloroacrylonitrile and 2-acetoxyacrylonitrile has shown that the former is a more reactive dienophile. D. A. Evans, W. L. Scott & L. K. Truesdale, *Tet. Lett.*, 121 (1972).
3. For a very early example of the use of 2-acetoxyacrylonitrile as a ketene equivalent in synthesis see: P. D. Bartlett & B. E. Tate, *J. Am. Chem. Soc.*, **78**, 2473 (1956).

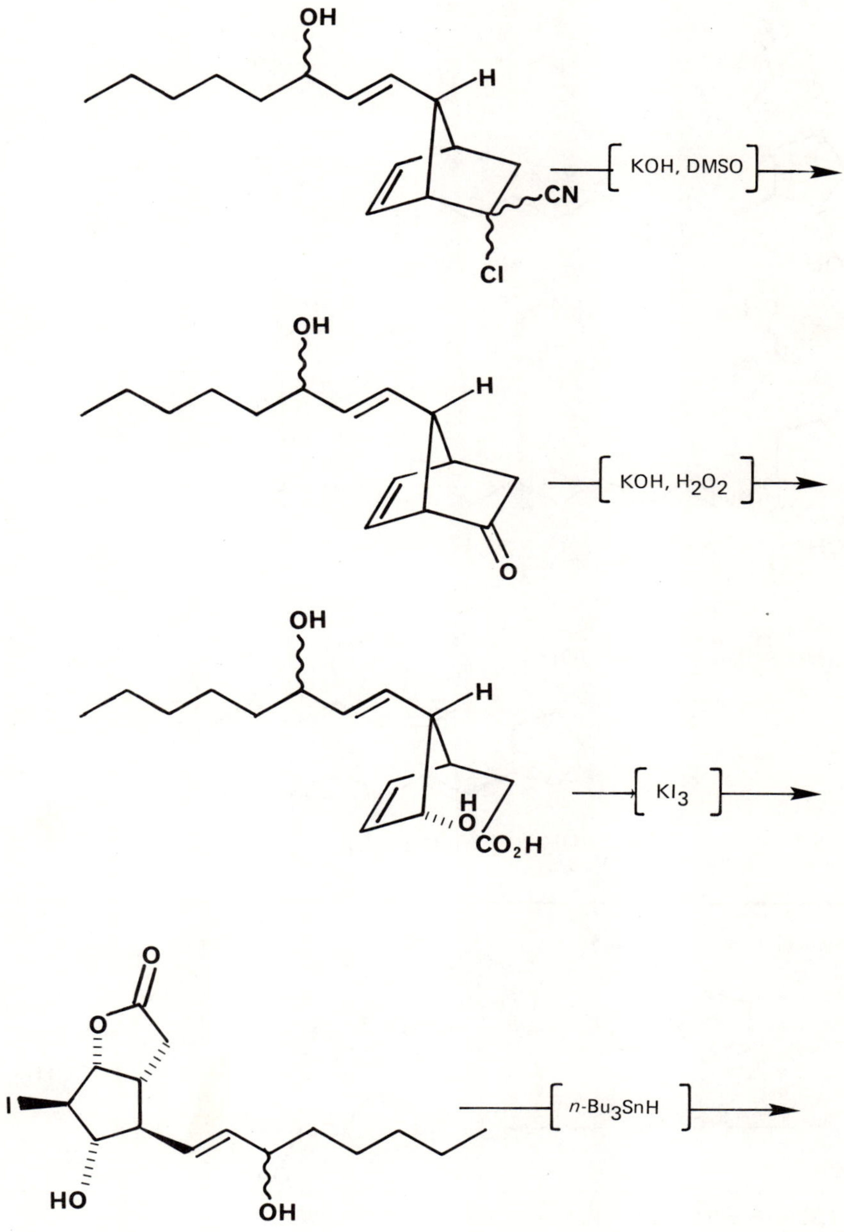
OH
H
CN
Cl
KOH, DMSO
OH
H
O
KOH, H2O2
OH
H
H
O
CO2H
KI3
O
O
I
HO
OH
n-Bu3SnH

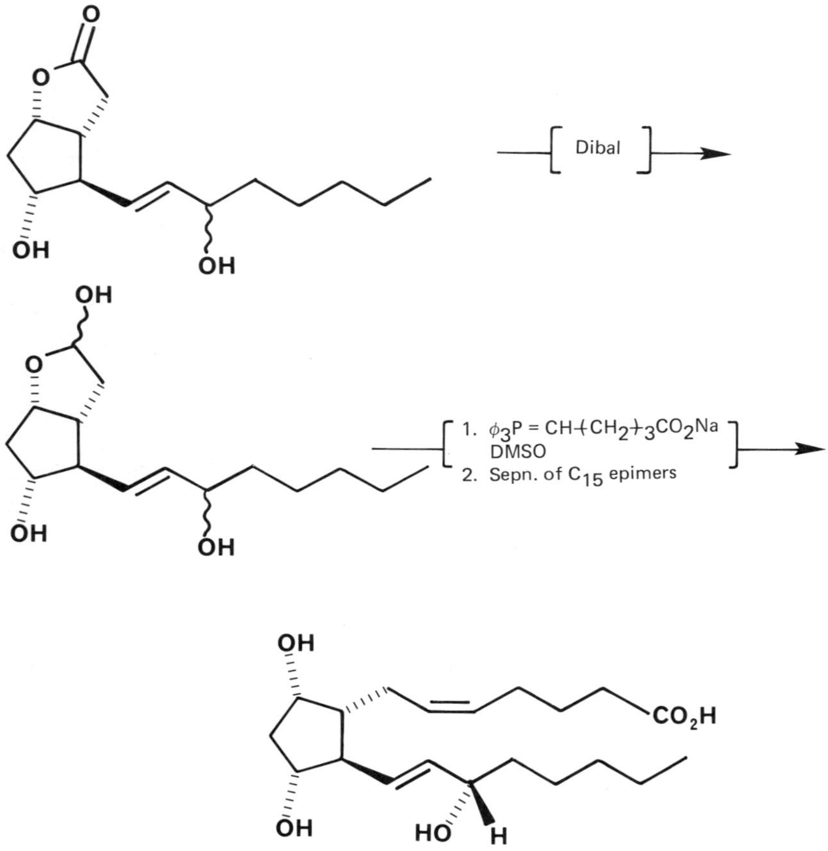

Synthesis of Acetoxyfulvene[4]

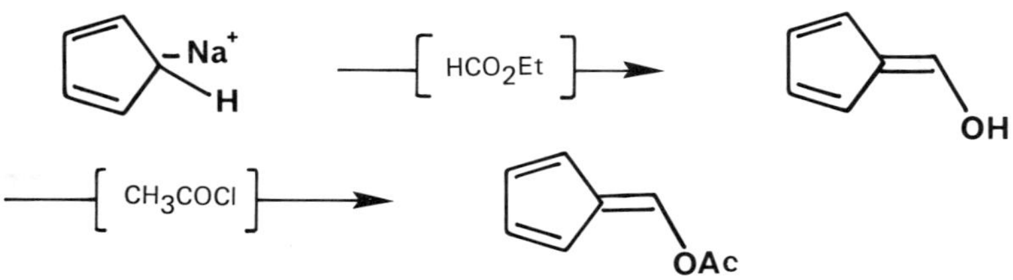

4. K. Haffner, G. Schulz & K. Wagner, *Annalen*, **678**, 39, (1964).

In a similar approach starting from acetoxyfulvene the introduction of the β-chain is postponed until a later stage.[5] So that in fact this is a synthesis of the Corey lactone.

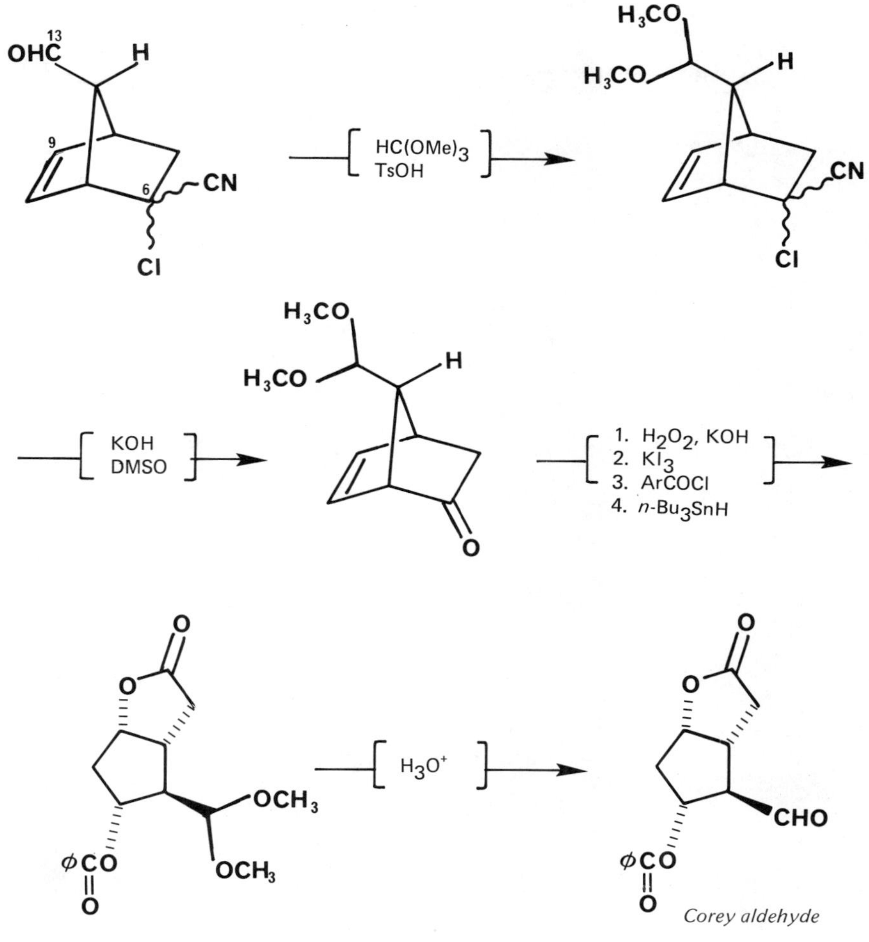

---

5. E. D. Brown, R. Clarkson, T. J. Leeney & G. E. Robinson, *Chem. Commun.*, 642 (1974).

12

Syntheses from Cyclopent-2-ene-1,4-diol

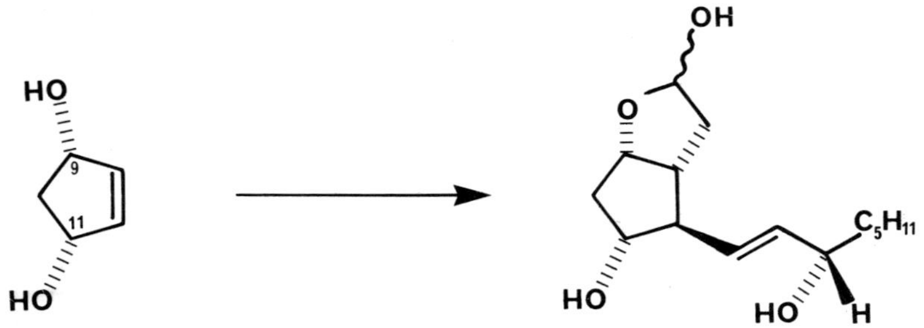

The opening of a protected epoxycyclopentanediol [1] with diallylcuprate followed by epoxidation and opening of the second epoxide with an alane introduces the α- and β- chains of the prostaglandins.[1,2,3] Lack of regiospecificity in the opening of the epoxide [2] led to the development of a modified approach.

---

1. J. Fried, M. Mehra, C. Lin, W. Kao & P. Dalven in "Prostaglandins," *Annals of New York Academy of Sciences*, P. Ramwell & J. E. Shaw (Eds.) **180**, 1971, p. 38.
2. J. Fried, C. H. Lin, J. C. Sih, P. Dalven & G. F. Cooper, *J. Am. Chem. Soc.*, **94**, 4342 (1972).
3. This principle was first successfully applied to the synthesis of 7-oxa-PGF$_{1\alpha}$. See p. 394 for further details. J. Fried, M. M. Mehra & W. L. Kao, *J. Am. Chem. Soc.*, **93**, 5594 (1971).

SYNTHETIC STRATEGY

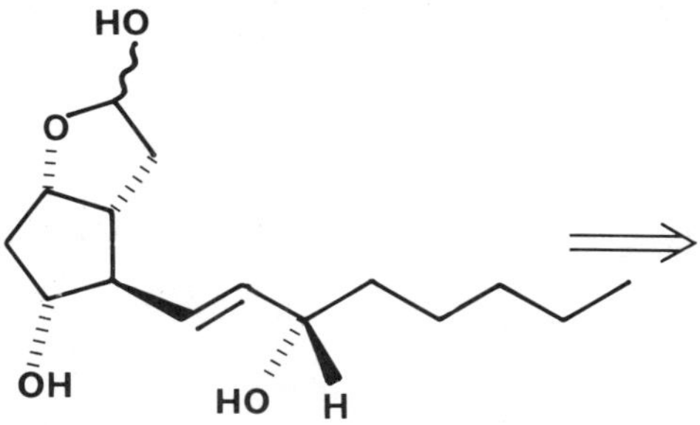

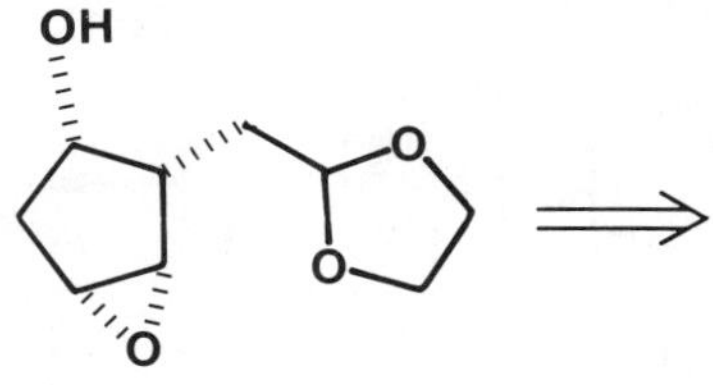

[2]

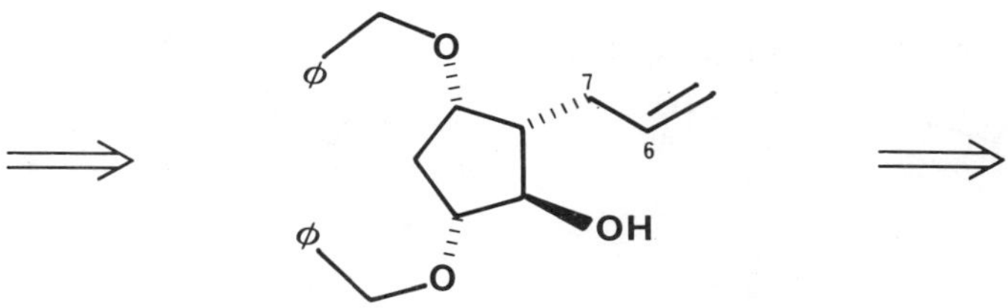

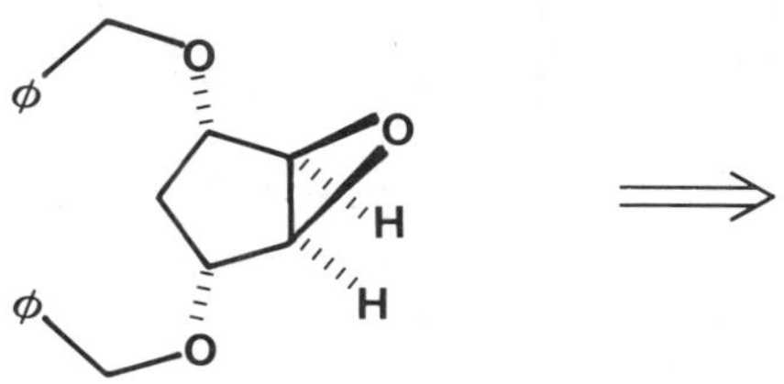

[1]

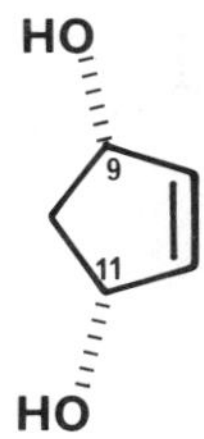

cis-*1,3-Cyclopent-4-enediol*[4]

---

4. This symmetric intermediate, *cis*-1,3-cyclopent-4-ene diol, has also been used by Corey & Fuchs in an another approach to prostaglandins, see p. 245. E. J. Corey & P. L. Fuchs, *J. Am. Chem. Soc.*, **94**, 4014 (1972).
5. Unlike in some other cases (see p. 138) here the epoxidation takes place from the least hindered side. Such a stereochemistry of this epoxide was necessary for the desired stereospecific introduction of the α- and β- chains.

SYNTHETIC PLAN[2]

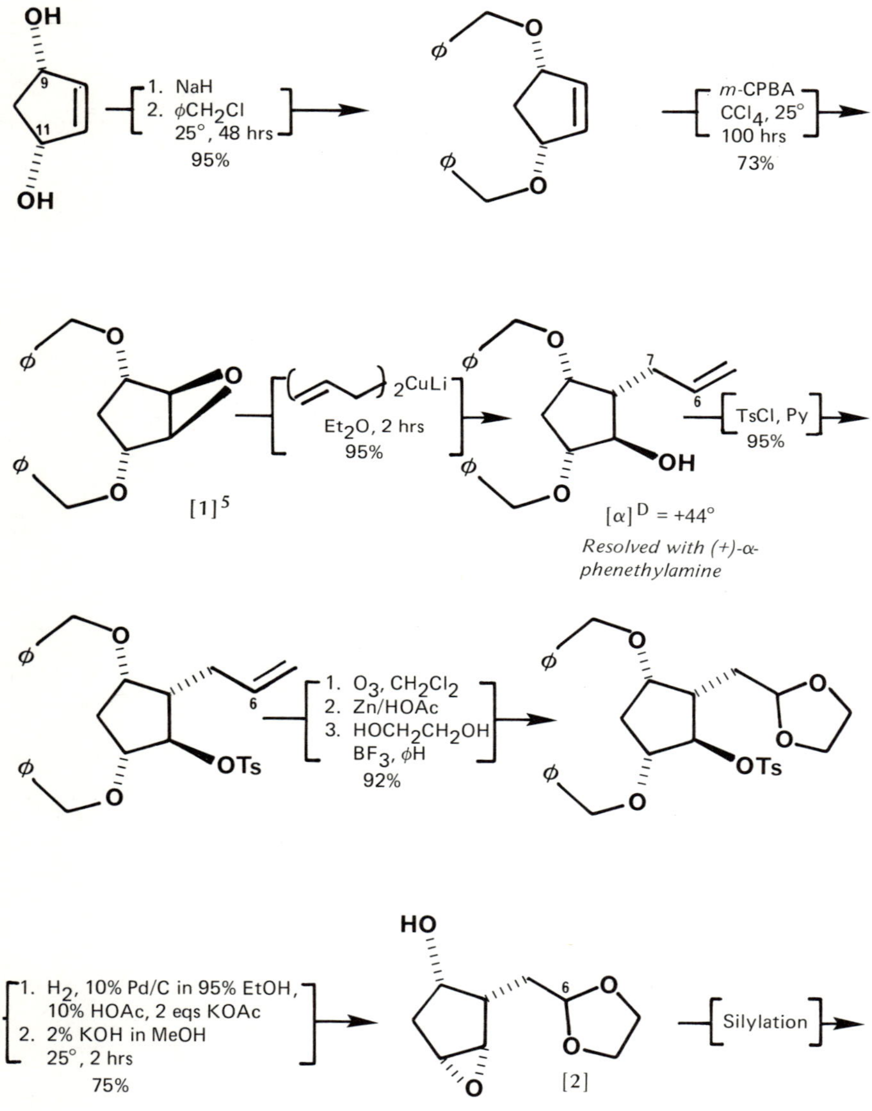

All cis

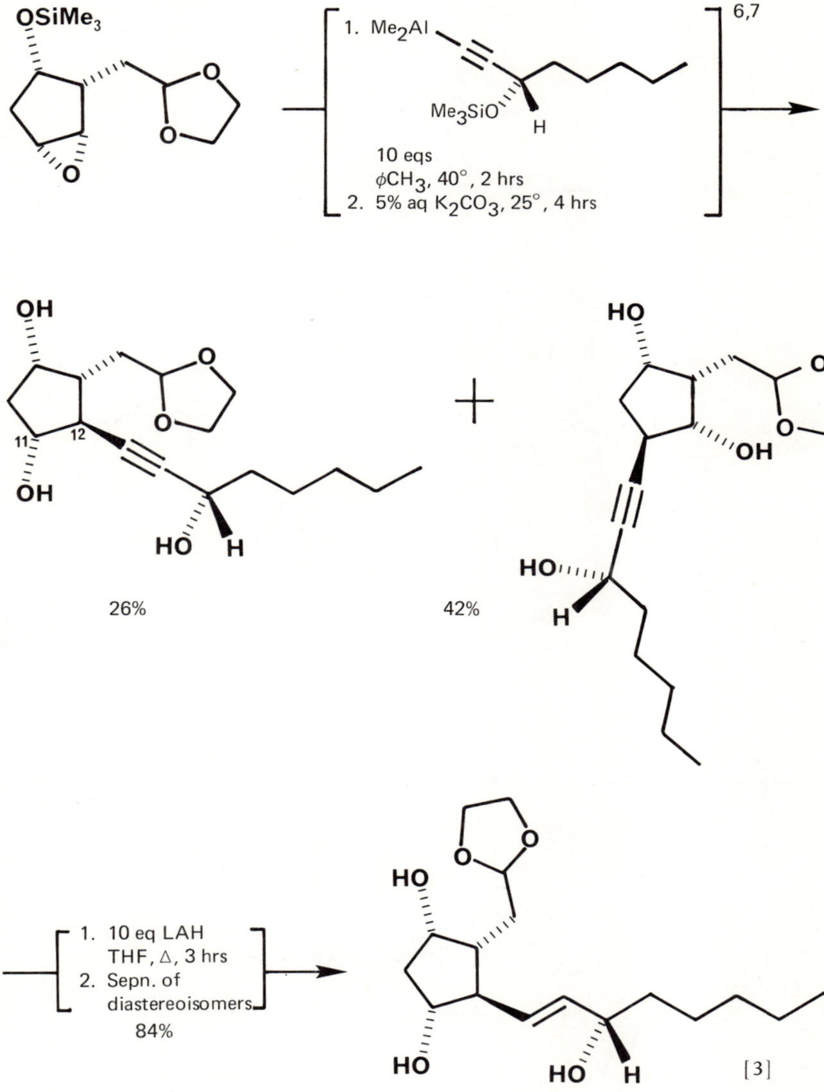

[3]

6. The alane was prepared from (*S*)-(−)-3-hydroxy-1-octynol by silylation followed by lithiation (*n*-BuLi in hexane) in toluene at −35° C and subsequent reaction with dimethylchloroalane in toluene at 0° C for 1 hr.

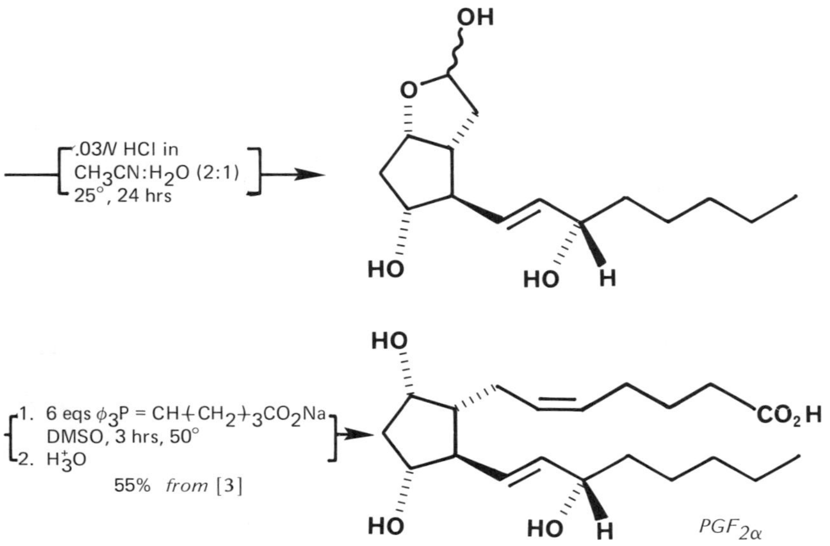

7. $PGF_{3\alpha}$ has also been made by opening the epoxide [4] with the alane as shown:

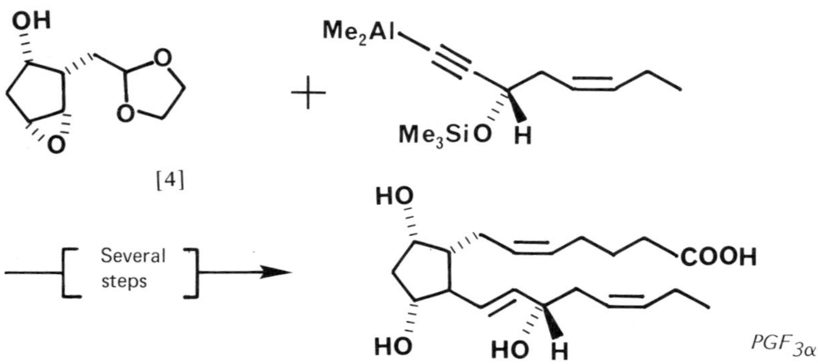

A suitably positioned alcohol function at C_6 [5] directs the opening of the epoxide by the alane.

SYNTHETIC PLAN[8]

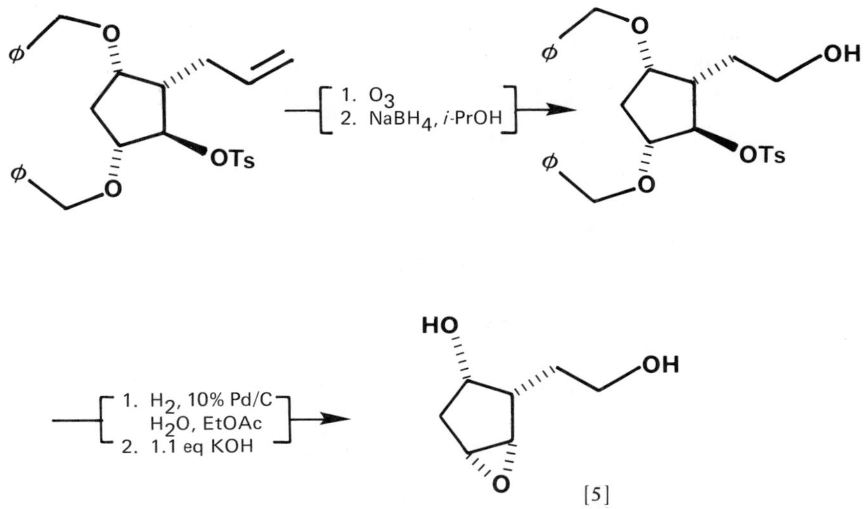

[5]

8. J. Fried, C. H. Lin, J. C. Sih, P. Dalven, G. F. Cooper, *J. Am. Chem. Soc.*, **94**, 4343 (1972).
9. Using *t*-Bu- as the protecting group one gets exclusively the C_{12} alkylated product, whereas using Me_3Si- as the protecting group one gets a regioselective opening, $C_{12}:C_{11}$ = 5:1. The observed regiospecificity in the opening of the epoxide [5] may be due to the preferred transition state complex formed between the epoxyalcohol [5] and two molecules of the alane reagent.

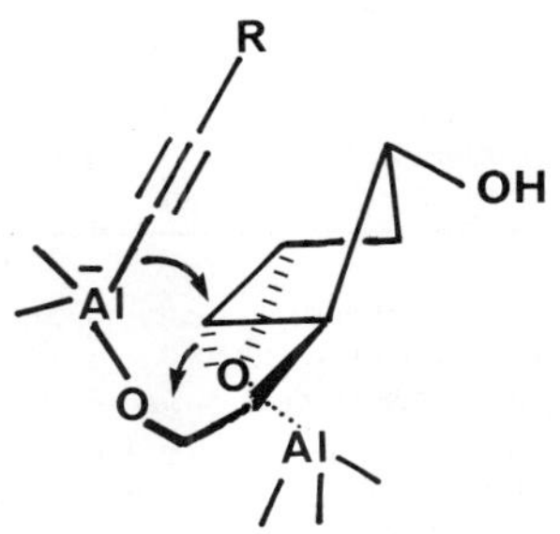

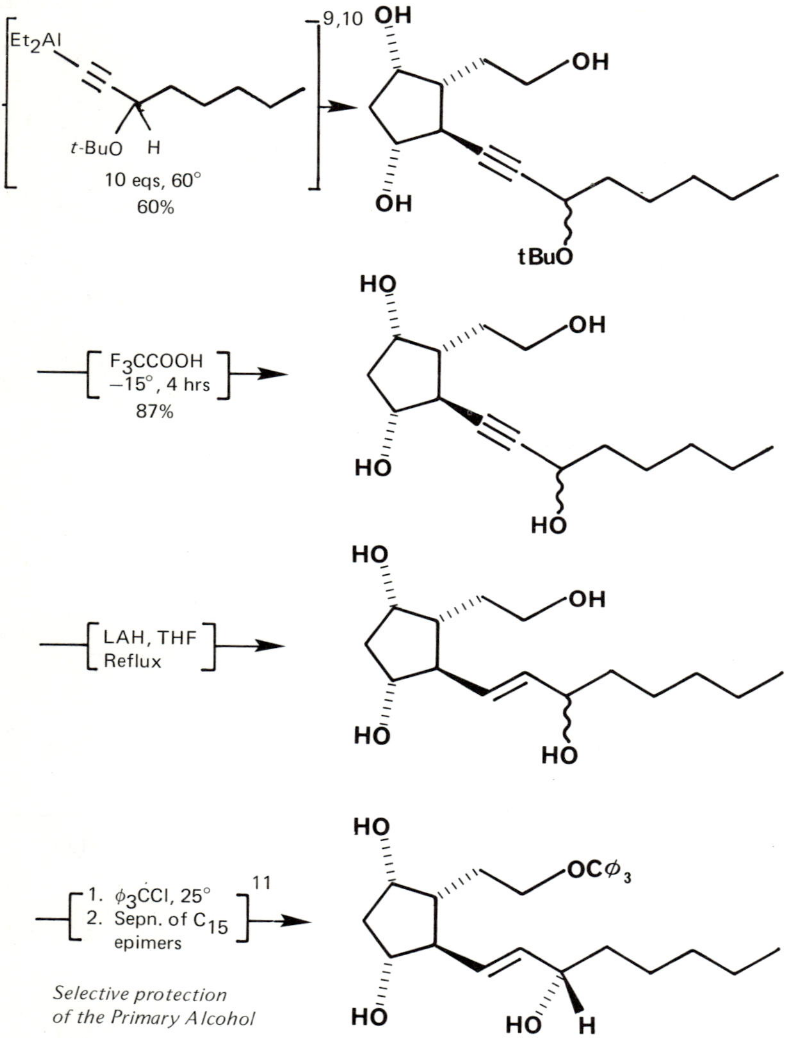

10. The lack of regiospecificity in the opening of a similar epoxide has also been observed by Corey. For further details see p. 139-140
E. J. Corey & R. Noyori, *Tet. Lett.*, 311 (1970) &
E. J. Corey, K. C. Nicolaou & D. J. Beames, *Tet. Lett.*, 2439 (1974).
11. In addition to 55% of monotrityl derivatives, 20% of secondary monotrityl and 25% of ditrityl compounds were also formed which were hydrolyzed and recycled.

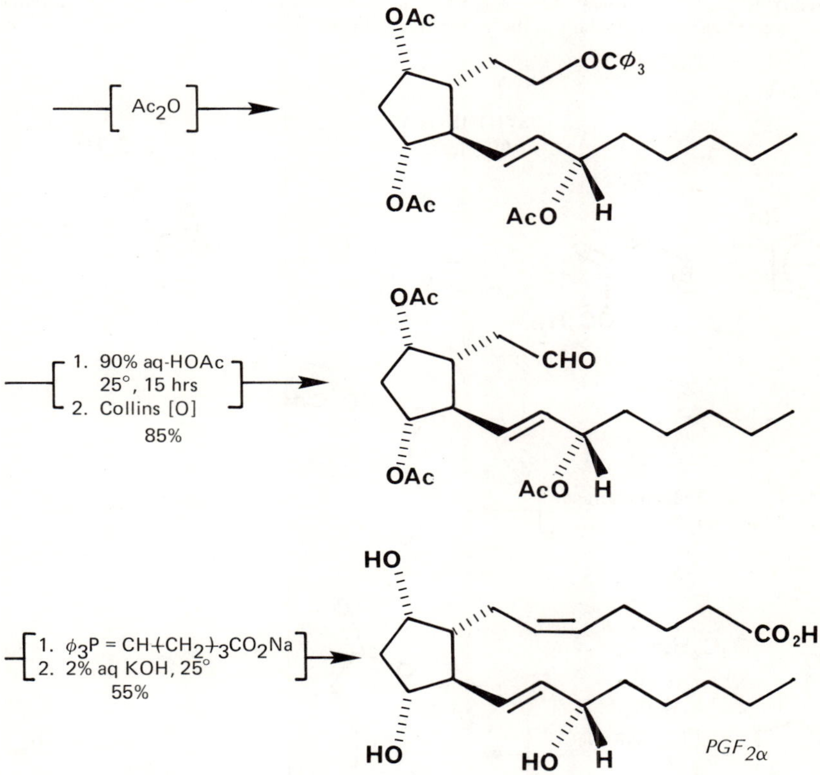
Ac2O
OAc
OCφ3
OAc
AcO
H
1. 90% aq-HOAc
25°, 15 hrs
2. Collins [O]
85%
OAc
CHO
OAc
AcO
H
1. φ3P = CH(CH2)3CO2Na
2. 2% aq KOH, 25°
55%
HO
CO2H
HO
HO
H
PGF2α

The epoxide (5, Fried's intermediate) has been made in chiral form by Partridge[12] by a simple route using (+) di-3-pinanylborane as the asymmetry inducing agent.

SYNTHETIC PLAN[12]

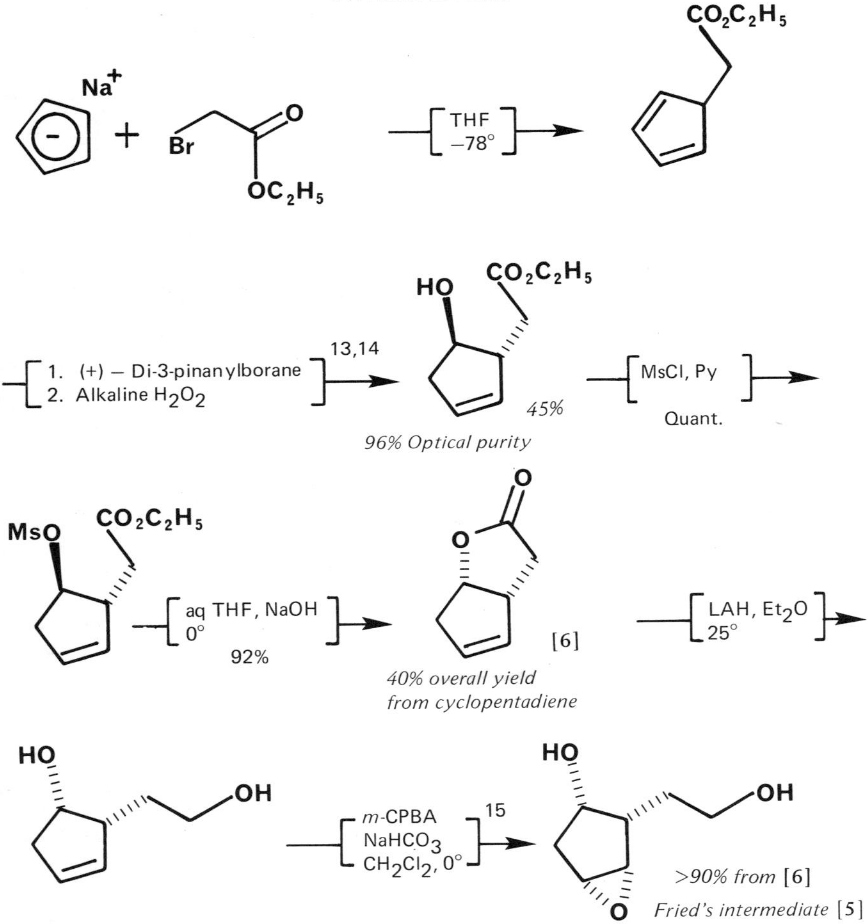

12. J. J. Partridge, N. K. Chadha & M. R. Uskokovic, *J. Am. Chem. Soc.*, **95**, 7171 (1973).
13. For a discussion on the hydroboration of various dienes, see Ch. 6, p.199, "Hydroboration of dienes and polyenes," in *Organoboranes in Organic Synthesis*, G. M. L. Cragg, M. Dekker, New York, 1973.

The chiral form of the bicyclic lactone [6] has also been made from 1,4-diacetoxycyclopent-2-ene by enzymatic hydrolysis followed by a Claisen rearrangement.[16] The resolution takes place during the enzymatic hydrolysis.

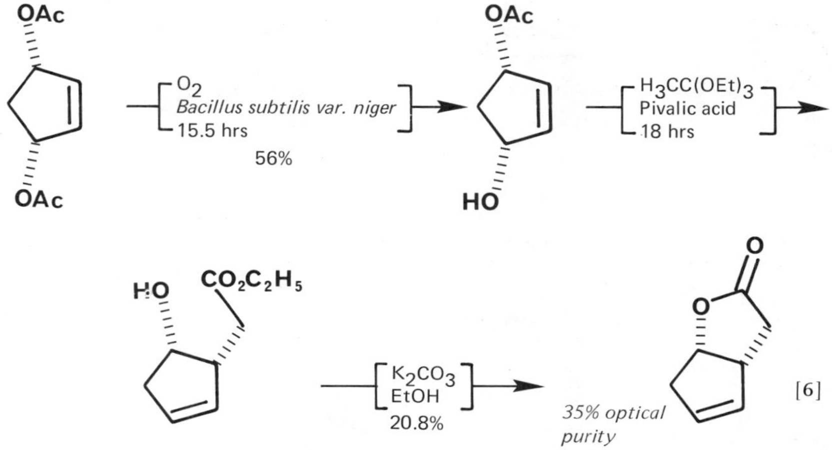

[6]

14. It is not obvious what controls the regioselectivity of the hydroboration reaction.

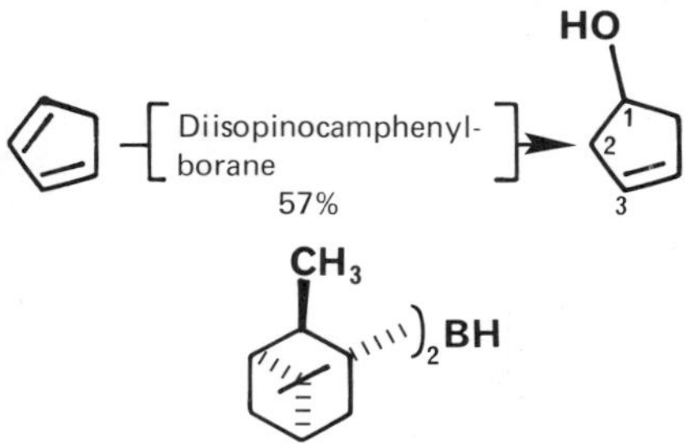

H. M. Hess & H. C. Brown, *J. Org. Chem.*, 32, 4138 (1967).

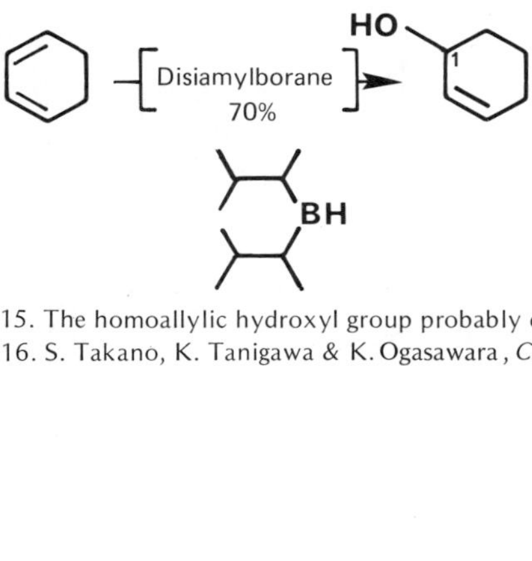

G. Zweifel, K. Nagase & H. C. Brown, *J. Am. Chem. Soc.*, **84**, 182, 190 (1962).

15. The homoallylic hydroxyl group probably directs the stereochemistry of epoxidation.
16. S. Takano, K. Tanigawa & K. Ogasawara, *Chem. Commun.*, 189 (1976).

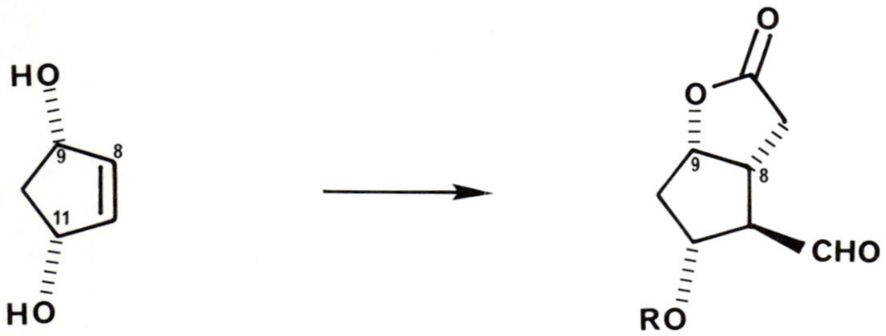

In this modification of the bicyclo[3.1.0]hexane[17] route the C_9-hydroxyl directs the intramolecular carbene addition[18,19] giving the ester bridged *endo*-bicyclo[3.1.0]hexane derivative. The β-chain is, then, introduced by a *trans (exo)* addition of divinylcuprate to the diacylcyclopropane.

SYNTHETIC STRATEGY

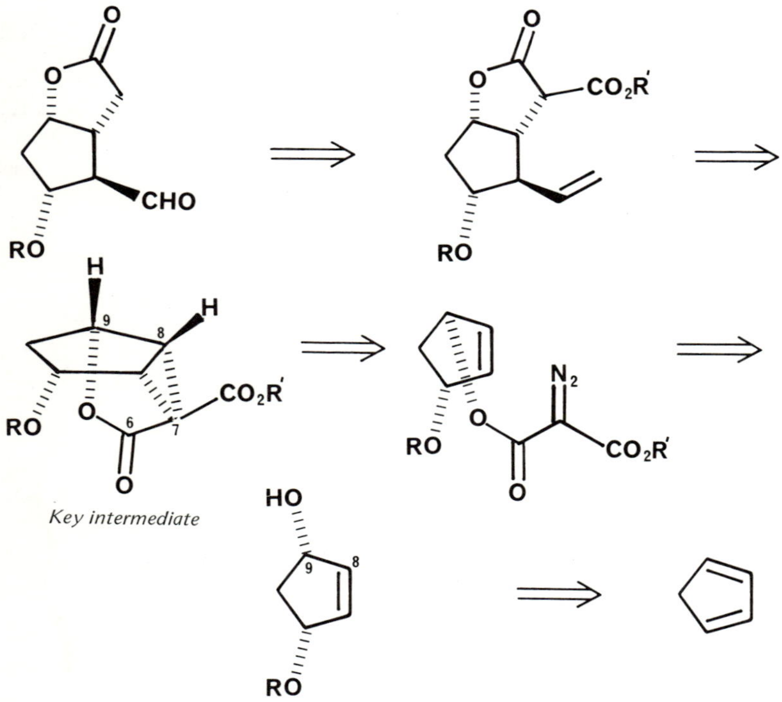

17. E. J. Corey & P. L. Fuchs, *J. Am. Chem. Soc.*, 94, 4014 (1972).

SYNTHETIC PLAN[17]

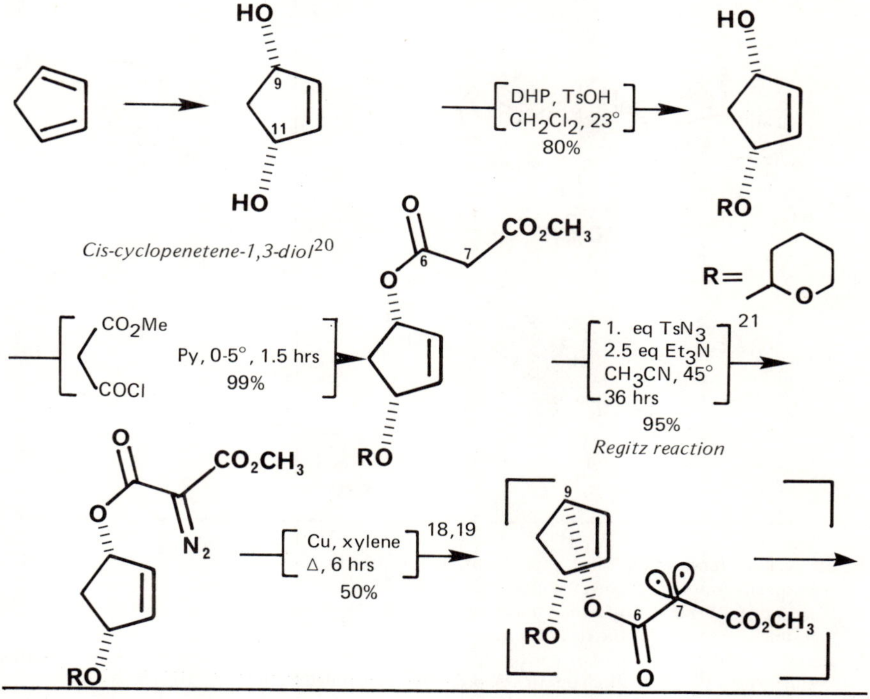

18. Intramolecular carbene addition of malonate esters of allylic alcohols via a diazo compound was first studied by French workers:
M. M. Sylvestre Julia, G. Cannic & G. Linstrumelle, *Comptes Rendus,* **264**, 1890 (1967).
G. Cannic, G. Linstrumelle & S. Julia, *Bull. Soc. Chim. Fr.,* 4913 (1968).

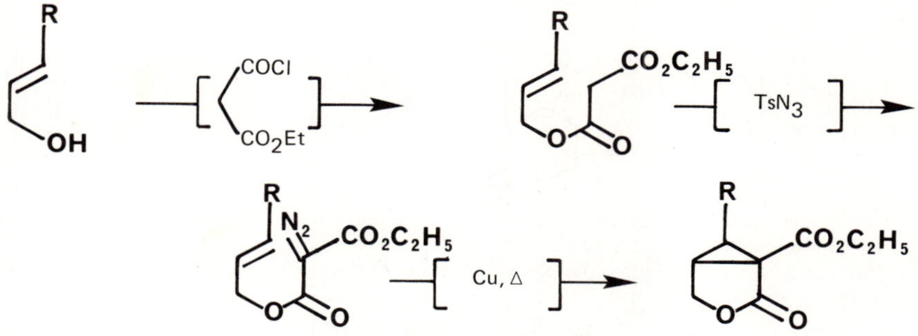

19. See also: L. Solomon, *Dissertation Abstr.,* **26**, 101 (1965) & H. O. House & C. J. Blankley, *J. Org. Chem.,* **33**, 53 (1968).

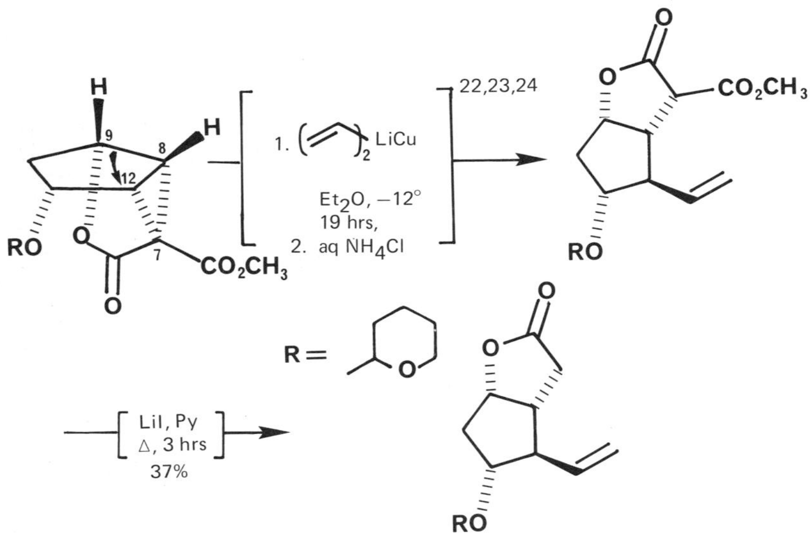

20. *Cis*-cyclopentene-1,3-diol has been used by Prof. J. Fried (University of Chicago) in the regiospecific opening of the cyclopentene epoxide by alanes. (*Vide supra.*)
21. "Recent synthetic methods in diazo chemistry," by M. Regitz, *Synthesis*, 351 (1972). For a plausible mechanism of the reaction, see p. 363.
22. Like the reductive opening of cyclopropyl ketones with Li/NH_3, the opening of cyclopropyl ketones (esters) with dialkylcuprates is, probably, controlled by stereoelectronic factors.
W. G. Dauben & R. E. Wolf, *J. Org. Chem.*, 35, 374, 2361 (1970).
J. D. White, S. Torii & J. Nogami, *Tet. Lett.*, 2879 (1974).
The bond that overlaps better with the carbonyl π system is usually cleaved with cuprates.
R. D. Clark & C. H. Heathcock, *Tet. Lett.*, 529 (1975).

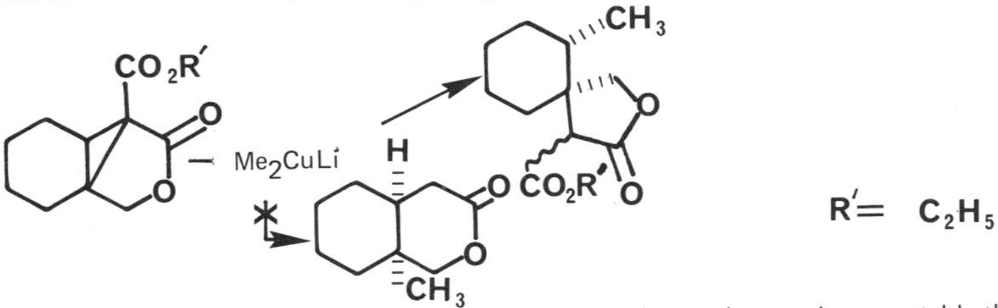

23. The opening may be controlled, in this case, because the resultant γ-lactone is more stable than the corresponding δ-lactone.
24. This was done as a model for the possible opening of the cyclopropane with the whole β-side chain.

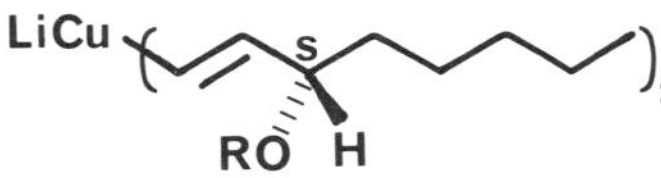

13

1,4-Addition Approach

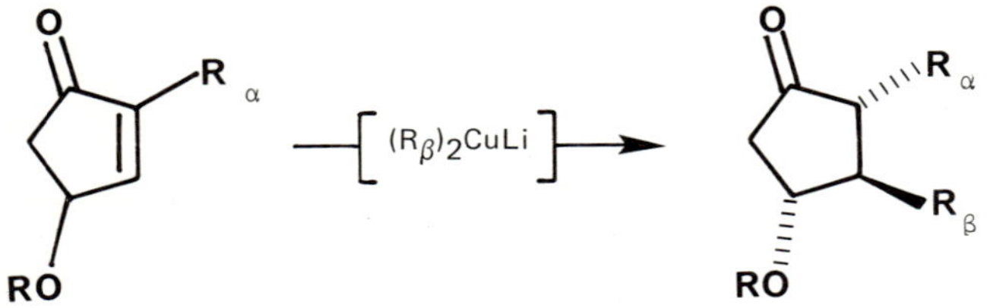

1,4-addition of a organometallic reagent to 2-alkyl-4-alkoxycyclopent-2-enones is an interesting concept for the direct convergent synthesis of PGs of the E series. The addition of divinylcuprates to substituted cyclopentenones has been studied independently by the Syntex[1,2] and the Wisconsin[3] groups. The method has been generalized by using different alcohol protecting groups and soluble cuprous iodide complexes. This approach has also led to the development of several syntheses of 4-alkoxycyclopentenones.

In such a synthesis the two units, the cyclopentenone and the vinyl group can be chiral, thus resulting in the formation of natural PGs. Alternatively, one of the pieces can be chiral and then by a kinetic or thermodynamic process the other piece can be resolved.

In the Sih[4,5] approach the chiral cyclopentenone was synthesized by a sequence involving an enzymatic reduction of the 2-alkyl-1,3,4-cyclopentanetrione. The resulting chiral alkoxycyclopentenone was then coupled with the chiral cuprate reagent.

---

1. F. S. Alvarez, D. Wren & A. Prince, *J. Am. Chem. Soc.*, **94**, 7823 (1972).
2. A. F. Kluge, K. G. Untch & J. H. Fried, *J. Am. Chem. Soc.*, **94**, 7827 (1972).
3. C. J. Sih, P. Price, R. Sood, R. G. Solomon, G. Peruzzotti & M. Casey, *J. Am. Chem. Soc.*, **94**, 3643 (1972).
4. C. J. Sih, H. B. Heather, R. Sood, P. Price, G. Peruzzotti, L.F. Hsu Lee & S. S. Lee, *J. Am. Chem. Soc.*, **97**, 865 (1975).
5. J. B. Heather, R. Sood, P. Price, G. P. Peruzzotti, S. S. Lee, L. F. Hsu Lee & C. J. Sih, *Tet. Lett.*, 2313 (1973).

SYNTHETIC STRATEGY

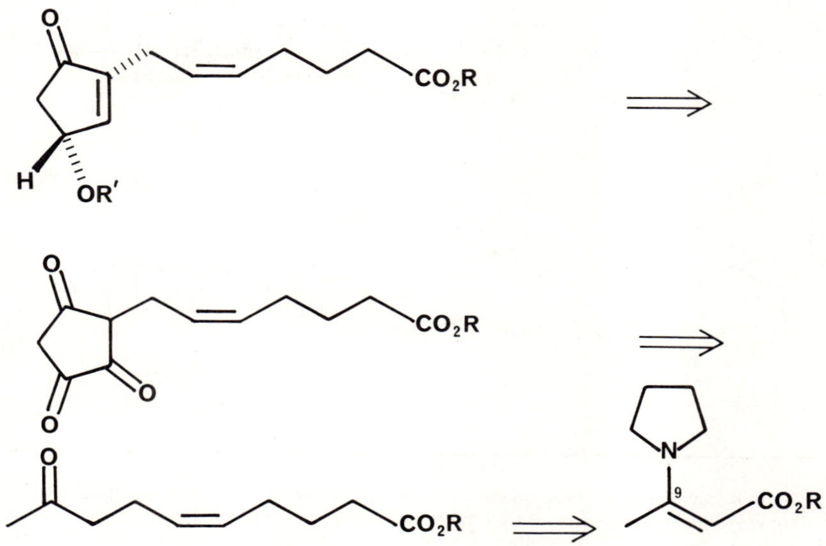

SYNTHETIC PLAN[4,5]

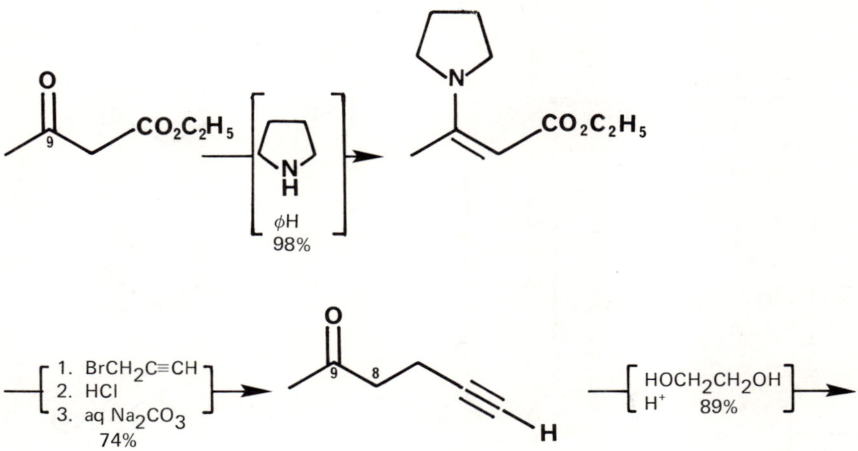

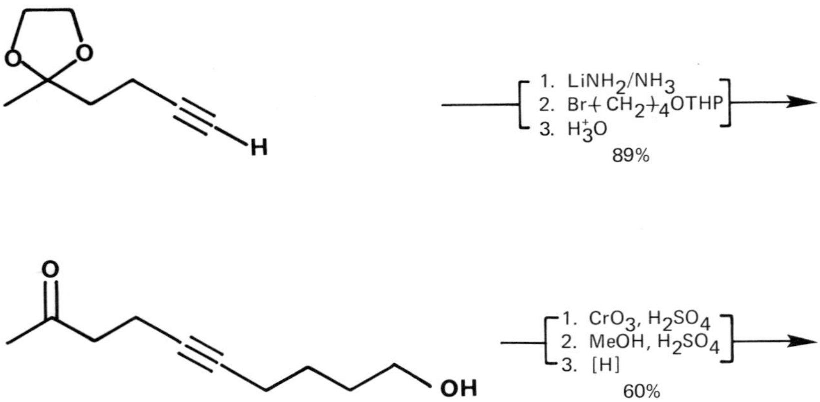

6. In a similar synthesis of PGs, the α-chain precursor required for the synthesis of the 4-alkoxycyclopentenone was made by a different route as shown in the following: M. Bruhn, C. H. Brown, P. W. Collins, J. R. Palmer, E. Z. Dajani & R. Pappo, *Tet. Lett.*, 235 (1976).

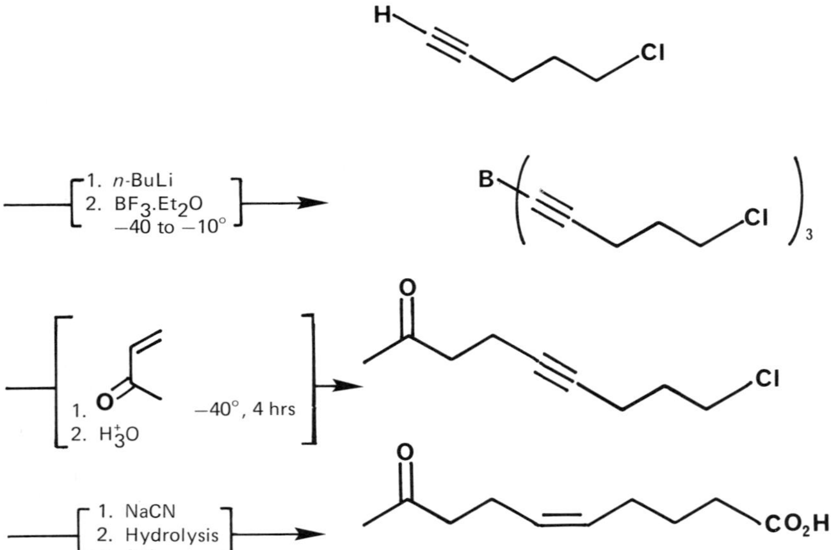

α-chain precursor

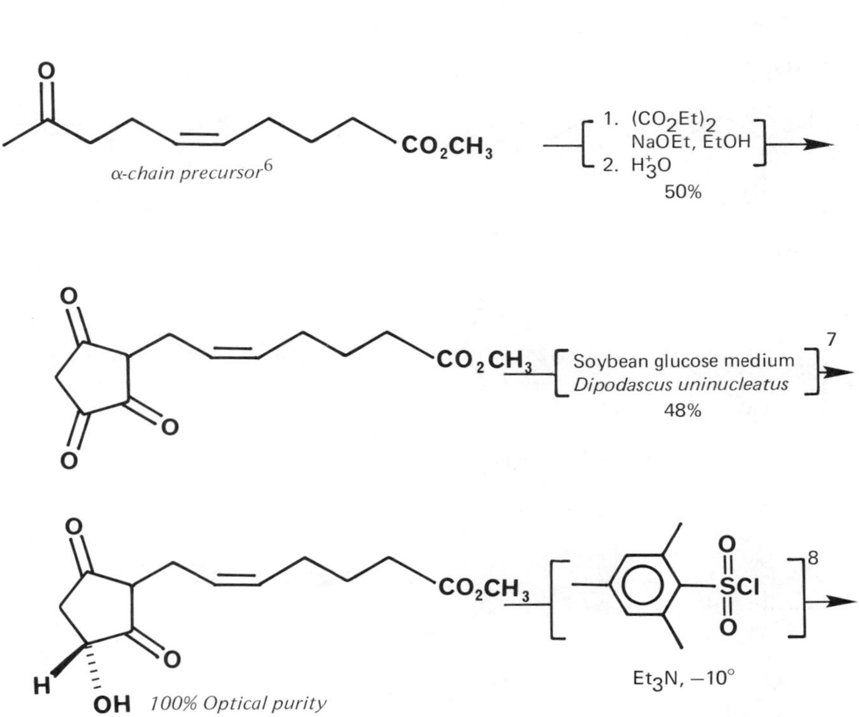

7. Catalytic reduction gives the alcohol in low optical purity.

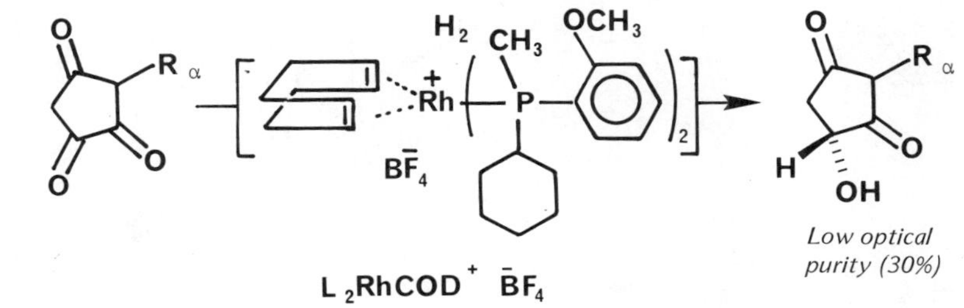

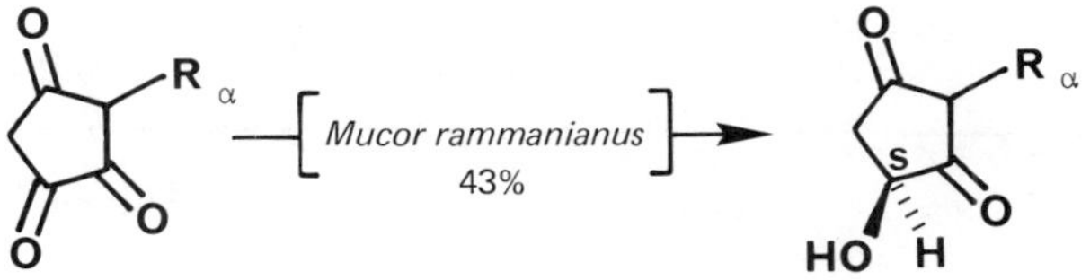

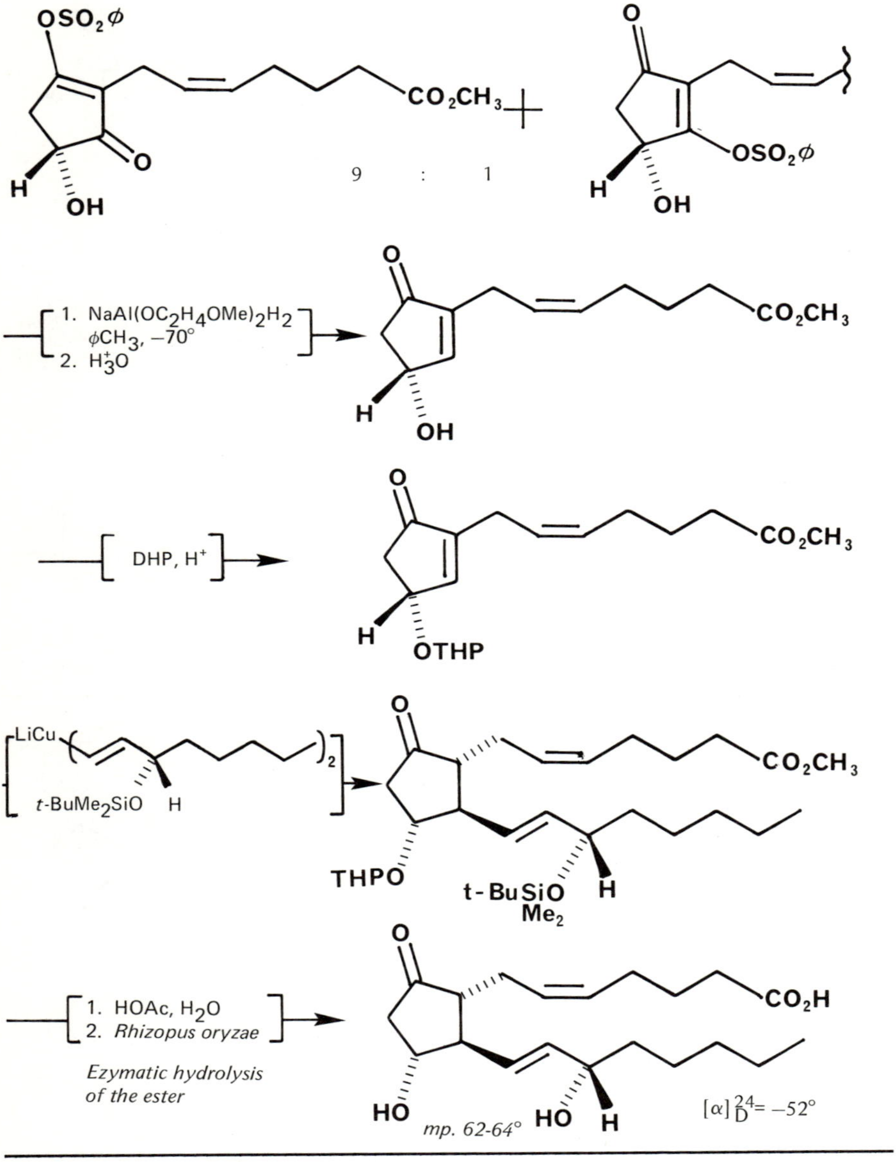

8. The size of the acylating or the alkylating agent determines the ratios of the resulting isomeric enolates.

Modified Hydroalumination Procedure for the Synthesis of Trans Vinyl Iodides [1]

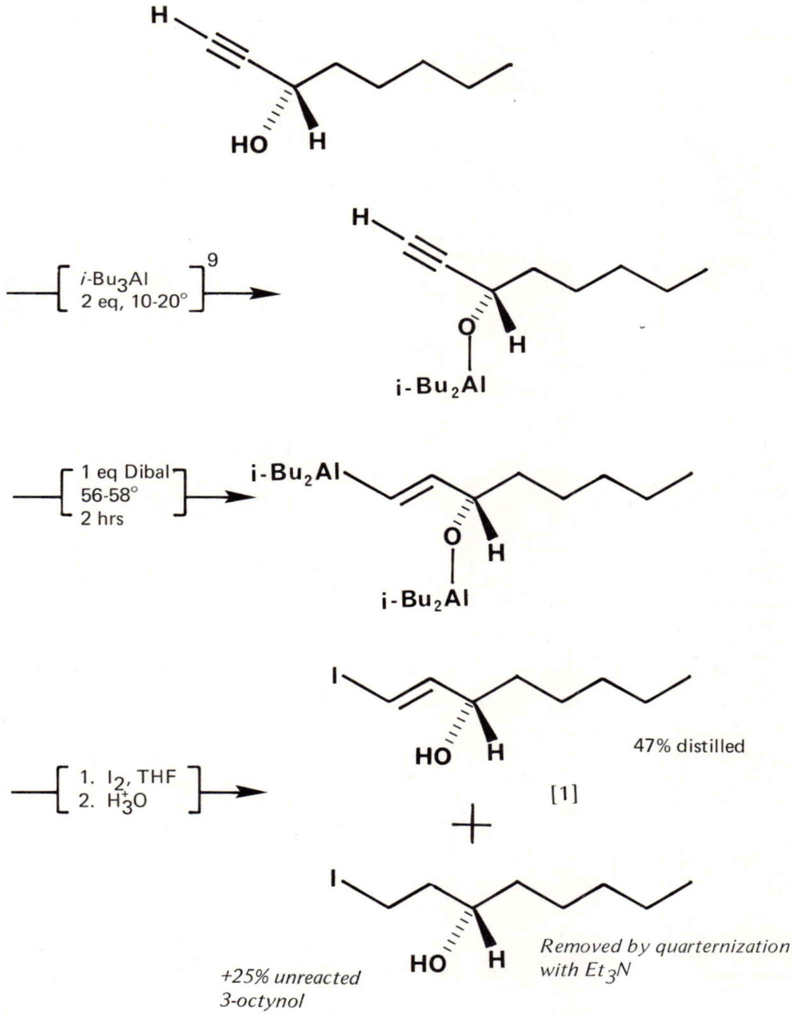

9. Direct hydroalumination with Dibal followed by iodination (Zweifel method) gives, only in poor yields, the *trans* vinyl iodide.
G. Zweifel & C. C. Whitney, *J. Am. Chem. Soc.*, 89, 2753 (1967).

The 4-alkoxycyclopentenone [3] required for the synthesis of PGE_1 was made from cyclopentadiene via the *endo*-peroxide [2]. The synthesis was then completed by the 1,4-addition of the chiral cuprate reagent.[10,11,12,13]

SYNTHETIC PLAN[12]

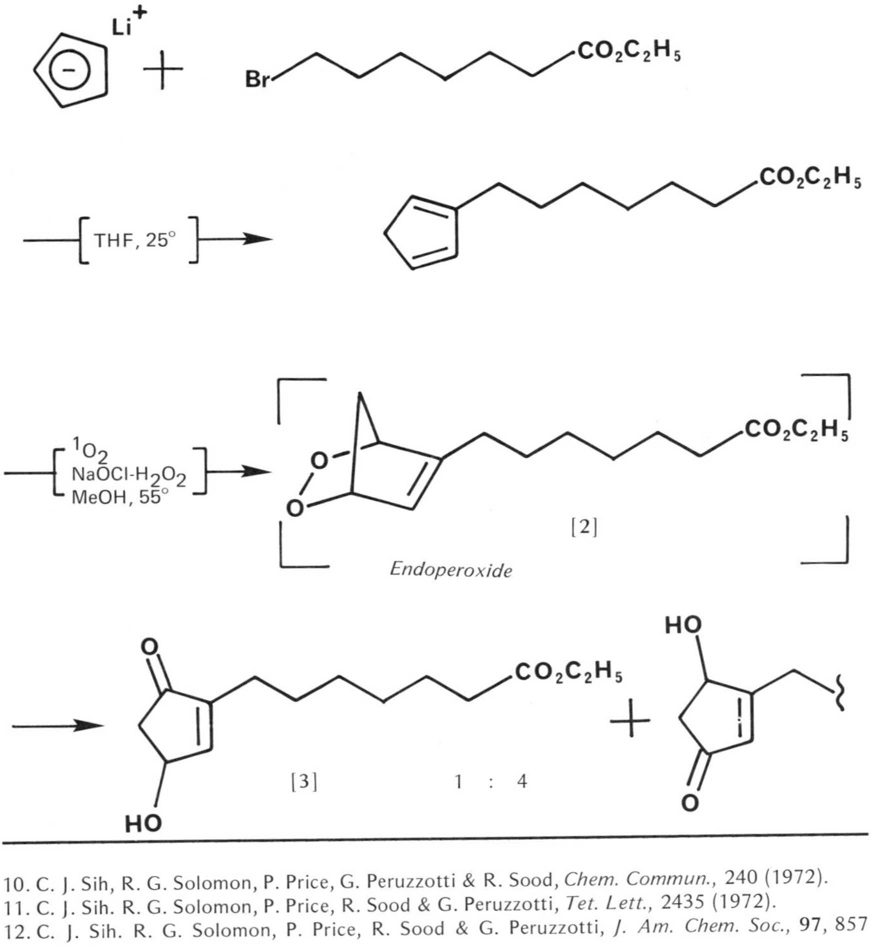

10. C. J. Sih, R. G. Solomon, P. Price, G. Peruzzotti & R. Sood, *Chem. Commun.*, 240 (1972).
11. C. J. Sih. R. G. Solomon, P. Price, R. Sood & G. Peruzzotti, *Tet. Lett.*, 2435 (1972).
12. C. J. Sih. R. G. Solomon, P. Price, R. Sood & G. Peruzzotti, *J. Am. Chem. Soc.*, **97**, 857 (1975).
13. C. J. Sih, J. B. Heather, G. P. Peruzzotti, P. Price, R. Sood, L. F. Hsu Lee, *J. Am. Chem. Soc.*, **95**, 1676 (1973).

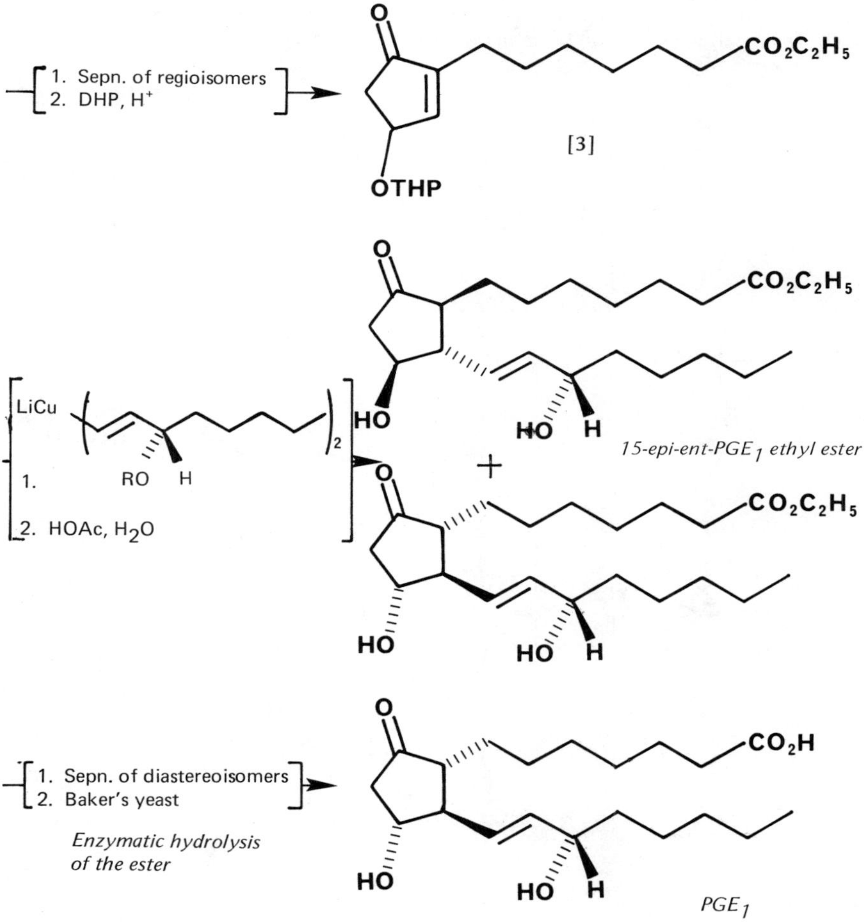
1. Sepn. of regioisomers
2. DHP, H+
O
CO2C2H5
OTHP
[3]
LiCu
1. RO H
2. HOAc, H2O
O
CO2C2H5
HO
HO H
15-epi-ent-PGE1 ethyl ester
+
O
CO2C2H5
HO
HO H
1. Sepn. of diastereoisomers
2. Baker's yeast
Enzymatic hydrolysis of the ester
O
CO2H
HO
HO H
PGE1

The Syntex group has shown that the 1,4-addition of *cis*-divinylcuprates[14] to the 4-alkoxycyclopentenones proceeds with higher stereoselectivity to give the prostanoids in higher yields. The chiral cuprate reagent has been used to resolve the 4-alkoxycyclopentenone.[15]

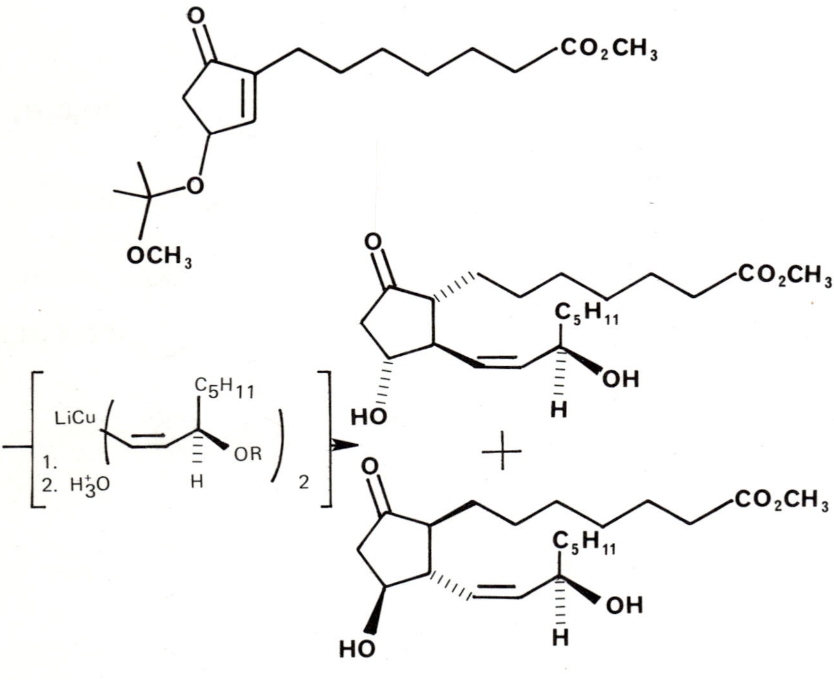

---

14. A. F. Kluge, K. G. Untch & J. H. Fried, *J. Am. Chem. Soc.*, 94, 9256 (1972).
15. In another approach a chiral alkoxycyclopentenone has been used to resolve the cuprate reagent. For further details see p. 295.

The *cis*-allylic alcohol with the wrong chirality at C_{15} was successfully converted to the *trans* allylic alcohol with the desired chirality at C_{15}.[16]

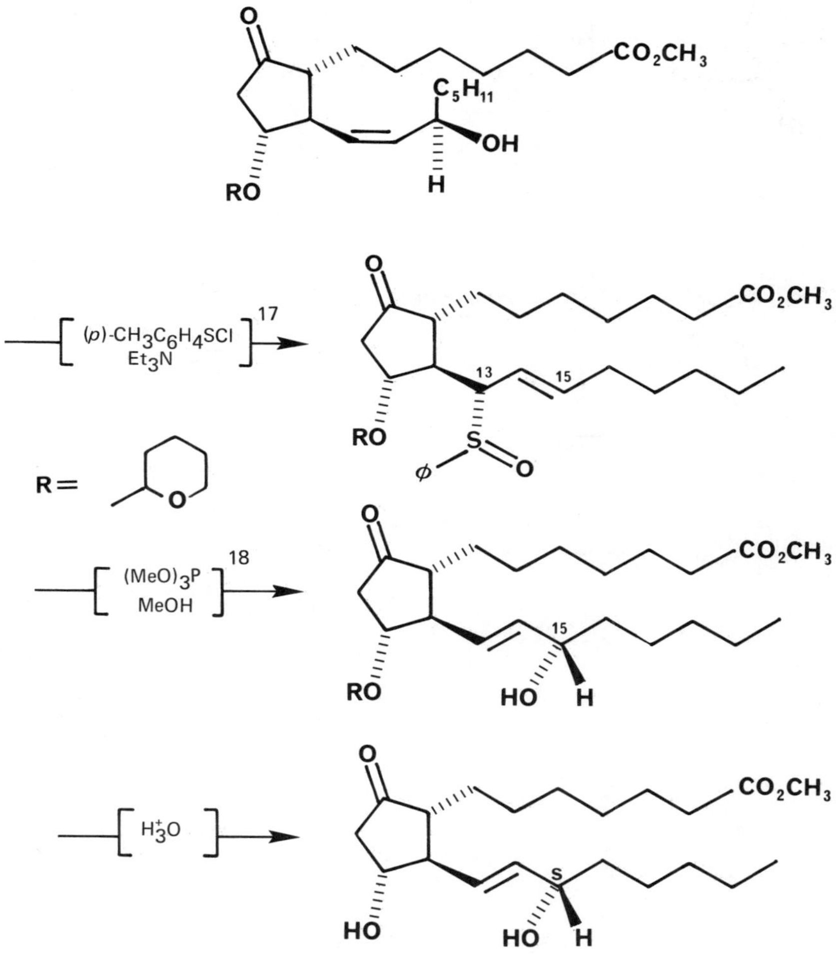

16. J. G. Miller, W. Kurz, K. G. Untch & G. Stork, *J. Am. Chem. Soc.*, **96**, 6774 (1974).
17. P. Bickart, F. W. Carson, J. Jacobus, E. G. Miller & K. Mislow, *J. Am. Chem. Soc.*, **90**, 4869 (1968).
18. D. A. Evans & G. C. Andrews, *Accounts Chem. Res.*, **7**, 147 (1974).

Mechanism of the Stork-Untch Inversion[17,18]

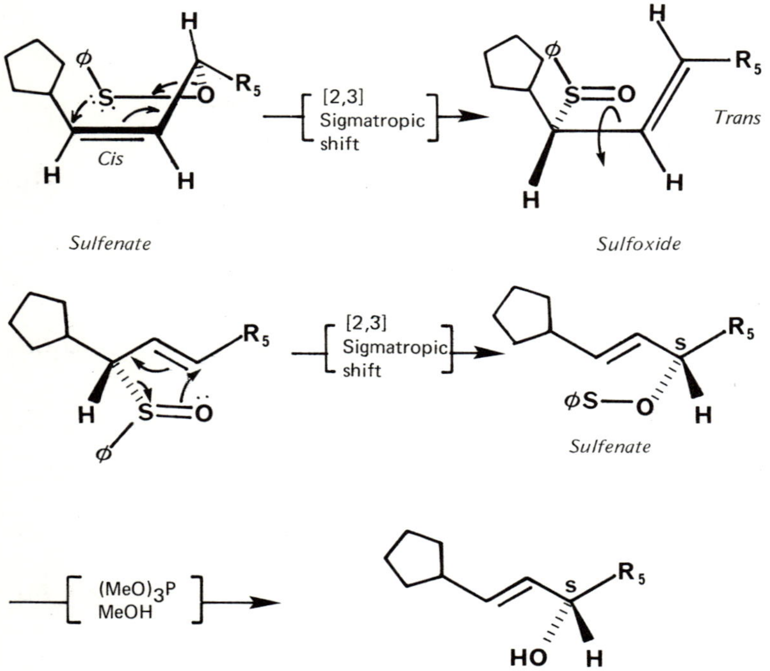

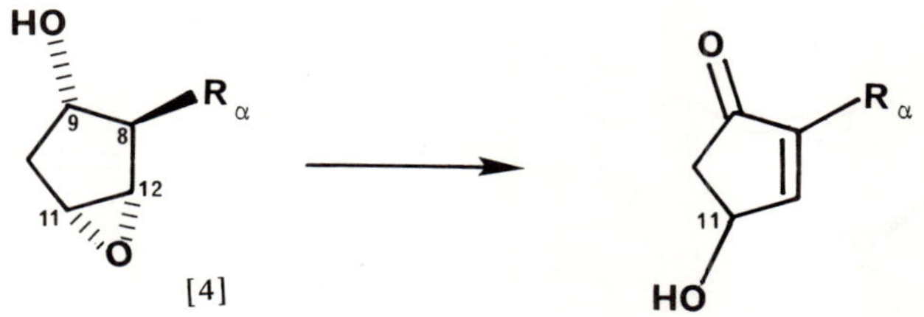

[4]

An interesting synthesis of the 4-alkoxycyclopentenone starting from the epoxycyclopentanol has been devised by Stork.[19]

Epoxycyclopentanols[20] [4] offer a conceptually very direct route to 4-hydroxycyclopentenones and could provide a more generally useful approach to the PGs of the E series. However, their practical use is limited because opening of the epoxide [4] by the incipient β-chain reagent requires very specialized conditions and also demands constraints on the nature of the α-chain.

---

19. G. Stork, C. Kowalski & G. Garcia, *J. Am. Chem. Soc.*, **97**, 3258 (1975).
20. Epoxycyclopentanols [4] have been used by Fried for the synthesis of PGs. For further details, see p. 236.

SYNTHETIC STRATEGY

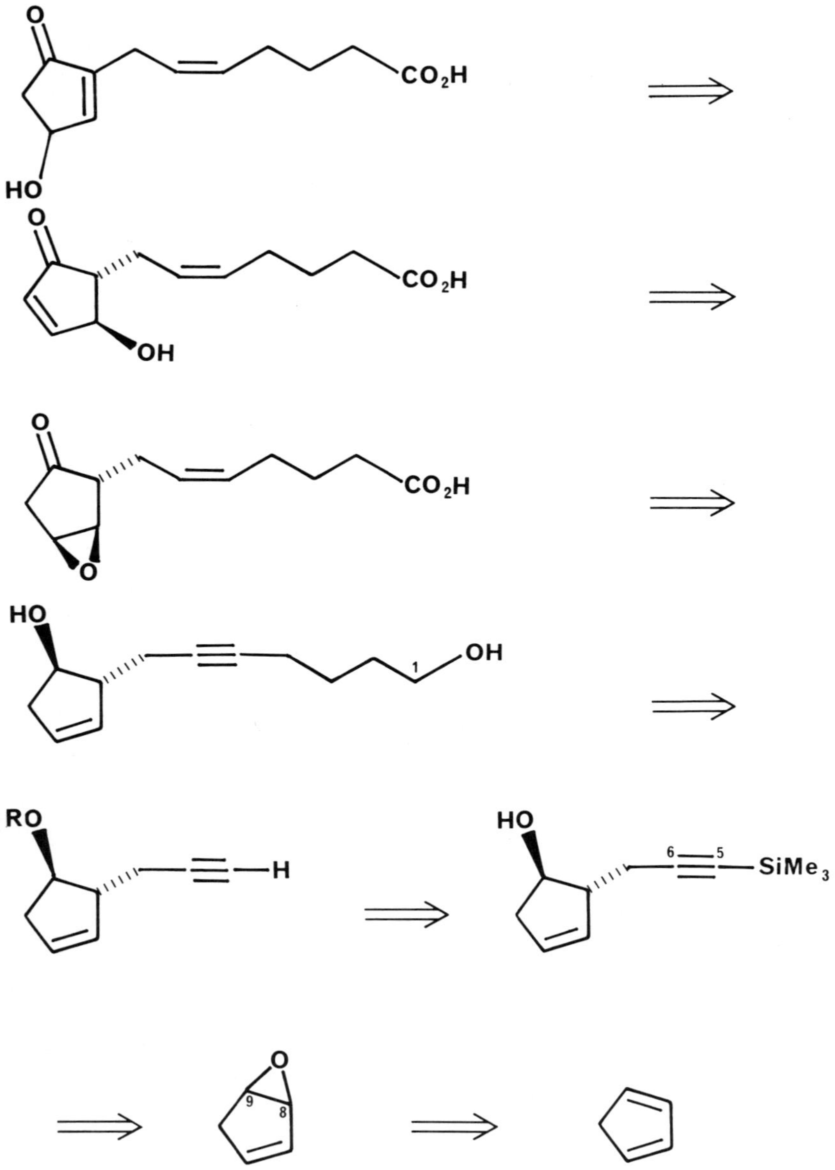

SYNTHETIC PLAN[19]

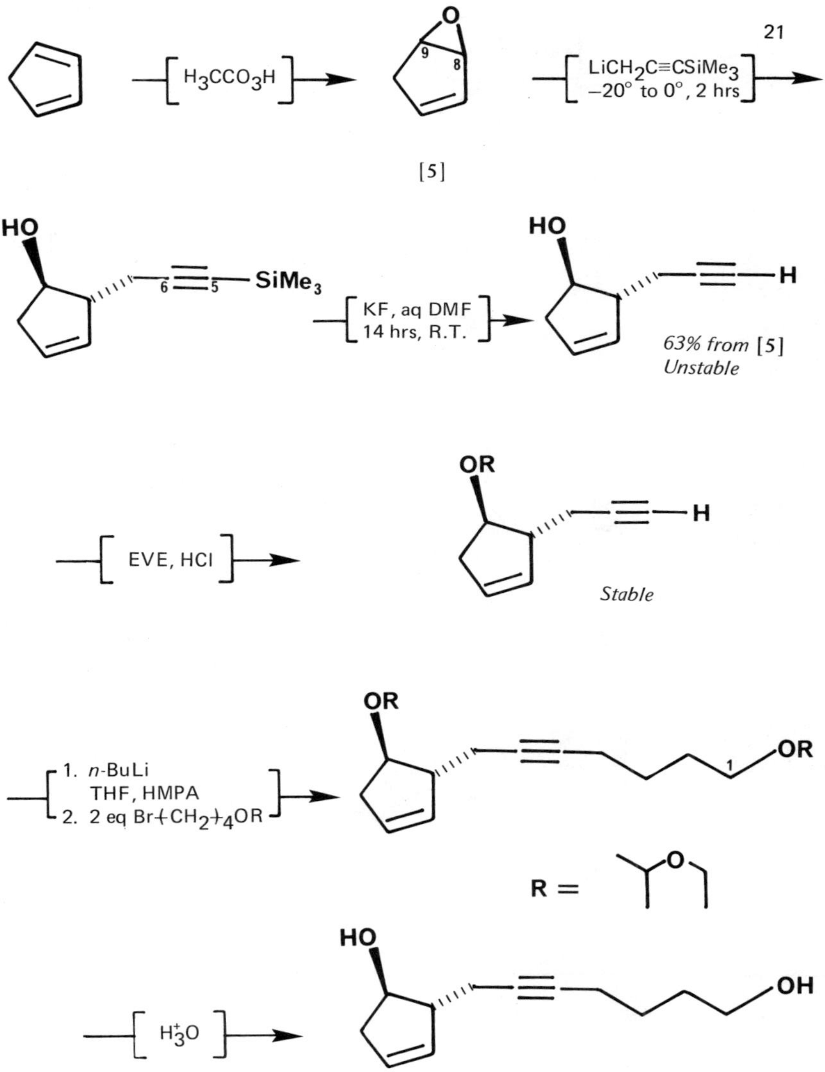

21. For a similar opening of the epoxide with 3-alkoxy-lithiumacetylide see p. 273.

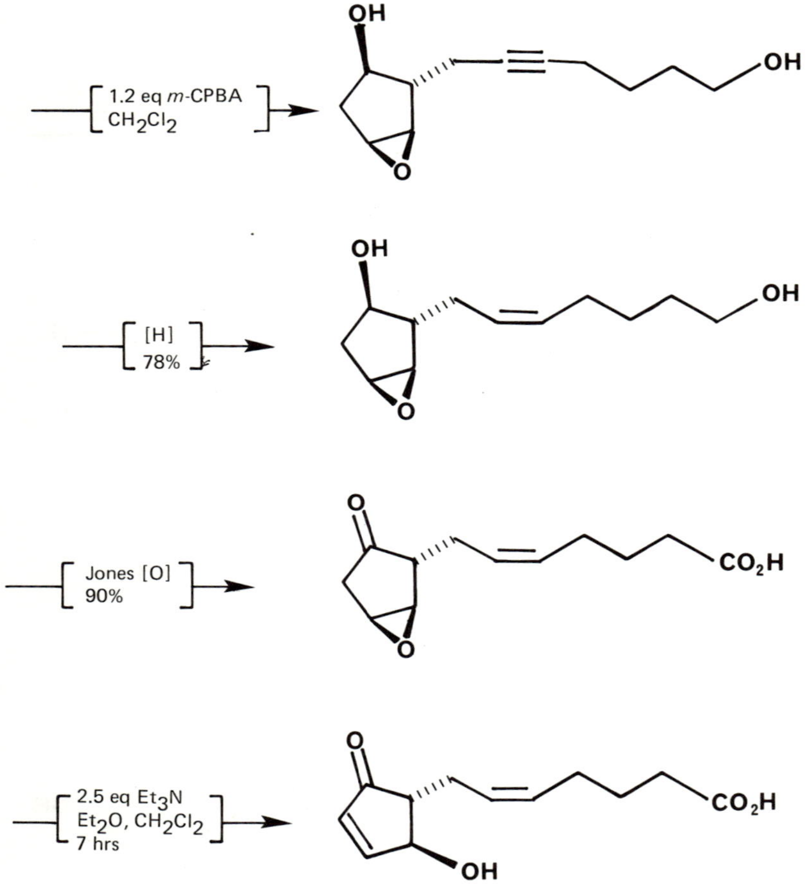

---

22. This mechanism is also supported by a recent report of the elimination of an isopropylidene analog of the acetal intermediate.
L. Gruber, I. Tomoskozi, E. Magor & G. Kovacs, *Tet. Lett.*, 3729 (1974).
When the rearrangement is carried out in $H_2{}^{18}O$, there was complete exchange of both the carbonyl and the hydroxyl oxygens with the solvent. The transformation proceeds, therefore, by the intermediate hydration to a glycol and not via an epoxide. G. Stork & C. Kowalski, in press (1977).

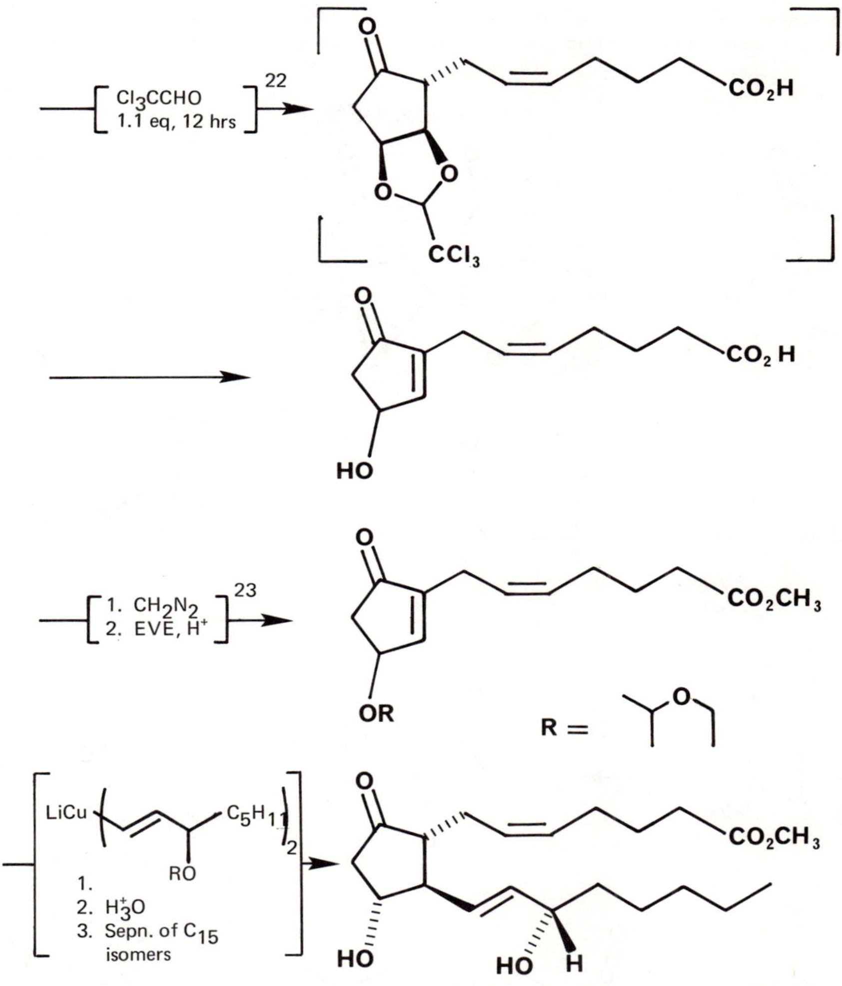

PGE$_2$ methyl ester

---

23. The drawback of using CH_2N_2 is that one gets PGE_2 methyl ester as the final product.

In a similar synthesis,[24] it was found that there is no difference (in terms of yields) in the rearrangement of the epoxycyclopentanols derived from the *cis-syn-cis* and *cis-anti-cis* epoxide.

SYNTHETIC PLAN[24]

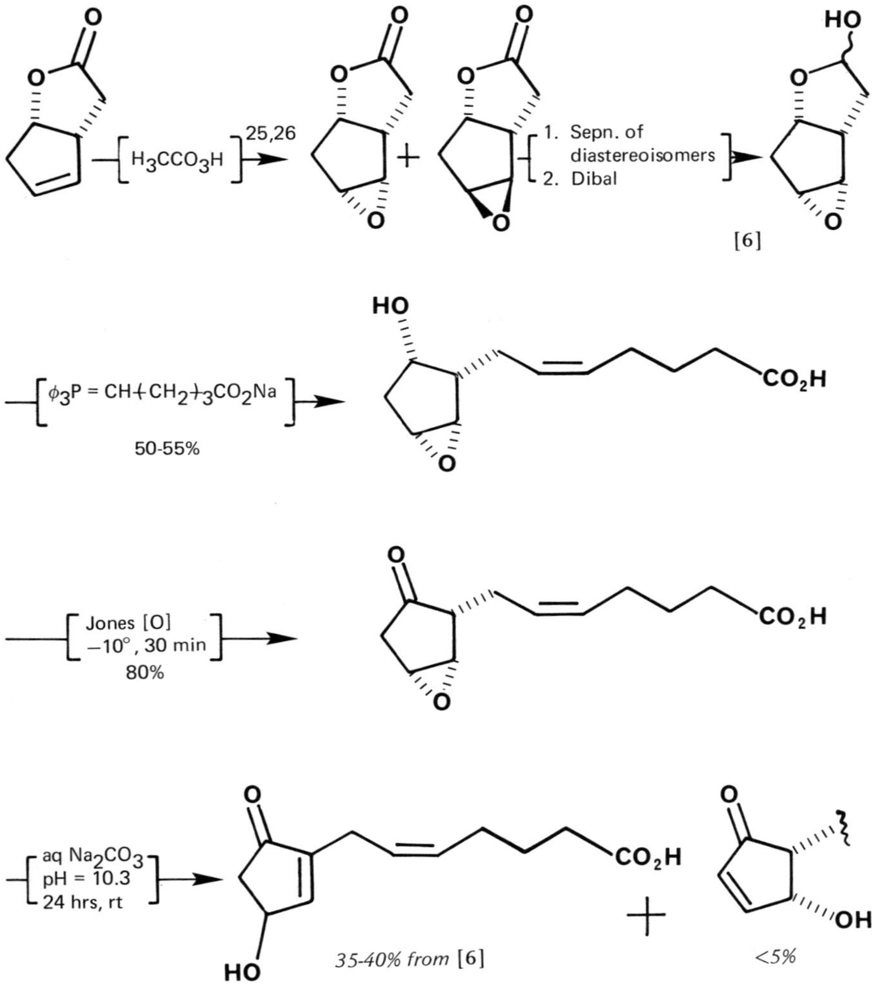

24. M. Brawner Floyd, *Syn. Commun.*, 4, 317 (1974).
25. E. J. Corey, Z. Arnold & J. Hutton, *Tet. Lett.*, 307 (1970).
26. E. J. Corey & R. Noyori, *Tet. Lett.*, 311 (1970).

Alanates and alanes, among other organometallic reagents, have also been added 1,4 to 4-alkoxycyclopentenones. The lithioalanate is made from the alane which in turn can be made by the reduction of the 3-alkoxyacetylenes. This hydroalumination procedure normally gives the *cis* olefin. But when there is a bulky C_{15} alcohol protecting group, only the *trans* olefin is formed. The hydroalumination at best proceeds in 40% yields. Reaction of the *trans* vinyllithium with R_3Al is an improved method of preparing the alanate reagent. There are other complications in the hydroalumination and the subsequent 1,4-addition of the alanate and this limits the usefulness of this particular approach.[27,28,29]

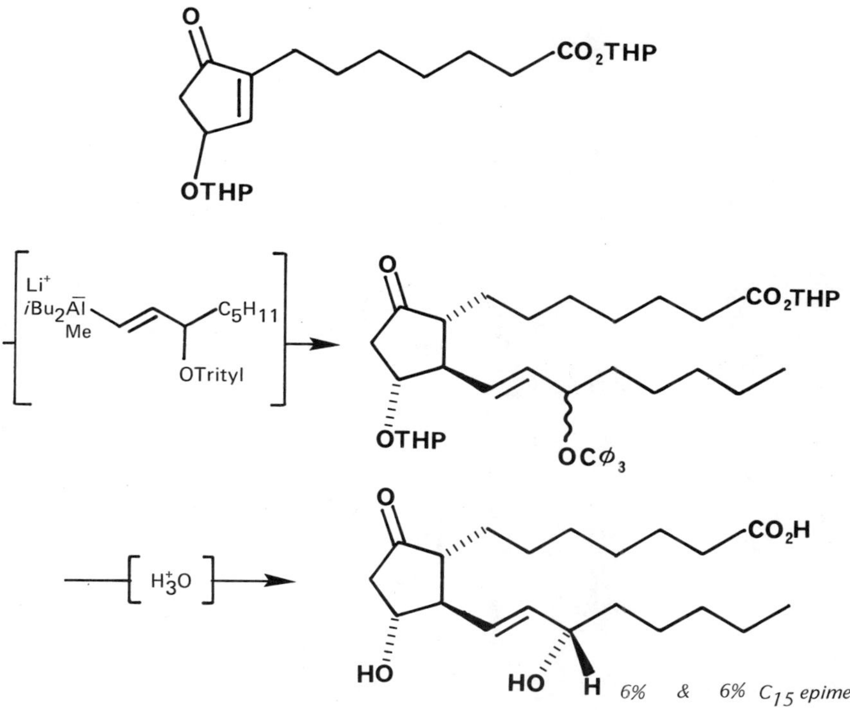

6% & 6% C_{15} epimer

27. M. Brawner Floyd & M. J. Weiss, *Prostaglandins*, 3, 921 (1973).
28. Various PG analogs have been made the 1,4-addition of alanates:
K. F. Bernady & M. J. Weiss, *Tet. Lett.*, 4083 (1972); K. F. Bernady, J. F. Poletto & M. J. Weiss, *Tet. Lett.*, 765 (1975); M. Brawner Floyd, R. E. Schaub & M. J. Weiss, *Prostaglandins*, **10**, 289 (1975).
29. Synthesis of PG analogs by the CuI catalyzed addition of appropriate Grignard reagents has also been carried out. R. E. Schaub & M. J. Weiss, *Tet. Lett.*, 129 (1973); K. F. Bernady & M. J. Weiss, *Prostaglandins*, 3, 505 (1973); J. F. Poletto, K. F. Bernady, D. Kupfer, R. Partridge & M. J. Weiss, *J. Med. Chem.*, **18**, 359 (1975).

Alanes have also been added to 4-alkoxycyclopentenones.[30] But unlike the alanates the alane approaches the cyclopentenone [7] *cis* to the C_{11} alkoxy group thus giving *cis* orientation of the substituents at C_{11} and C_{12}.

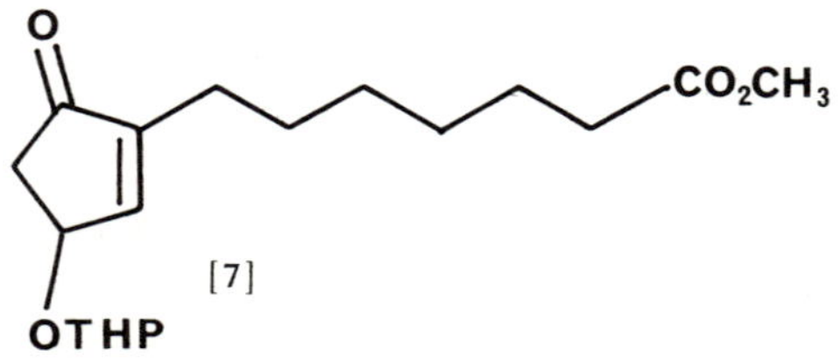

[7]

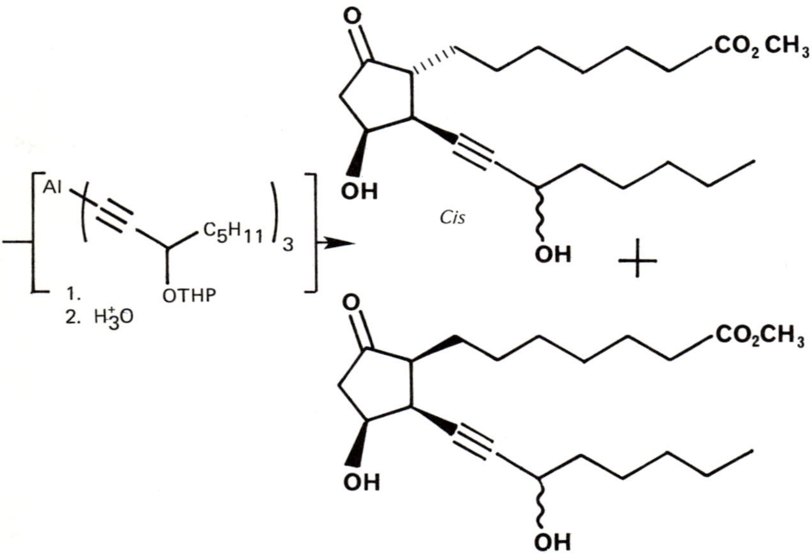

30. Similarly R_3Ga and RCu have also been added. R. Pappo & P. W. Collins, *Tet. Lett.*, 2627 (1972).

14

Trapping of Regiospecific Enolates

One of the shortest and simplest routes to prostaglandins involves the 1,4-addition of the β-chain to 4-alkoxycyclopent-2-enone and the trapping of the resulting enolate with either the whole α-chain or a potential α-chain. In the Michael addition the β-chain approaches *trans* to the C_{11} alkoxy group and the subsequent trapping of the enolate gives the all *trans* orientation of the three substituents about the cyclopentanone ring.

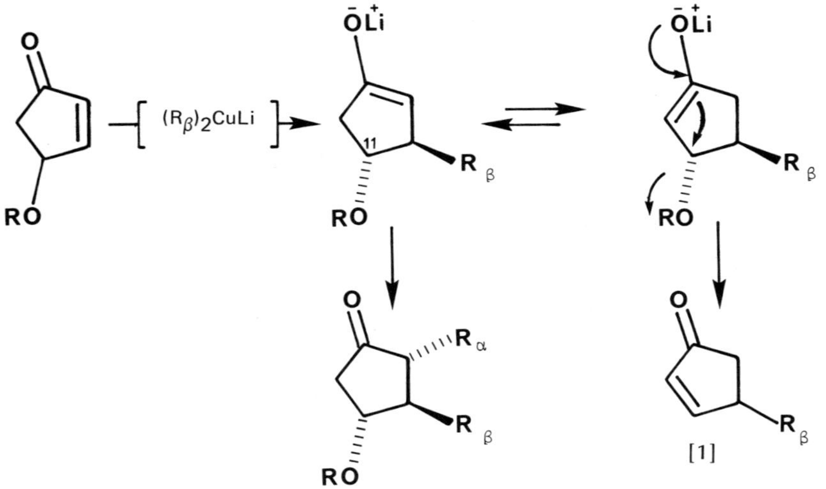

[1]

The choice of suitable electrophilic trapping reagents is crucial to the success of this approach. A slow rate of enolate trapping of the 4-alkoxycyclopent-2-enone leads to the equilibration of the enolate followed by the elimination of alkoxide to give the cyclopentenone [1]. For example, alkylation even with such reactive electrophiles as allylic halides is slow enough to allow equilibration of the enolate. Only interesting solution[1] to this problem was to use the highly reactive electrophile, formaldehyde, to give the aldol [2] which is then converted to the exocyclic enone [3]. The subsequent 1,4-addition of the remainder of the α-side chain to this enone [3] completes the synthesis. Thus two consecutive 1,4-additions are used to introduce the α- and β-chains.

---

1. G. Stork & M. Isobe, *J. Am. Chem. Soc.*, **97**, 6260 (1975)

SYNTHETIC PLAN[1]

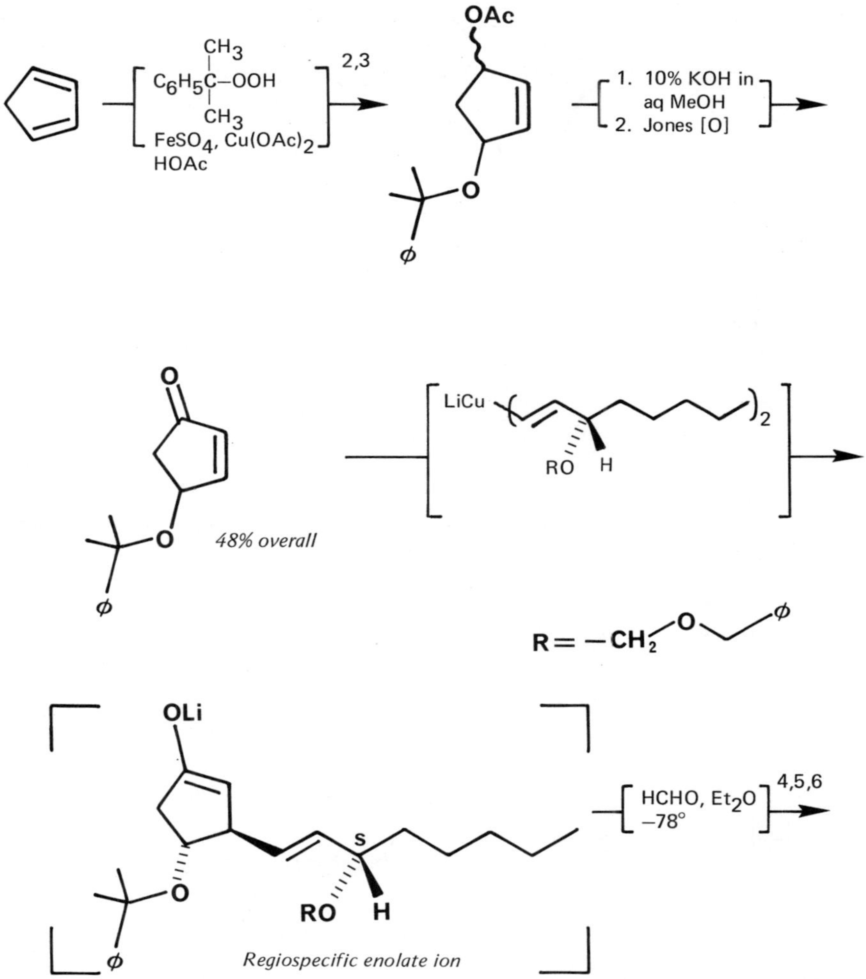

---

2. H. Haubenstock, P. G. Monnitt & P. E. Butler, *J. Org. Chem.*, **35**, 3208 (1970).
3. The cumyl group is a suitable alcohol protecting group, cleavable by Li/NH_3, which can be put on directly starting with cumylhydroperoxide. The benzyl or benzyloxymethyl group, though suitable, cannot be put on directly by an oxidation process.
4. The successful trapping of regiospecific enolates with formaldehyde has been earlier shown by G. Stork & J. D'Angelo, *J. Am. Chem. Soc.*, **96**, 7114 (1974).

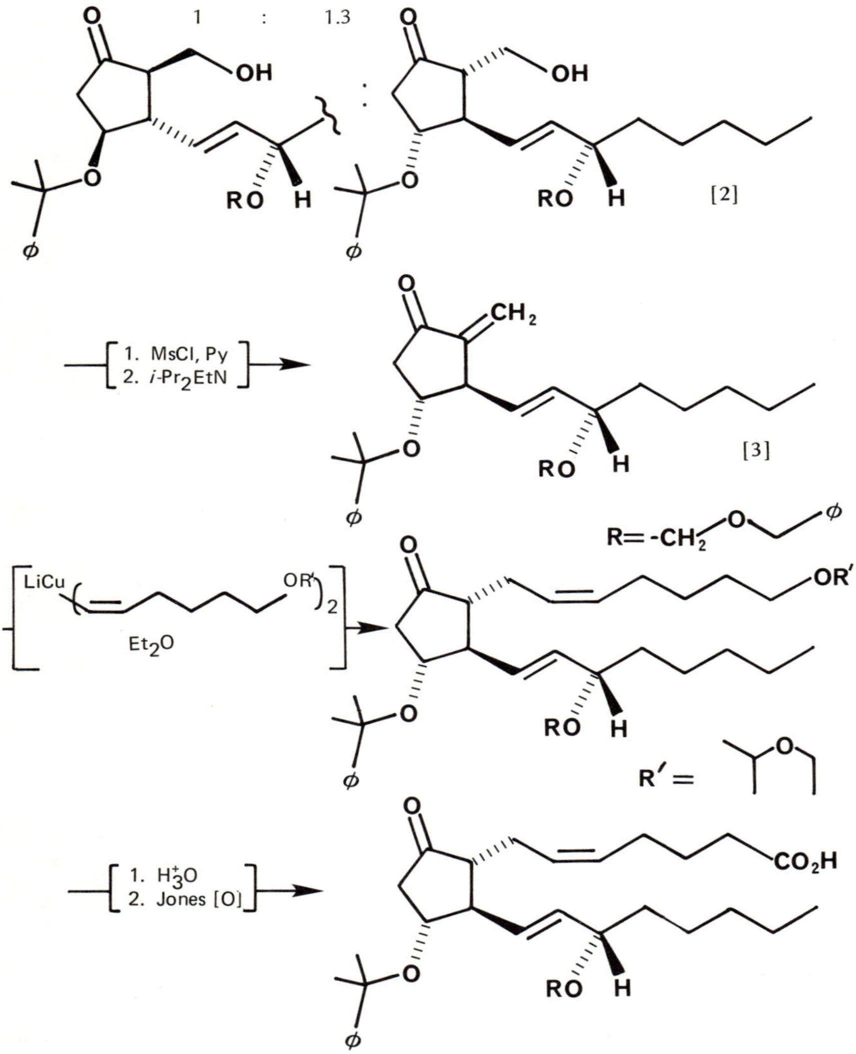

[2]

[3]

5. It has been shown that in the 1,4 addition of lithium dimethylcuprate to an enone, the enolate formed is a lithium enolate. H. O. House & J. M. Wilkins, *J. Org. Chem.*, 41, 4031 (1976).
6. The separation is postponed until the end.
7. Stork + Isobe, JACS, 97, 4745 (1975)

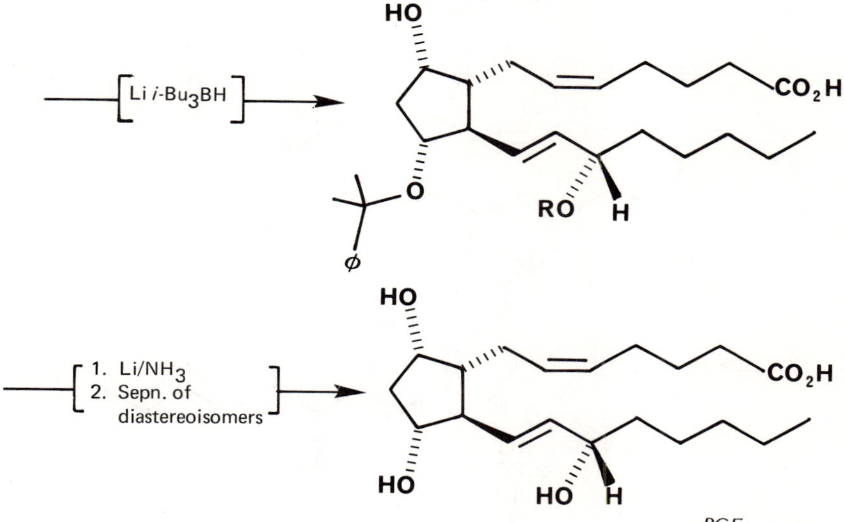

$PGF_{2\alpha}$

In an earlier approach[7] the regiospecific enolate was generated via a different reaction sequence. The formation of the desired enolate is based on the regiospecific formation of the bromohydrin from the cyclopentene [4].

Complementary Strategies

Stork-Kowalski (p. 261) *Stork-Isobe*[7]

SYNTHETIC STRATEGY

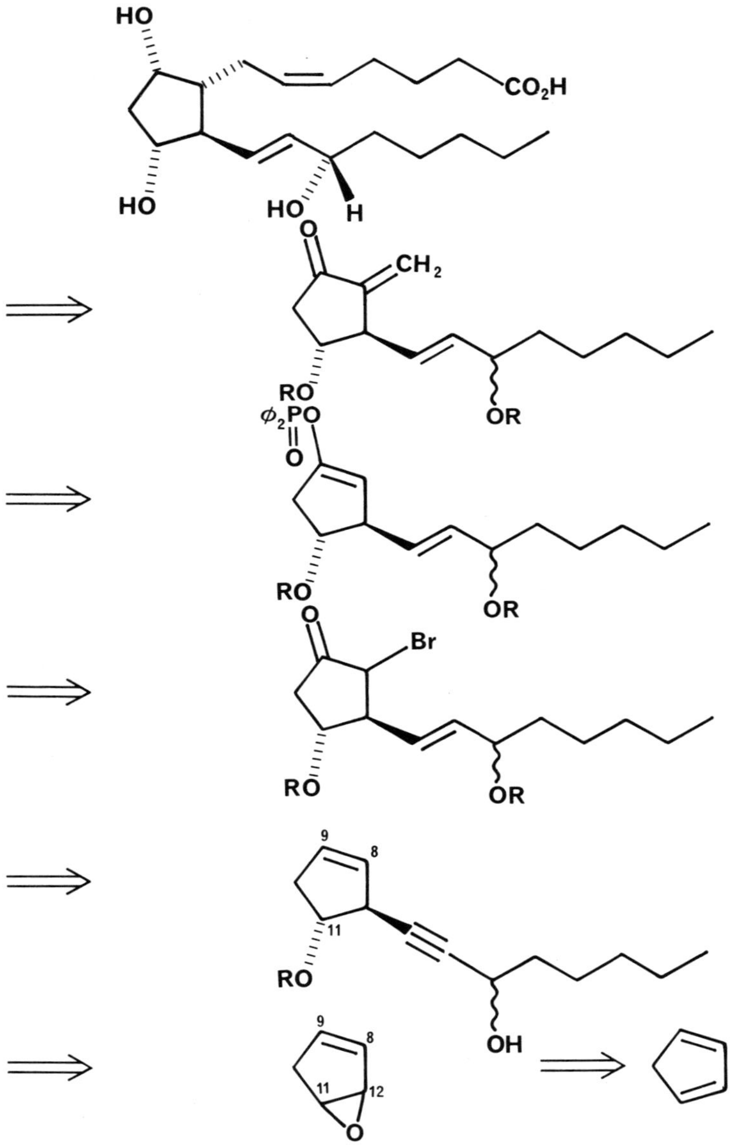

SYNTHETIC PLAN[7]

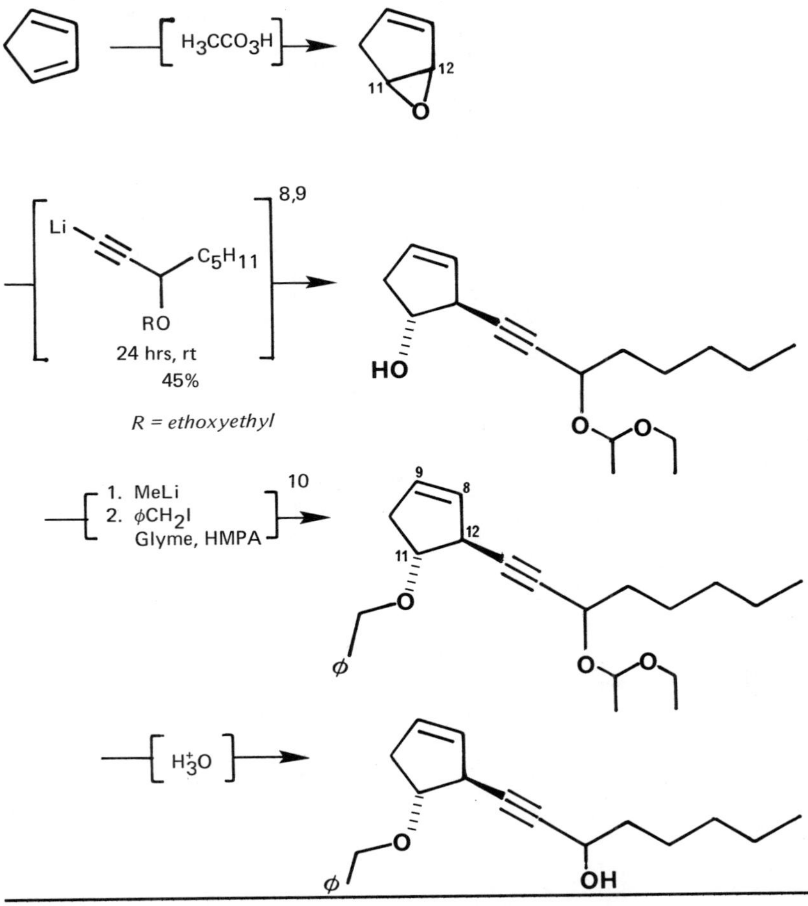

8. The epoxide is opened at the desired position (C_{12}) with this reagent. The reaction gives more complex results with Grignard reagents.
   G. Stork, K. Utimoto & C. Kowalski, in preparation.
9. Opening of 3,4-epoxycyclopentene with diethylhex-1-ynyl aluminum has also been studied. G. A. Crosby & R. A. Stephenson, *Chem. Commun.*, 287 (1975).
10. Acetal type protecting groups are sufficiently more electron withdrawing to lead to some elimination during the generation and subsequent trapping of the eventual cyclopentanone enolate. On the other hand, protection of the allylic alcohol function by an electron withdrawing group is helpful in preventing electrophilic attack on the adjacent (C_{13}-C_{14}) double bond.

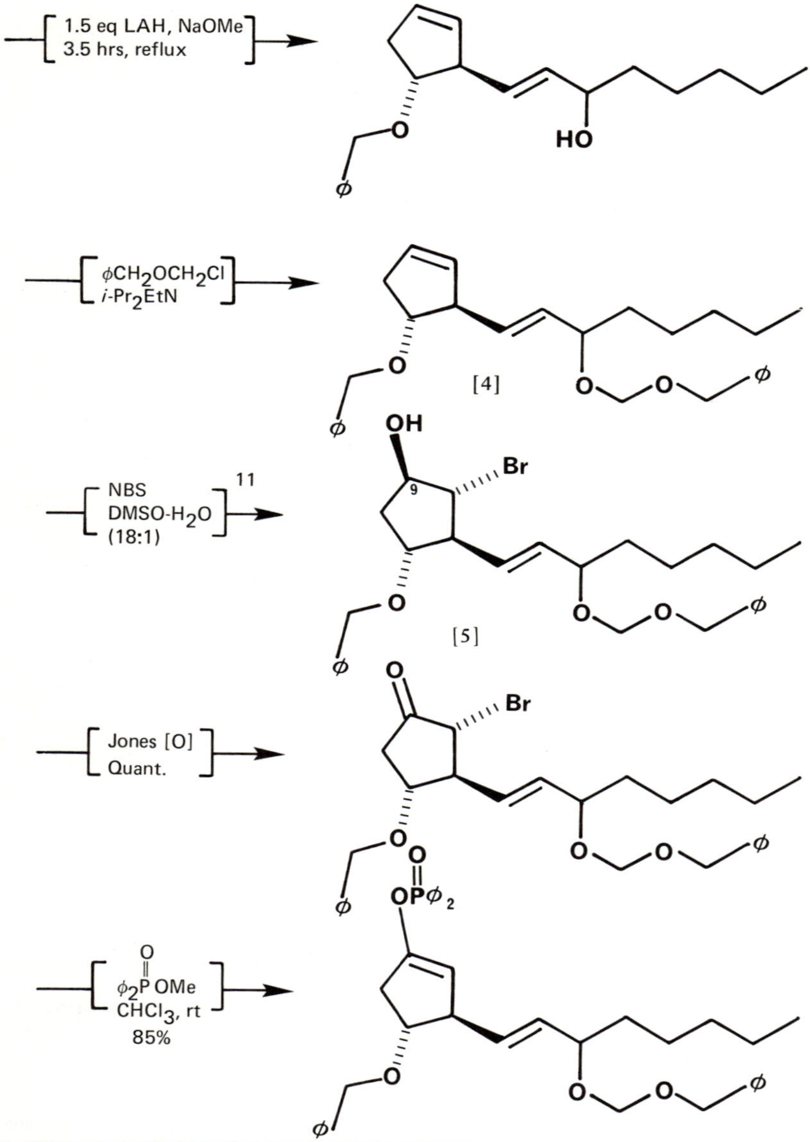

11. The intermediate kinetic bromonium ion is displaced at the less hindered site (C_9, further from the β-side chain) to give the desired bromohydrin.

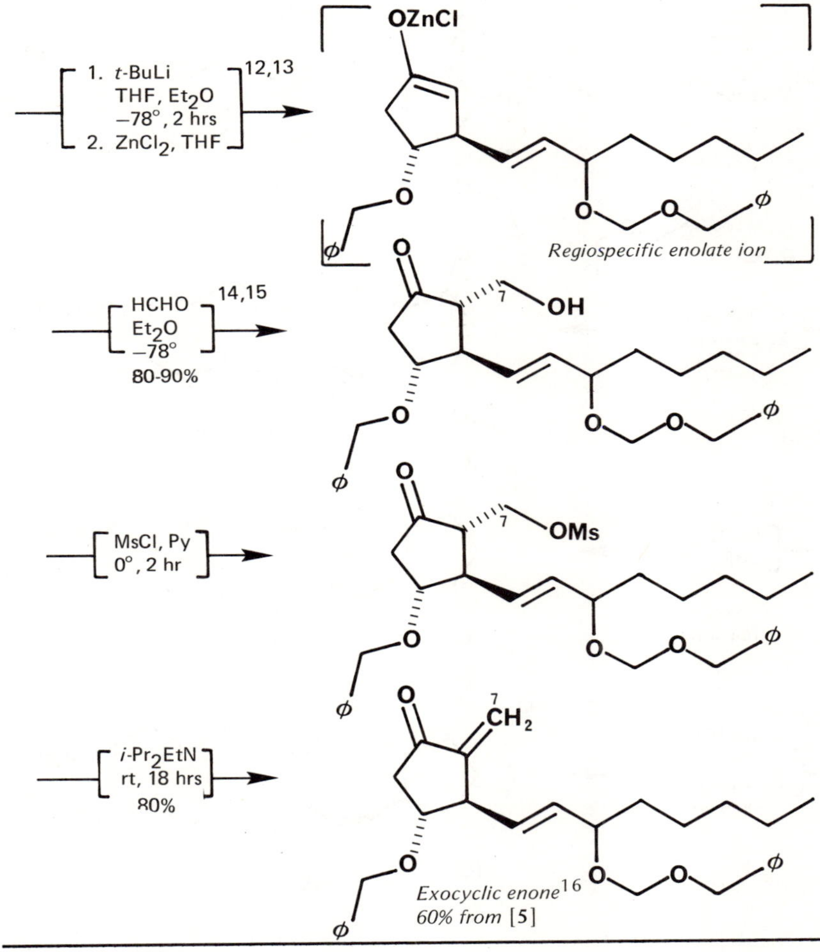

12. Unlike enol phosphates, enol phosphinates can be cleaved at sufficiently low temperatures to allow the survival of this regiospecific enolate. Generation of enolates from derivatives of this type was introduced by I. J. Borowitz, E. W. R. Casper, R. K. Crouch & K. C. Yee, *J. Org. Chem.*, **37**, 3873 (1972).
13. Use of the Zn-enolate may prevent the retro-aldol reaction. G. Stork & P. Tardella, (unpublished results) (1967); H. O. House, D. S. Crumrine, A. Y. Teranishi & H. D. Ohmstead, *J. Am. Chem. Soc.*, **95**, 3310 (1973).
14. Attempted trapping of the lithium enolate with allyl iodide at −20° C gave only 15% of the desired alkylation product.
15. The regiospecific enolate trapping method leads directly to the synthesis of $PGF_{2\alpha}$. The synthesis of the E prostaglandins would require juggling of protecting groups.

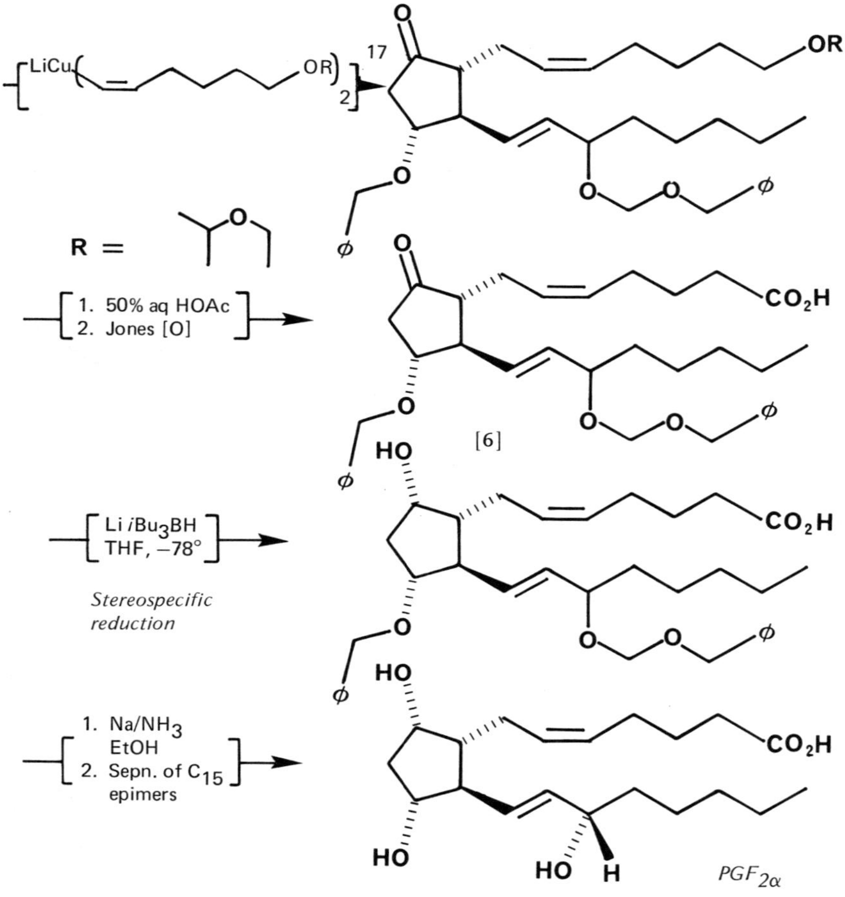

60% from [6]

---

16. This key intermediate has also been made by a different route. For further details see p. 46.
17. The synthesis of the ω -alkoxy-*cis*-vinyliodide used the method developed by K. Untch et. al. A. F. Kluge, K. G. Untch & J. H. Fried, *J. Am. Chem. Soc.*, **94**, 9256 (1972).

The chiral form of the cyclopentenone [7] has been synthesized from D (—) tartaric acid.[18] This may be an useful intermediate for the Stork-Isobe synthesis if a suitable protecting group is found for the secondary alcohol.

SYNTHETIC PLAN[18]

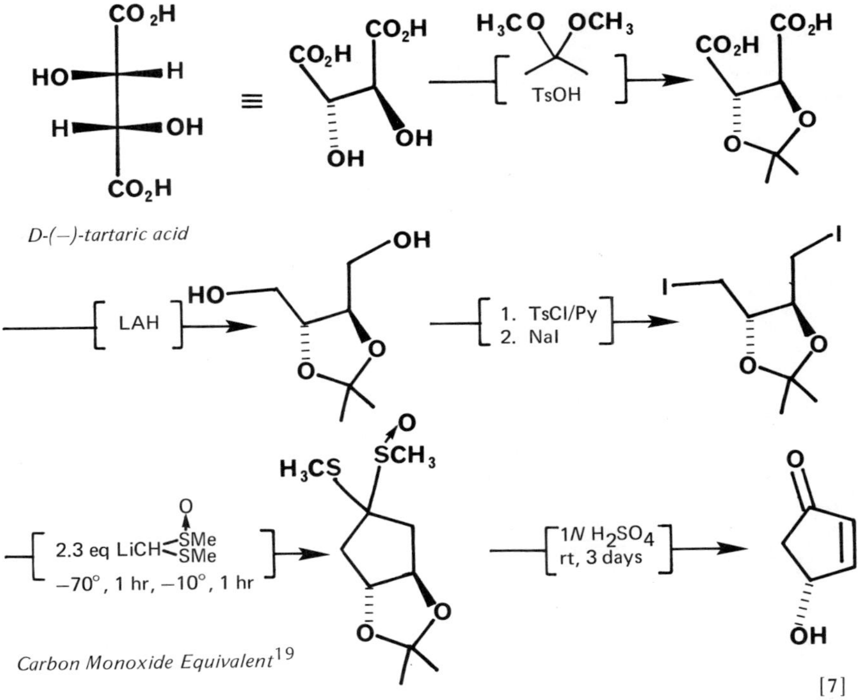

[7]

$[\alpha]_D^{28} = 81^\circ$

For another carbon moxide equivalent see G. Stork, A. Leong & A. M. Touzin, *J. Org. Chem.*, **41**, 3491 (1976)

---

18. K. Ogura, M. Yamashita & G. Tsuchihashi, *Tet. Lett.*, 759 (1976).
19. K. Ogura, M. Yamashita, S. Furukawa, M. Suzuki, & G. Tsuchihashi, *Tet. Lett.*, 2767 (1975).

15

Syntheses from Chiral Precursors

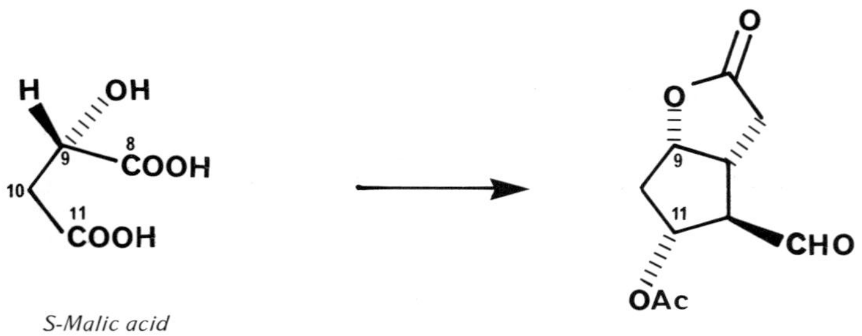

S-Malic acid

Several syntheses of natural prostaglandins have been reported in the recent past which circumvent resolution. Such syntheses start with chiral precursors and the asymmetry at the other centers is induced by various methods.

The first such synthesis reported by Johnson,[1] starts from optically active malic acid. The carbon atom bearing the secondary alcohol function in *S*-malic acid becomes the C_9 atom of the prostaglandins. This C_9 asymmetry is then used to induce asymmetry at C_{12} in a catalytic hydrogenation step. This is followed by a stereospecific reduction of the C_{11} ketone to give the desired configuration of the hydroxyl group at C_{11}.

1. K. G. Paul, F. Johnson & D. Favara, *J. Am. Chem. Soc.*, 98, 1285 (1976).

SYNTHETIC STRATEGY

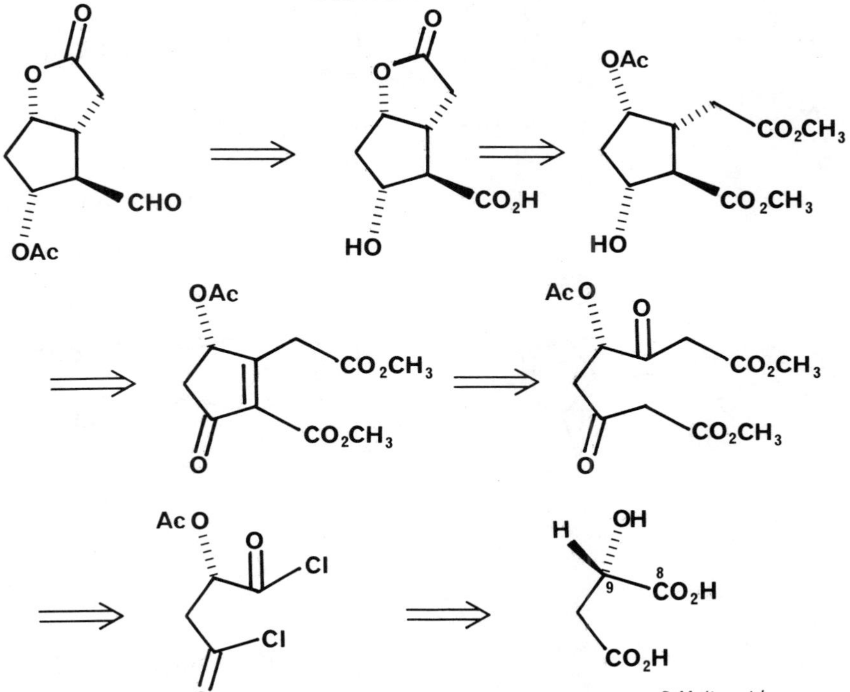

S-Malic acid

SYNTHETIC PLAN[1]

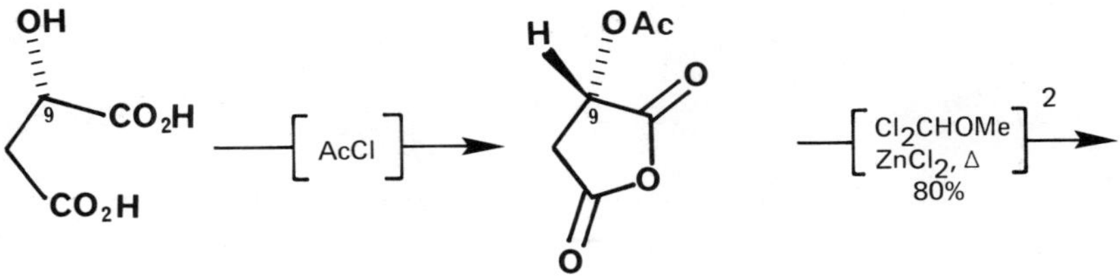

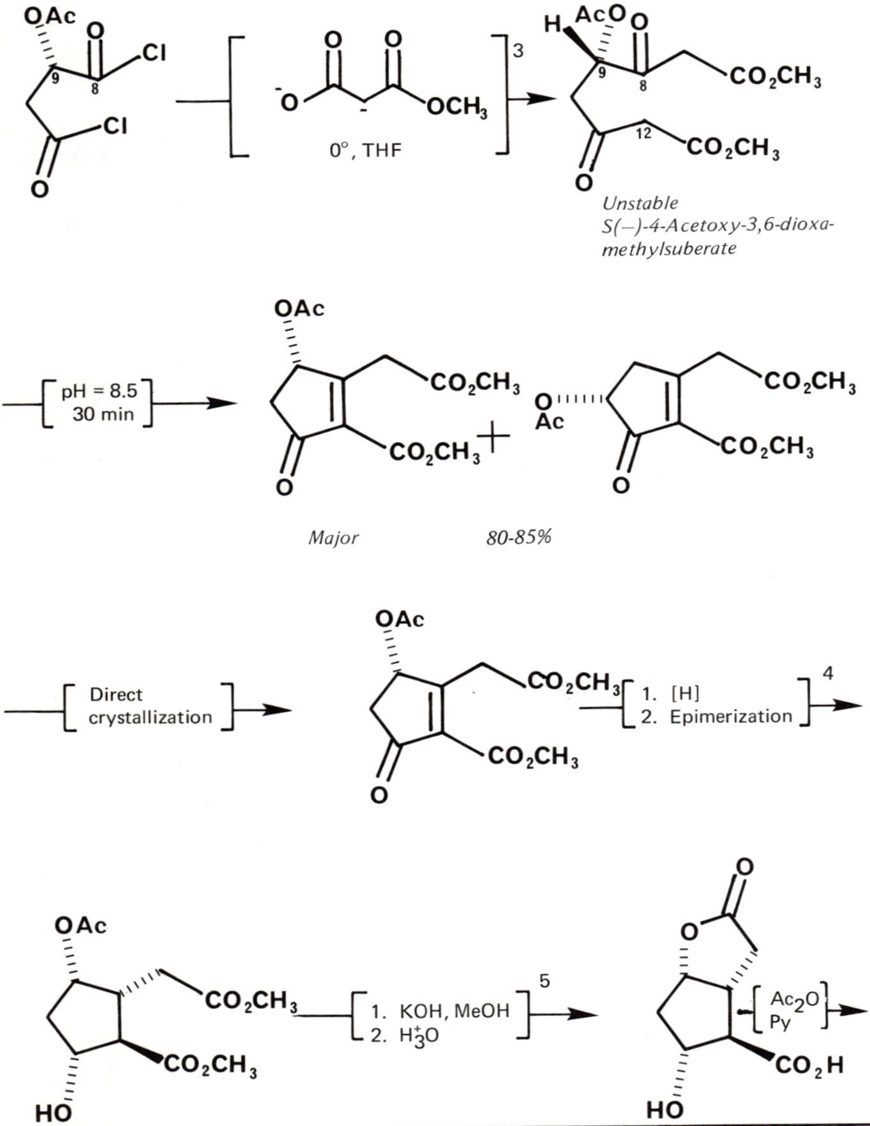

2. A. Rieche & H. Gross, *Chem. Ber.*, **92**, 83 (1959).

3. This dianion is a $\overline{C}H_2CO_2R$ equivalent. R. E. Ireland & J. A. Marshall, *J. Am. Chem. Soc.*, **81**, 2907 (1959).

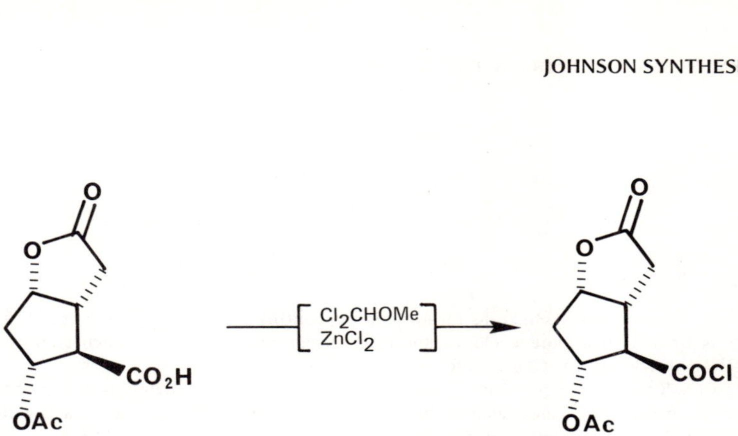

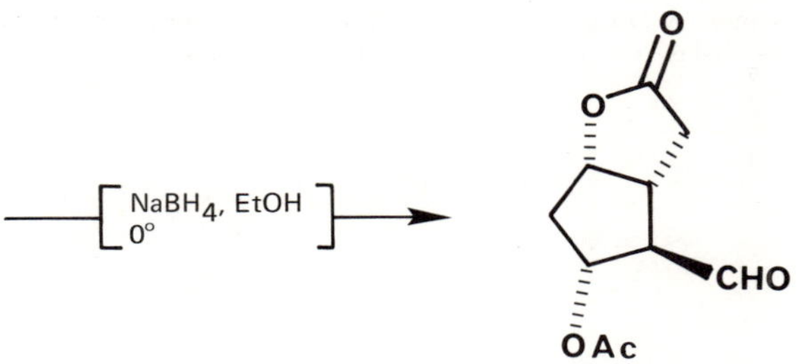

30% overall yield from S-malic acid

Corey lactone

---

4. The hydrogenation takes place from the less hindered side. Thus the acetoxy group controls the stereochemistry of the adjacent center. Contrast, however, reduction of 2-cyclopentylidene-1-methoxy cyclopentane which gives 92% of the *trans* isomer of 2-cyclopentylcyclopentanol. T. J. Howard, *Recl. Trav. Chim. Pays-Bays,* **83**, 992 (1964).
5. The two ester functions are thus distinguished.

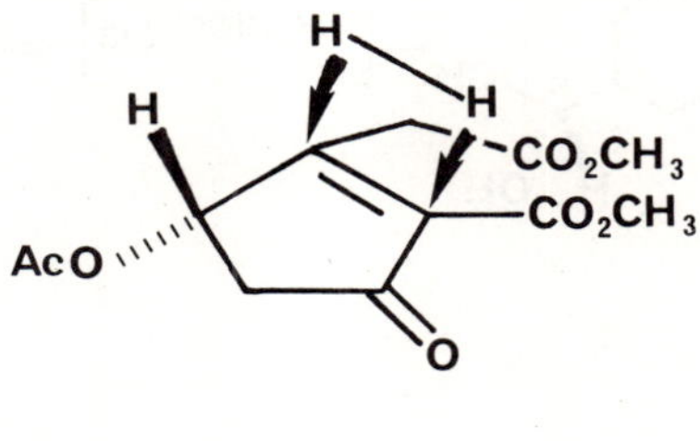

There are very few syntheses which demonstrate steric control over the C_{15} asymmetric center, that which is isolated from the cyclopentane ring, except that by Corey, which employs the stereoselective reduction of the C_{15} ketone with hindered borohydrides.[6]

An elegant solution to the problem of steric control at C_{15} has been demonstrated by Stork[7] whose approach makes use of the available chirality of natural sugars. The synthesis starts with the appropriate carbohydrate, L-rhamnose, having the desired asymmetry at C_{14} and the C_{15} alcohol center. The chirality at C_{14} is then transferred to C_{12}, via a Claisen rearrangement to give the correct chirality.[8,9,10] The asymmetry at C_8 is easily attained by virtue of the more stable *trans* configuration of the α- and β- chains. The first synthesis of PGA_2 utilizing this principle was reported by Stork and Raucher.[7]

---

6. E. J. Corey, K. B. Becker, &. R. K. Varma, *J. Am. Chem. Soc.*, **94**, 8616 (1972). For syntheses controlling the C_{15} asymmetric center see: J. Martel, E. Toromanoff, J. Mathieu & G. Nomine, *Tet. Lett.*, 1491 (1972). (See p. 61); K. Kondo, T. Umemoto, Y. Takahatake & D. Tunemoto, *Tet. Lett.*, 113 (1977) & D. F. Taber, *J. Am. Chem. Soc.*, **99**, 3513 (1976).See p.79
7. G. Stork & S. Raucher, *J. Am. Chem. Soc.*, **98**, 1583 (1976).
8. For previous examples of synthesis using a C-O chiral center to induce chirality at a C-C center see:
   T. M. Dawson, J. Dixon, P. S. Littlewood & B. Lythgoe, *J. Chem. Soc., C,* 2960 (1971). (Synthesis of $Precalciferol_3$).
9. R. K. Hill & A. G. Edwards, *Tet. Lett.*, 3239 (1964).
10. M. Uskokovic et al., personal communication.:

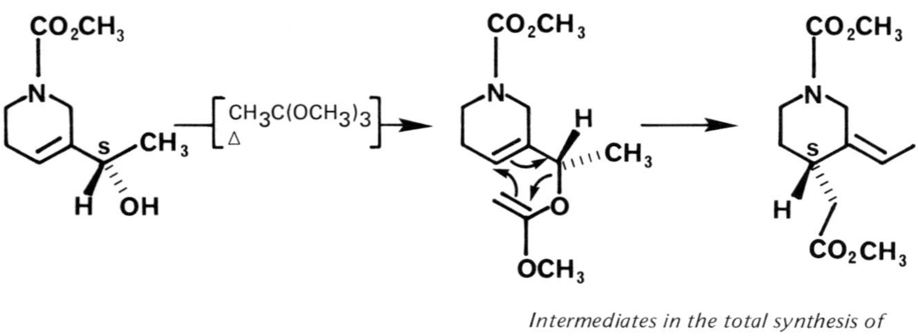

Intermediates in the total synthesis of cinchona and heteroyohimbine alkaloids.

SYNTHETIC STRATEGY[11]

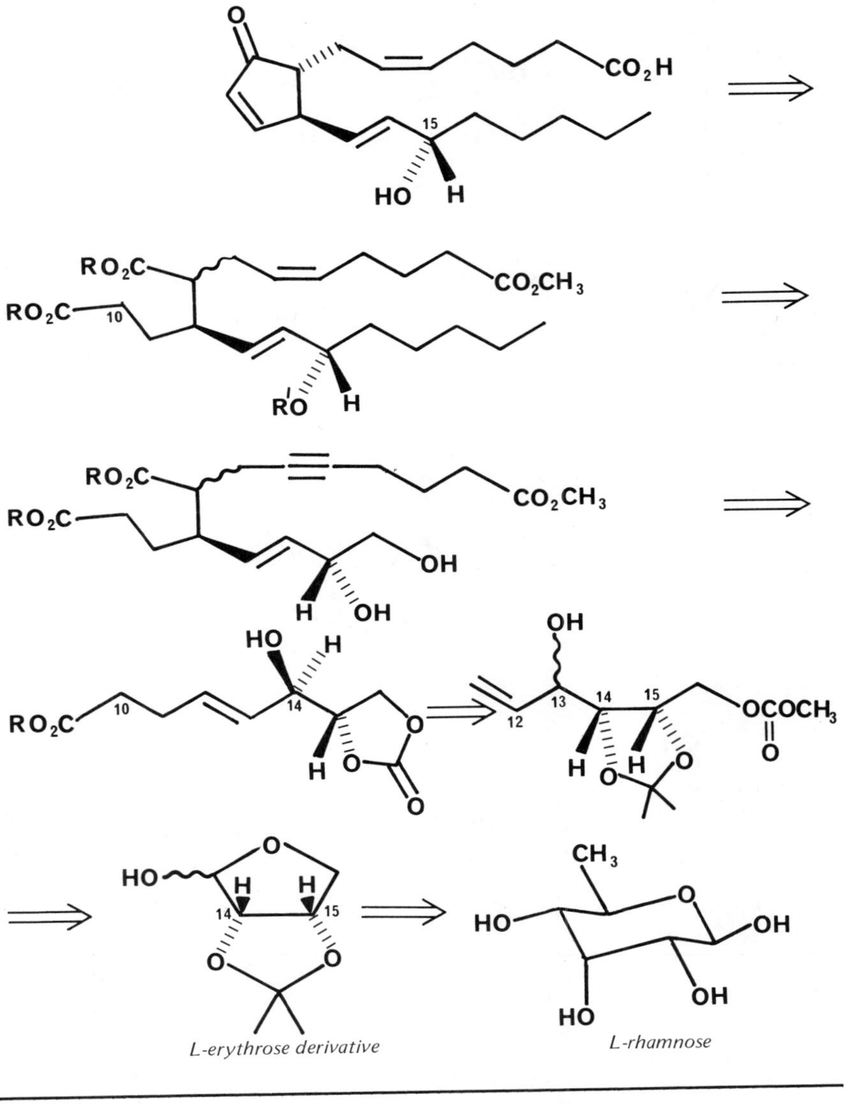

11. For an interesting discussion on the use of carbohydrates in synthesis, see B. Fraser-Reid, *Accounts Chem. Res.*, 8, 192 (1975).

SYNTHETIC PLAN[7]

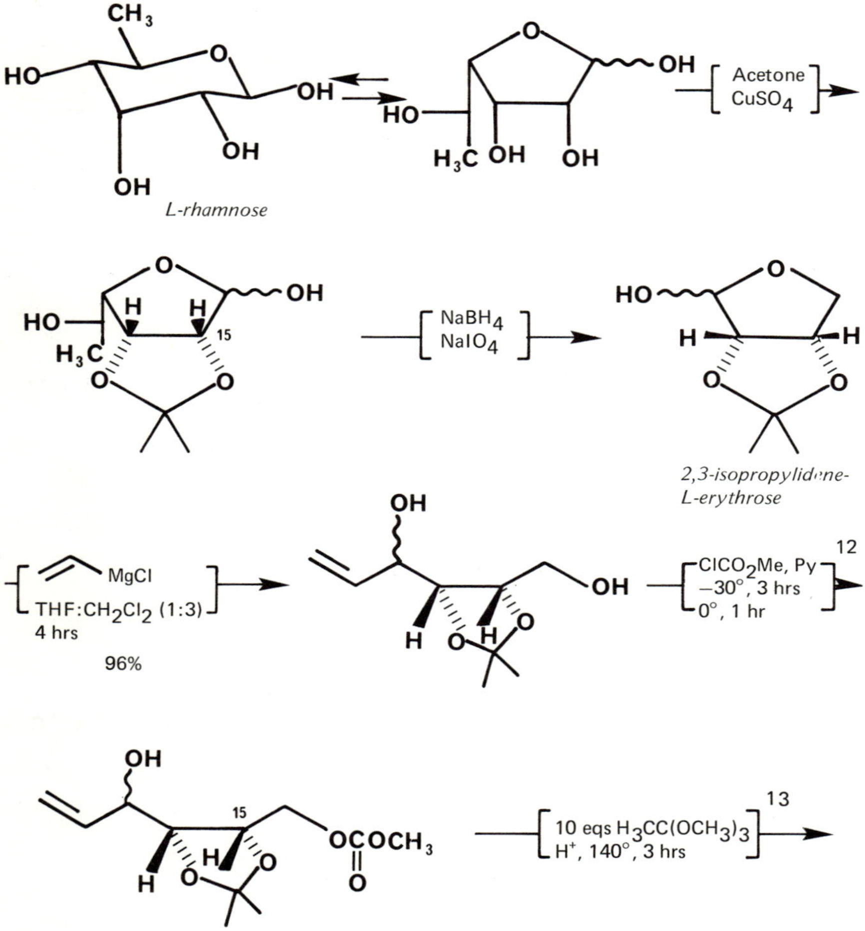

---

12. Attempts to do Claisen rearrangement on the diol led to the formation of the cyclic orthoester:

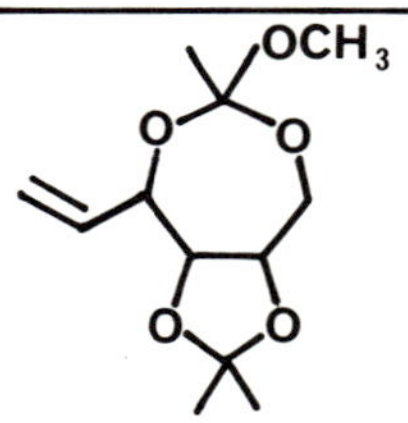

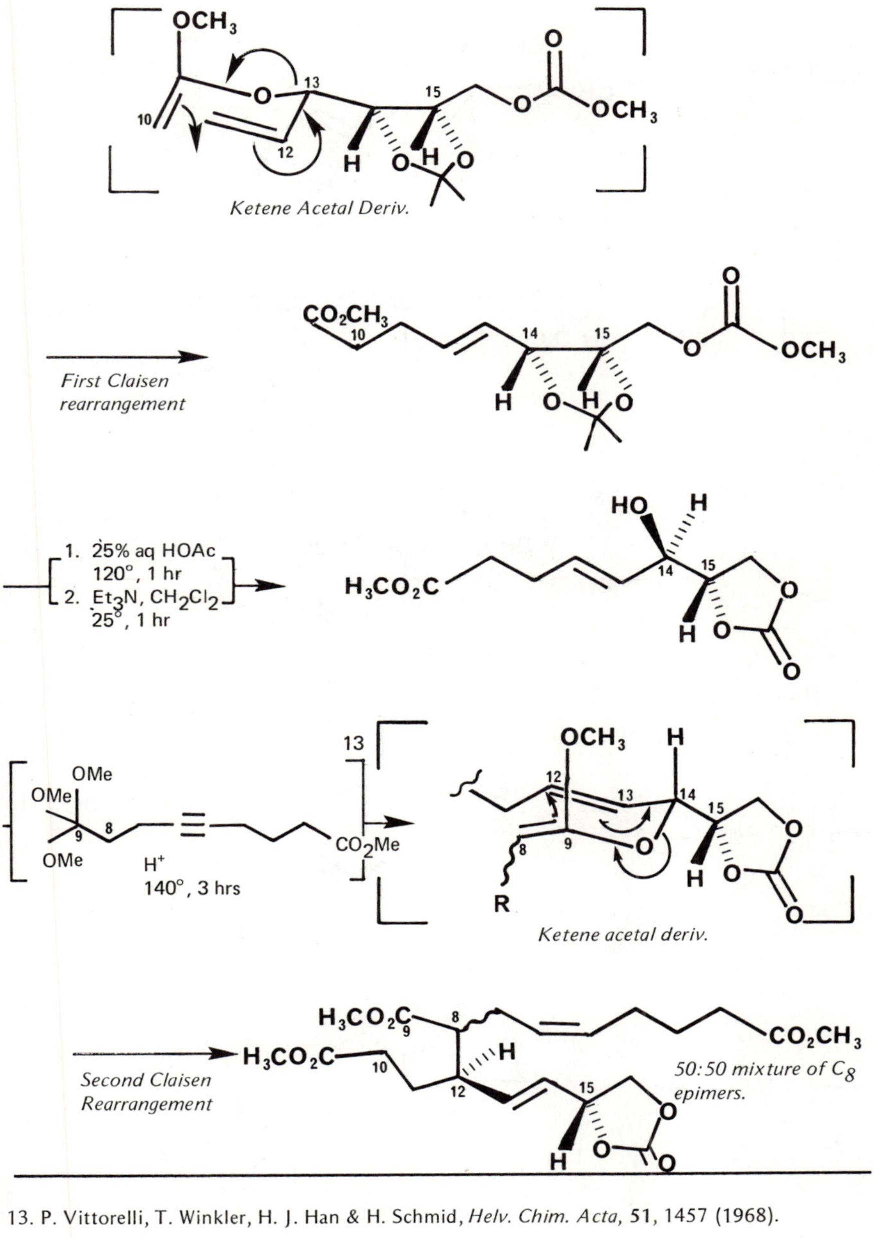

13. P. Vittorelli, T. Winkler, H. J. Han & H. Schmid, *Helv. Chim. Acta*, **51**, 1457 (1968).

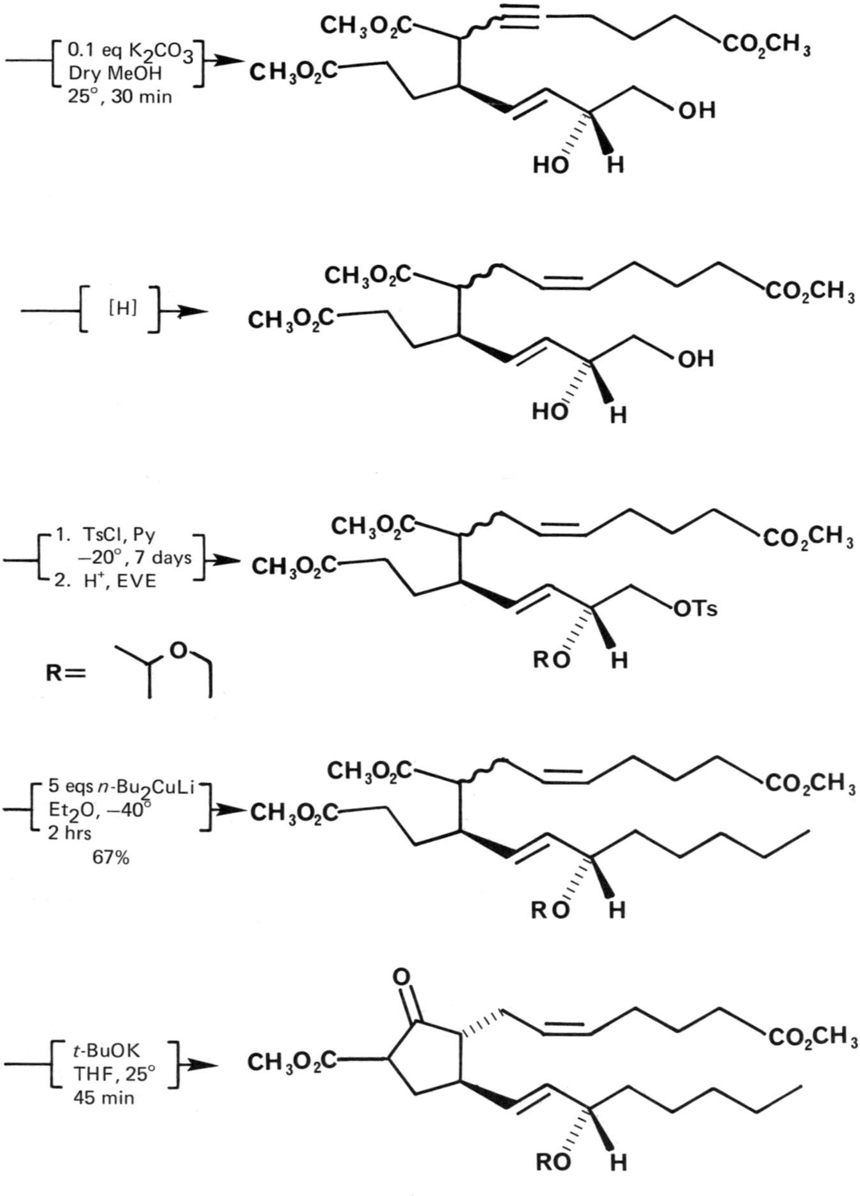
0.1 eq K_2CO_3
Dry MeOH
25°, 30 min
CH_3O_2C
CO_2CH_3
OH
HO
H
[H]
1. TsCl, Py
−20°, 7 days
2. H⁺, EVE
OTs
RO
R=
O
5 eqs n-Bu_2CuLi
Et_2O, −40°
2 hrs
67%
t-BuOK
THF, 25°
45 min
O

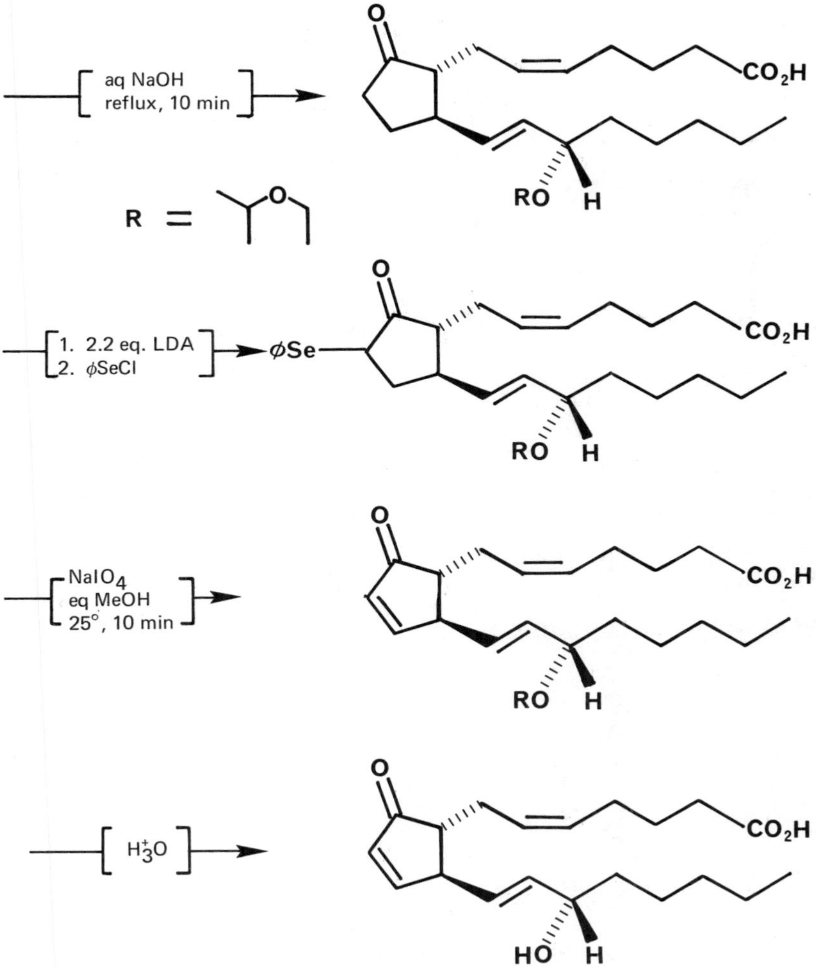

$[\alpha]_D^{20} = +130°$ *(+)-PGA$_2$*

7.7% Overall yield from
2,3-isopropylidene
L-erythrose

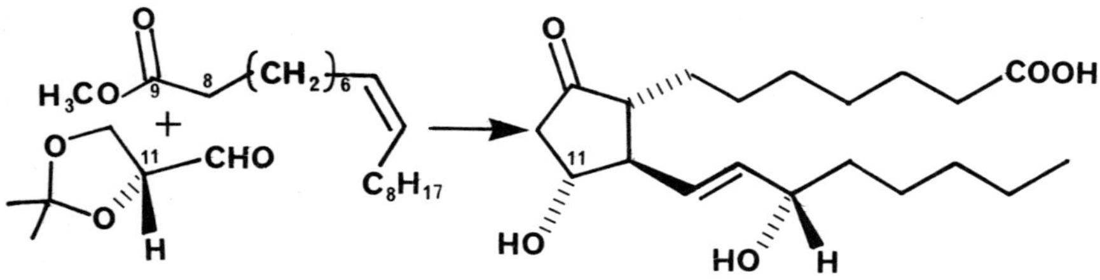

In this synthesis of PGE_1,[14,15] the correct absolute configuration at C_{11} is produced from D-glyceraldehyde via the chiral enone [1]. This center serves to control the chirality of the rest of the PGE_1 molecule by means of an efficient kinetic resolution.

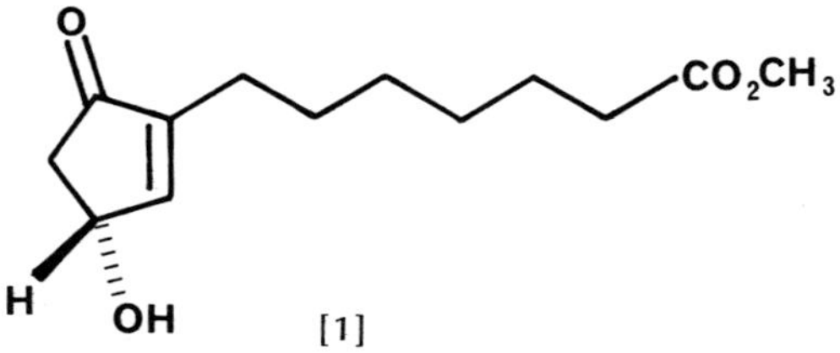

[1]

14. G. Stork & T. Takahashi,, *J. Am. Chem. Soc.*, 99, 1275 (1977).
15. T. Takahashi, Ph.D. Dissertation Thesis, Columbia University (1976).

SYNTHETIC STRATEGY

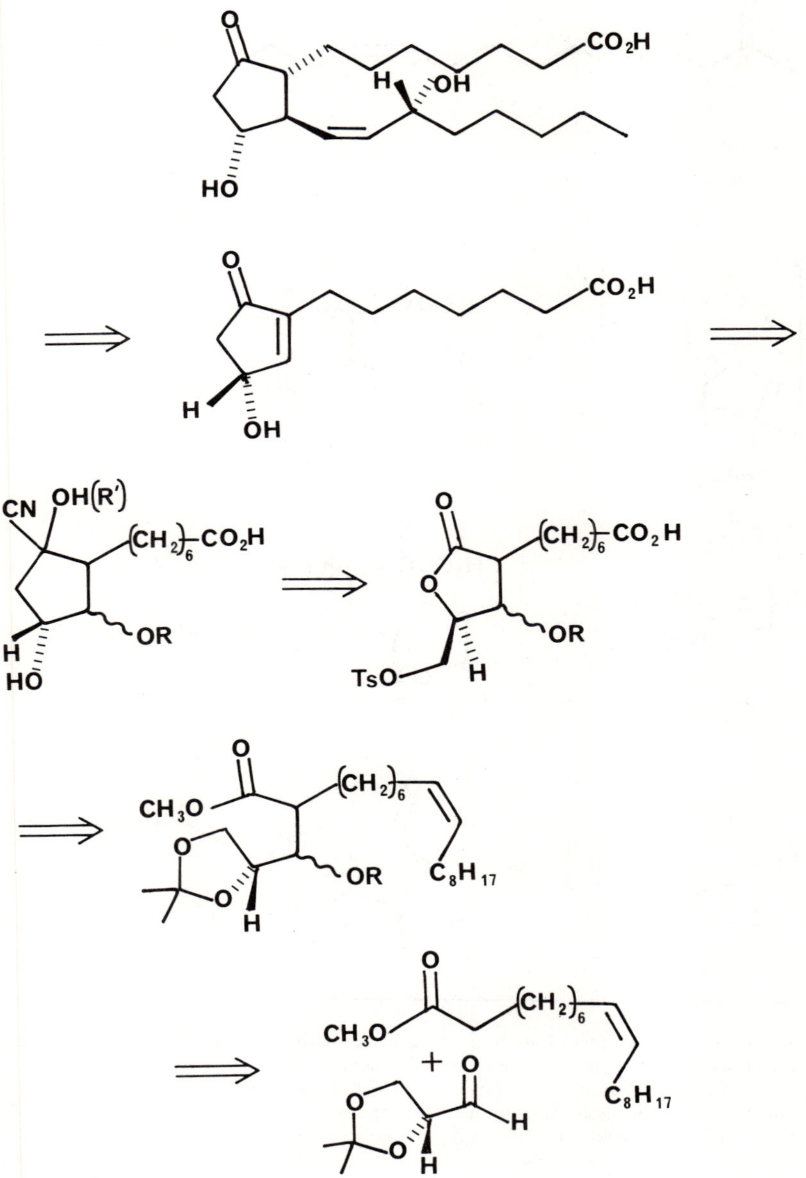

SYNTHETIC PLAN[14,15]

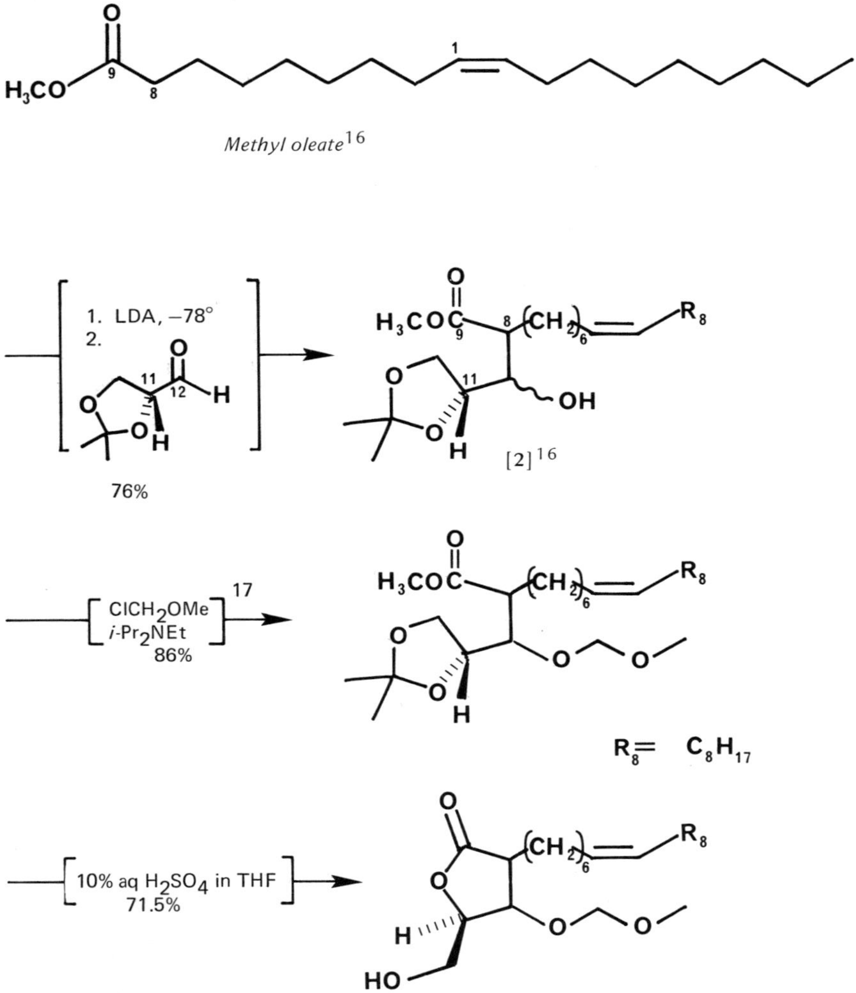

---

16. The double bond of methyl oleate becomes so placed in the aldol [2] as to become the latent carboxyl in the eventual heptanoic acid chain (α-chain).
17. The correct choice of protecting group was crucial because stability to acidic conditions used in the selective hydrolysis of isopropylidene and ethoxyethyl groups was necessary and furthermore the subsequent elimination required a good departing group. Thus methoxymethyl group was chosen.

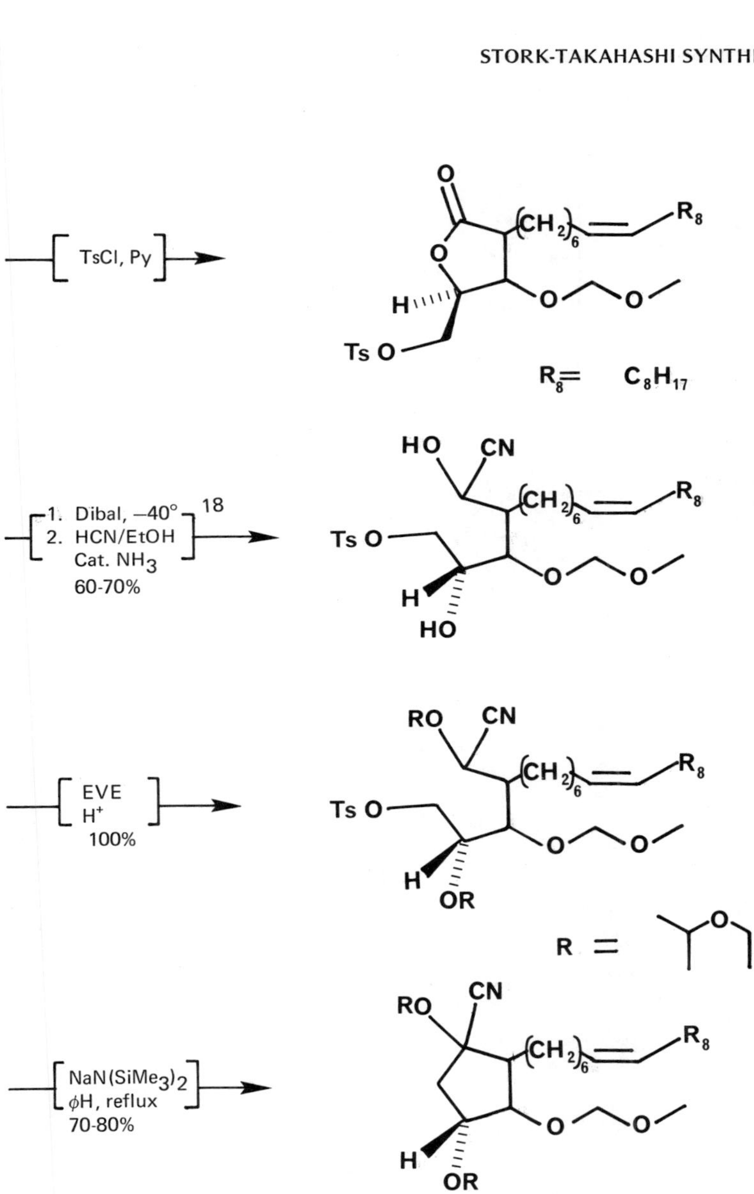

18. The use of cyanohydrin as an acyl carbanion equivalent is advantageous because they are stable to subsequent acid treatment thereby maintaining the integrity of the latent β-ketol system. In addition, the cyanohydrin moiety is compatible with the oxidizing conditions required to transform the olefin to the carboxylic acid.
For a recent review on acyl carbanion equivalents see: "New Horizons in Carbonyl Chemistry: Reagents for Nucleophilic Acylation." O. William Lever, Jr., *Tet.*, 32, 1943 (1976).

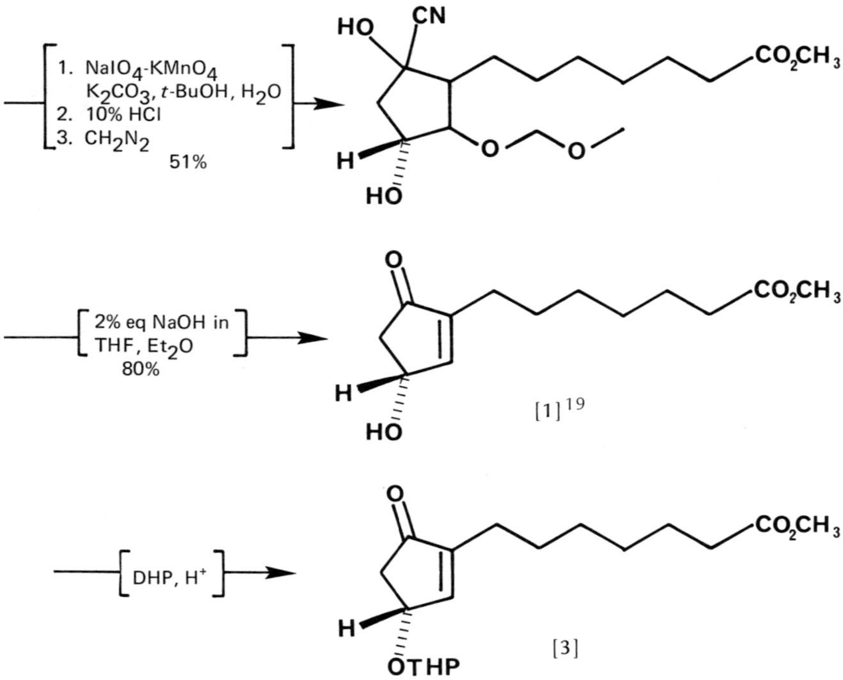

19. This cyclopentenone [1] has been made previously by a combination of chemical and microbiological methods: C. J. Sih, R. G. Salomon, P. Price, R. Sood & G. Peruzzotti, *J. Am. Chem. Soc.*, **97**, 857 (1975).
20. The Syntex group observed that the (+) component of the dl-cyclopentenone (**4**, 1 equiv.) as its THP ether, reacts considerably faster than its antipode with the optically active divinyl cuprate (**5**, 3 equivs.) derived from the *cis*-vinyliodide.
A. F. Kluge, K. G. Untch & J. H. Fried, *J. Am. Chem. Soc.*, **94**, 9256 (1972).

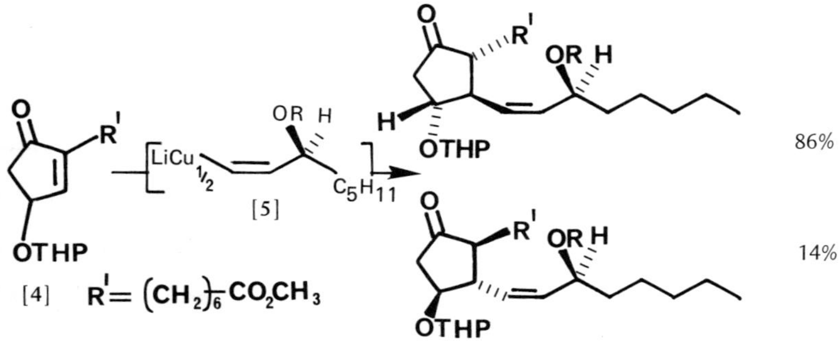

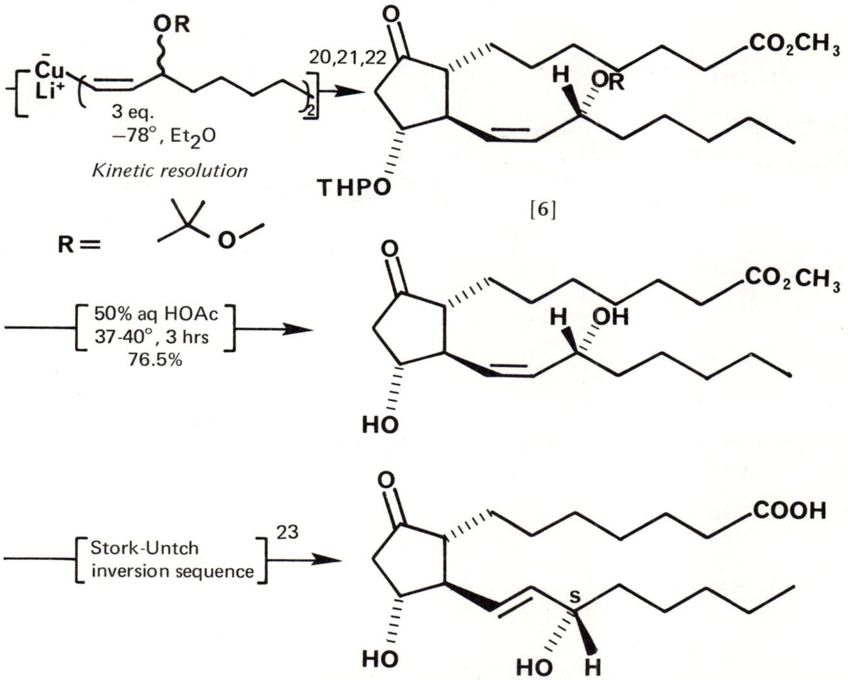

21. As a first approximation, the maximum kinetic resolution should be obtained by the reversal of the Syntex process, that is, by the reaction of 1 equiv. of (*R*)-cyclopentenone [3] with 3 equivs. of the dl-side chain. This is because there would be none of the wrong enantiomer of the enone to react with the excess of divinyl cuprate. The extent of kinetic resolution obtained by such an operation should either be equal to or higher than the Syntex observation. Indeed, only the desired isomer [**6**] was obtained.

22. The ratio 86:14 of the two diastereoisomers obtained in the Syntex experiment suggests a difference of 2-3 K cal/mole between the two diastereomeric transition states.

Syntex:	AA*	+	B	→	AB	+	A*B
Columbia:	A	+	BB*	→	AB	+	B*

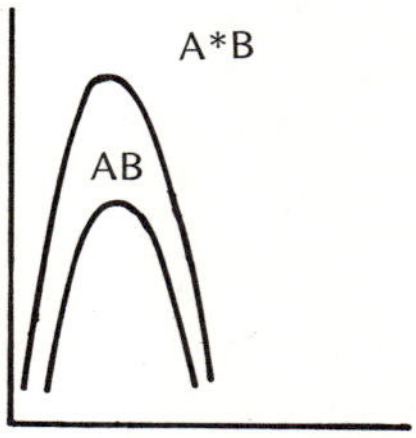

A = optically active cyclopentenone
AA* = *dl*-cyclopentenone
B = optically active divinyl cuprate
BB* = *dl*-divinyl cuprate

23. J. G. Miller, W. Kurz, K. G. Untch & G. Stork, *J. Am. Chem. Soc.*, **96**, 6774 (1974).

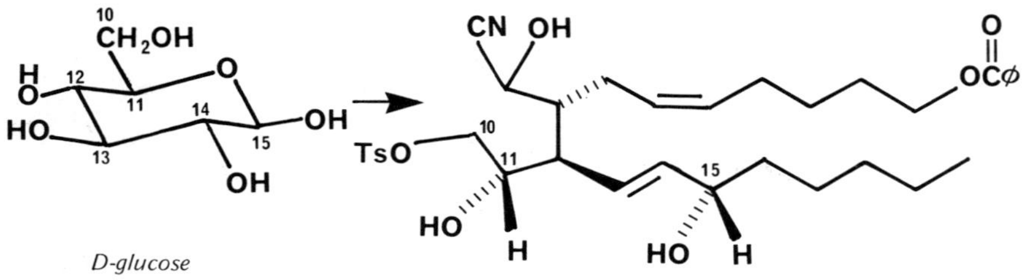

Subsequently the carbohydrate, D-glucose, was so chosen such that the chirality at both C_{11} and at C_{15} were correct.[24,25]

24. T. Takahashi, Ph.D. Dissertation Thesis, Columbia University (1976).
25. G. Stork & T. Takahashi, (unpublished results).

SYNTHETIC STRATEGY

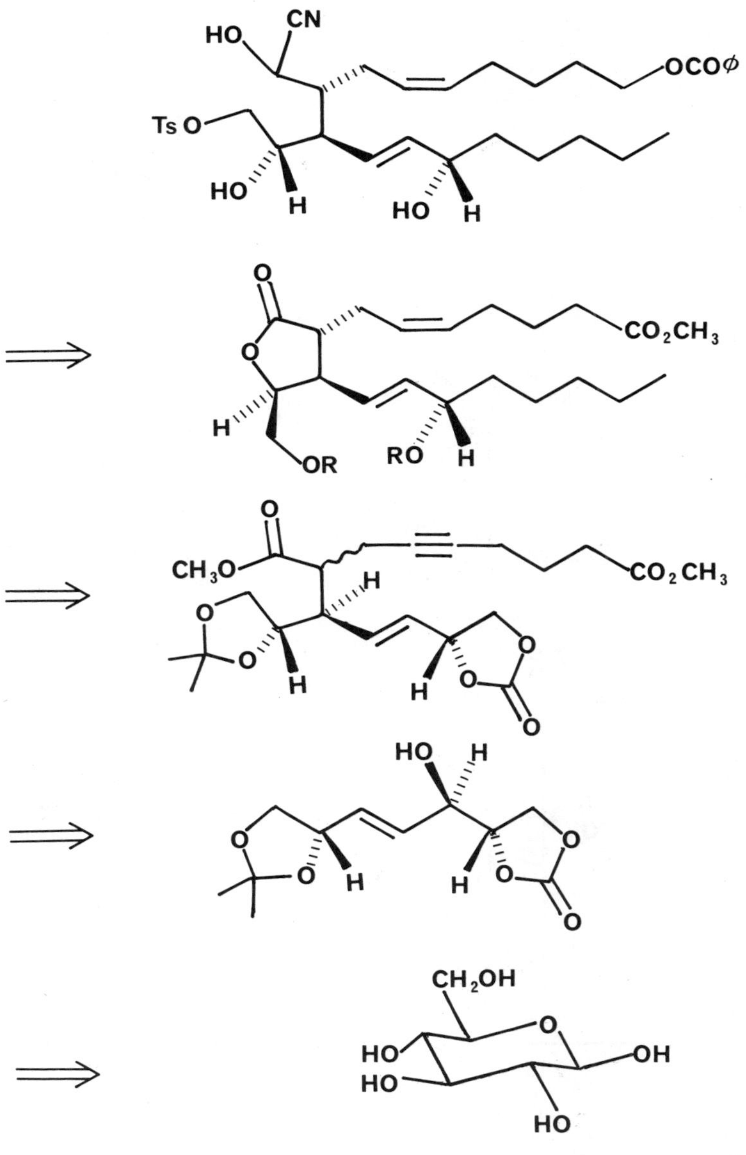

SYNTHETIC PLAN[24,25]

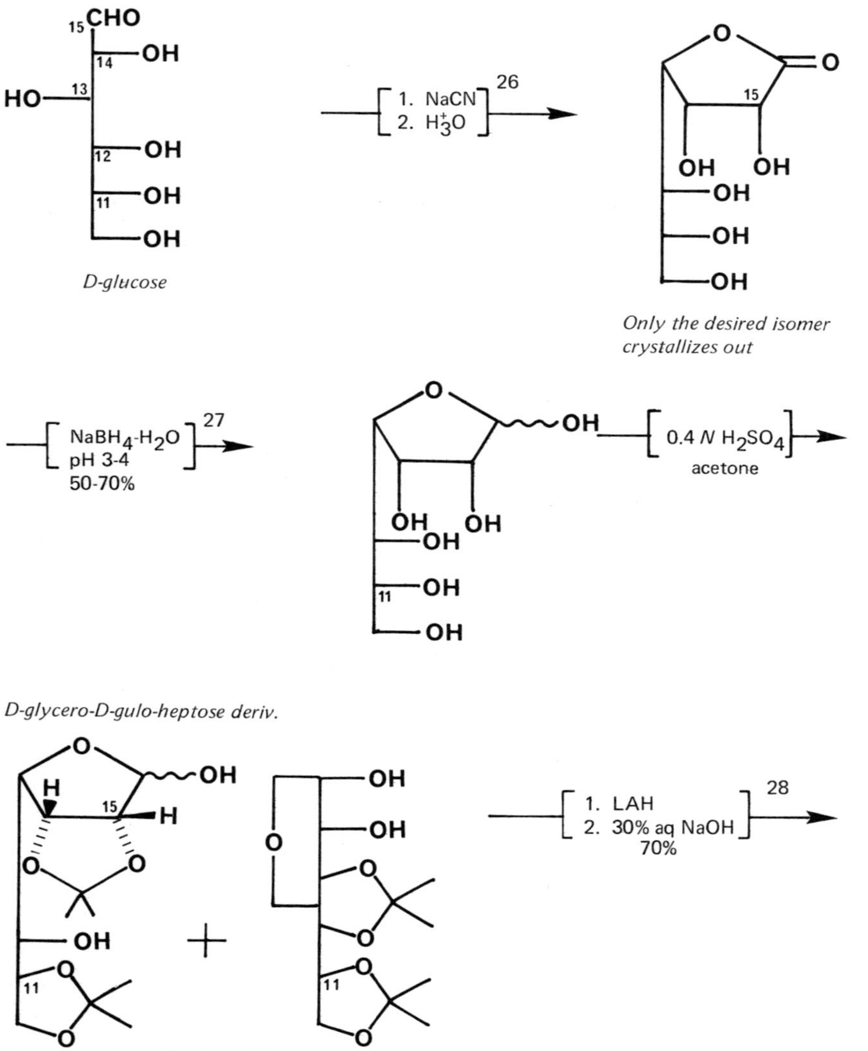

26. H. Kiliani, *Ber.*, 19, 767 (1886).
27. The separation of the two acetonides was postponed to a later stage.
28. When the reduction was carried out with $NaBH_4$ the isolated yield of the triol [7] was as low as 30%. This may be due to the borate complexation of the resulting triol.

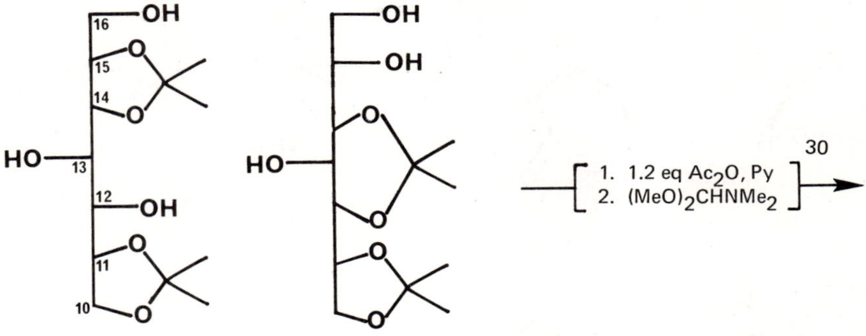

[7] 29

Threo vicinal diol.

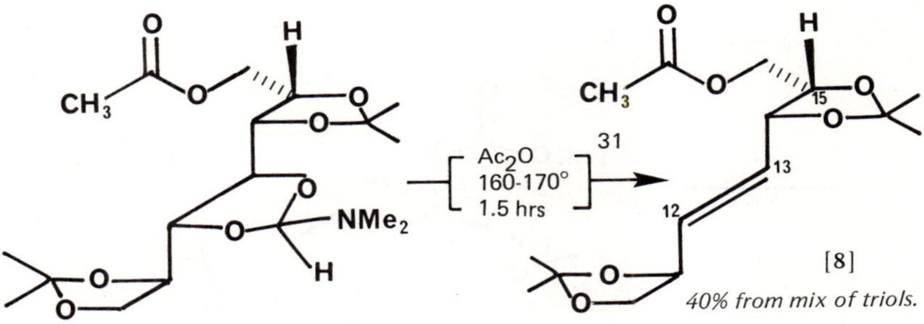

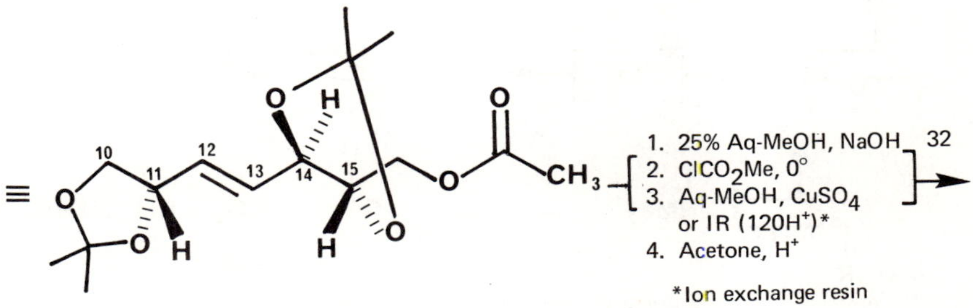

---

29. Only this vicinal glycol could form the *trans* olefin [8].
30. F. W. Eastwood, K. J. Harrington, J. S. Josan & J. L. Pura, *Tet. Lett.*, 5223 (1970).

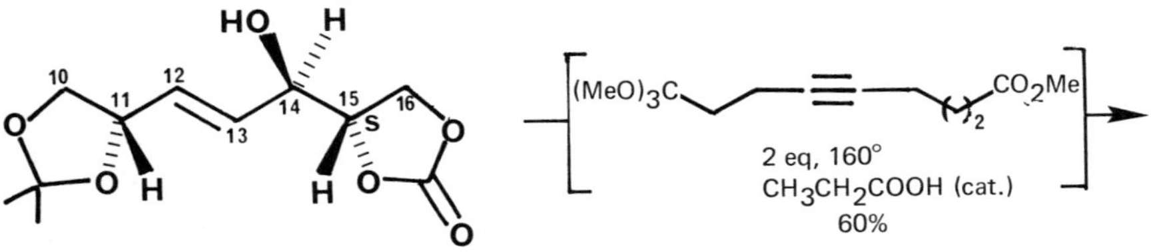

Key intermediate

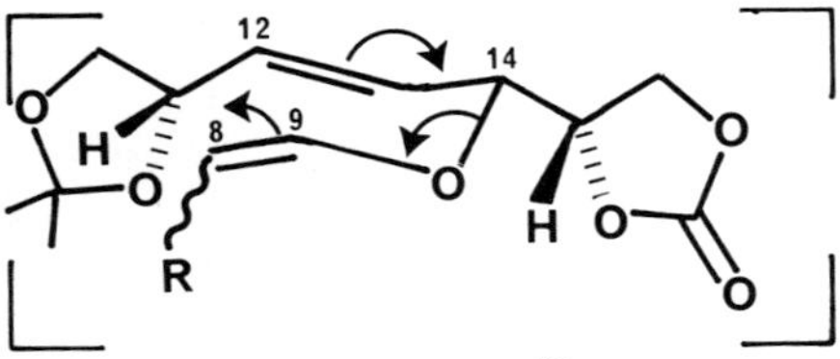

Ketene acetal deriv.[33]

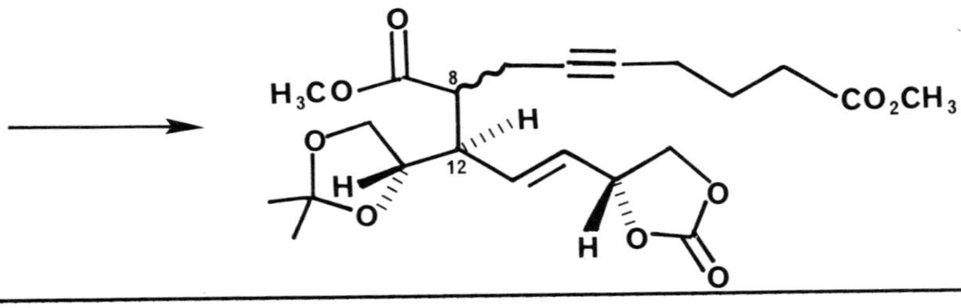

31. The mechanism of the elimination is unknown. But one could propose a plausible pathway as shown below:

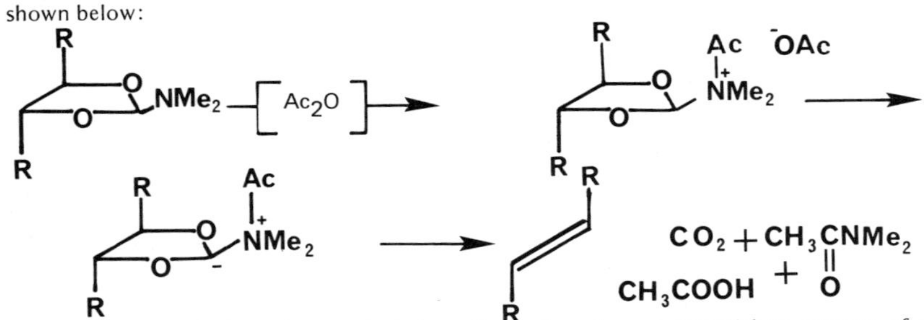

32. The protection of the primary alcohol as the carbonate was essential to success of the subsequent Claisen rearrangement which requires a free allylic alcohol function at C_{14}. The other secondary alcohol (C_{15}) must be protected to avoid cyclic orthoester formation during the Claisen rearrangement.
33. There is special steric preference of the acetylenic side chain R_{α} in the ketene, that is, it could be axial or equatorial. Thus the Claisen rearrangement product is epimeric at C_8.

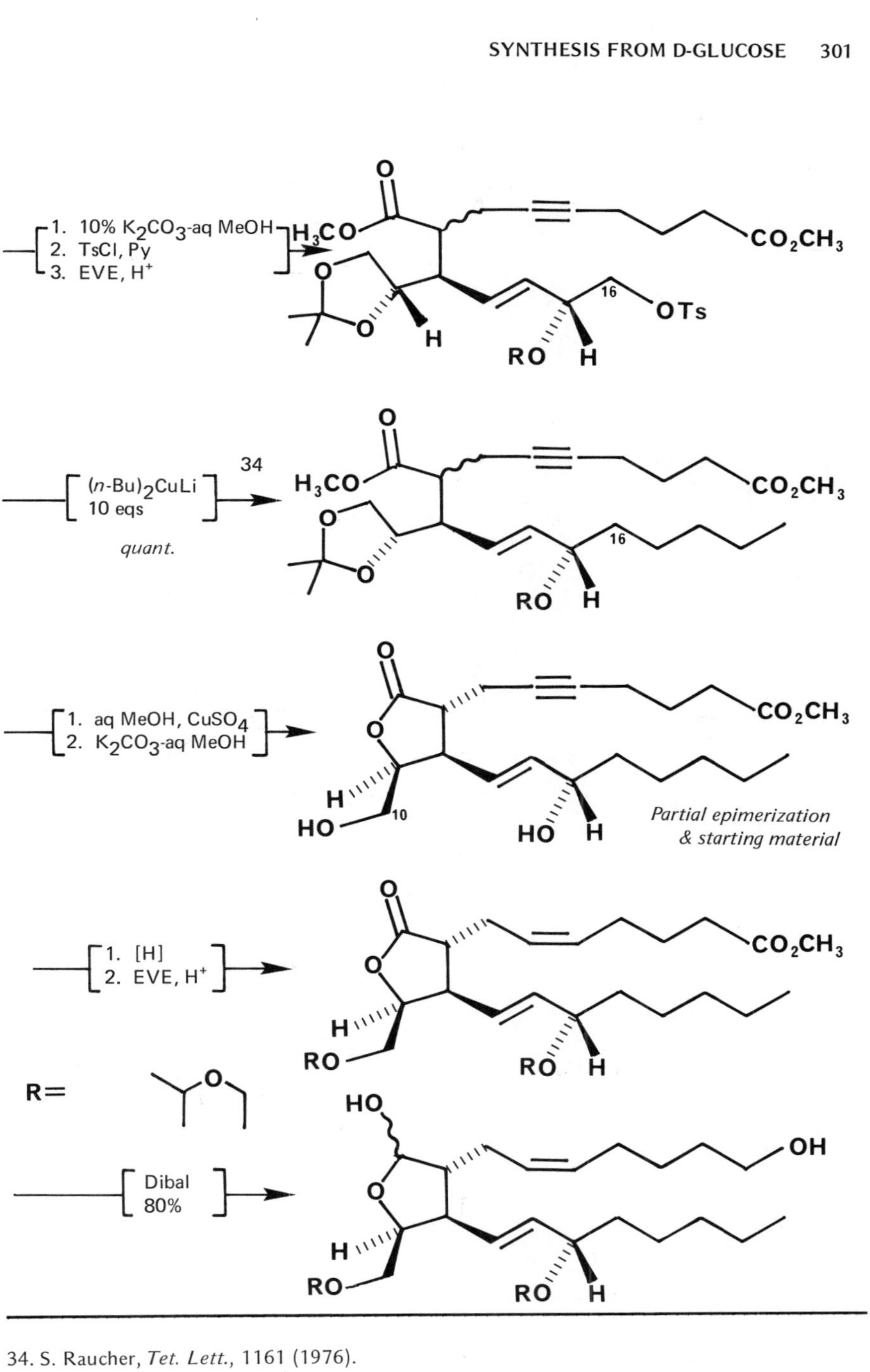

34. S. Raucher, *Tet. Lett.*, 1161 (1976).

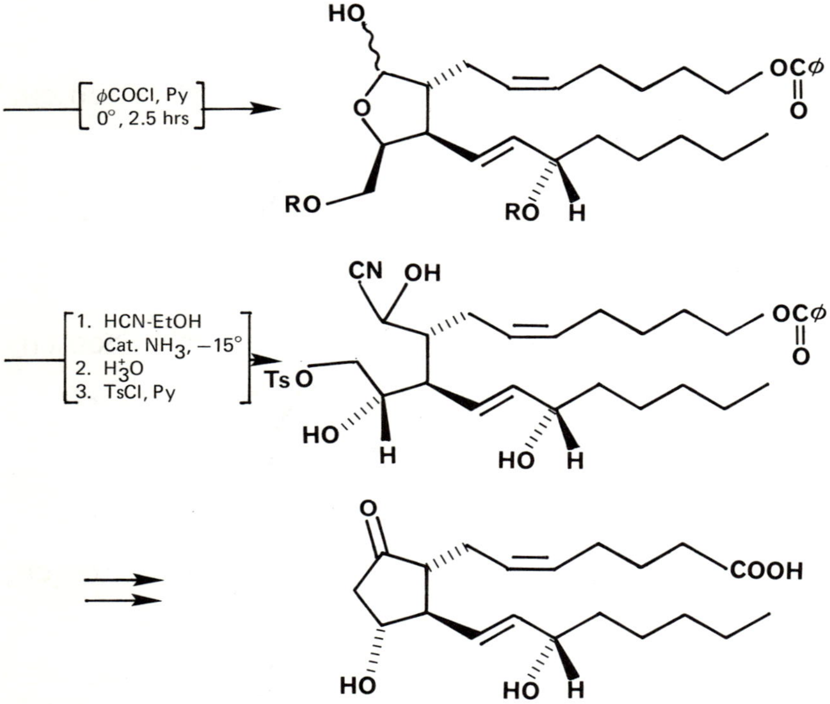
φCOCl, Py
0°, 2.5 hrs
HO
O
RO
RO H
OCφ
O
1. HCN-EtOH
Cat. NH3, −15°
2. H3O+
3. TsCl, Py
CN OH
Ts O
HO
H
HO H
O
COOH
HO
HO H

16

Syntheses of Thromboxanes

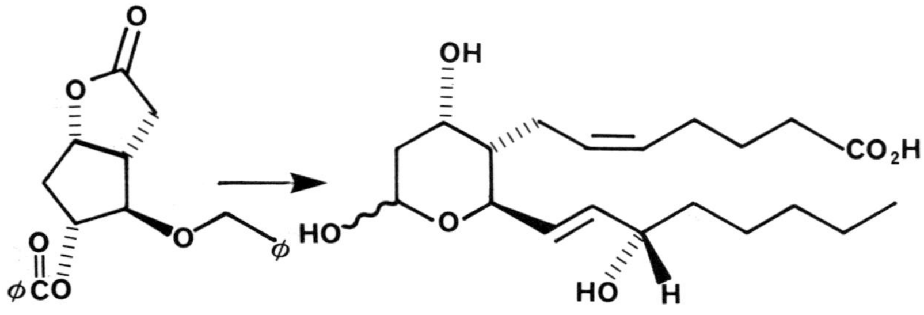

Corey lactone *Thromboxane B_2*

Recently, a new class of compounds closely related to prostaglandins have been discovered and shown to be potentially biologically active. These compounds have been named **THROMBOXANES** because they were found in the thrombocytes. Several syntheses of thromboxanes have been reported.

The syntheses reported by the Upjohn group start with the bicyclic Corey lactone. Different scission reactions of the C_{11}-C_{12} bond have been used and followed by cyclization, that is, acetal formation.

The synthesis reported by Nelson & Jackson[2] involves a periodic acid cleavage of the diol [1] followed by an acetalization of the aldehyde.

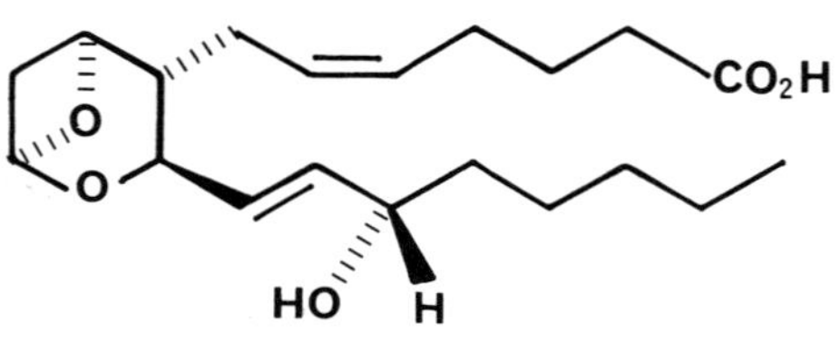

Thromboxane A_2

---

1. M. Hamberg, J. Svenson & B. Samuelsson, in *Advances in Prostaglandin and Thromboxane Research*, Vol. I, B. Samuelsson & R. Paoletti, (Eds.), Raven, New York, 1976, p. 19.

SYNTHETIC STRATEGY

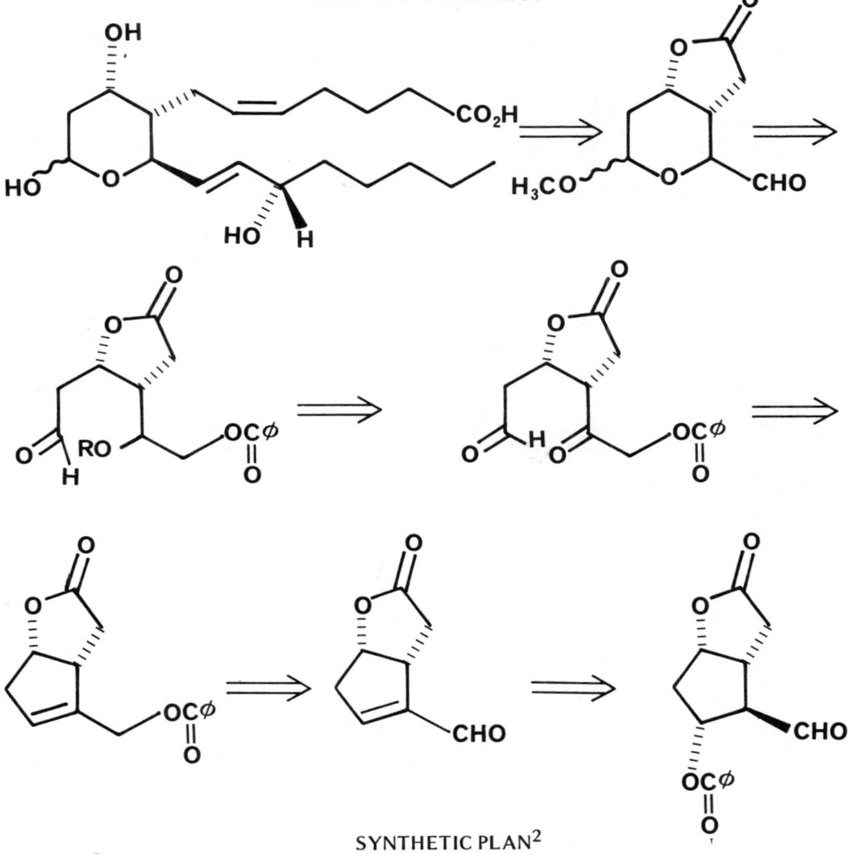

SYNTHETIC PLAN[2]

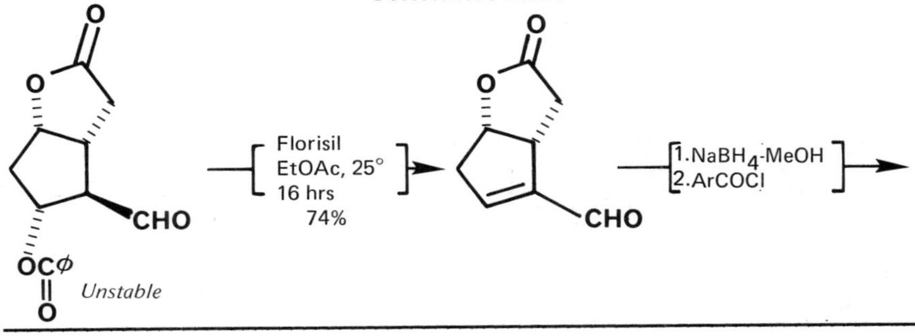

2. N. A. Nelson & R. W. Jackson, *Tet. Lett.*, 3275 (1976).

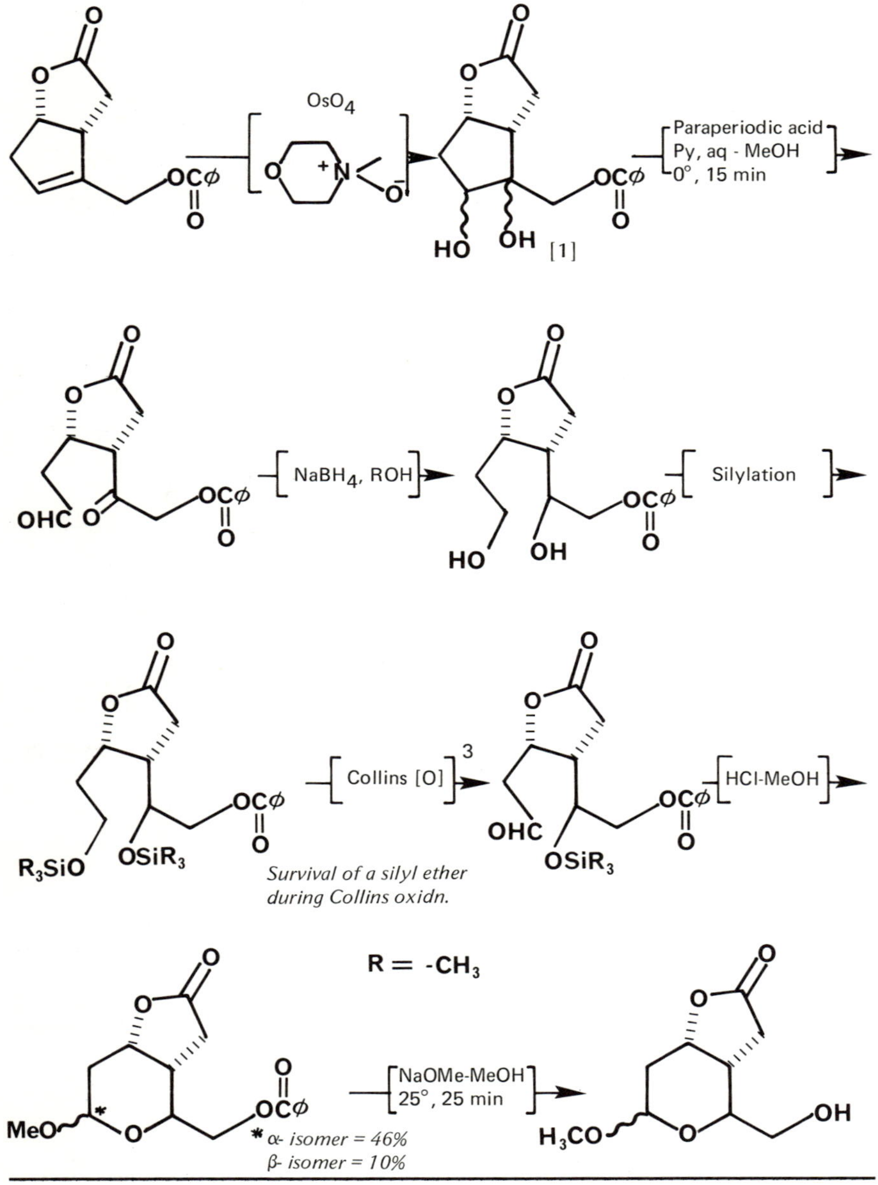

3. The Pfitzner-Moffatt oxidation gives a better yield (54%).

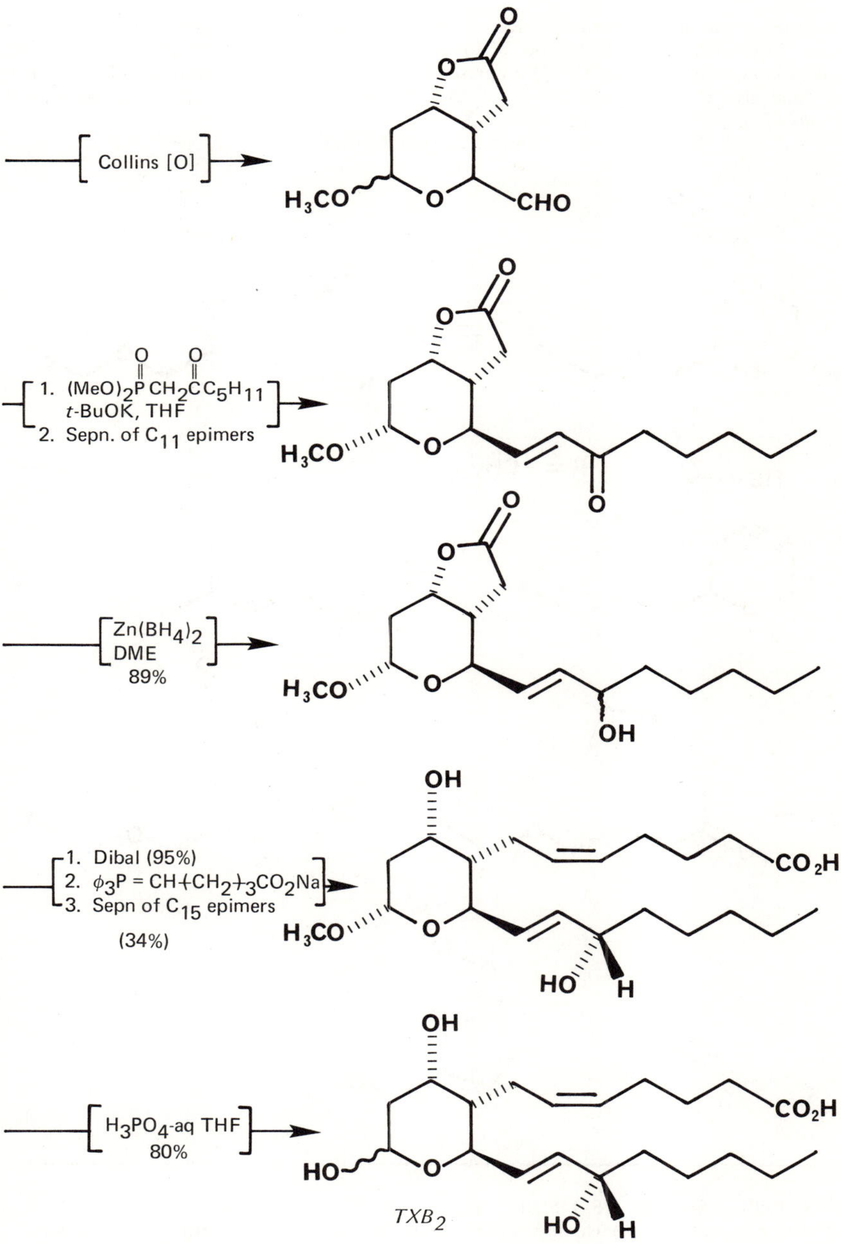
Collins [O]
H$_3$CO
O
CHO
1. (MeO)$_2$P(O)CH$_2$C(O)C$_5$H$_{11}$
t-BuOK, THF
2. Sepn. of C$_{11}$ epimers
Zn(BH$_4$)$_2$
DME
89%
OH
1. Dibal (95%)
2. ϕ_3P = CH(CH$_2$)$_3$CO$_2$Na
3. Sepn of C$_{15}$ epimers
(34%)
CO$_2$H
HO
H
H$_3$PO$_4$-aq THF
80%
TXB$_2$

In another synthesis reported by Kelly[4] the hemiacetal function was introduced by a Baeyer-Villiger oxidation of the ketone [2] followed by reduction to give [3]. The hemiacetal [3] was then converted to the acetal [4] to preserve the required *cis*-stereochemistry of the double bond[5] and also to differentiate the C_{12} aldehyde from the C_{13} aldehyde in the subsequent reactions.

SYNTHETIC STRATEGY

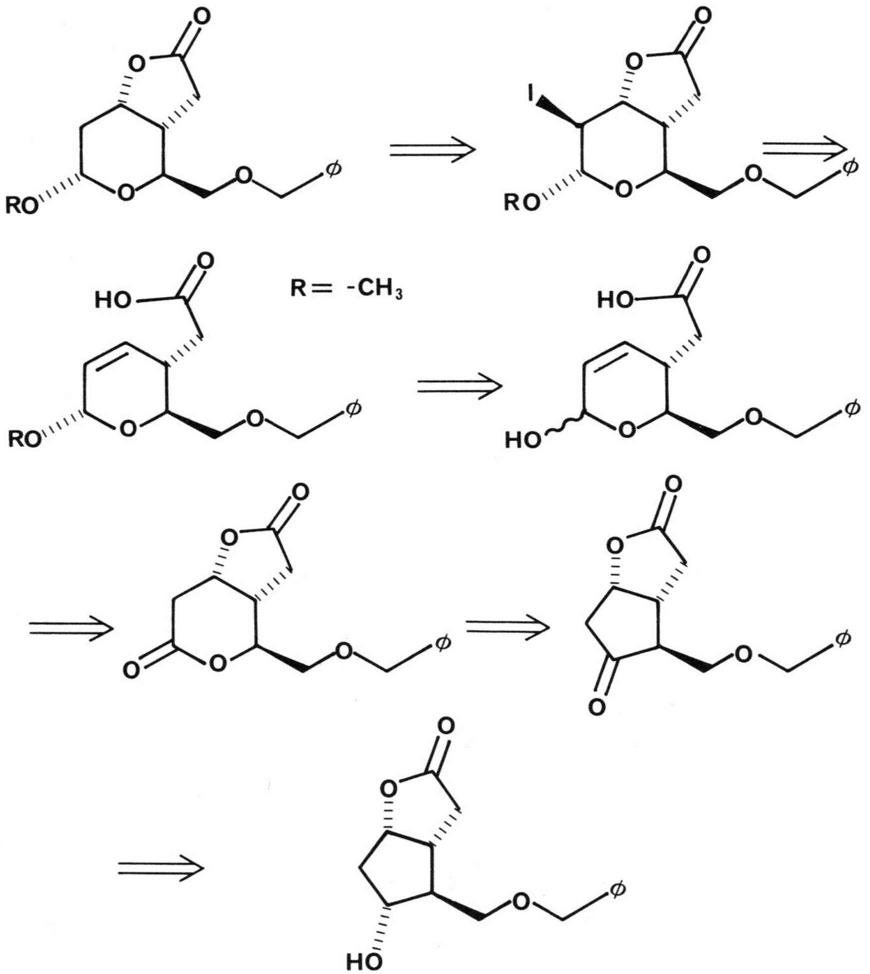

4. R. C. Kelly, I. Schletter & S. J. Stein, *Tet. Lett.*, 3279 (1976).
5. The *cis*-α,β-unsaturated aldehyde can isomerize to the *trans*-aldehyde which then gives [5].

SYNTHETIC PLAN[4]

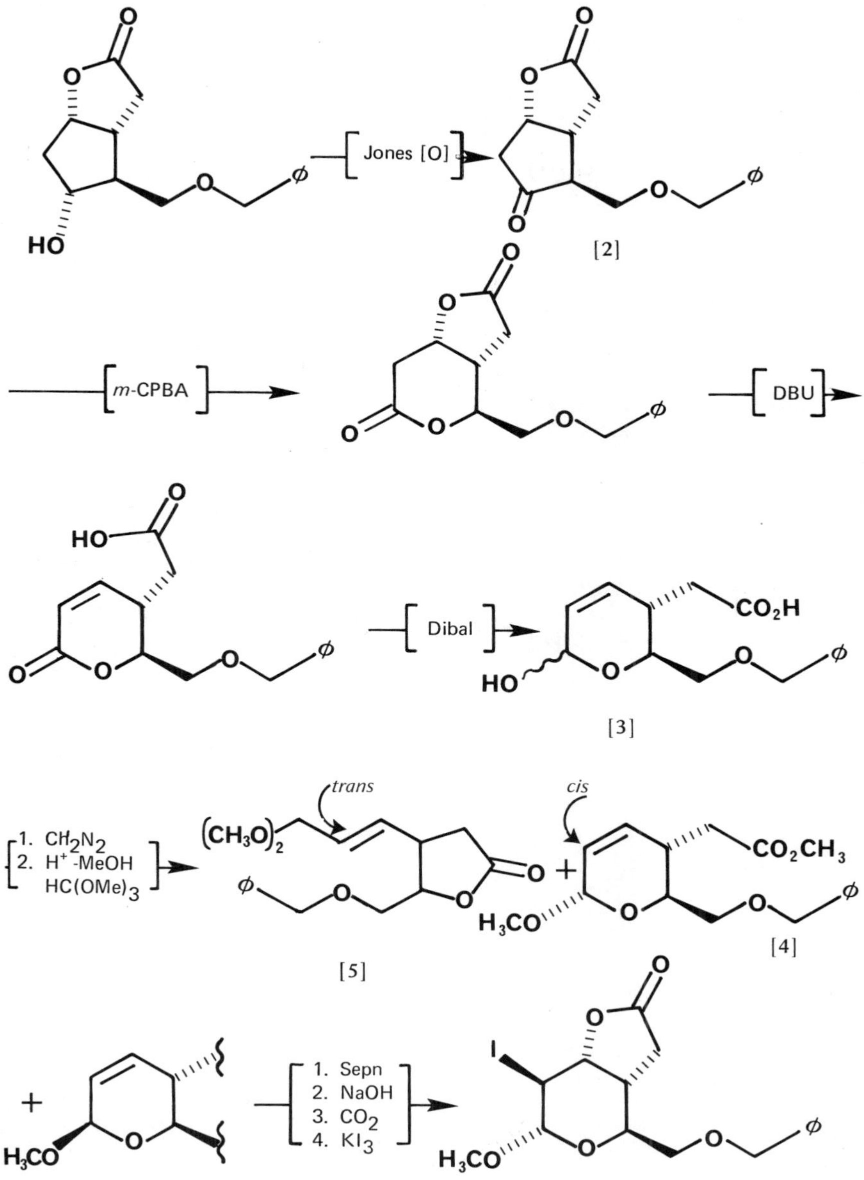

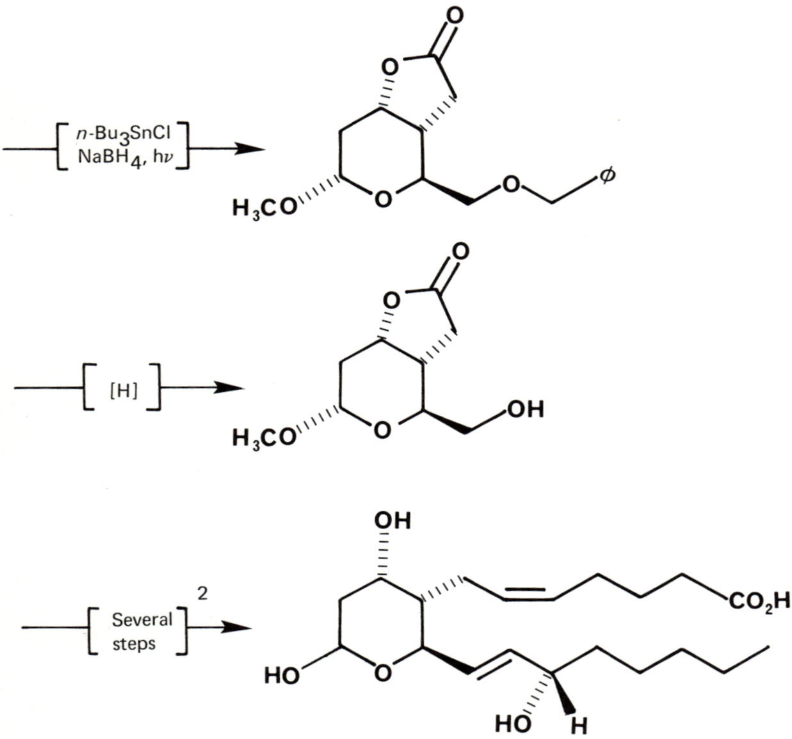
n-Bu3SnCl
NaBH4, hν
O
O
H3CO
O
O
φ
[H]
O
O
H3CO
O
OH
Several steps
2
OH
CO2H
HO
O
HO
H

Transformation of $PGF_{2\alpha}$ into Thromboxane B_2[6]

The cleavage of homoallylic alcohols, known previously in steroids, with lead tetraacetate to give aldehedo-acetate[7] has been used in the following transformation of $PGF_{2\alpha}$ to thromboxane B_2.[6]

SYNTHETIC PLAN[6]

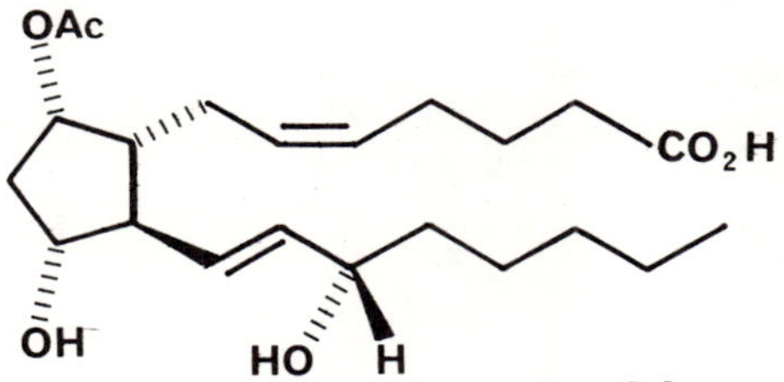

[6]

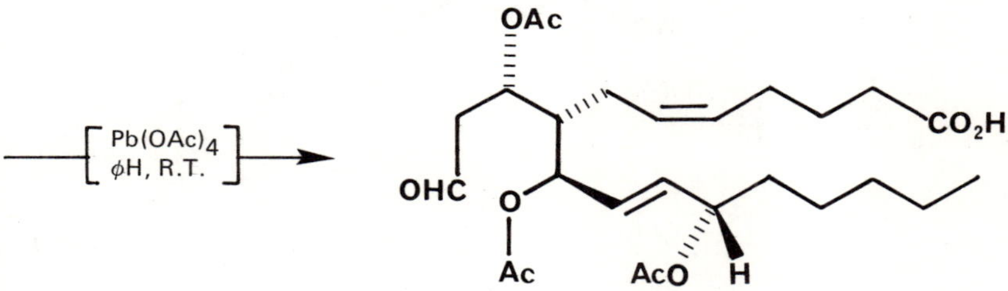

---

6. W. P. Schneider & R. A. Morge, *Tet. Lett.*, 3283 (1976).
7. M. Amorosa, L. Caglioti, G. Cianelli, H. Immer, J. Keller, H. Wehrli, M. Lj. Mihlaiovic, K. Schaffner, D. Arigoni & O. Jeger, *Helv. Chim. Acta.*, 45, 2674 (1973).

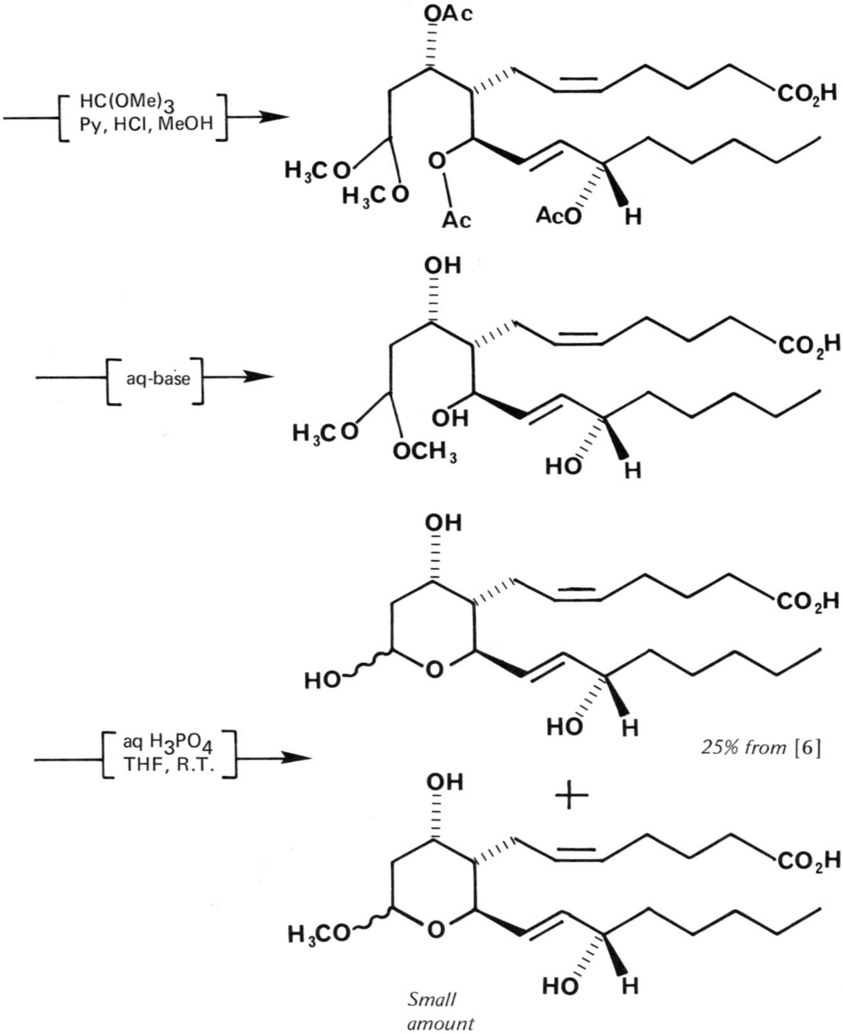
HC(OMe)3
Py, HCl, MeOH
OAc
CO2H
H3CO
H3CO
O
Ac
AcO
H
aq-base
OH
CO2H
H3CO
OH
OCH3
HO
H
OH
CO2H
HO
O
HO
H
25% from [6]
aq H3PO4
THF, R.T.
OH
+
CO2H
H3CO
O
HO
H
Small amount

Unlike the Upjohn syntheses[2,4,6] the Corey synthesis of thromboxane B_2[8] does not involve the intermediacy of a prostanoid. The β-chain is introduced by an aldol reaction followed by an intramolecular Michael reaction to give the pyran [7] which is subsequently elaborated to thromboxane B_2.

SYNTHETIC STRATEGY

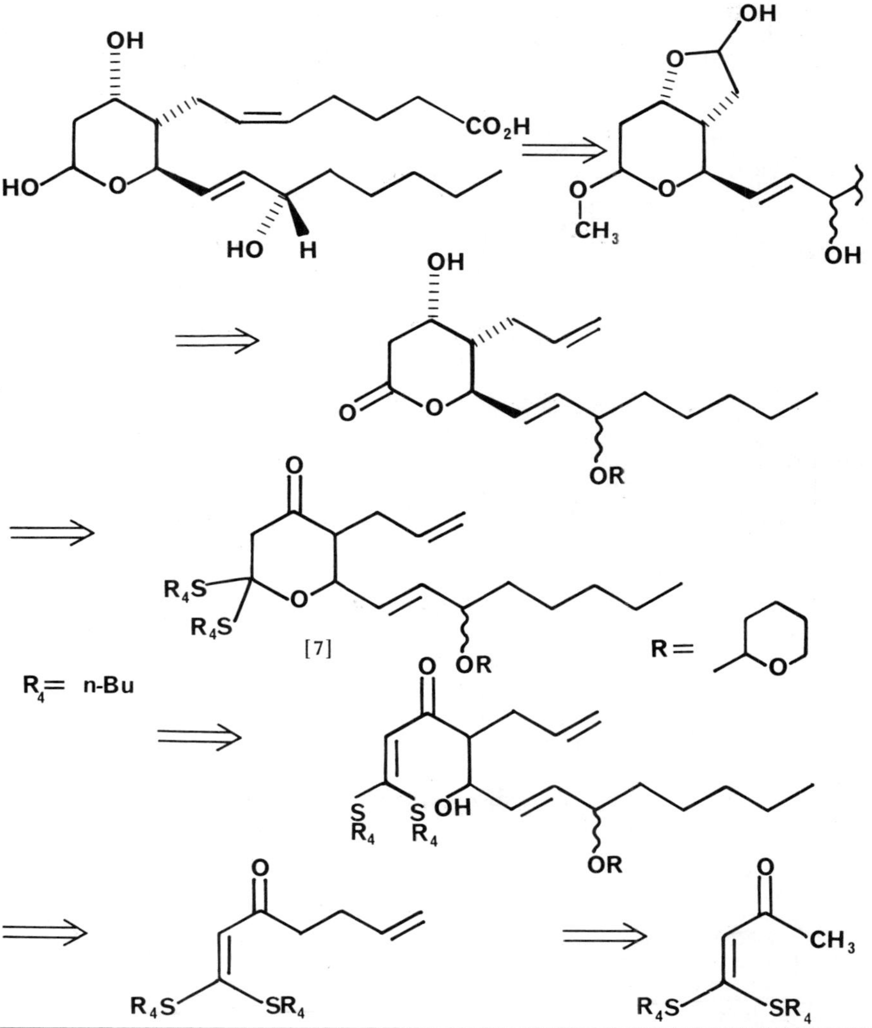

8. E. J. Corey, M. Shibasaki, J. Knolle & T. Sugahara, *Tet. Lett.*, 785 (1977).

SYNTHETIC PLAN[8]

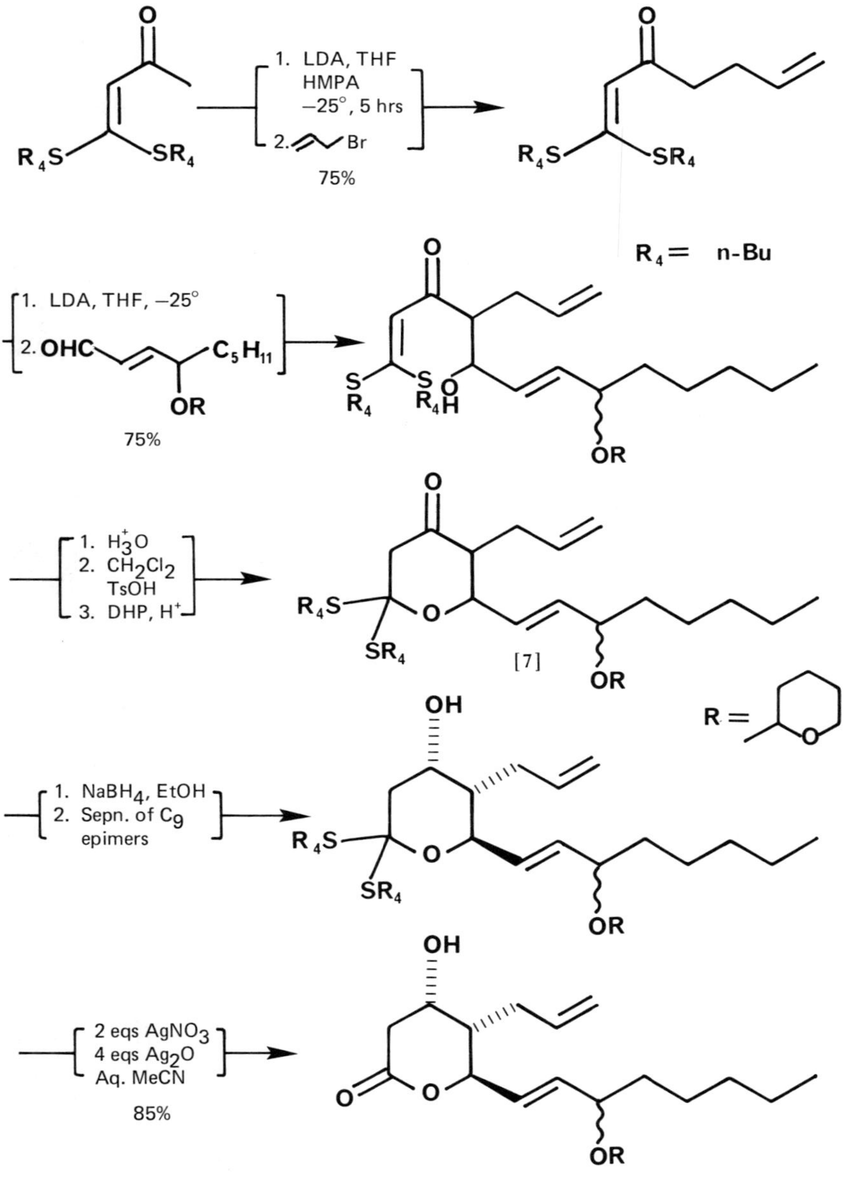

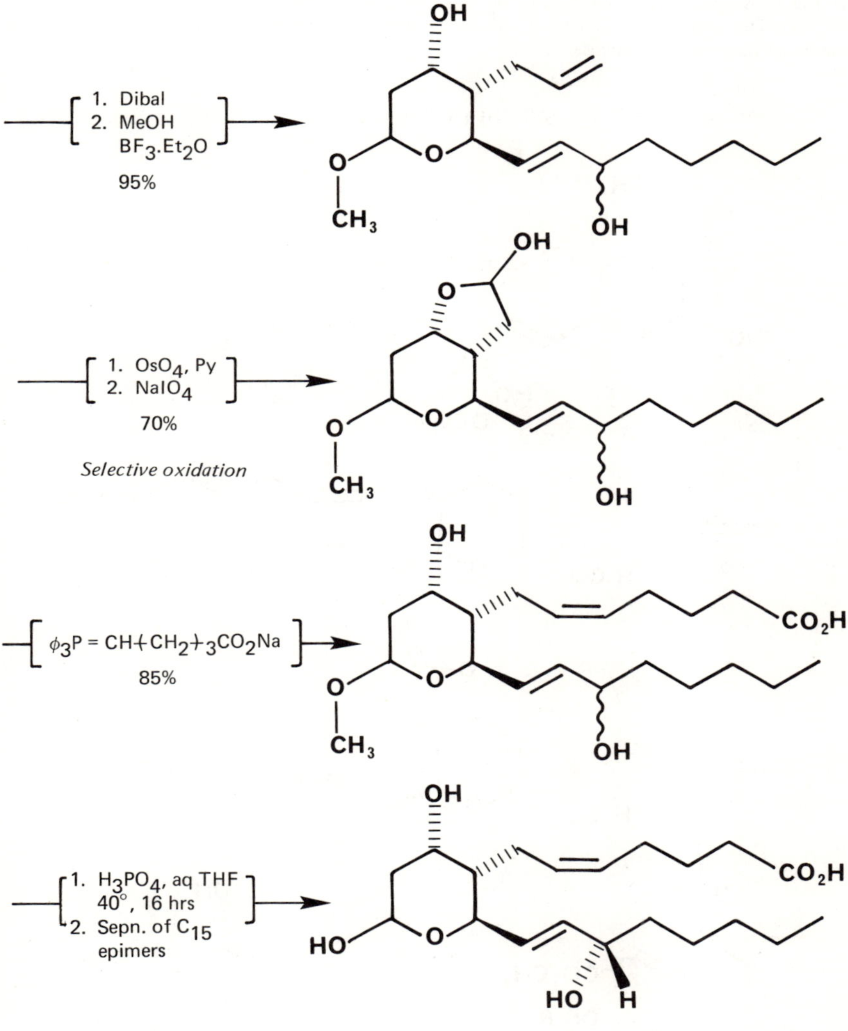
1. Dibal
2. MeOH
BF3.Et2O
95%
OH
O
CH3
OH
1. OsO4, Py
2. NaIO4
70%
Selective oxidation
OH
O
O
CH3
OH
φ3P = CH(CH2)3CO2Na
85%
OH
CO2H
O
CH3
OH
1. H3PO4, aq THF
40°, 16 hrs
2. Sepn. of C15
epimers
OH
CO2H
HO
O
HO
H

Like the prostaglandins, thromboxane B_2 has also been synthesized from a sugar[9] (a chiral precursor). The synthesis of Hanessian and Lavalle starts from 2,4,6-trideoxy-D-*ribo*-hexose which is readily available from D-glucose.

SYNTHETIC STRATEGY

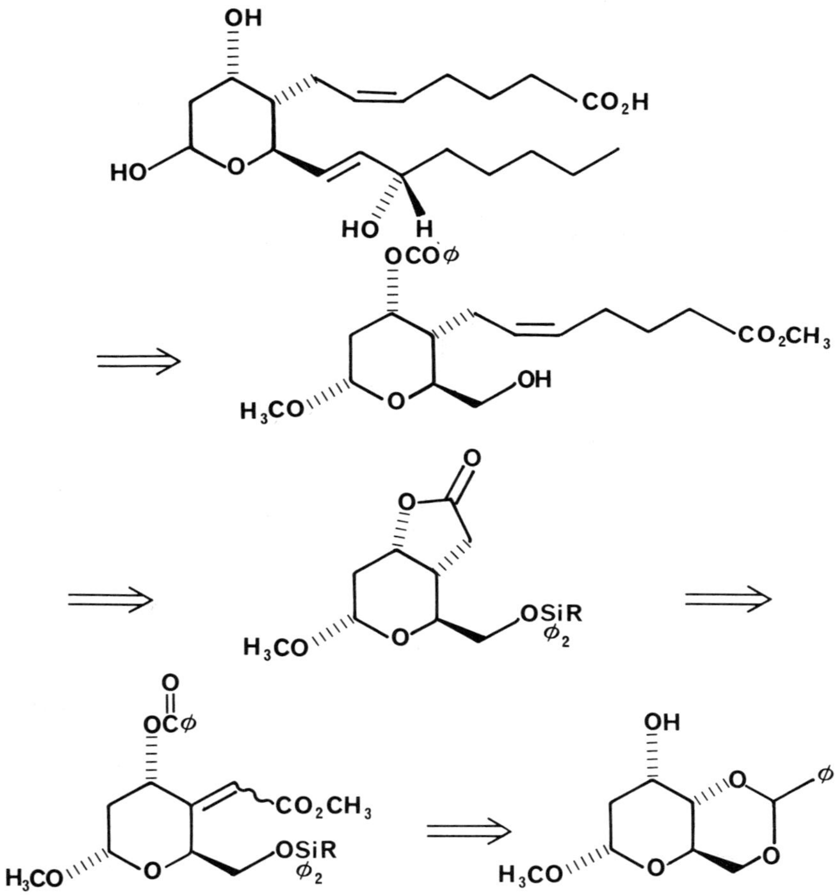

9. The first synthesis of a prostaglandin from a sugar was reported by G. Stork & S. Raucher, *J. Am. Chem. Soc.*, **98**, 1583 (1976).
10. S. Hanessian & P. Lavalle, *Can. J. Chem.*, **55**, 562 (1977).

SYNTHETIC PLAN[10]

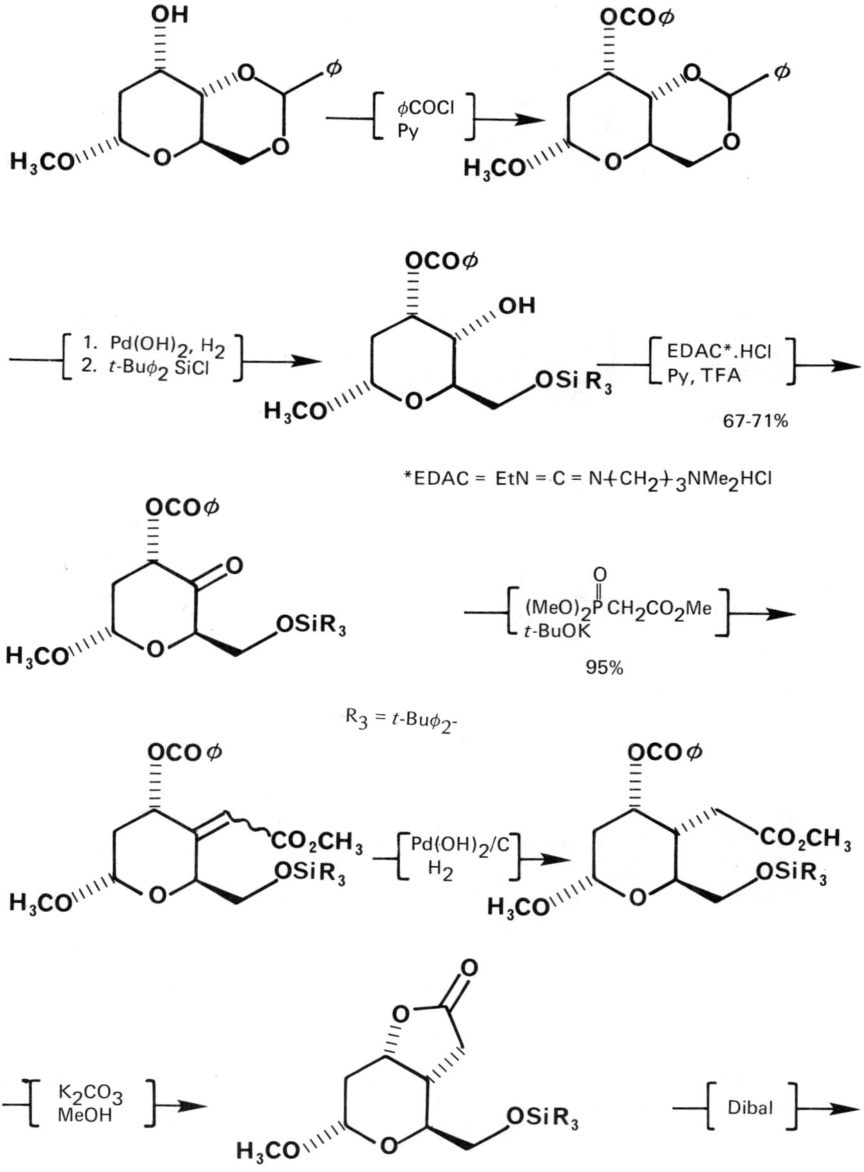

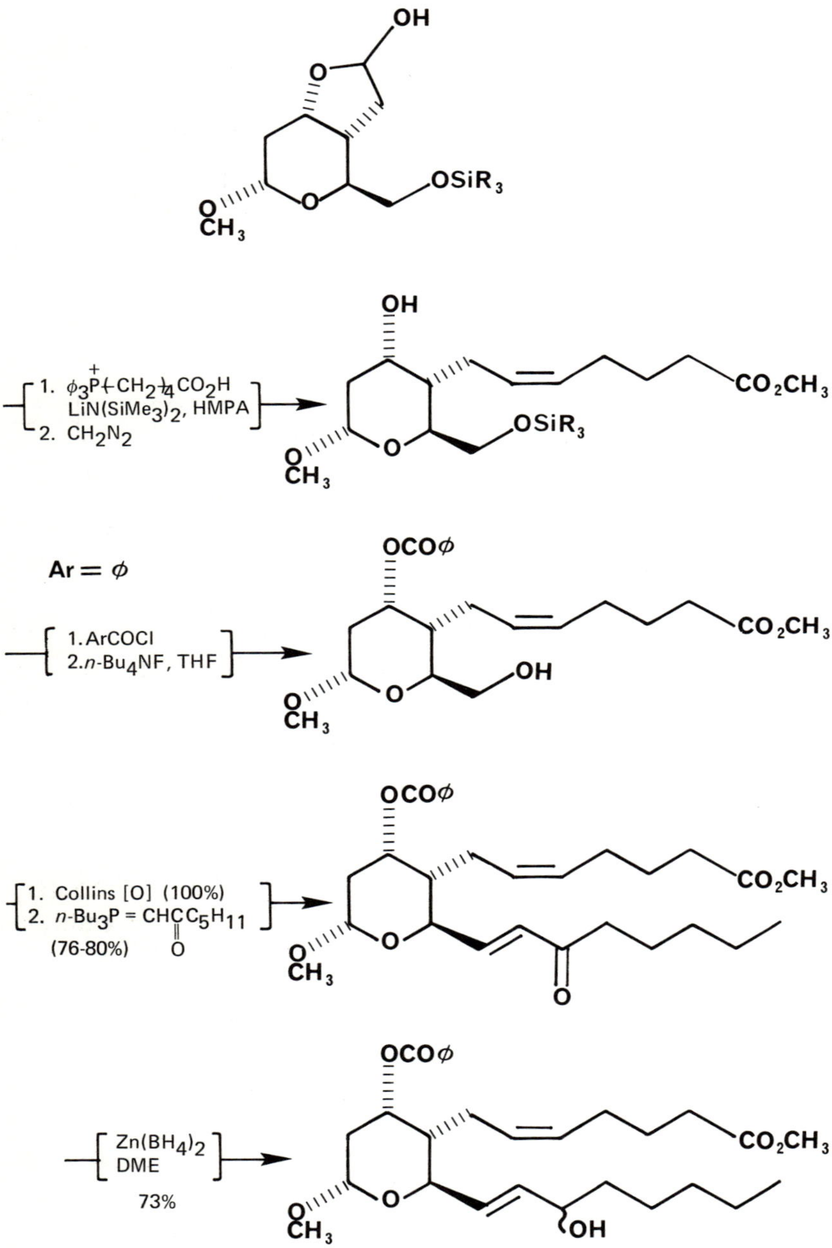

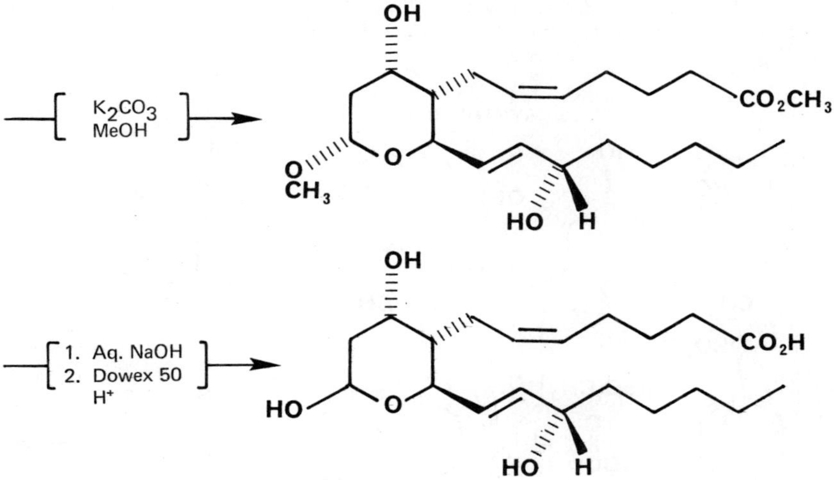

m. p. 91-93°

$[\alpha]_D^{25} = 57.4°$

After the publication of the Hanessian synthesis[10] of TXB_2, Corey reported a synthesis[11] of TXB_2 starting from *D*-glucose involving a Claisen rearrangement.[14]

SYNTHETIC PLAN[11]

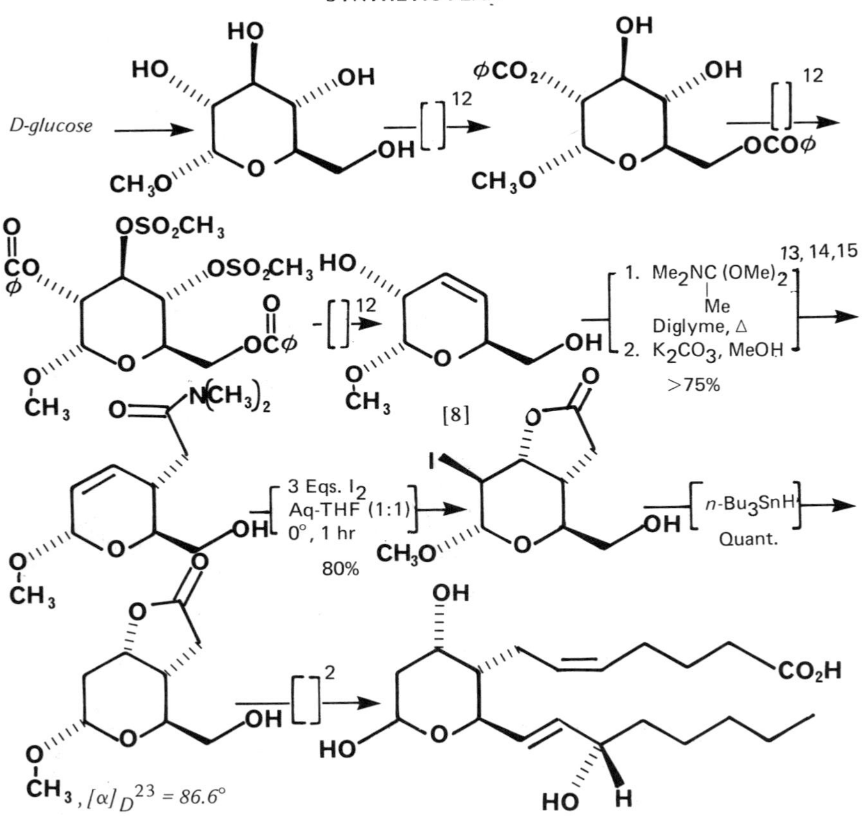

11. E. J. Corey, M. Shibasaki & J. Knolle, *Tet. Lett.*, 1625 (1977).
12. N. L. Holder & B. Fraser-Reid, *Can. J. Chem.*, **51**, 3357 (1973).
13. A. E. Wick, D. Felix, K. Steen and A. Eschenmoser, *Helv. Chim. Acta*, **47**, 2425 (1964) and **52**, 1030 (1969).
14. Only low yields of Claisen rearrangement product were obtained using the ortho ester precursor method of W. S. Johnson, L. Werthemann, W. R. Bartlett, T. J. Brockson, T-t. Li, D. J. Faulkner and M. R. Petersen, *J. Am. Chem. Soc.*, **92**, 741 (1970).
15. The carboxylic acid corresponding to the dimethylamide was readily obtained by the trimethylsilyl enol ether Claisen method starting from the diacetate of [**8**]; see, R. E. Ireland and A. K. Willard, *Tetrahedron Lett.*, 3975 (1975).

17

Syntheses of PGA_2

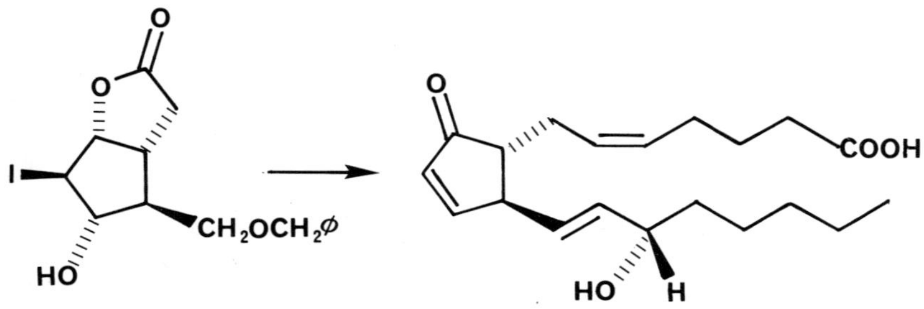

Iodohydrin

One of the first synthesis of the PGA compounds was carried out via the bicyclo[2.2.1]heptane route.[1] Reductive elimination of a suitable derivative of the intermediate iodohydrin gives the C_{10}-C_{11} double bond present in the prostaglandins of the A series. The unsaturated lactone [1] is then converted by standard procedures[2] to PGA$_2$. Introduction of the C_{10}-C_{11} double bond at an early stage of the sequence suffers from the lack of a directing group at C_{11} to control the reduction of the C_{15} ketone.

---

1. E. J. Corey & P. A. Grieco, *Tet. Lett.*, 107 (1972).
2. E. J. Corey, N. M. Weinshenker, T. K. Schaaf & W. Huber, *J. Am. Chem. Soc.*, **91**, 5675 (1969).

SYNTHETIC PLAN[1]

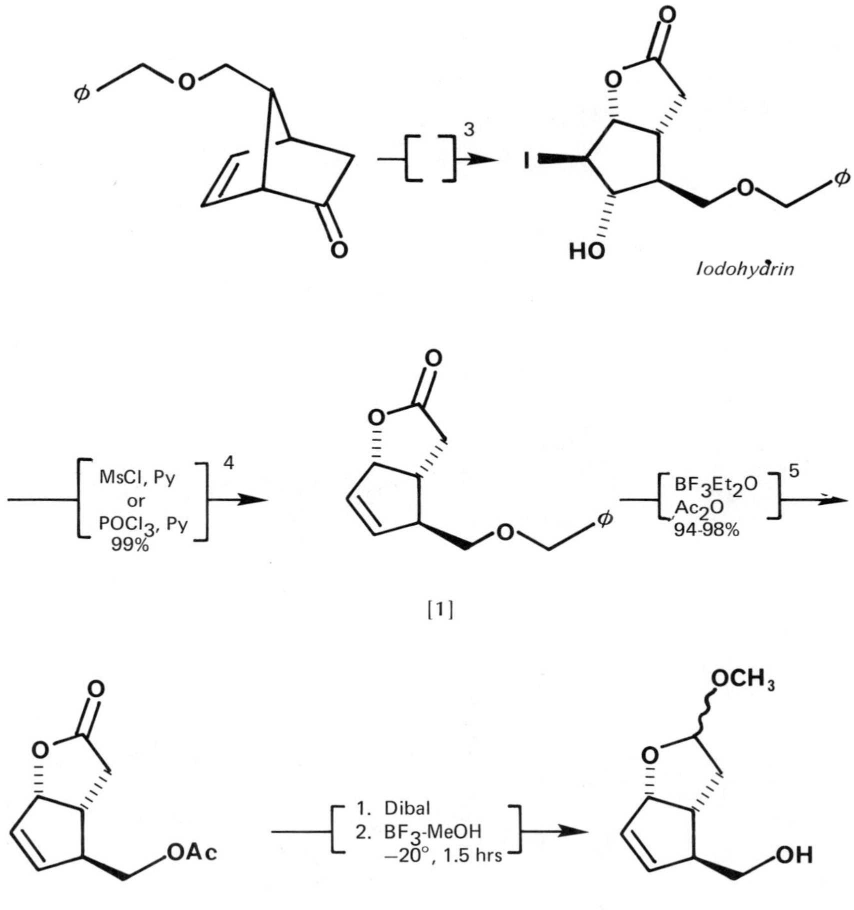

3. E. J. Corey, T. Ravindranathan & S. Terashima, *J. Am. Chem. Soc.*, **93**, 4326 (1971).
4. The one step conversion of the iodohydrin to the olefin [1] is mechanistically related to the Cornforth procedure for the conversion of epoxides to olefins. R. H. Cornforth & K. K. Mathew, *J. Chem. Soc.*, **112**, 2539 (1959).
   For an interesting study on the conversion of the iodohydrin to the cyclopentene using formate and oxalate as nucleophile see E. J. Corey & S. Terashima, *Tet. Lett.*, 111 (1972).
5. Removal of the benzyl group by the usual catalytic hydrogenation procedure is incompatible with the presence of the cyclopentene double bond. So a Lewis acid catalyzed hydrolytic method had to be used.

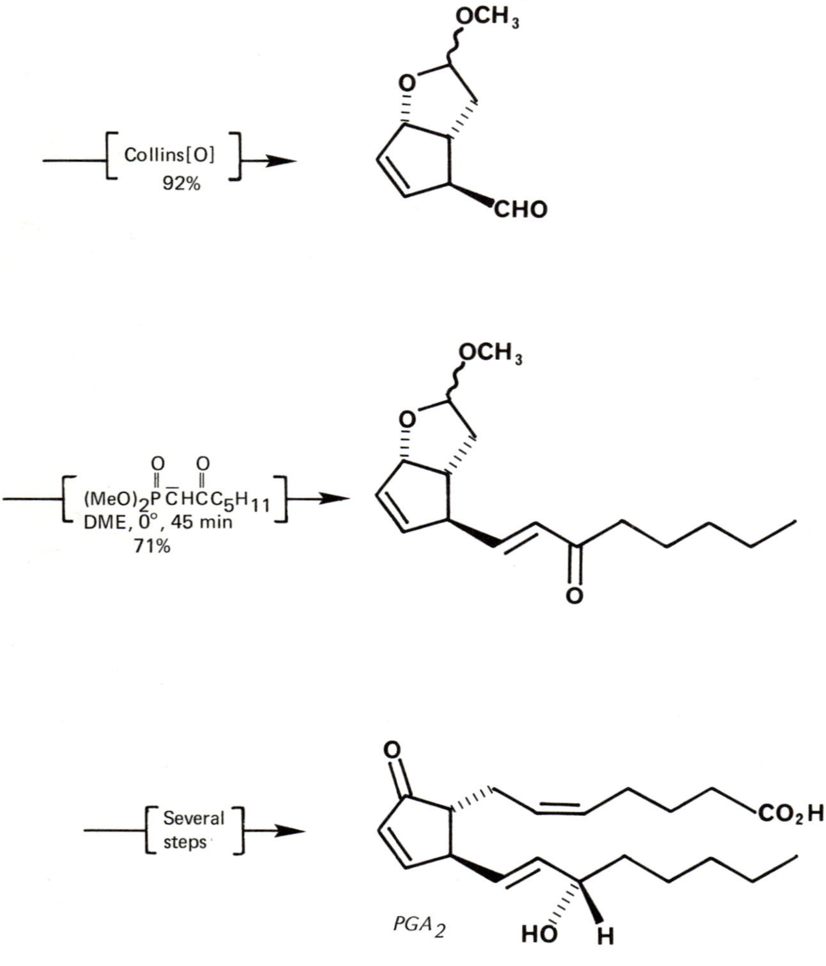

This modification postpones the introduction of the C_{10}-C_{11} double bond to a later stage in the sequence.[6] A C_{11} substituent, as shown earlier, is used to stereoselectively reduce the C_{15} ketone. A subsequent allylic displacement of the urethane [2] by the internal carboxylate nucleophile introduces the C_{10}-C_{11} cyclopentene double bond and simultaneously generates the desired *cis* lactone [3].

---

6. E. J. Corey & J. Moinet, *J. Am. Chem. Soc.*, **95**, 6831 (1973).

SYNTHETIC STRATEGY

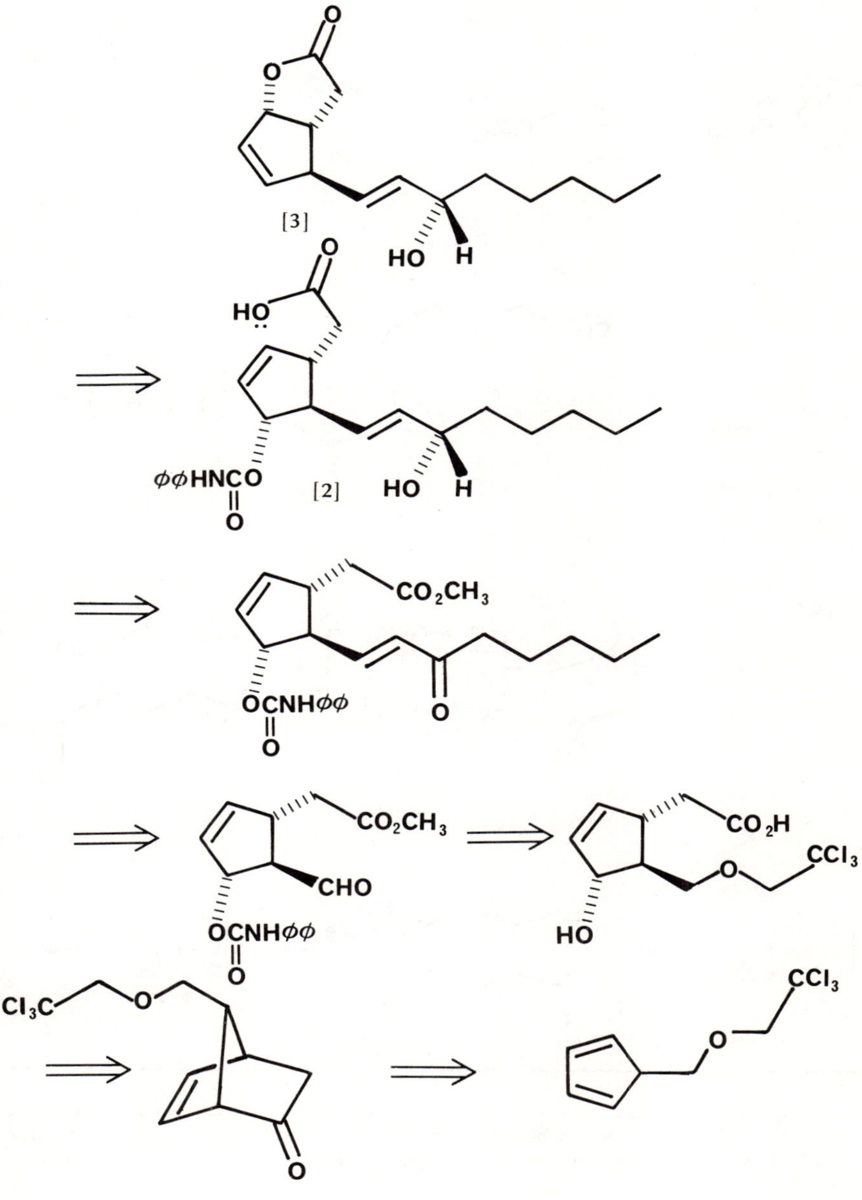

SYNTHETIC PLAN[6]

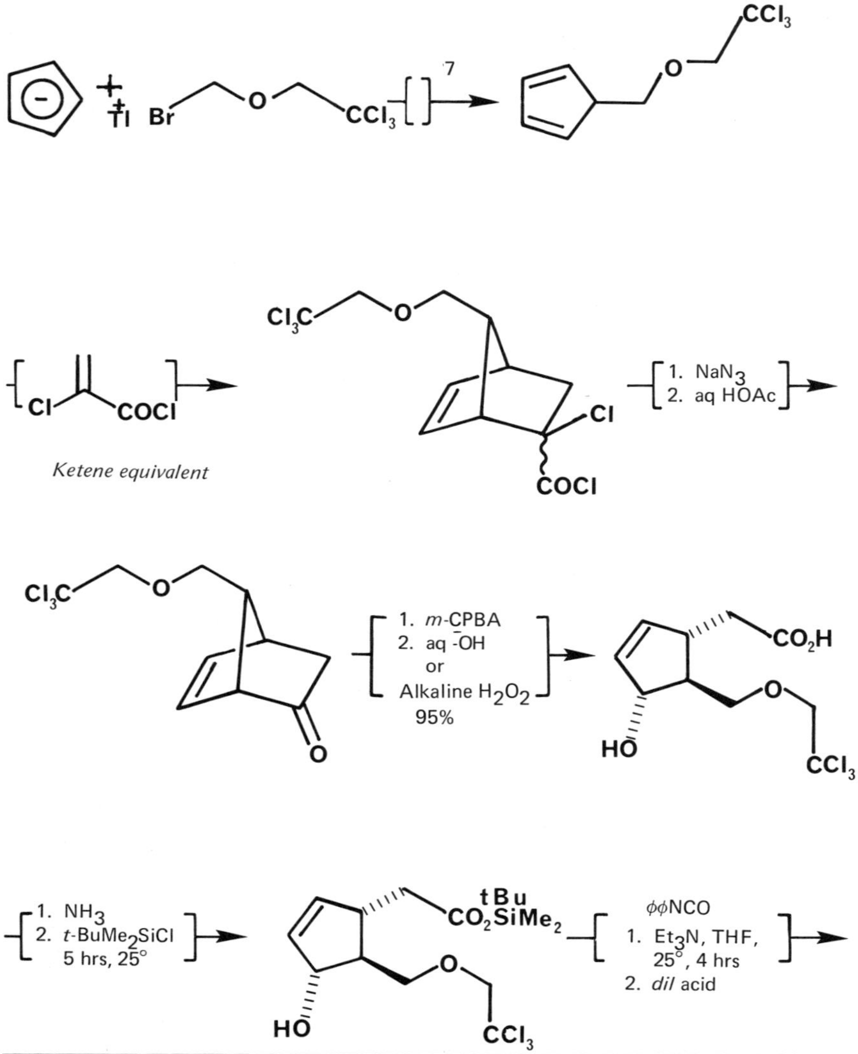

7. The commonly used benzyl protecting group cannot be used in this case since its removal by catalytic hydrogenation would be incompatible with the cyclopentene double bond. The β,β,β-trichloroethyl group is suitable protecting group because it can be reductively cleaved by Zn/H^+.

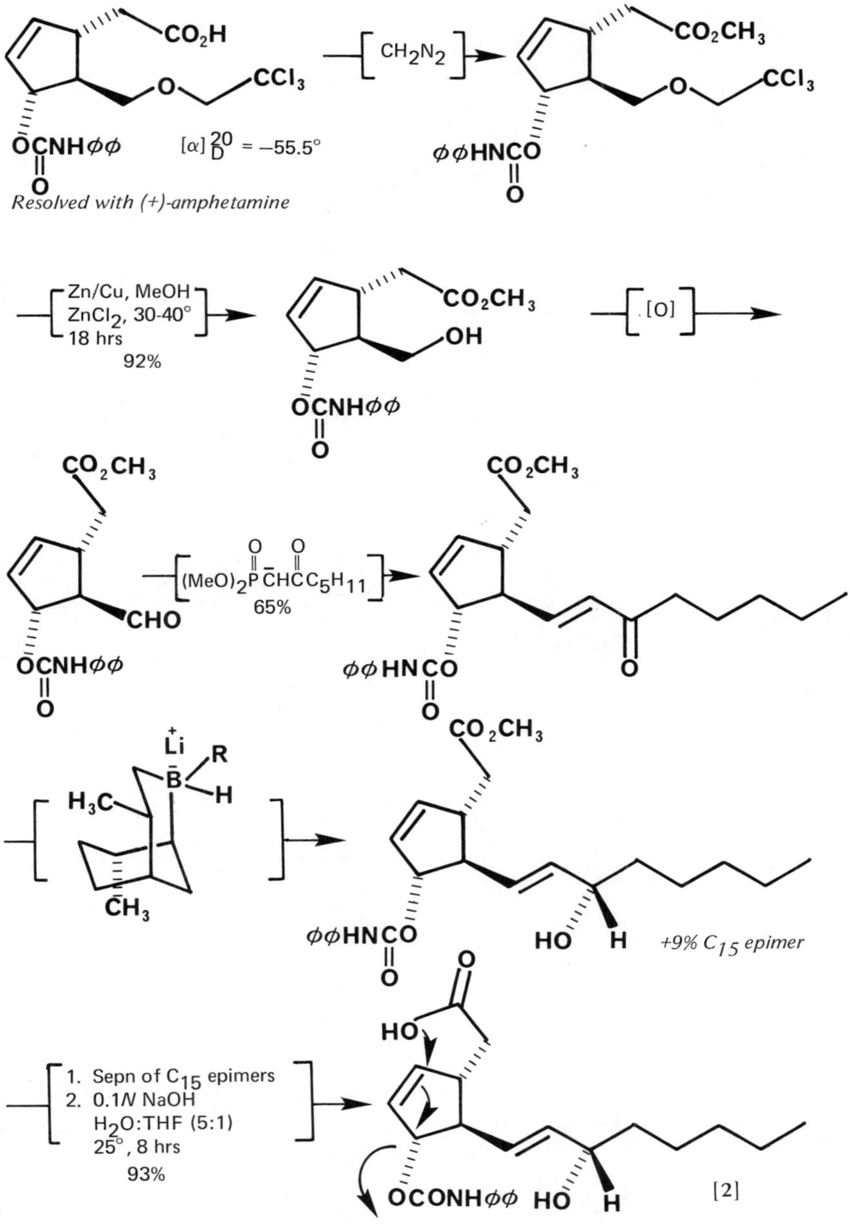
CO2H
CCl3
OCNHφφ
[α]20D = −55.5°
Resolved with (+)-amphetamine
CH2N2
CO2CH3
CCl3
φφHNCO
Zn/Cu, MeOH
ZnCl2, 30-40°
18 hrs
92%
CO2CH3
OH
OCNHφφ
[O]
CO2CH3
CHO
OCNHφφ
(MeO)2PCHCC5H11
65%
CO2CH3
φφHNCO
Li
R
B
H
H3C
CH3
CO2CH3
φφHNCO
HO
H
+9% C15 epimer
1. Sepn of C15 epimers
2. 0.1N NaOH
H2O:THF (5:1)
25°, 8 hrs
93%
HO
OCONHφφ
HO
H

[2]

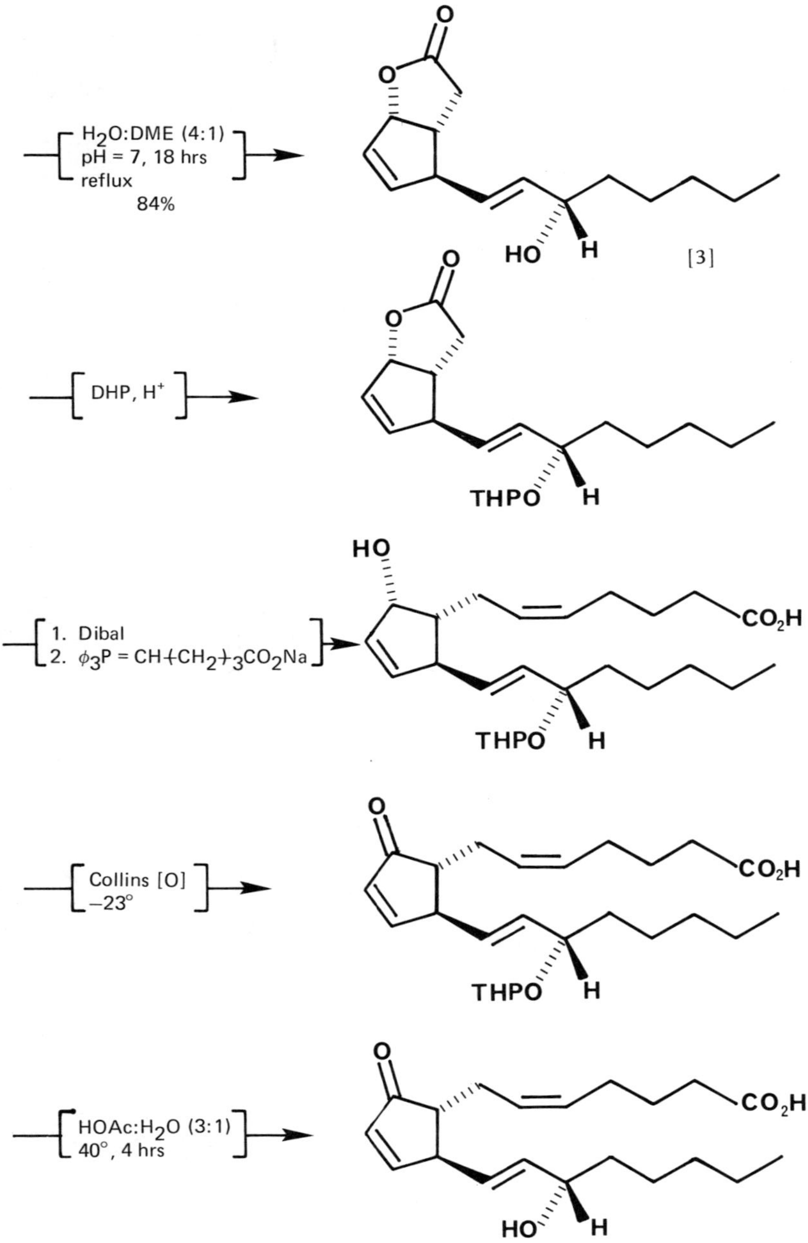
H2O:DME (4:1)
pH = 7, 18 hrs
reflux
84%
HO
H
O
DHP, H+
THPO
H
1. Dibal
2. φ3P = CH(CH2)3CO2Na
HO
CO2H
Collins [O]
−23°
HOAc:H2O (3:1)
40°, 4 hrs

[3]

The most recent Corey approach to the synthesis of PGA_2, the complete β-chain is introduced via a cuprate addition to the bicyclic lactone [4].[8]

SYNTHETIC PLAN[8]

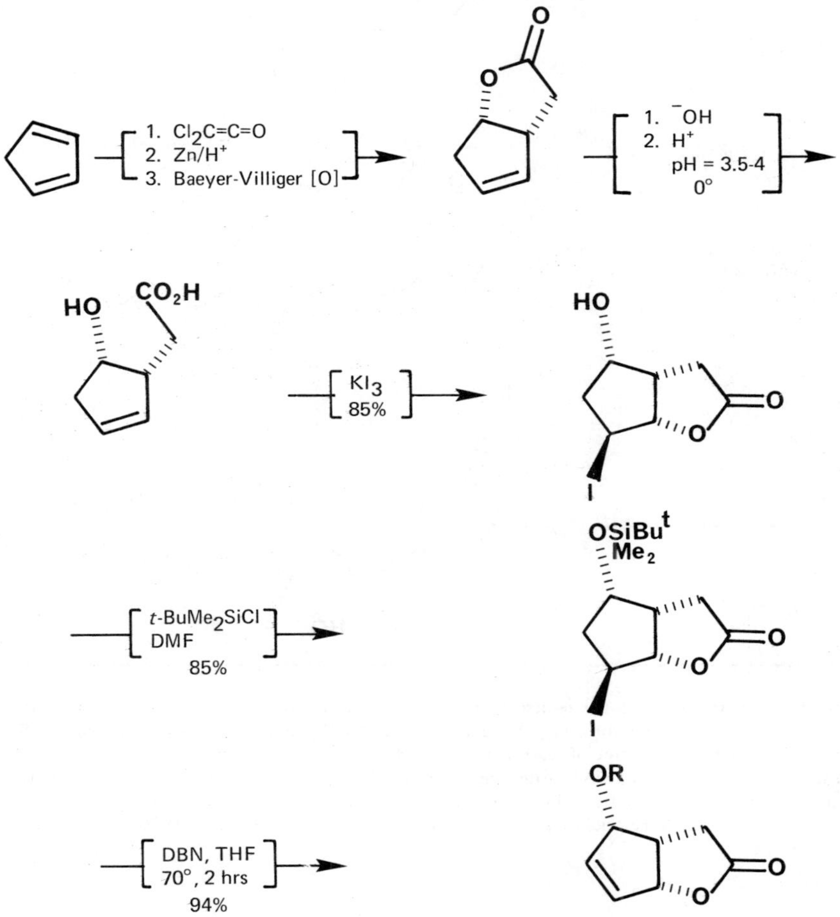

R = t-BuMe$_2$Si

[4]

8. E. J. Corey & J. Mann. *J. Am. Chem. Soc.*, **95**, 6832 (1973).
9. For the synthesis of the chiral cuprate reagent [5] see p. 331.

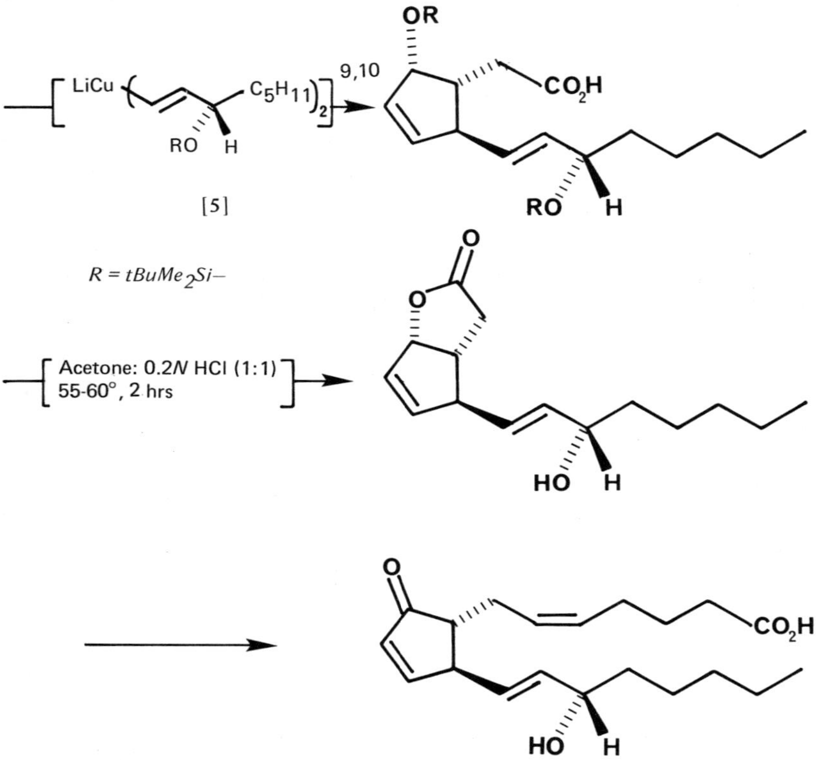

10. It is interesting to note the course of reaction of the divinylcuprate with the unsaturated lactone [4]. It has been shown by Andersen[11] that dimethylcuprates react with acyclic allylic acetates with varying degree of rearrangement. In this case rearrangement may be prevented by the bulky *t*-butyldimethylsilyl protecting group of the C_9 alcohol. With a different protecting group, both the products from direct displacement and rearrangement are obtained.[12]
11. R. J. Andersen, C. A. Henrick & J. B. Siddall, *J. Am. Chem. Soc.*, **92**, 735 (1970).

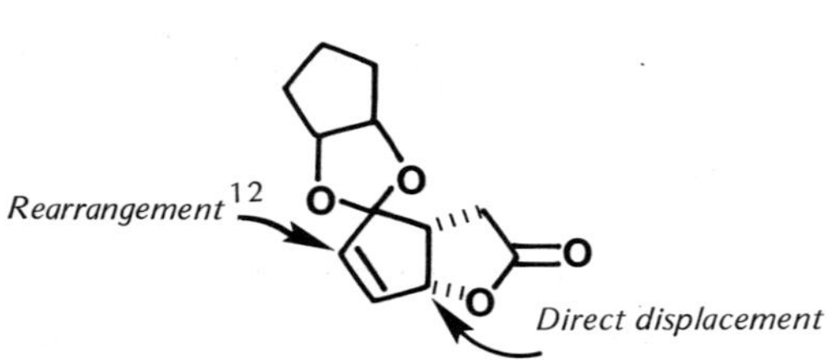

12. For further studies see Anthony Kreft, Ph.D., Dissertation Thesis, Columbia University (1976).

Synthesis of the Chiral Cuprate Reagent [5][8]

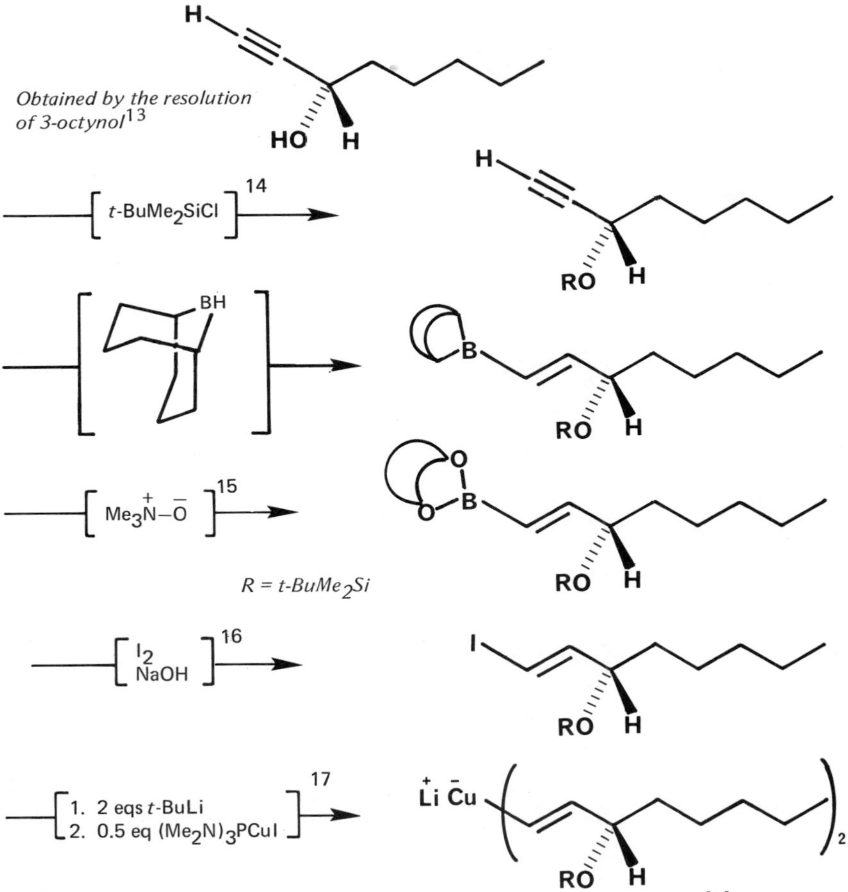

[5]

---

13. J. Fried, M. Mehra, C. Lin, W. Kao & P. Dalven in "Prostaglandins," *Annals of the New York Academy of Sciences*, P. Ramwell & J. E. Shaw (Eds.), **180**, 38 (1971).
14. E. J. Corey & A. Venkateswarlu, *J. Am. Chem. Soc.*, **94**, 6190 (1972).
15. R. Koster & Y. Morita, *Angew. Chem. [Int. Ed. Engl.]*, **5**, 580 (1966).
16. For a proposed mechanism of the reaction see H. C. Brown, T. Hamaoka & N. Ravindran, *J. Am. Chem. Soc.*, **95**, 5786, 6456 (1973).
17. E. J. Corey & D. J. Beames, *J. Am. Chem. Soc.*, **94**, 7210 (1972).

18

Syntheses of PGC_2

The highly unstable PGC_2 has been synthesized by controlled isomerization of the C_{10}-C_{11} double bond to the C_{11}-C_{12} (1→2) position with an iron carbonyl derivative from a known precursor [1] of PGA_2.[1]

SYNTHETIC PLAN[1]

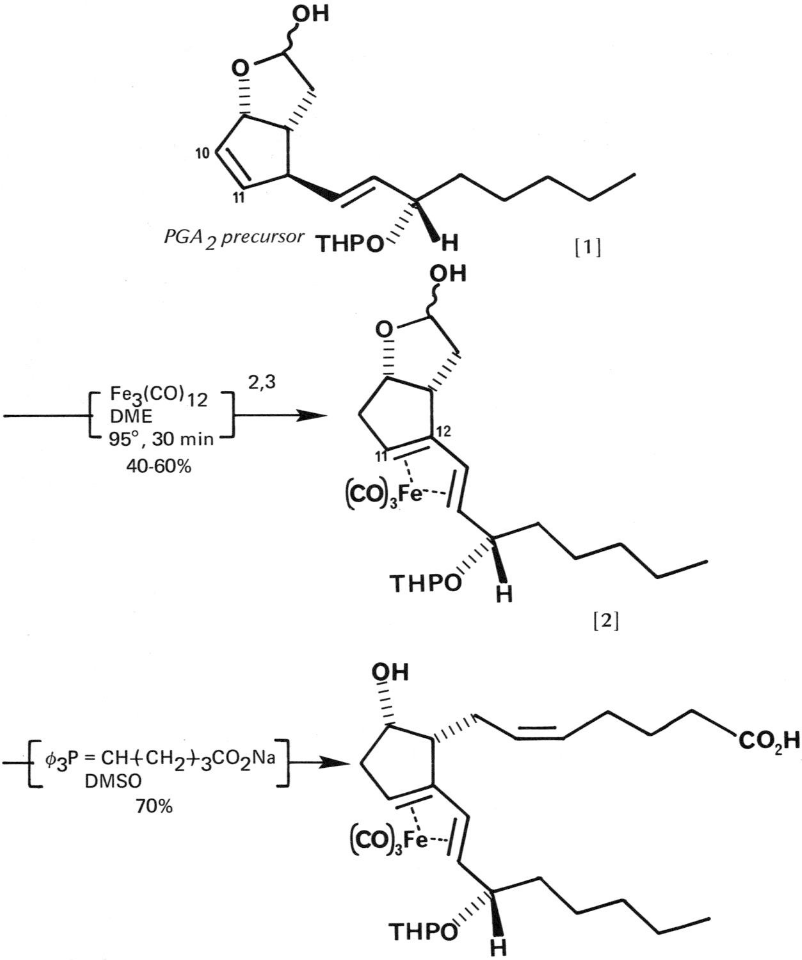

1. E. J. Corey & G. Moinet, *J. Am. Chem. Soc.*, 95, 7185 (1973).

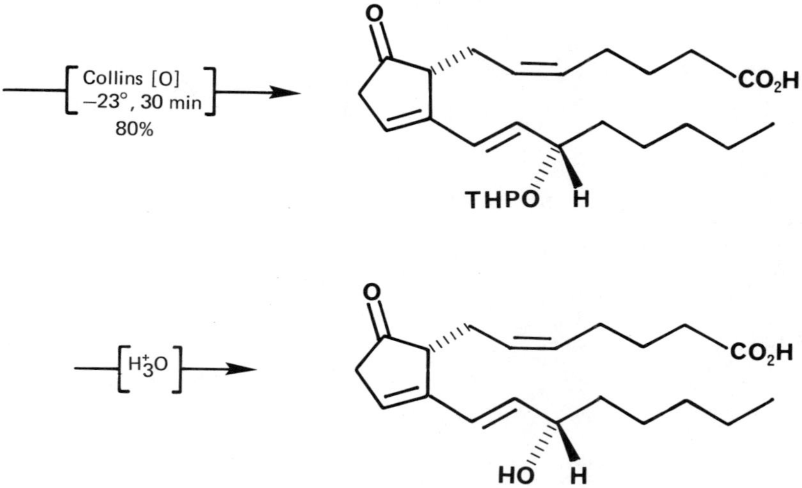

PGC₂

---

2. The lactone [3] does not form the diene complex [4].

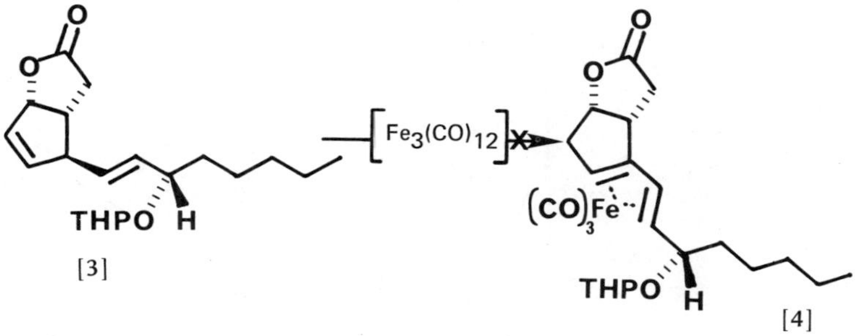

[3] [4]

3. Attempted isomerization of the C_{15} unprotected alcohol [5] leads to the satured ketone [6].

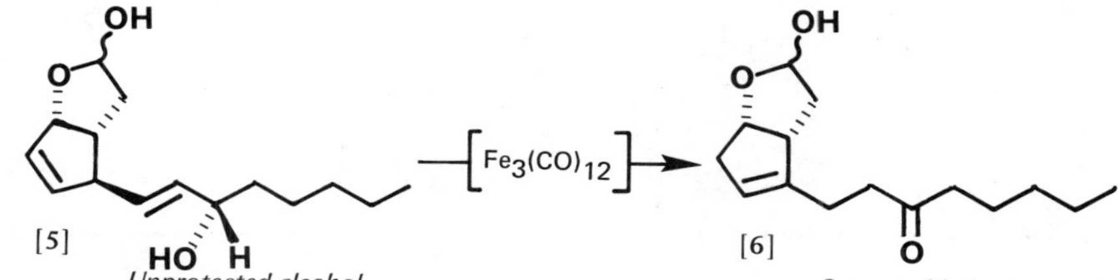

[5] *Unprotected alcohol* [6] *Saturated ketone*

SYNTHETIC PLAN[4]

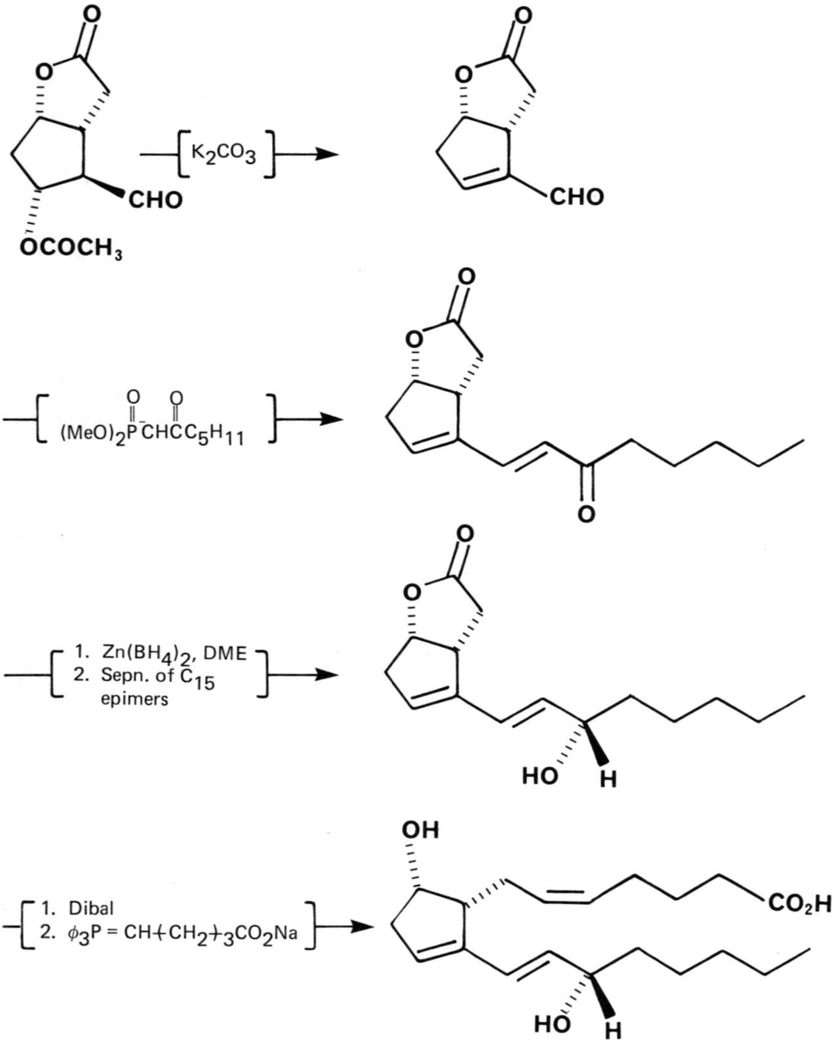

4. P. Crabbe, A. Guzman & M. Vera, *Tet. Lett.*, 3021 (1973).

19

Syntheses of PG Analogs

11-DEOXY-PROSTAGLANDINS

The first application of a ring contraction method for the construction of the prostanoid nucleus was made by the Ayerst group.[1] A Buchi ring contraction[2] was followed by Michael addition with a one-carbon synthon. Further, elaboration of the β-chain gives 11-deoxy PGE_2 methyl ester.

SYNTHETIC PLAN[1]

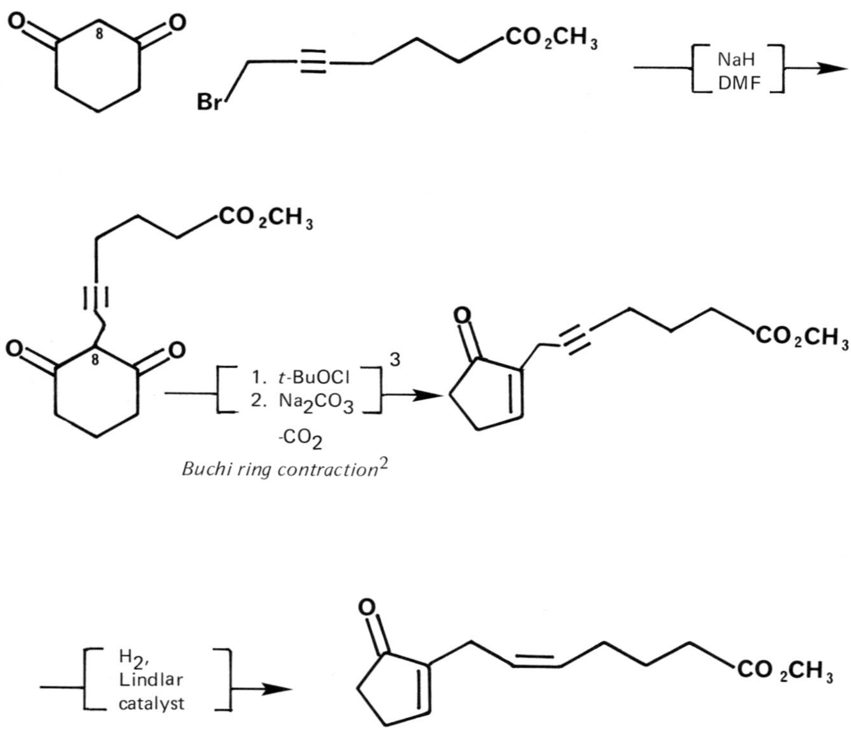

1. J. Bagli & T. Bogri, *Tet. Lett.*, 3815 (1972).
2. G. Buchi & B. Egger, *J. Org. Chem.*, **36**, 2021 (1971).
3. Similar ring contraction method was later applied to the synthesis of $PGF_{2\alpha}$ by the Hoffmann-La Roche group. F. Kienzle, G. W. Holland, J. L. Jernow, S. Kwoh & Perry Rosen, *J. Org. Chem.*, **38**, 3440 (1973).

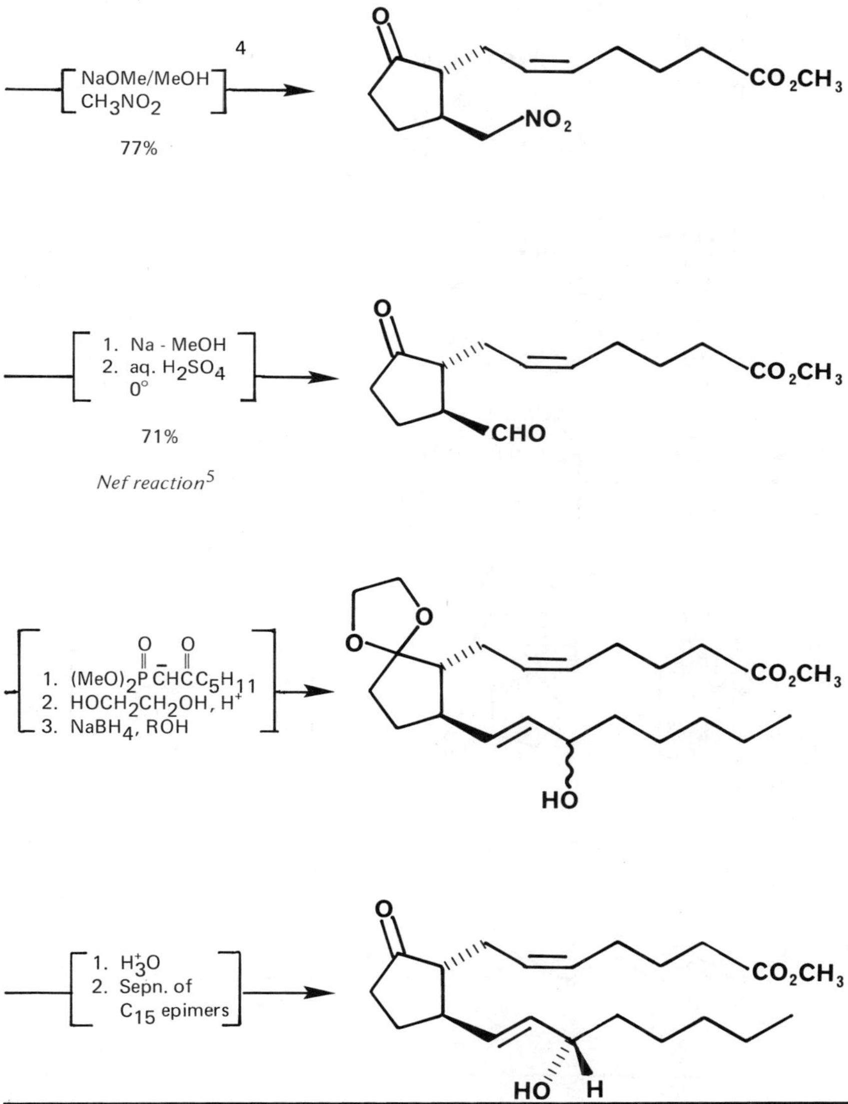

4. A similar synthesis has since been reported by the Syntex group. F. S. Alvarez & D. Wren, *Tet. Lett.*, 569 (1973).

5. See p. 180 for further references on Nef reaction. For recent work on Nef reaction see J. E. McMurry, J. Melton & H. Padgett, *J. Org. Chem.*, 39, 259 (1974).

The Corey approach involves the ring contraction of the cyclohexene [1] with thallic nitrate.[6]

SYNTHETIC PLAN[6]

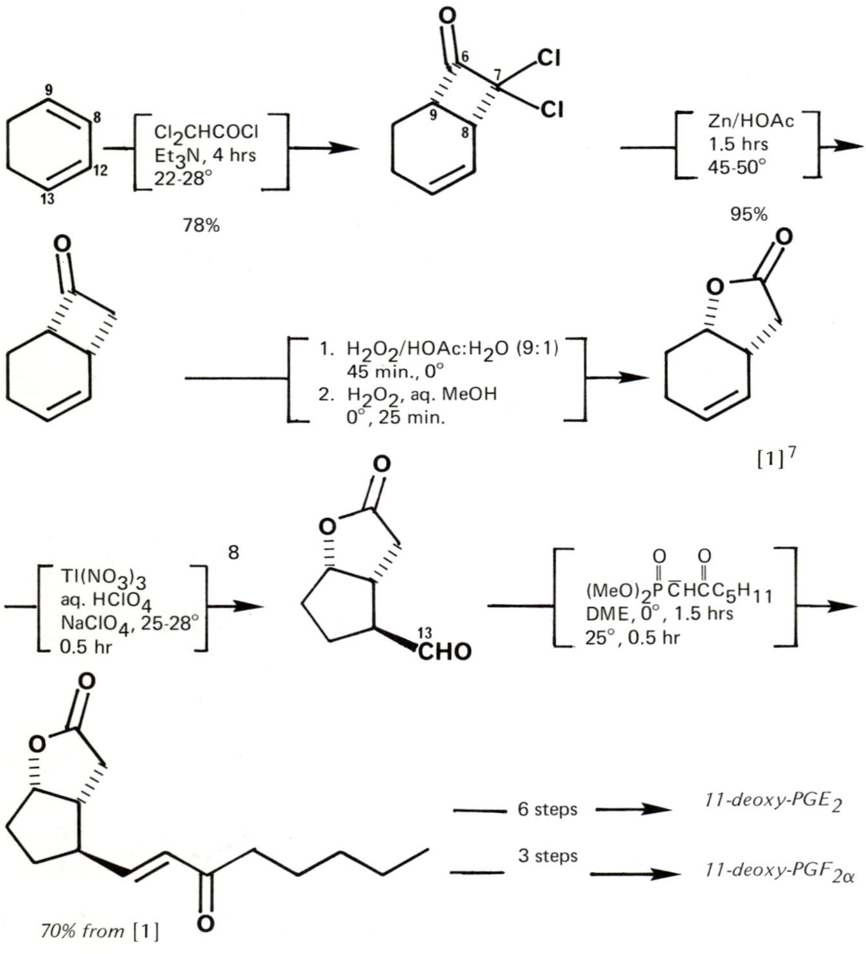

---

6. E. J. Corey & T. Ravindranathan, *Tet. Lett.*, 4753 (1971).
7. This intermediate has been used in the synthesis of the natural prostaglandins. E. J. Corey & B. B. Snider, *Tet. Lett.*, 3091 (1973). For further details see p. 174.
8. This ring contraction method with thallium nitrate was not applicable in the Woodward synthesis. I. Ernest, *Angew. Chem. [Int. Edit.]*, 15, 207 (1976). See p. 172.

A malonate can react with a cyclopropanedicarboxylate to give a cyclopentanone derivative. Such a ring expansion approach has been used by Abraham in the synthesis 11-deoxy prostaglandin.[9,10]

SYNTHETIC PLAN[9,10]

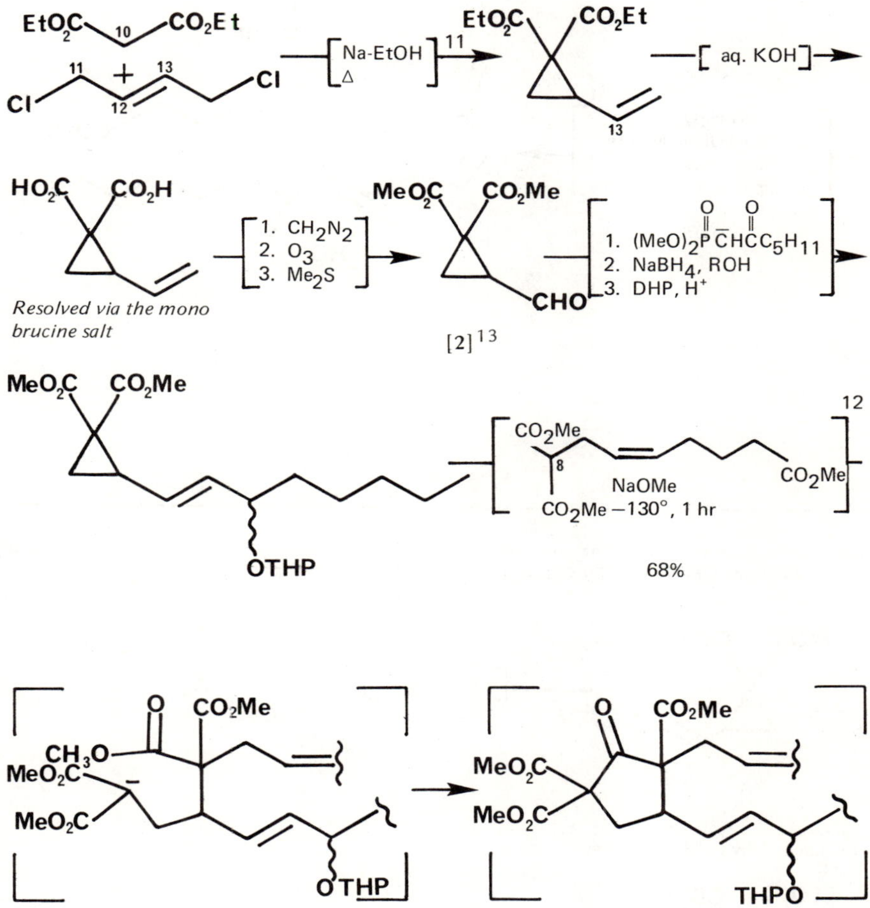

9. N. A. Abraham, *Tet. Lett.*, 1393 (1974).
10. N. A. Abraham, *Tet. Lett.*, 451 (1973).
11. R. W. Kirstead, R. P. Linstead & B. C. L. Weedon, *J. Chem. Soc.*, 3610 (1952).

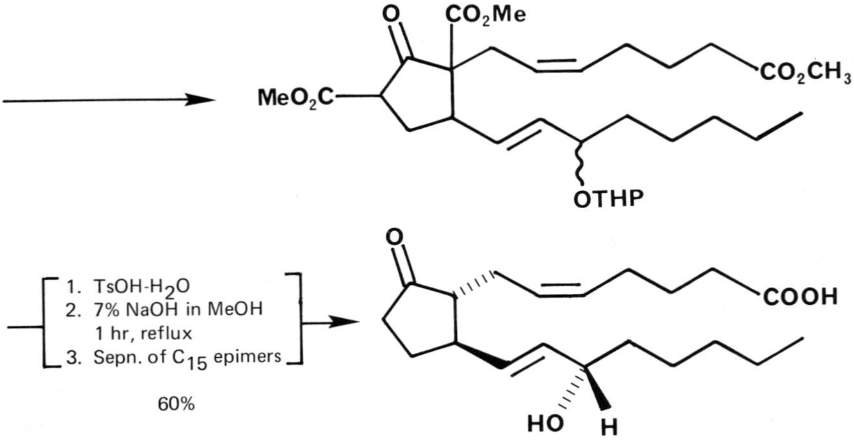

---

12. Dimethylcuprate opens the vinylcyclopropanecarboxylate [3] via allylic displacement as shown. P. A. Grieco & R. Finkelhor, *J. Org. Chem.*, **38**, 2100 (1973).

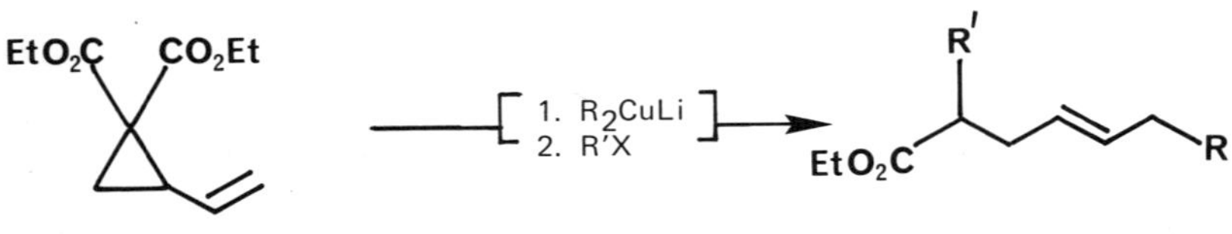

[3]

13. The aldehyde [2] can also be made directly from acrolein.

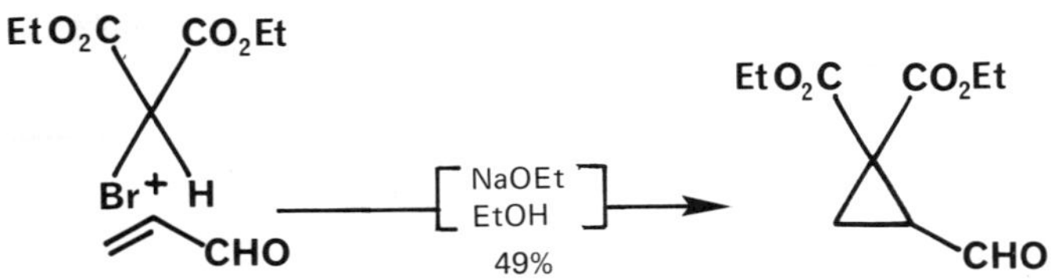

In this straightforward convergent synthesis of 11-deoxy-PGE_2 the α- and β-chains are introduced by 1,4-addition of the β-chain and alkylation of the α-chain unit with a regiospecifically generated enolate.[14,15] This can be viewed, formally, as a conjugate addition–enolate trapping sequence.

SYNTHETIC PLAN[14]

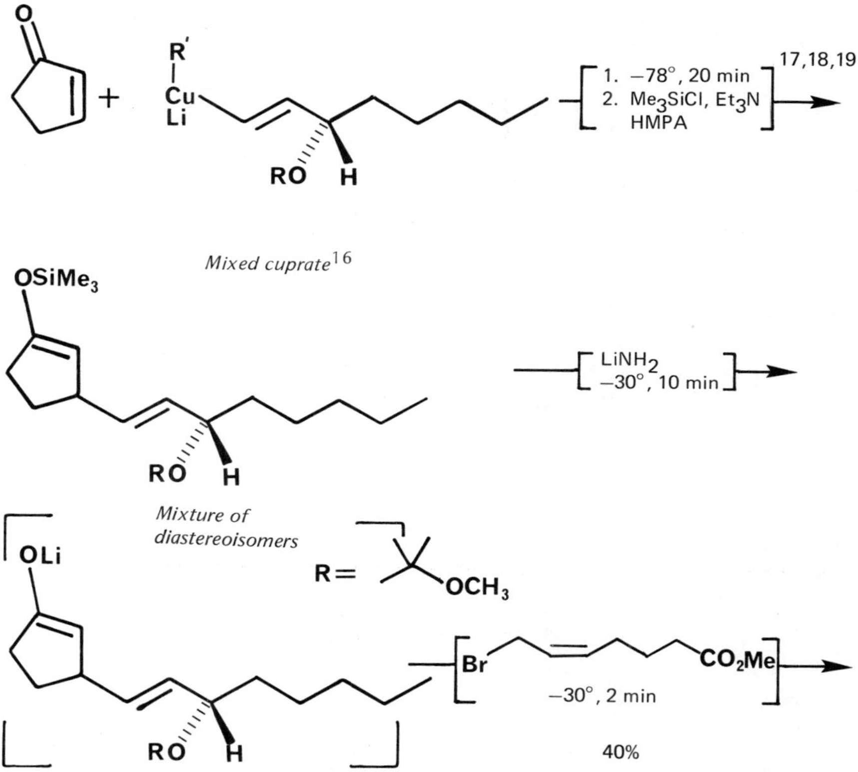

---

14. J. W. Patterson Jr. & J. H. Fried, *J. Org. Chem.*, **39**, 2406 (1974).
15. A similar approach has been used in the more complicated case by Stork and Isobe for the synthesis of $PGF_{2\alpha}$. For details see p. 268.
16. The mixed cuprate ($R' = C \equiv C\text{-}C_3H_7$) was used. E. J. Corey & D. J. Beames, *J. Am. Chem. Soc.*, **94**, 7210 (1972).
17. The trapping of enolates as trialkylsilyl enol ethers was first demonstrated by Stork & Hudrlik. Subsequent regeneration of the enolate and its alkylation has been shown to be a viable synthetic operation. G. Stork & P. F. Hudrlik, *J. Am. Chem. Soc.*, **90**, 4462, 4464 (1968).
18. The *t*-$BuMe_2Si$- enol ethers are comparatively more stable than the Me_3Si- enol ethers. See P. F. Hudrlik, Ph.D. Dissertation Thesis, Columbia University, 1968.

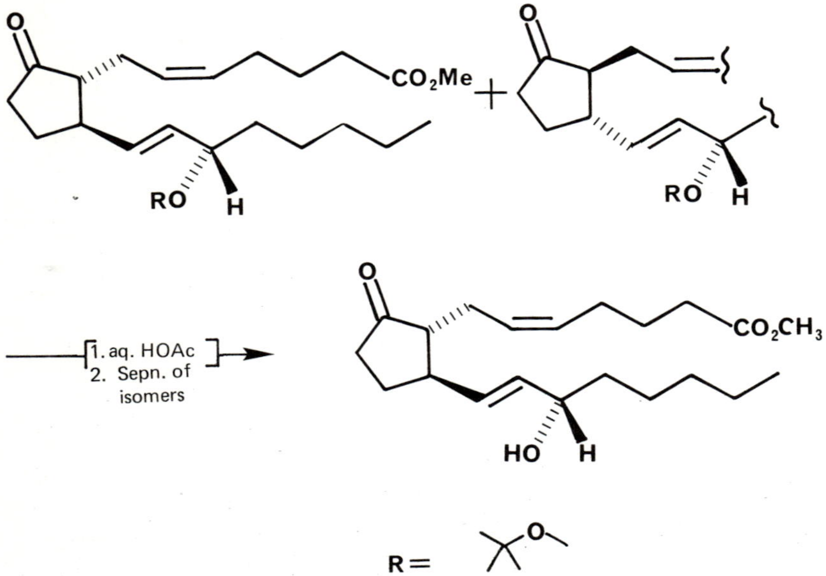

---

19. The other enol ether is not formed. This may reflect some difference in properties between the simple cyclopentenone and the 4-alkoxycyclopentenone (see Chapter 14).

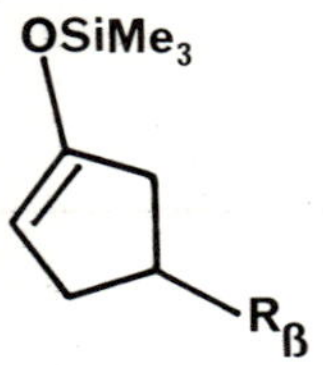

Not formed

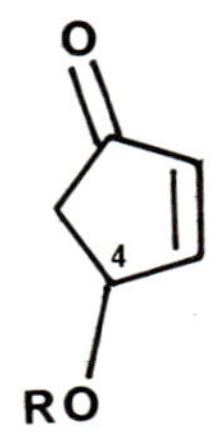

4-Alkoxycyclopentenone

This method of trapping a regiospecifically generated enolate of cyclopentanone has been applied to the synthesis of other prostaglandin derivatives. See S. Kurozumi, T. Toru, T. Tanaka, M. Kobayashi, S. Miura & S. Ishimoto, *Tet. Lett.*, 4087, 4091 (1976).

The cyclopentene system of the bicyclo[3.3.0]octenone [5], made via a vinylcyclopropane rearrangement, serves as the latent aldehyde units required for the elaboration into the α- and β-chains.[20]

SYNTHETIC PLAN[20]

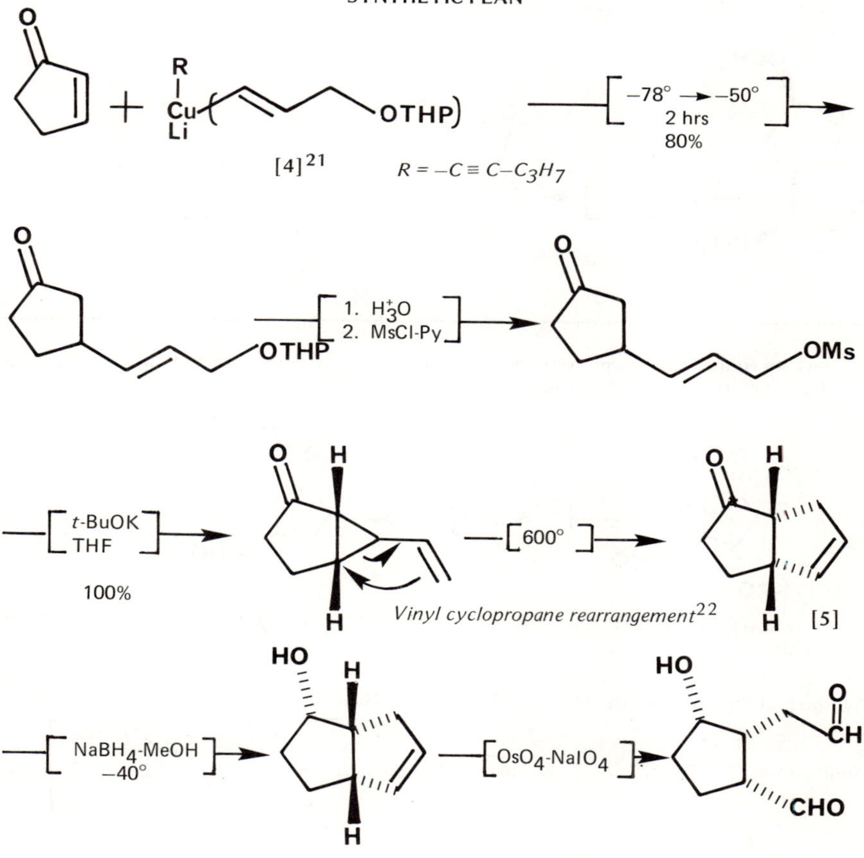

---

20. E. J. Corey & R. H. Wollenberg, *J. Org. Chem.*, **40**, 2265 (1975).
21. For the synthesis of this reagent see p. 346.
22. For a recent review on vinylcyclopropane rearrangement see B. M. Trost, *Accounts Chem. Res.*, 7, 85 (1974). For the stereochemistry of the vinyl cyclopropane rearrangement see G. D. Andrews & J. E. Baldwin, *J. Am. Chem. Soc.*, **98**, 6705 (1976).

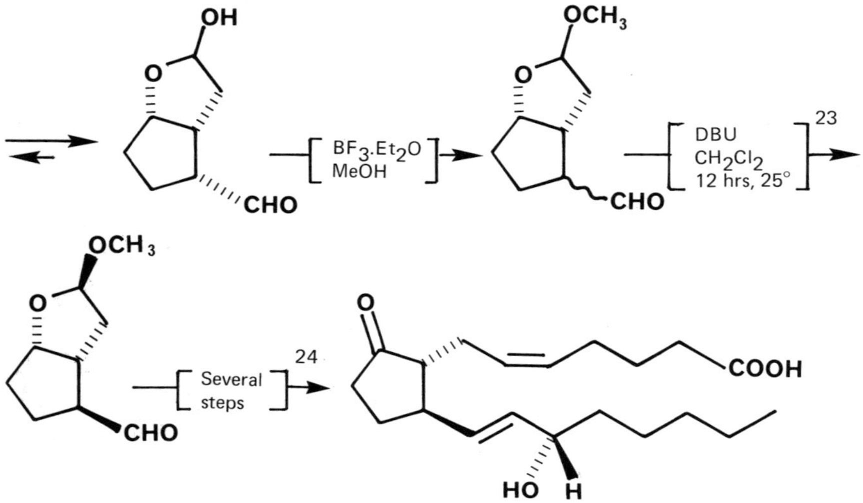

23. Such an epimerization is probably possible in the 11-deoxy series. In the 11-alkoxy compound elimination to the unsaturated aldehyde may be a serious problem:

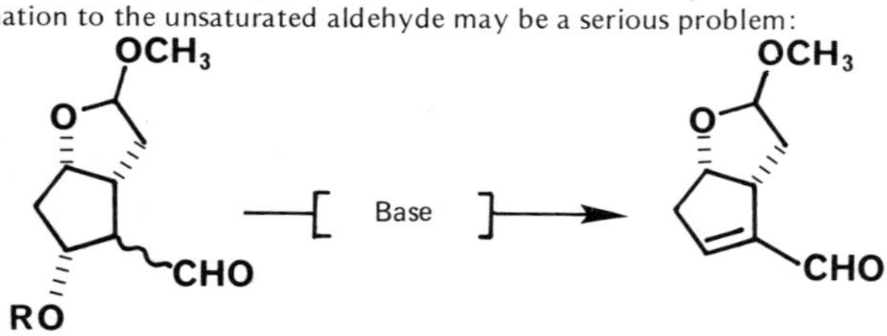

24. E. J. Corey, N. M. Weinshenker, T. K. Schaaf & W. Huber, *J. Am. Chem. Soc.*, **40**, 2565 (1975).

Synthesis of the Vinylcuprate Reagent [4] Via the Tin Hydride Reduction[20]

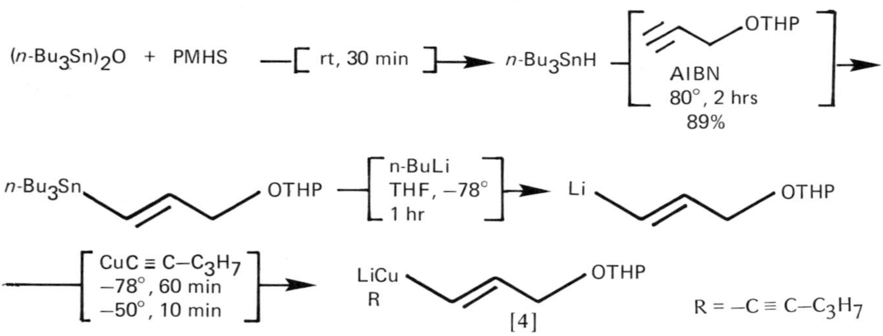

The known ring contraction of α-tropolone methyl ether via photochemical valence tautomerization[25] has been successfully utilized by Crabbe[26,27] in the synthesis of 11-deoxy-PGE_1. The olefin in the bicyclic intermediate serves as the latent C_{13} aldehyde functionality.

SYNTHETIC PLAN[26,27]

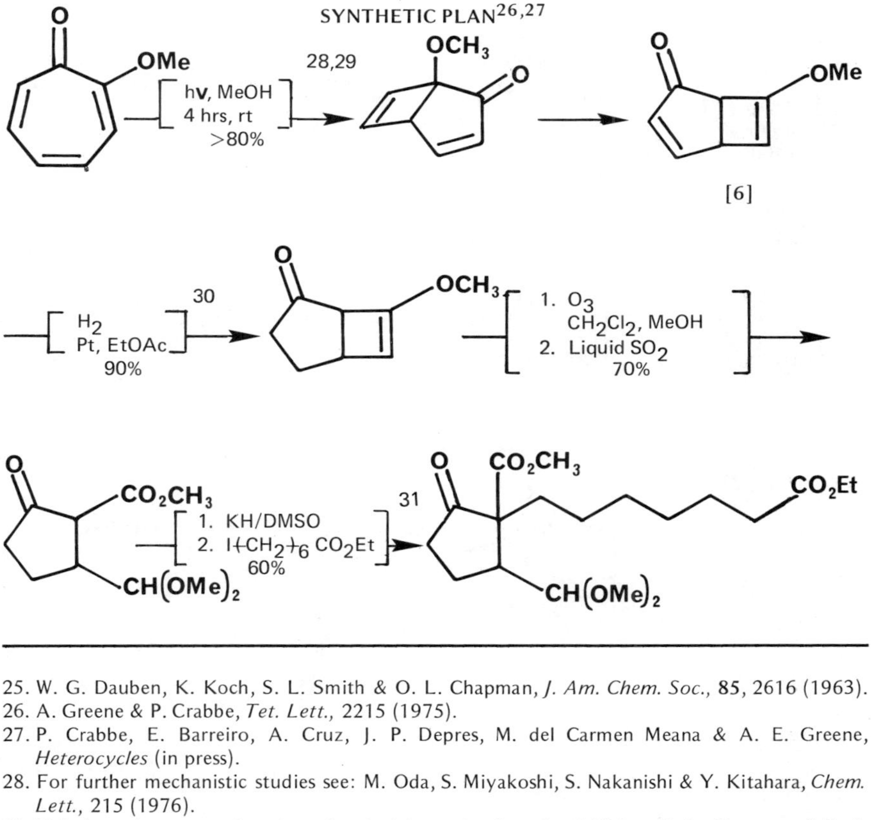

---

25. W. G. Dauben, K. Koch, S. L. Smith & O. L. Chapman, *J. Am. Chem. Soc.*, **85**, 2616 (1963).
26. A. Greene & P. Crabbe, *Tet. Lett.*, 2215 (1975).
27. P. Crabbe, E. Barreiro, A. Cruz, J. P. Depres, M. del Carmen Meana & A. E. Greene, *Heterocycles* (in press).
28. For further mechanistic studies see: M. Oda, S. Miyakoshi, S. Nakanishi & Y. Kitahara, *Chem. Lett.*, 215 (1976).
29. This is analogous to the photochemical isomerization of colchicine. O. L. Chapman & D. J. Pasto, *J. Am. Chem. Soc.*, **82**, 3642 (1960).
30. This intermediate [6] can be epoxidized under known conditions to lead ultimately to the 11-oxygenated natural prostaglandins. P. Crabbe & A. Greene in *Advances in Prostaglandin and Thromboxane Research*, B. Samuelsson and R. Paoletti (Eds.), Vol. 1, Raven Press, New York, 1976, p. 205.
31. Dimsylpotassium (DMSO-KH, 25°, <5 min.) is easier to prepare than dimsylsodium (DMSO-NaH, 70°, 1 hr.). A. E. Greene, J. P. Depres, M. C. Meana & P. Crabbe, *Tet. Lett.*, 3755 (1976).

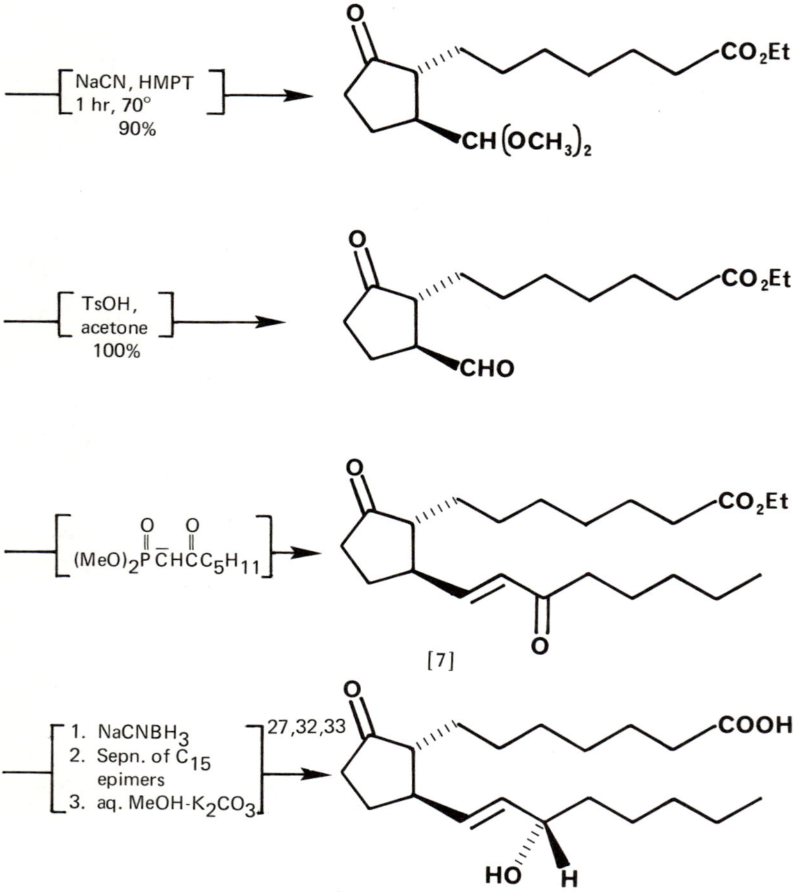

32. Thexyllimonyl borohydride has been used for the selective reduction of the enone [7] to the allylic alcohol in the E_1 series. M. Miyano & M. A. Stealey, *J. Org. Chem.*, **40**, 1748 (1975). But in the 11-deoxy series the 15α:15β alcohol ratio is 1:2 and the yield is only 40%.

33. Some diol is formed which is oxidized back to the dione and reduced. The C_{15} epimeric alcohols are formed in equal amounts.

In this synthesis of 11-deoxy PGE_2 starting from the bicyclic lactol [8] the C_{11}-C_{12} double bond is isomerized to the conjugated enone [9] after the oxidation of the C_9 alcohol.[34]

SYNTHETIC PLAN[34]

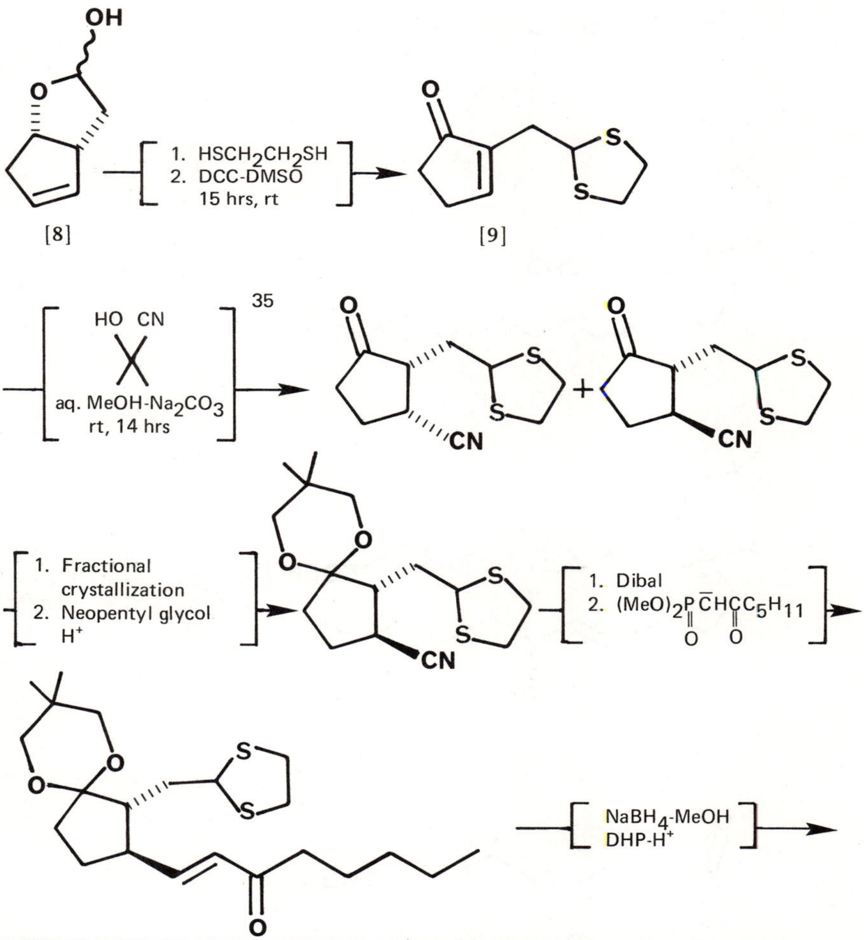

34. W. Bartmann, G. Beck & U. Lerch., *Tet. Lett.*, 2441 (1974).
35. It is interesting to note that Nagata's reagent Et_2AlCN is not used for the 1,4-addition of cyanide.

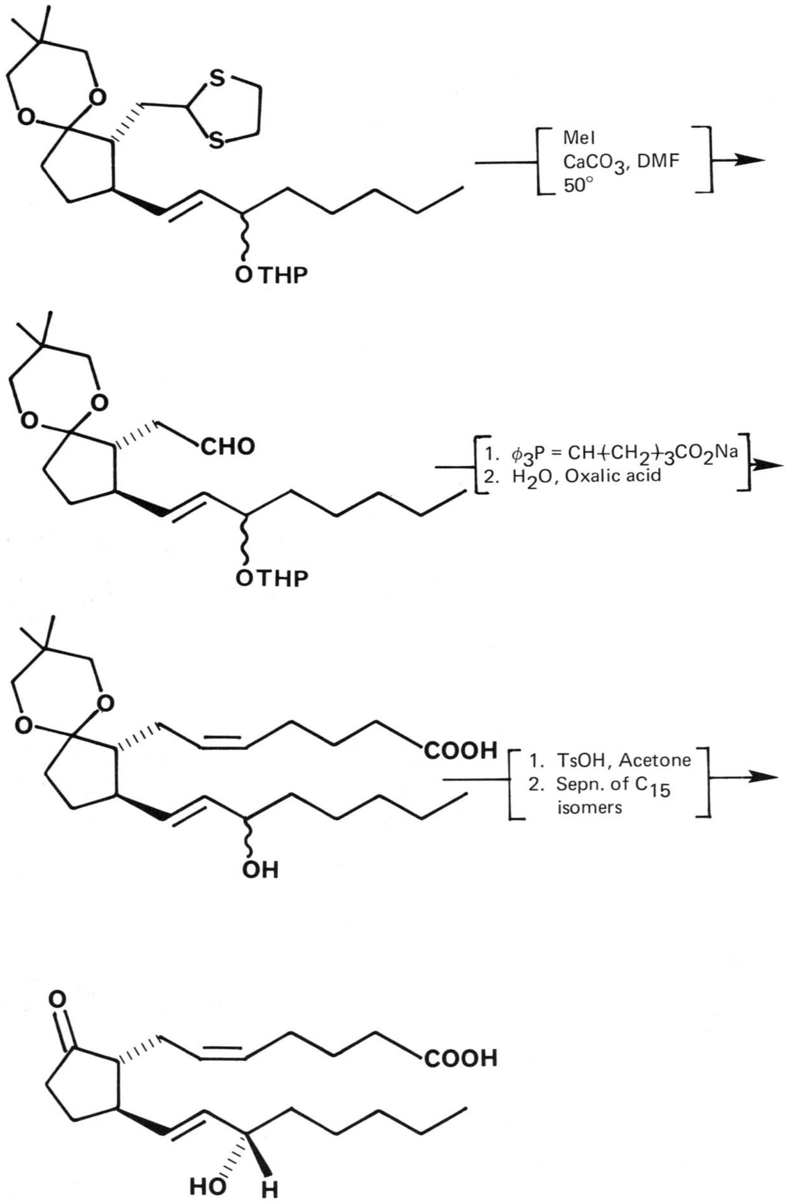
S
S
O
O
OTHP
MeI
CaCO3, DMF
50°
CHO
1. φ3P = CH(CH2)3CO2Na
2. H2O, Oxalic acid
COOH
OH
1. TsOH, Acetone
2. Sepn. of C15 isomers
O
COOH
HO
H

An intermediate [11] for the synthesis of 11-deoxy-PGE$_1$[36] has been synthesized by nucleophilic ring opening reaction of the activated bicyclo[3.1.0]hexane derivative.[37]

SYNTHETIC PLAN[37]

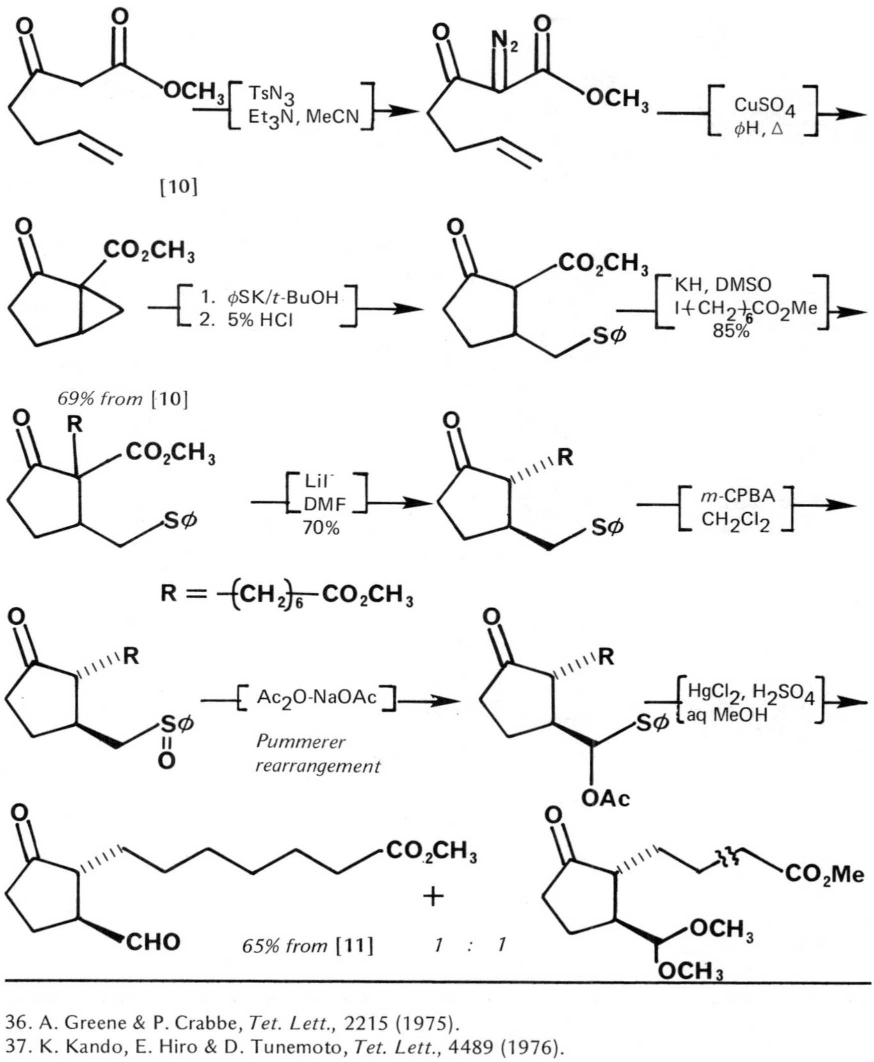

36. A. Greene & P. Crabbe, *Tet. Lett.*, 2215 (1975).
37. K. Kando, E. Hiro & D. Tunemoto, *Tet. Lett.*, 4489 (1976).

A convenient synthesis of an 11-deoxy-PG intermediate [14] from [13] has been reported by Sakai.[38]

SYNTHETIC PLAN[38]

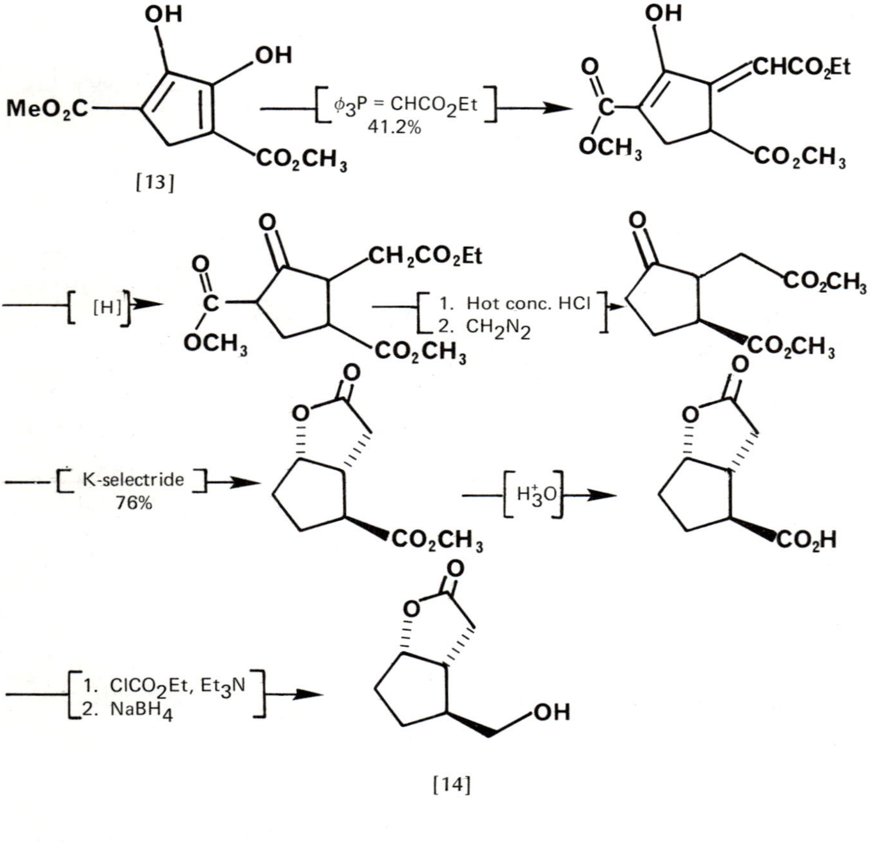

[14]

38. K. Inoue & K. Sakai, *Tet. Lett.*, 4107 (1976).

12-SUBSTITUTED PROSTAGLANDINS

The bicyclo[2.2.1]heptane approach has been used in the following synthesis of 12-α-methyl-PGA_2.[1] Reductive elimination of cyclopropyliodide [1] gives the vinyl group necessary for the elaboration of the β-chain.

SYNTHETIC PLAN[1]

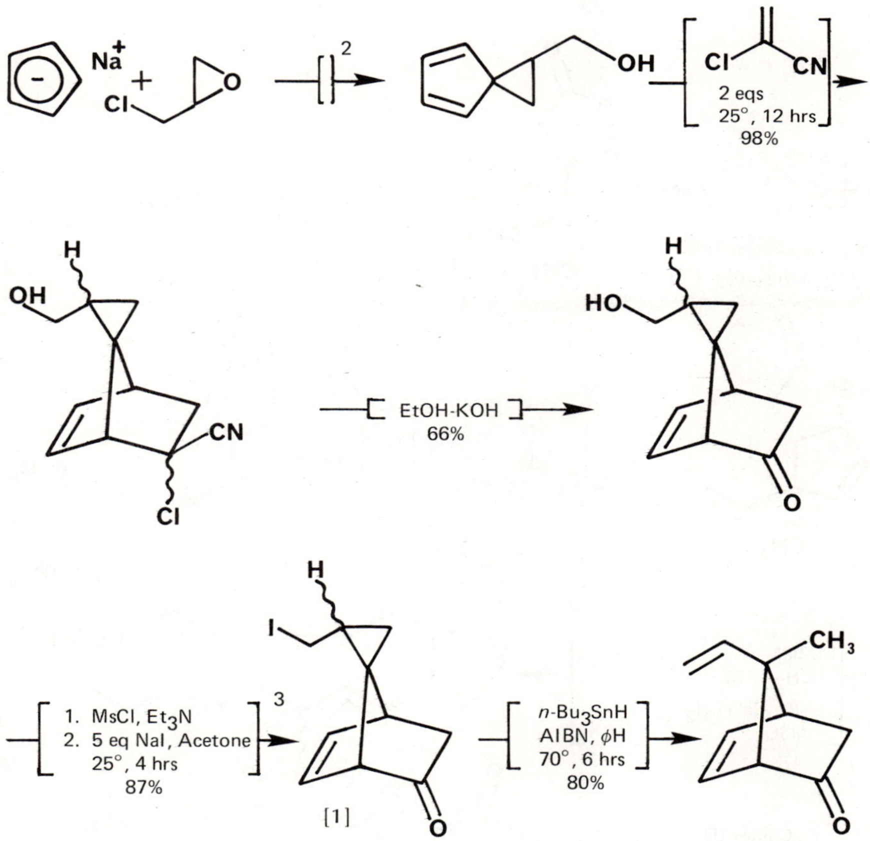

1. E. J. Corey, C. Shiner, R. P. Volante & C. R. Cyr, *Tet. Lett.*, 1161 (1975).
2. K. Bangert & V. Boekelhide, *Tet. Lett.*, 1119 (1963).
3. This method of mesylation is superior to the original Tipson procedure. R. K. Crossland & K. L. Servis, *J. Org. Chem.*, **35**, 3195 (1970).

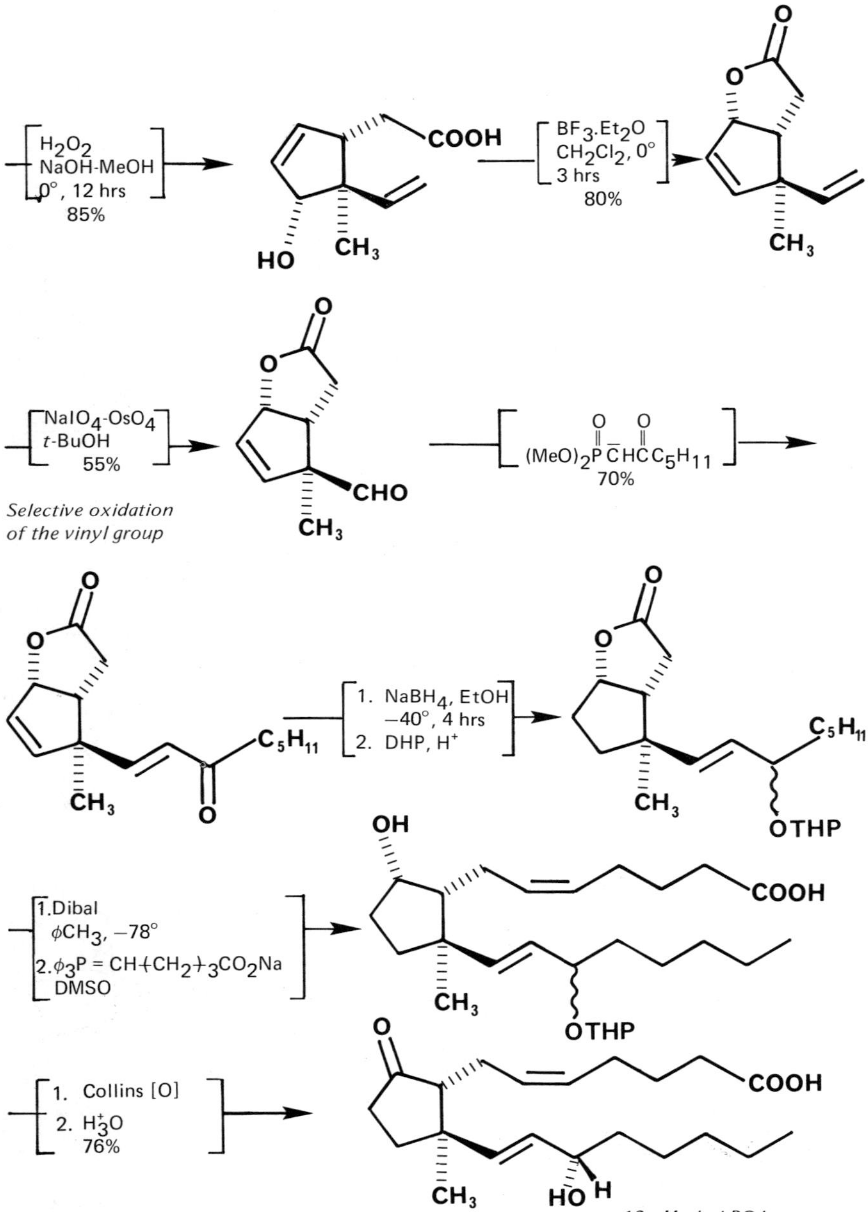

12α-Methyl PGA 2

Grieco's synthesis of 12α-methyl PGA_2 involves the alkylation of the bicyclo[2.2.1]heptane carboxylate to introduce the C_{12}-Me group stereospecifically.[4]

SYNTHETIC PLAN[4]

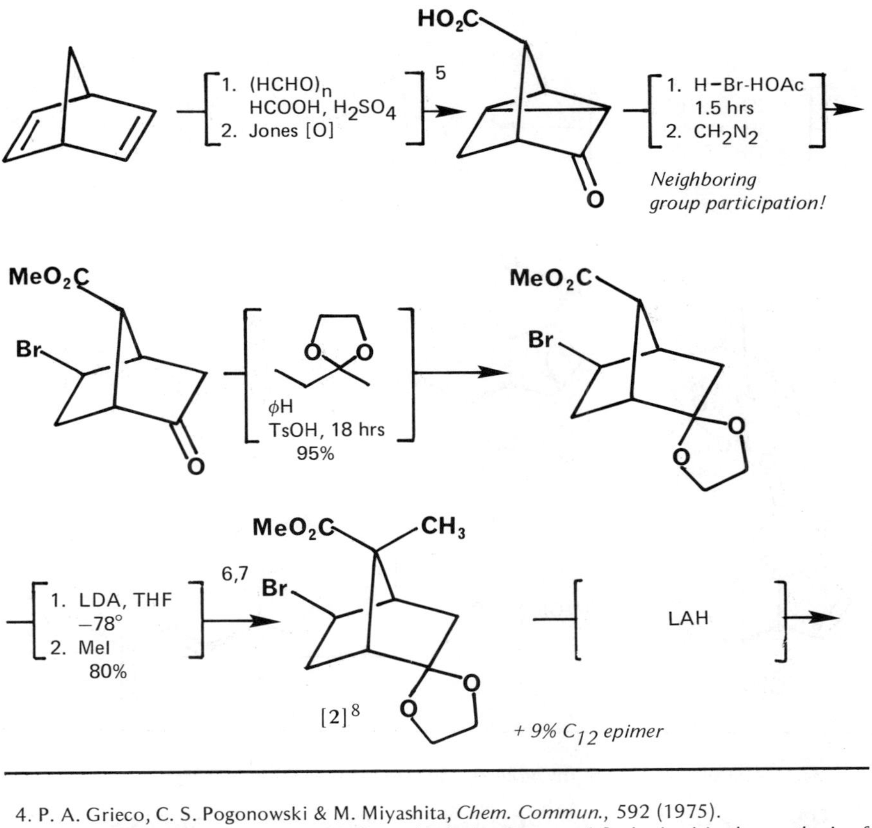

4. P. A. Grieco, C. S. Pogonowski & M. Miyashita, *Chem. Commun.*, 592 (1975).
5. This reaction sequence was used independently by Corey and Sutherland in the synthesis of prostaglandins. For details see p. 216.
6. The electrophile comes in from the less hindered side.
7. With a smaller electrophile like F^+ a mixture, containing both the epimers in equal amounts, is obtained. The fluorinated compound has been used in the synthesis of 12-fluoro-PG analog. For details see p. 360.
8. This intermediate [2] has been used in the synthesis of sesquifenchene. P. A. Grieco & Y. Masaki, *J. Org. Chem.*, **40**, 150 (1975).

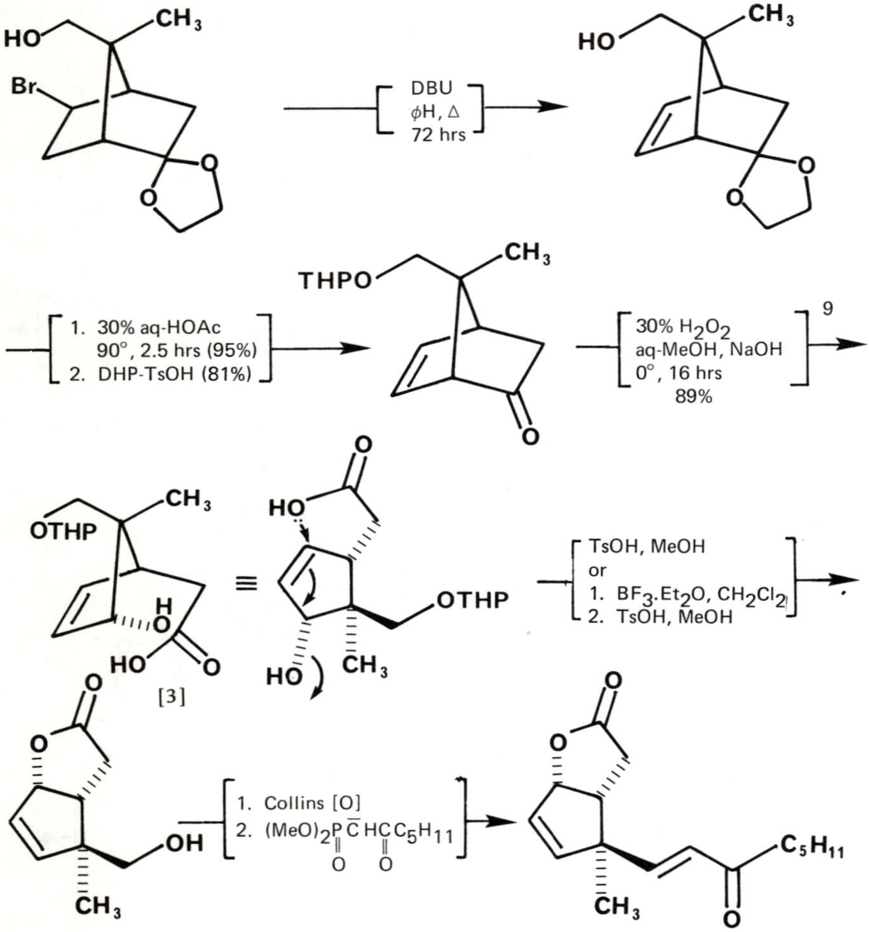

9. Baeyer-Villiger oxidation of the bromo-ketone gives undesirable products.

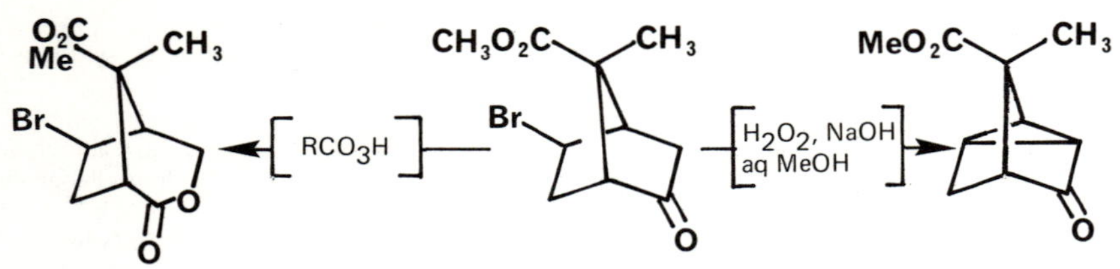

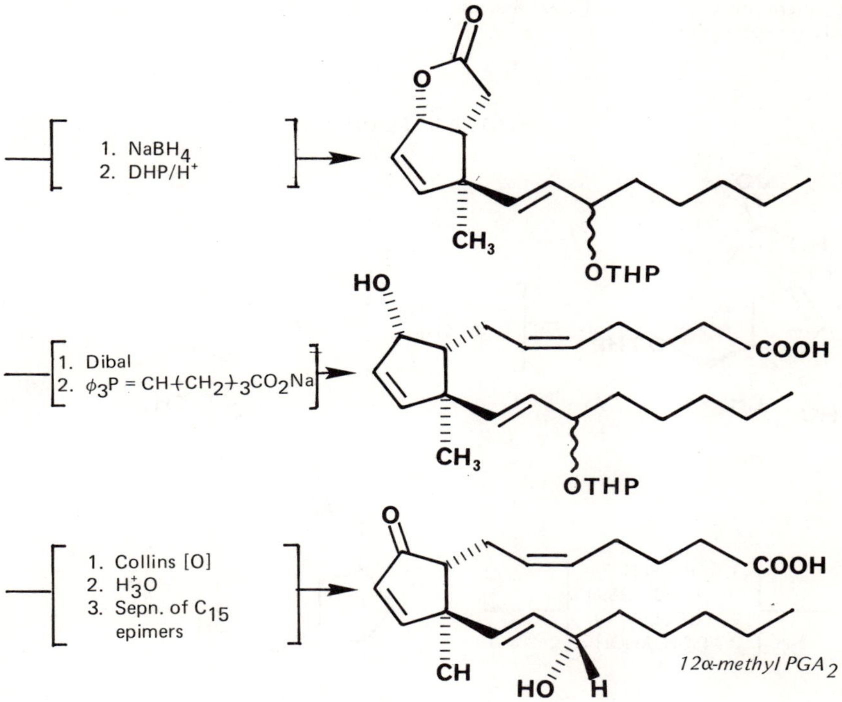

---

10. The phosphonate reagent was made by the alkylation of the dianion of β-keto phosphonate. This new method was developed by: P. A. Grieco & C. S. Pogonowski, *J. Am. Chem. Soc.*, **95**, 3071 (1973).

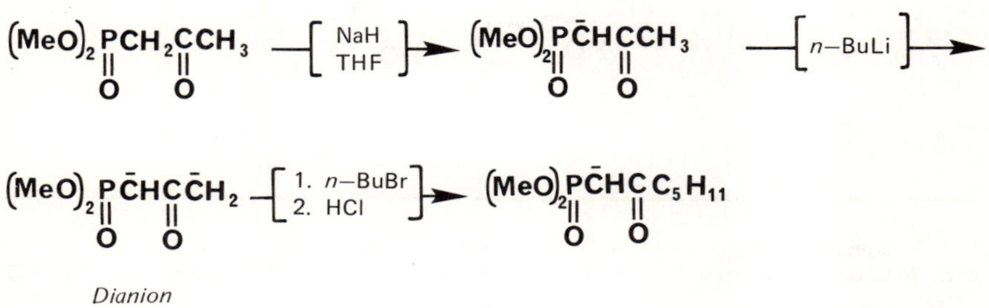

The intermediate hydroxyacid [3] has also been converted to 12α-methyl-$PGF_{2\alpha}$ via the iodolactonization route.[11]

SYNTHETIC PLAN[11]

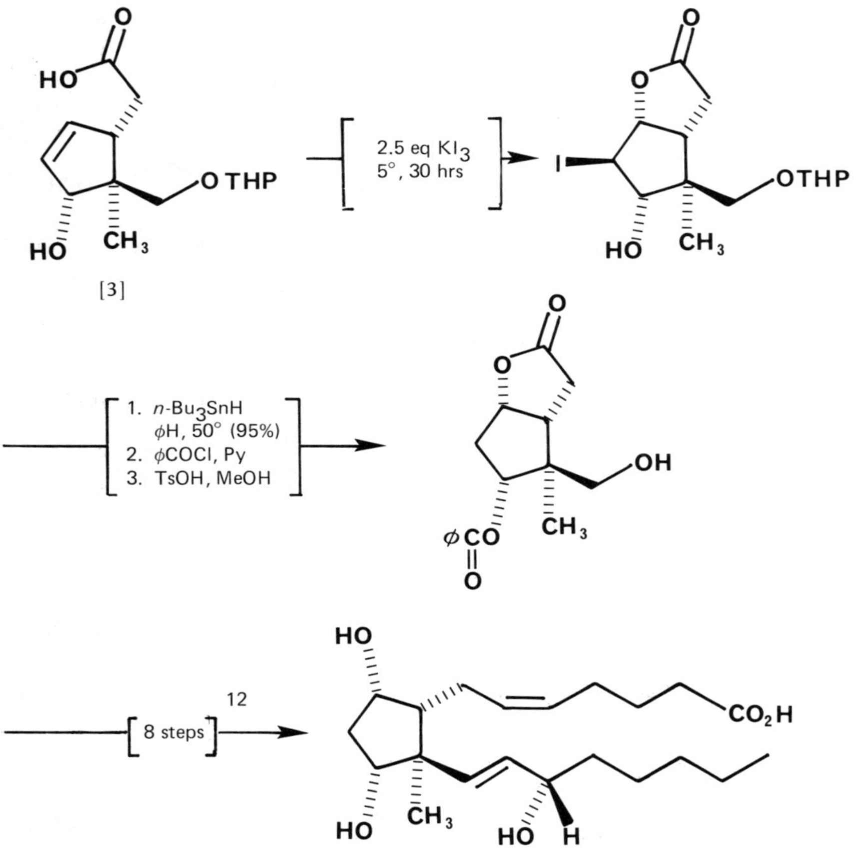

12α-methyl $PGF_{2\alpha}$

---

11. P. A. Grieco, C. S. Pogonowski, M. Nishizawa & C. L. J. Wang, *Tet. Lett.*, 2541 (1975).
12. E. J. Corey, N. M. Weinshenker, T. K. Schaaf & W. Huber, *J. Am. Chem. Soc.*, 91, 5675 (1969).

Grieco has reported an asymmetric approach to the synthesis of 12-methyl prostaglandins.[13]

SYNTHETIC PLAN[13]

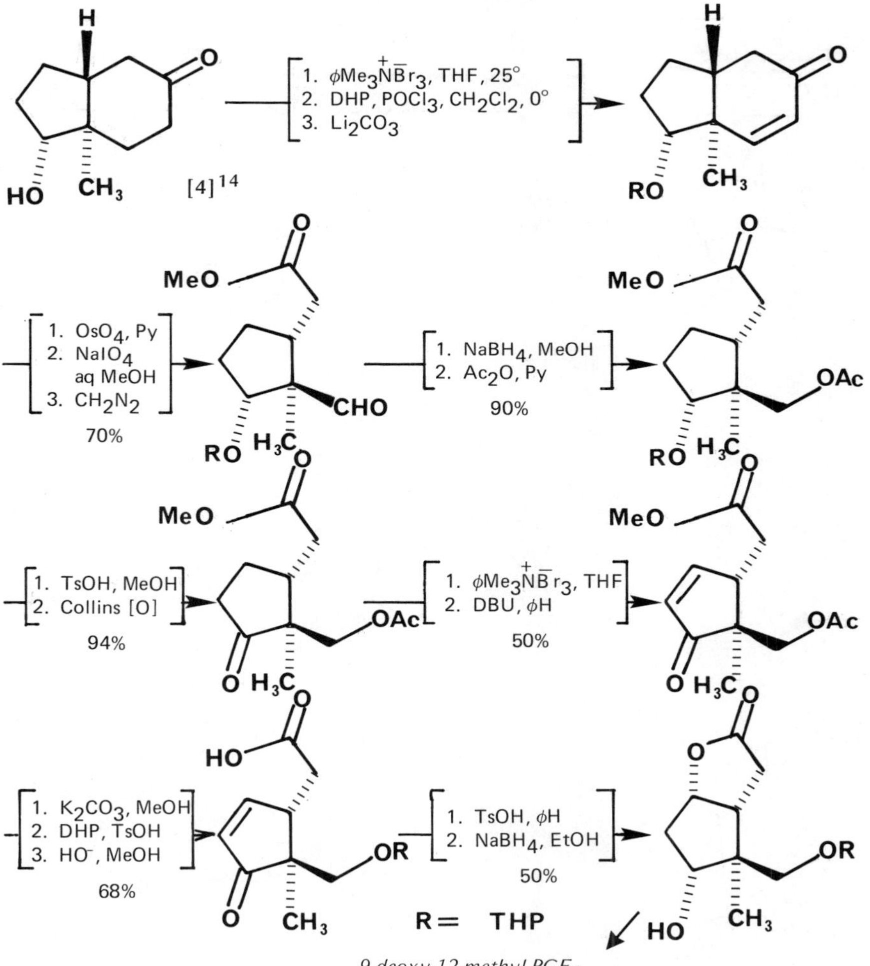

9-deoxy-12-methyl PGF$_{2\alpha}$

13. P. A. Grieco, N. Fukamiya, M. Miyashita, *Chem. Commun.*, 573 (1976).
14. For a review on the asymmetric aldol condensation used in the preparation of [4] see N. Cohen, *Accounts Chem. Res.*, 9, 412 (1976).

The synthesis of the highly potent 12-α-fluoro-$PGF_{2\alpha}$ involves the fluorination of the common bicyclo[2.2.1]heptane carboxylate intermediate[15] [5]. It should be noted that unlike the methylation the fluorination of [5] is not stereospecific.[15]

SYNTHETIC PLAN[15]

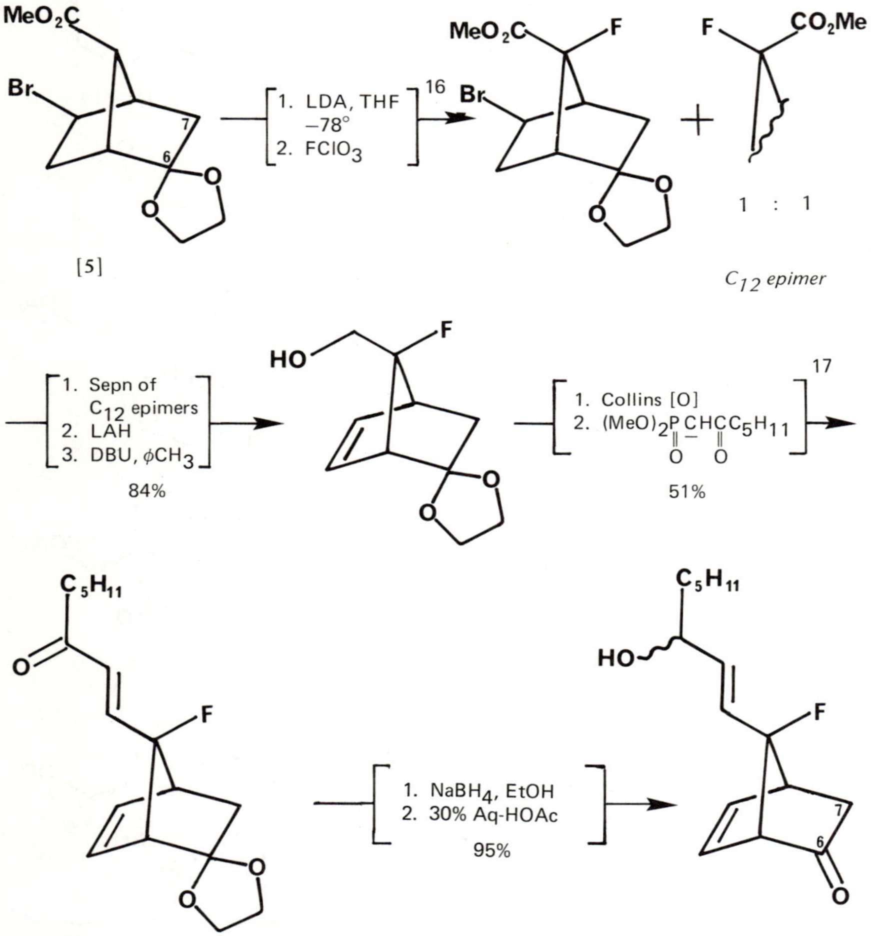

15. C. L. J. Wang, P. A. Grieco & F. J. Okuniewicz, *Chem. Commun.*, 468 (1976).
16. For discussion see footnote 7, p. 355.

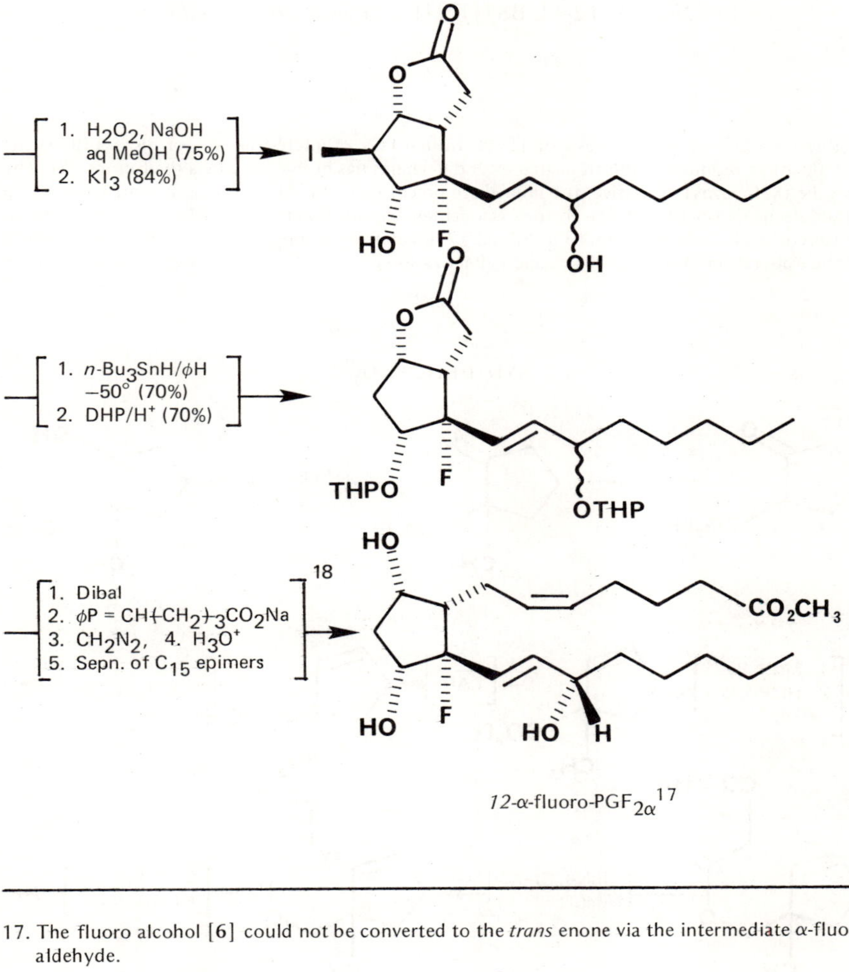

12-α-fluoro-$PGF_{2\alpha}$[17]

17. The fluoro alcohol [6] could not be converted to the *trans* enone via the intermediate α-fluoro aldehyde.

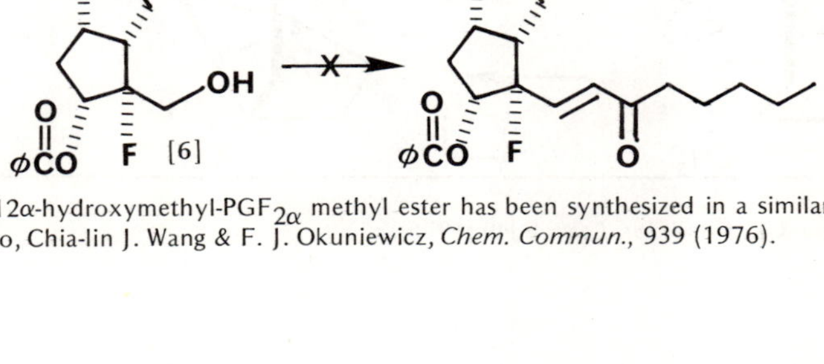

18. The 12α-hydroxymethyl-$PGF_{2\alpha}$ methyl ester has been synthesized in a similar manner. P. A. Grieco, Chia-lin J. Wang & F. J. Okuniewicz, *Chem. Commun.*, 939 (1976).

11-DEOXY-12-SUBSTITUTED PROSTAGLANDINS

In this approach to the synthesis of 12-substituted PGs an interesting way of distinguishing the two aldehyde residues of the truncated α- and β- chains has been realized via the lactone [2]. The tricyclic cyclopropyl derivative, the immediate precursor of the lactone [1], is synthesized by an intramolecular carbene addition to the cyclopentene double bond. This unfortunately gives the all *cis* stereochemistry at the carbons 9, 8, and 12. Oxidative opening of the cyclopropane followed by the elaboration of the side chains and epimerization gives the C_{12}-substituted prostaglandin.

SYNTHETIC PLAN[1]

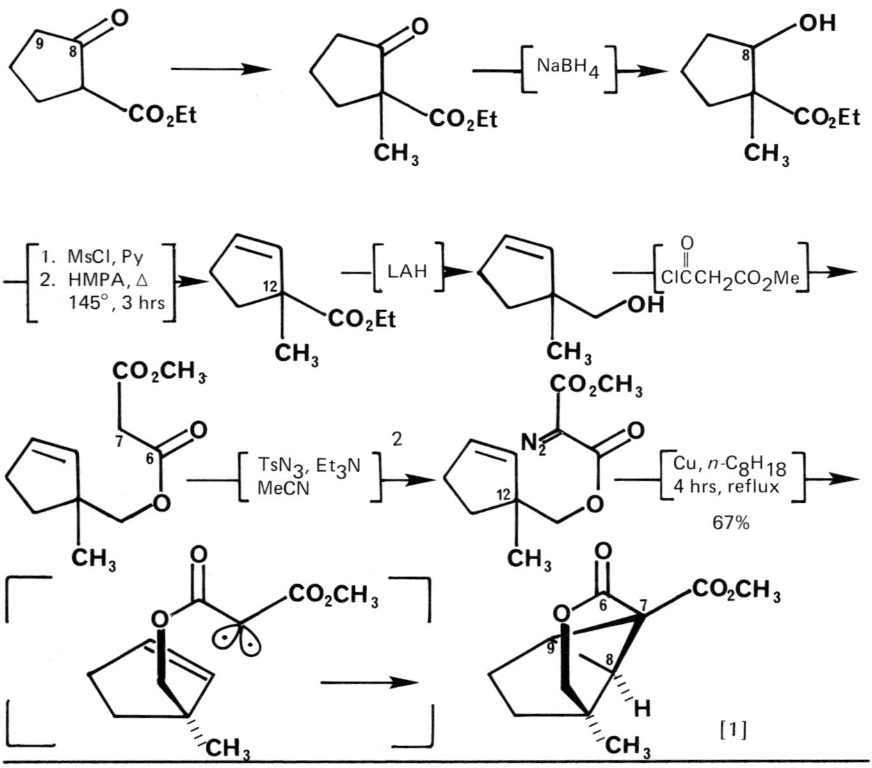

[1]

1. N. Nakamura & K. Sakai, *Tet. Lett.*, 2049 (1976).

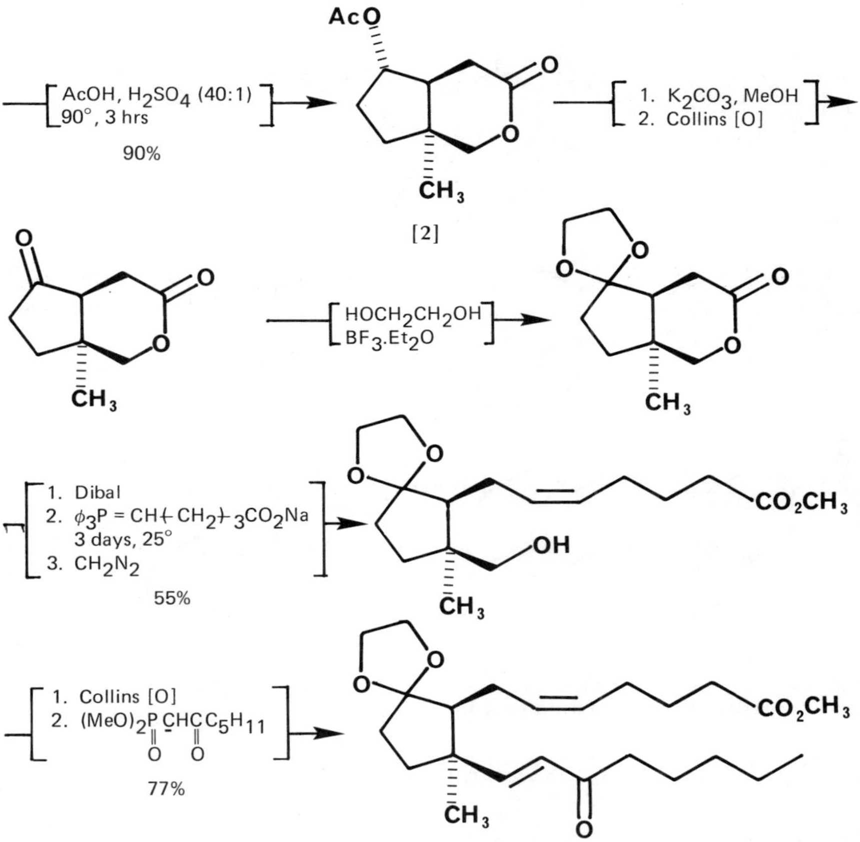

2. "Recent Synthetic Methods in Diazo Chemistry" by M. Regitz, *Synthesis*, 351 (1972).

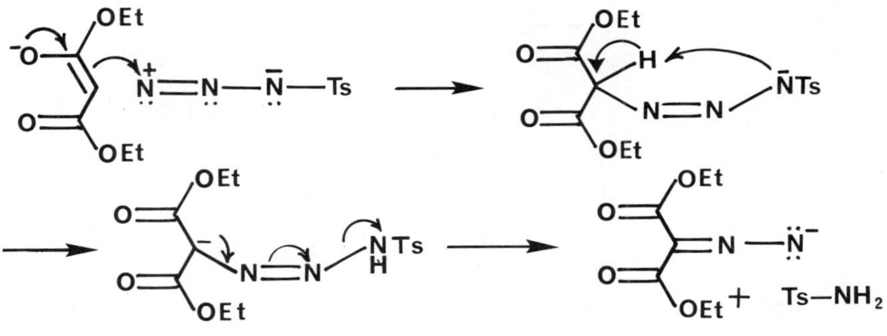

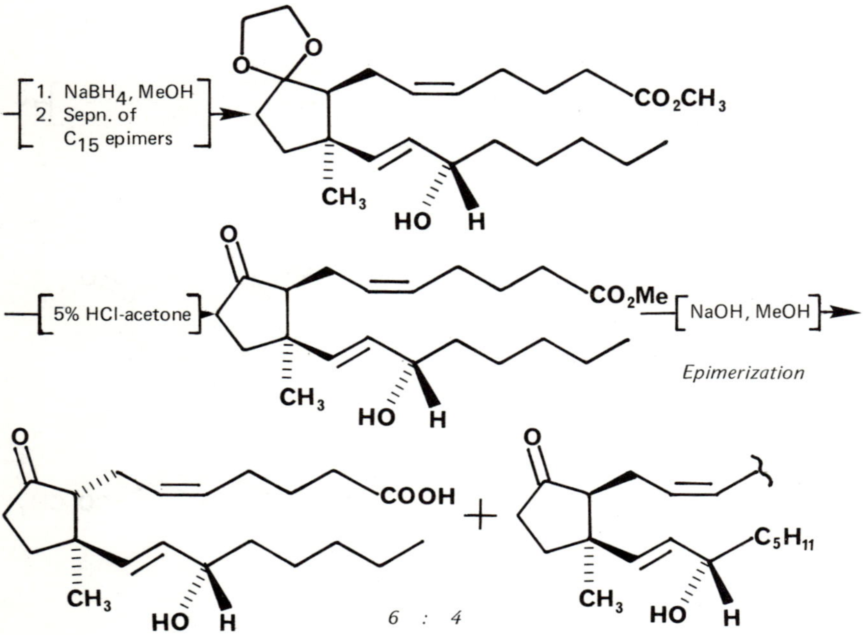

The lactone [3] gives rise to the correct C_8, C_{12} *trans* stereochemistry. Further elaboration leads to the synthesis of 11-deoxy-12-hydroxymethyl PGE_2.[1]

SYNTHETIC PLAN[1]

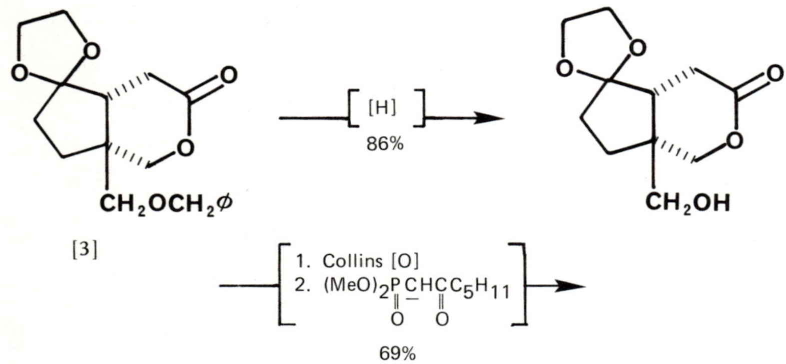

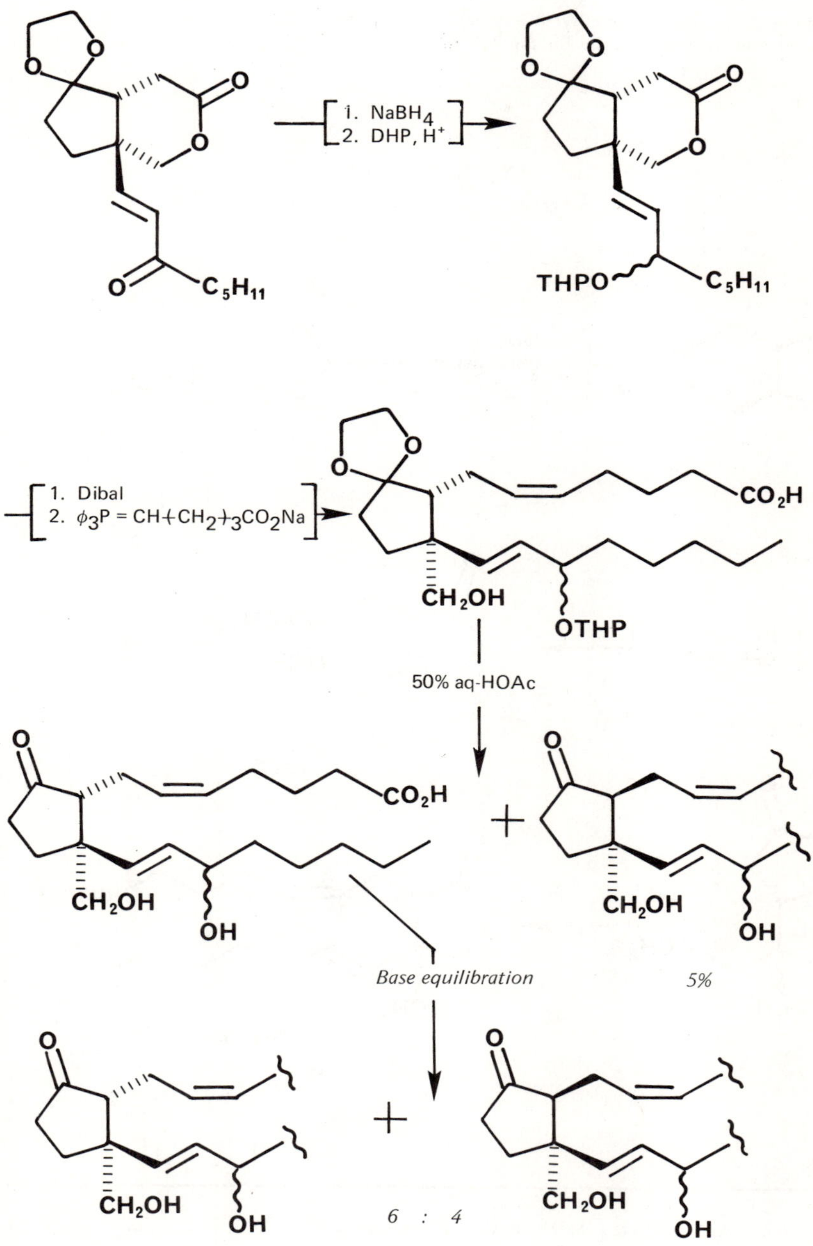

1. $NaBH_4$
2. DHP, H^+
THPO
C_5H_{11}
1. Dibal
2. $\phi_3P = CH(CH_2)_3CO_2Na$
CO_2H
CH_2OH
OTHP
50% aq-HOAc
OH
Base equilibration
5%
6 : 4

A synthesis of 11-deoxy-12-methyl PGA_2 has been reported where the 12-methyl substituent is introduced non-stereospecifically by the 1,4-addition of dimethylcuprate to the cyclopentenone [4].[3]

SYNTHETIC PLAN[3]

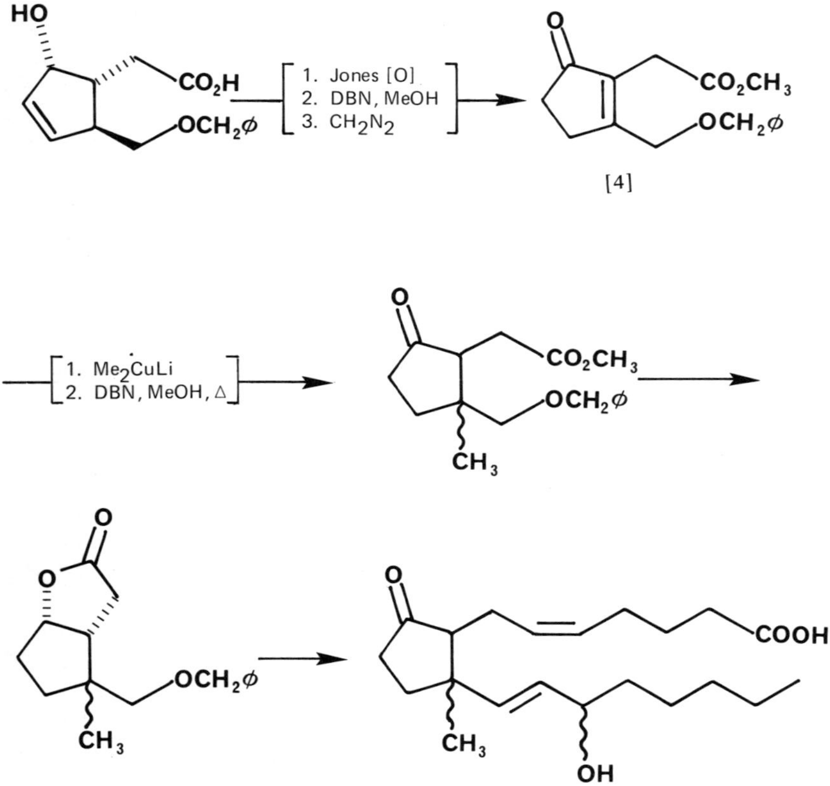

[4]

3. L. Godoy, A. Guzman & J. M. Muchowski, *Chem. Lett.*, 327 (1975).

8-METHYL-PGC$_2$

The unstable PGC$_2$ is very easily converted to PGB$_2$ by the conjugation of the double bond. Such a conjugation can be prevented by substituting an alkyl group at C$_8$. Such a concept has been realized by the synthesis of 8-methyl-PGC$_2$ starting from 2-methylcyclopentane-1,3-dione.[1,2]

SYNTHETIC PLAN[1]

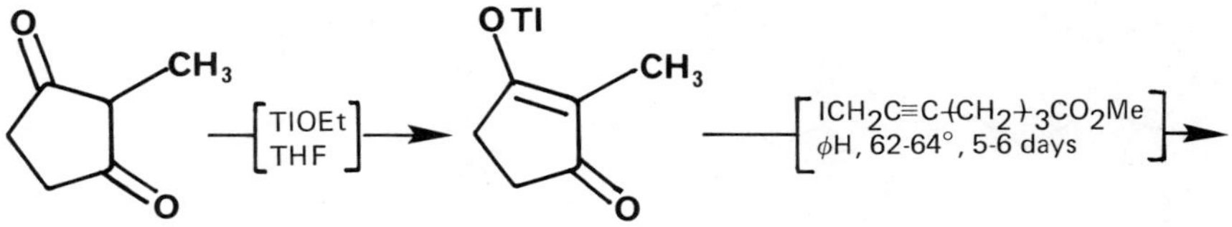

2-Methylcyclopenta-1,3-Dione[2]

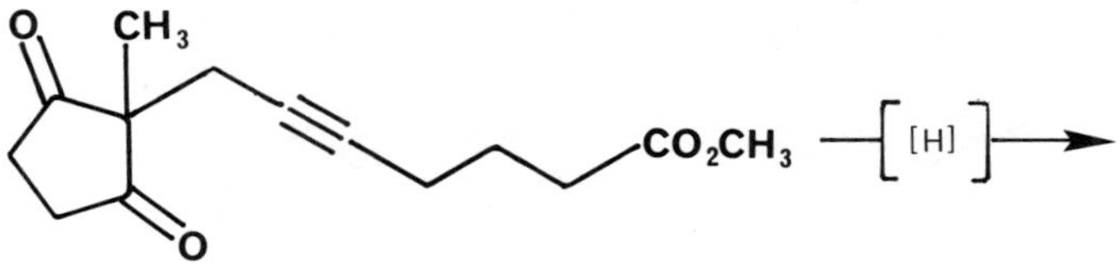

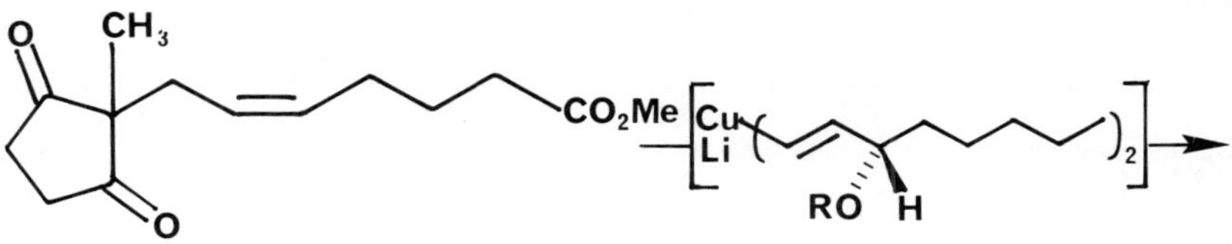

---

1. E. J. Corey & H. S. Sachdev, *J. Am. Chem. Soc.*, **95**, 8483 (1973).
2. For the problems in the synthesis of this steroid D-ring synthon see: V. J. Grenda, G. W. Lindberg, N. L. Wendler & S. H. Pines, *J. Org. Chem.*, **32**, 1236 (1967); H. Schik, G. Lehnmann & G. Hilgetag, *Angew. Chem. [Int. Ed.]*, **6**, 80 (1967).

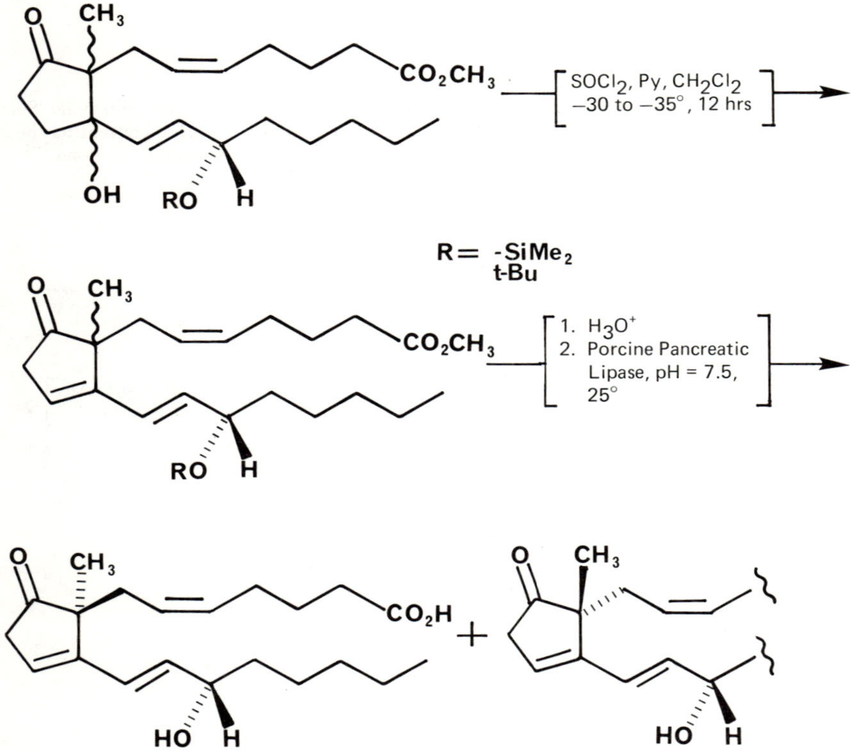

[1] [2]

1/30th as active as PGE_2 in the smooth muscle test.

[2] is 10-30 times more active than [1] in the contraction of smooth muscle (guinea pig uterus).

Both the esters were found to have 60% of the activity of PGE_2 or PGA_2 in inhibiting gastric acid secretion in rats.

10,10-DIMETHYL-PGE$_1$

The 10,10-dimethyl PGE$_1$ analog has been synthesized starting from 2,2-dimethylcyclopentane-1,3-dione.[1,2] The selective reduction of the C_{11} carbonyl group differentiates it from the C_9 carbonyl group. Subsequent reduction of the C_{12} carboethoxy group has been achieved by the protection of the C_9 carbonyl group as the oxime, as shown by Finch.[3]

SYNTHETIC PLAN[1]

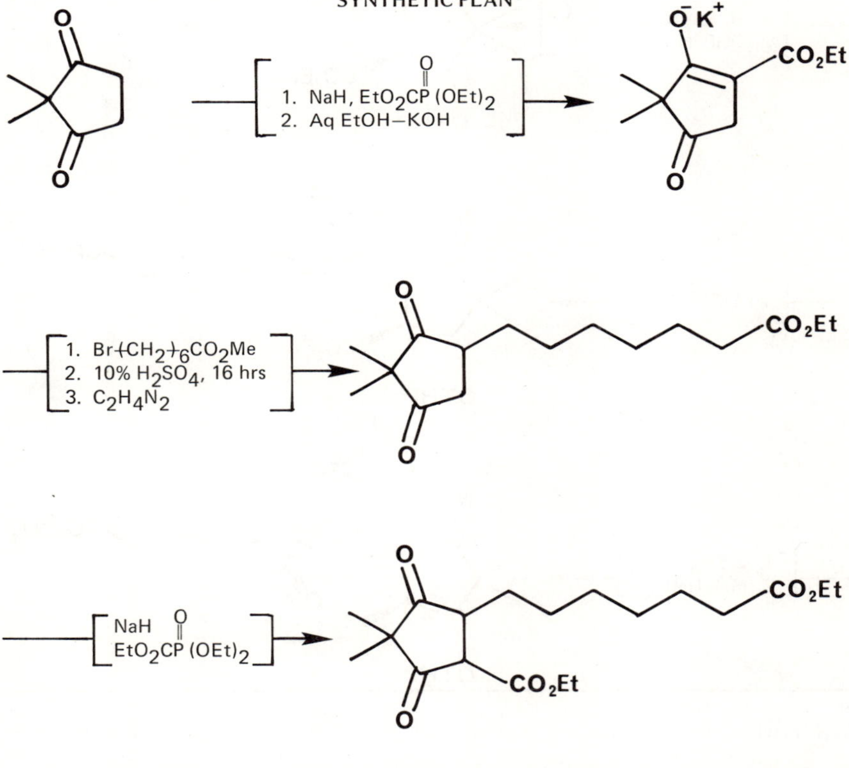

---

1. O. G. Plantema, H. de Koning & H. O. Huisman, *Tet. Lett.*, 4595 (1975).
2. For further details see: O. G. Plantema, Ph.D. Dissertation Thesis, University of Amsterdam (1975), "Synthesis of 10,10-Dimethyl Prostaglandins."

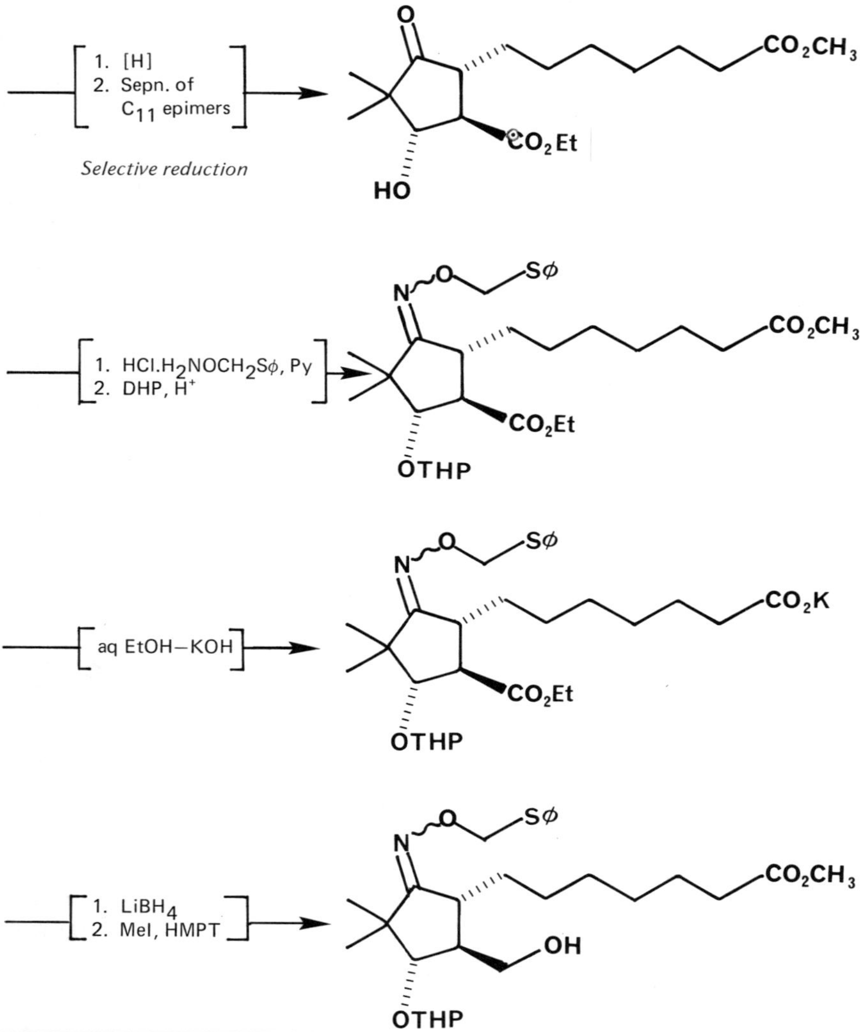

3. N. Finch, L. Della Vecchia, J. J. Fitt, R. Stephani, I. Vlattas, *J. Org. Chem.*, **38**, 4412 (1973).

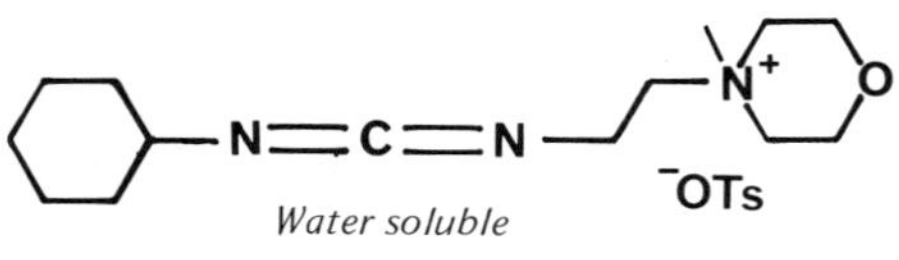

1-Cyclohexyl-3-(2-morpholinoethyl)-carbodiimide metho-p-toluenesulfonate

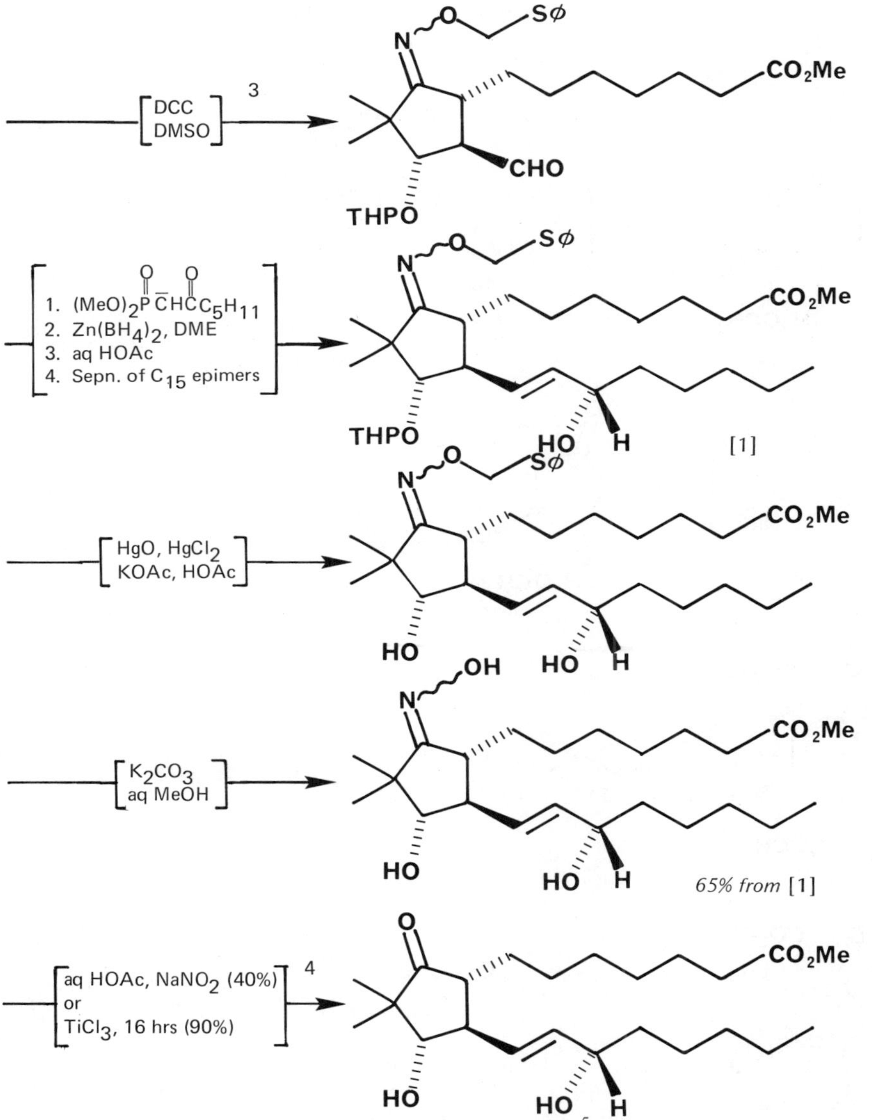

10,10-Dimethyl-PGE$_1$ methyl ester[5]

4. G. H. Timms & E. Wildsmith, *Tet. Lett.*, 195 (1971).
5. O. G. Plantema, H. de Koning & H. O. Huisman, *Tet. Lett.*, 2945 (1975) (for PGF derivative).

11-HYDROXYMETHYL-PGE₁

SYNTHETIC PLAN[1]

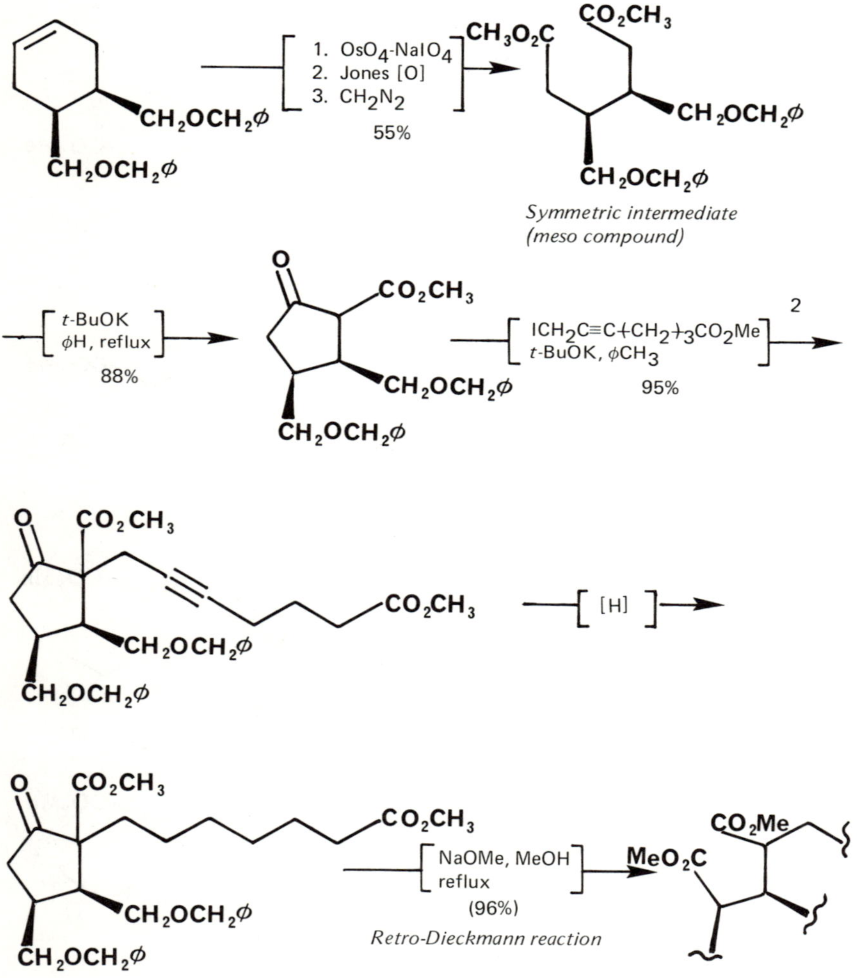

1. J. Ide & K. Sakai, *Tet. Lett.*, 1367 (1976).
2. Alkylation with 7-iodoheptanoate gave a mixture of O- and C- alkylated products.

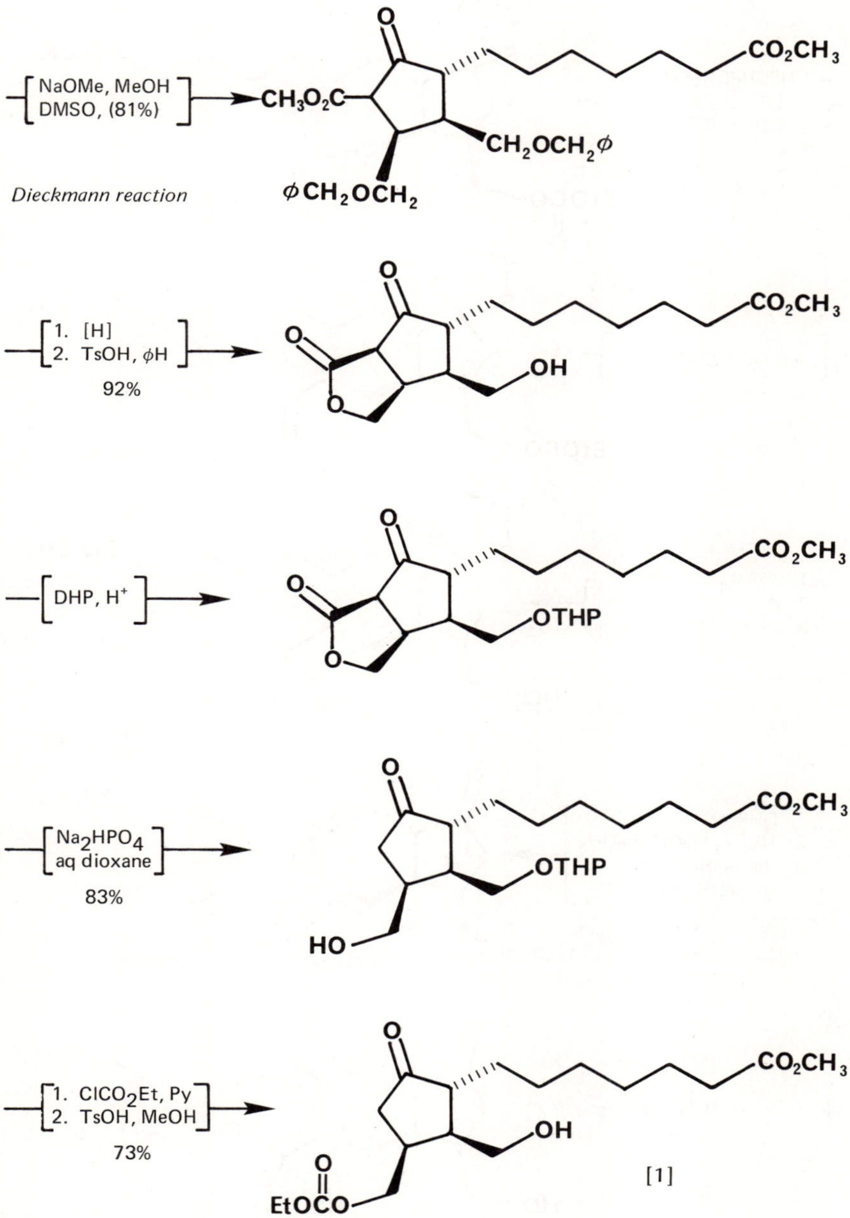

NaOMe, MeOH
DMSO, (81%)
CH3O2C
CO2CH3
CH2OCH2φ
φCH2OCH2
Dieckmann reaction
1. [H]
2. TsOH, φH
92%
OH
DHP, H+
OTHP
Na2HPO4
aq dioxane
83%
HO
1. ClCO2Et, Py
2. TsOH, MeOH
73%
EtOCO

[1]

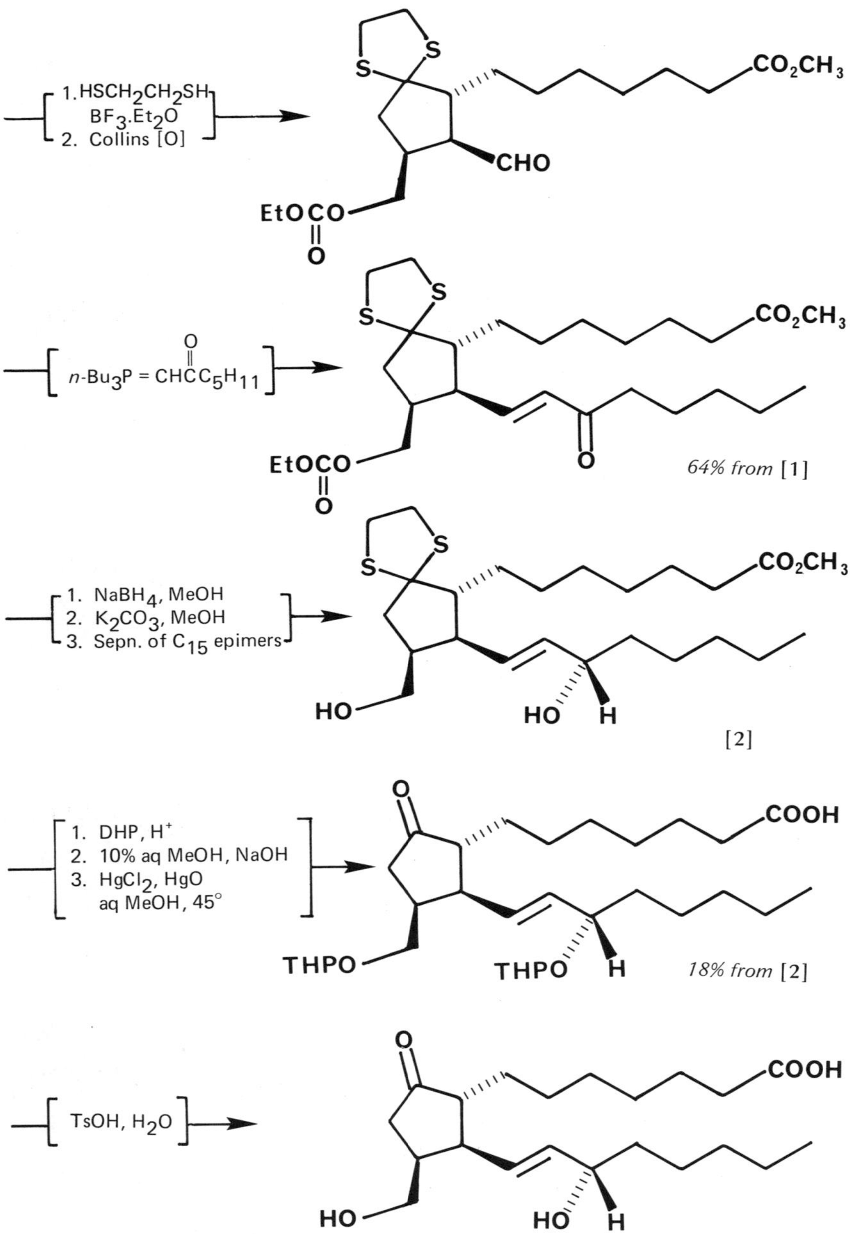
1. HSCH2CH2SH
BF3.Et2O
2. Collins [O]
S
S
CO2CH3
CHO
EtOCO
O
O
n-Bu3P = CHCC5H11
S
S
CO2CH3
EtOCO
O
O
64% from [1]
1. NaBH4, MeOH
2. K2CO3, MeOH
3. Sepn. of C15 epimers
S
S
CO2CH3
HO
HO
H
[2]
1. DHP, H+
2. 10% aq MeOH, NaOH
3. HgCl2, HgO
aq MeOH, 45°
O
COOH
THPO
THPO
H
18% from [2]
TsOH, H2O
O
COOH
HO
HO
H

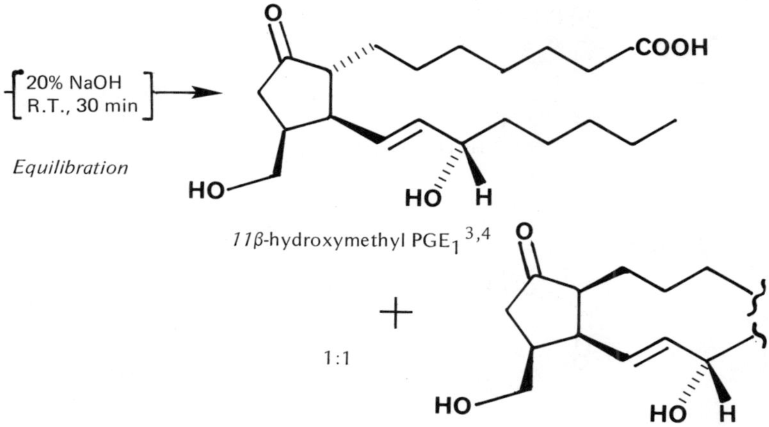

3. The 11α-hydroxymethyl PGE$_1$ which shows strong uterus contraction activity in guinea pigs has also been synthesized. K. Sakai, J. Ide & O. Oda, *Tet. Lett.,* 3021 (1975).
4. The corresponding PGE$_2$ has also been synthesized: A. Guzman & J. M. Muchowski, *Tet. Lett.,* 2053 (1975); G. L. Bundy, *Tet. Lett.,* 1957 (1975).

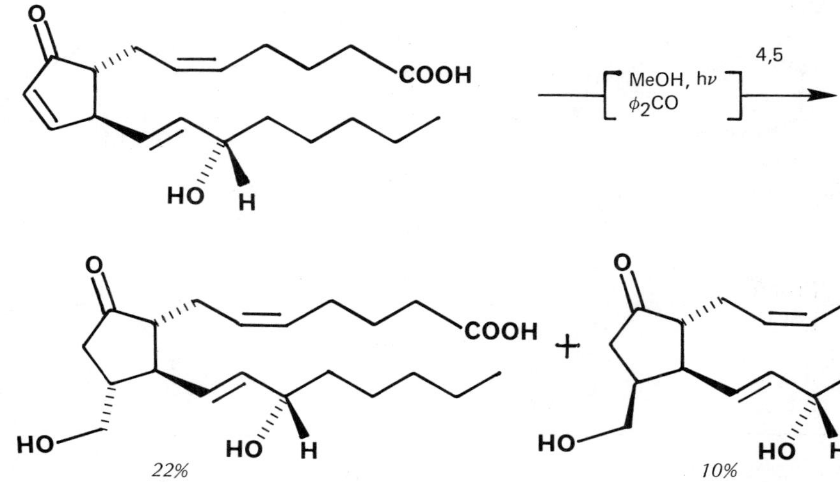

5. For other examples of 1,4-photoaddition of oxycarbinyl species to enones see B. Fraser-Reid, D. R. Hicks, D. L. Walker, D. E. Iley, M. B. Yunker, S. Yik-Kai Tam & R. C. Anderson, *Tet. Lett.,* 297 (1975).

9-HYDROXYMETHYL-PGF$_{2\alpha}$

SYNTHETIC PLAN[1]

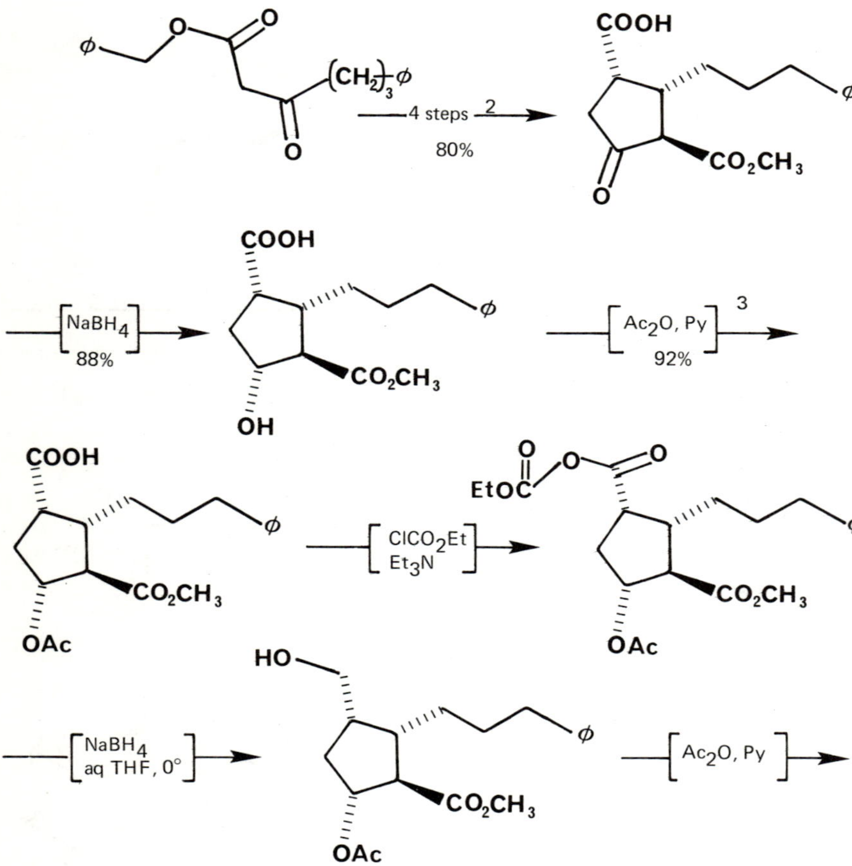

1. K. Kojima & K. Sakai, *Tet. Lett.*, 101 (1976).
2. K. Kojima & K. Sakai, *Tet. Lett.*, 3333 (1972).
3. Some of the lactone [1] is formed.

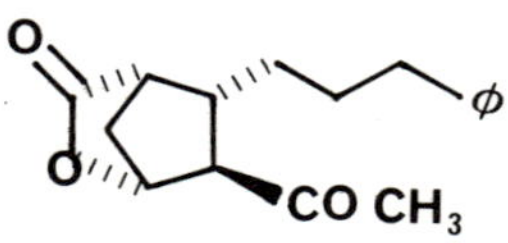

[1]

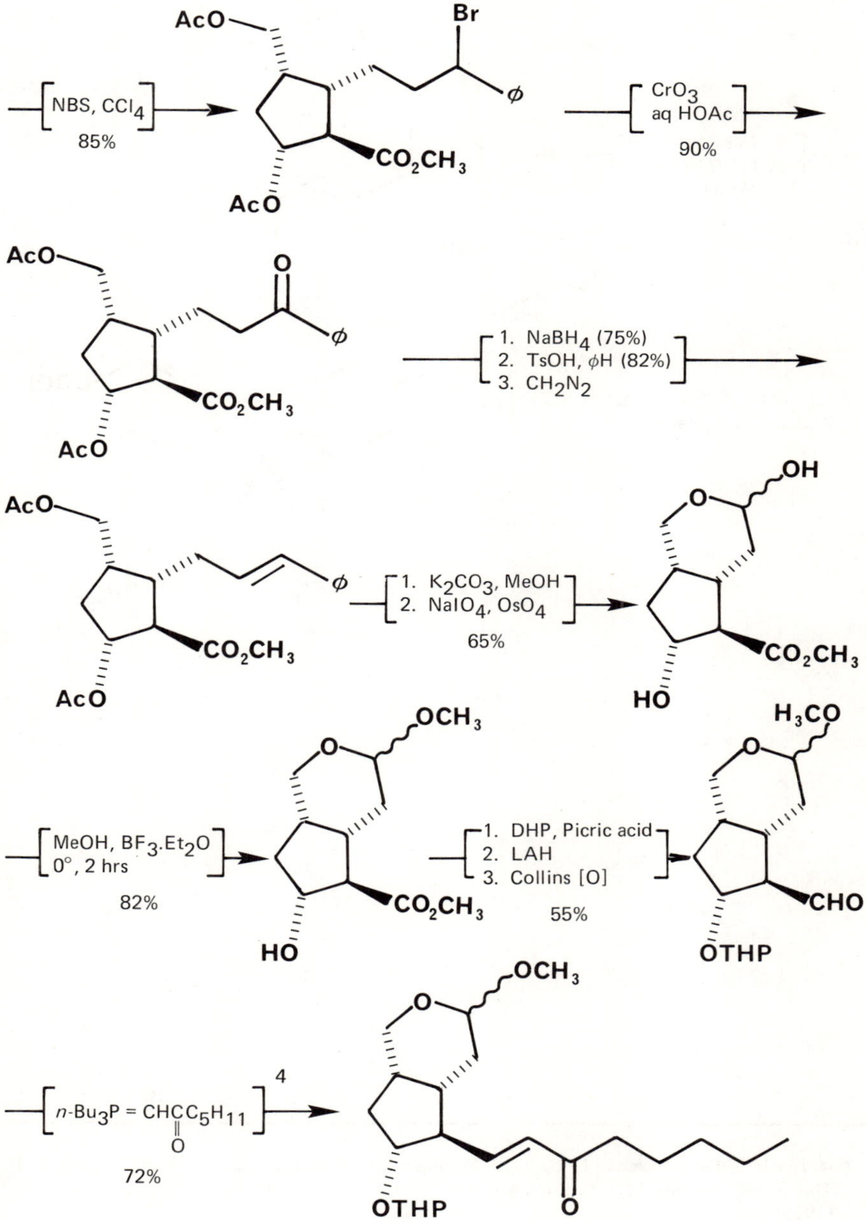
NBS, CCl4
85%
AcO
Br
ϕ
CO2CH3
AcO
CrO3
aq HOAc
90%
O
1. NaBH4 (75%)
2. TsOH, ϕH (82%)
3. CH2N2
1. K2CO3, MeOH
2. NaIO4, OsO4
65%
OH
HO
OCH3
MeOH, BF3.Et2O
0°, 2 hrs
82%
1. DHP, Picric acid
2. LAH
3. Collins [O]
55%
H3CO
CHO
OTHP
n-Bu3P = CHCC5H11
4
72%

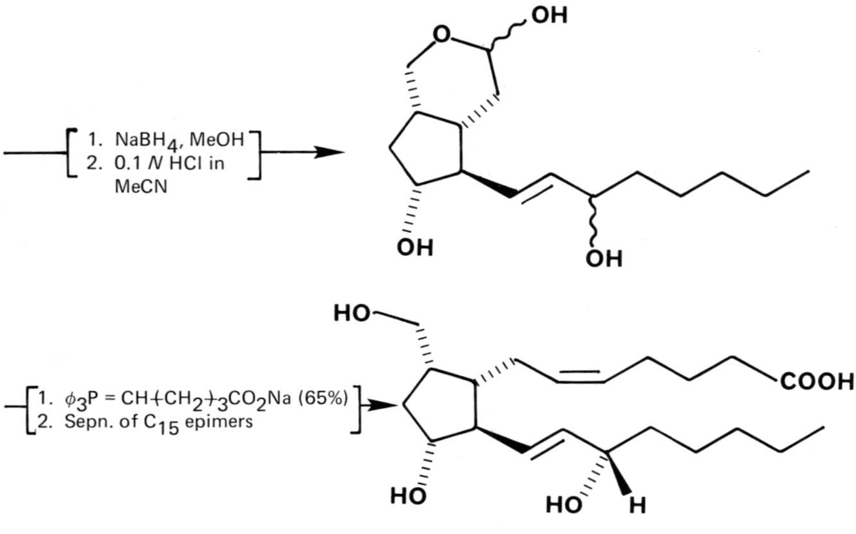

9-deoxy-9α-hydroxymethyl $PGF_{2\alpha}$[5]

4. N. Finch, L. Della Vecchia, J. J. Fitt, R. Stephani & I. Vlattas, *J. Org. Chem.*, **38**, 4412 (1973).
5. This analog has also been synthesized by a different route by G. L. Bundy, *Tet. Lett.*, 1957 (1975).

13-DEHYDRO-PGF$_{2\alpha}$

Several 13-dehydro-PG analogs have been made by Fried and Gandolfi. The synthetic approach of Gandolfi[1,2,3,4] is interesting. Horner-Emmons reaction of the bromophosphonate derivative [**1**] with the Corey aldehyde gives the α-bromoenone [**2**]. The bromine is eliminated during the subsequent Wittig reaction (for the introduction of the α-chain) to give the 13-dehydro PG.

SYNTHETIC PLAN[2,3,4]

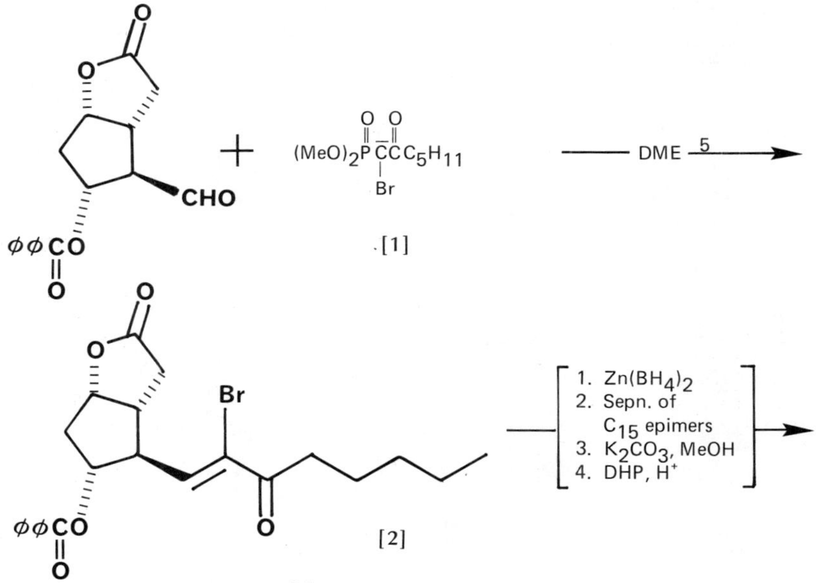

[1]

[2]

Trans bromoenone[5,6]

---

1. Presented at the International Conference on Prostaglandins, Florence, May 26-30, 1975.
2. C. Gandolfi, R. Pellegata, E. Dradi, A. Forgione & E. Pella, *Il Farmaco, Ed. Sc.* (1976), (in press) (personal communication).
3. C. Gandolfi, G. Doria & P. Gaio, *Il Farmaco, Ed. Sc.*, **27**, 1255 (1972).
4. C. Gandolfi, R. Pellegata, R. Ceserani, G. Agresta, G. Orsini & M. M. Usardi, *Advances in Prostaglandin and Thromboxane Research*, B. Samuelsson & R. Paoletti (Eds.), Raven, New York, 1976, p. 209.
5. Some of the *cis*-enone is also formed (5%).

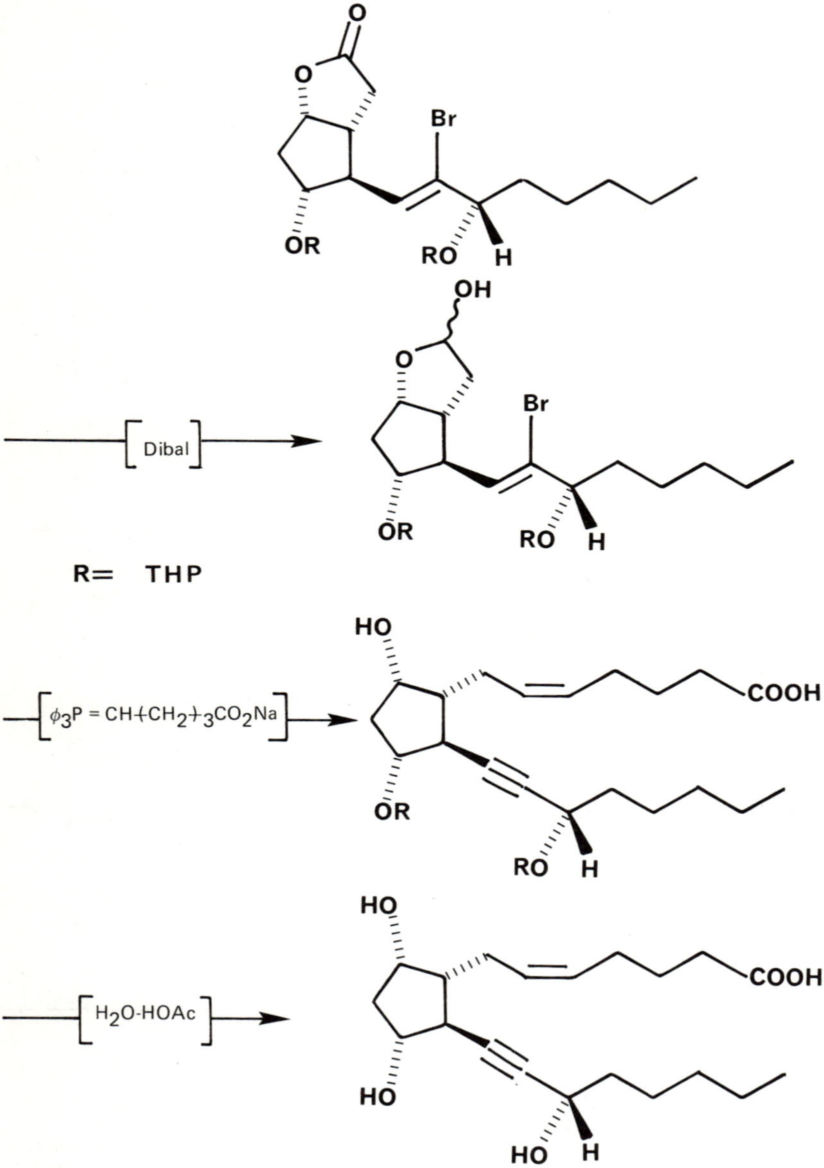

13-dehydro-$PGF_{2\alpha}$

Modified Synthesis of the Bromo-Phosphonate [1][2,3,4]

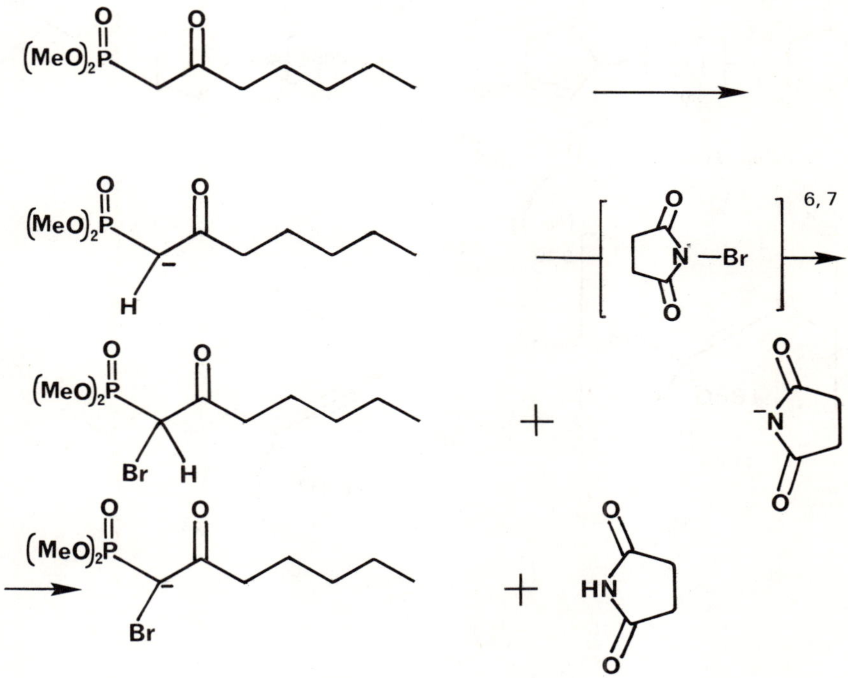

[1]

6. The corresponding chlorolactol (made by the reaction of the enone with sulfuryl chloride) gives a mixture of 13-dehydro- and 14-chloro- PGs in a ratio which varies depending on the base used to form the ylid and the reaction time.
7. Originally the bromination was done with molecular bromine. W. S. Wadsworth & W. D. Emmons, *J. Am. Chem. Soc.*, **83**, 1733 (1961).
   Use of NBS gave higher yields of the resulting bromo-enone [2].

The Fried method of synthesizing 13-dehydro-PGs involves the usual method of opening of the cyclopentane epoxide [3] with suitable alanes.[8]

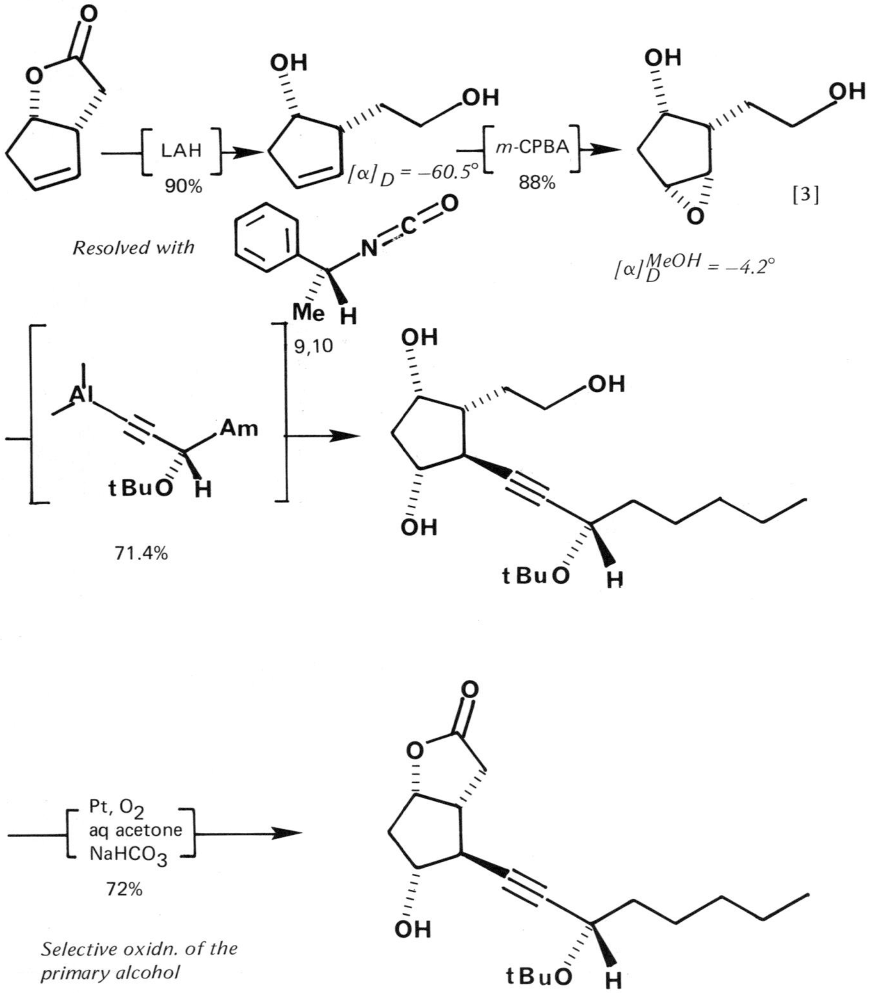

---

8. J. Fried, M. S. Lee, B. Gaede, J. C. Sih, Y. Yoshikawa & J. A. McCracken, *Advances in Prostaglandin and Thromboxane Research*, Vol. 1, B. Samuelsson & R. Paoletti (Eds.), Raven, New York 1976, p. 183.

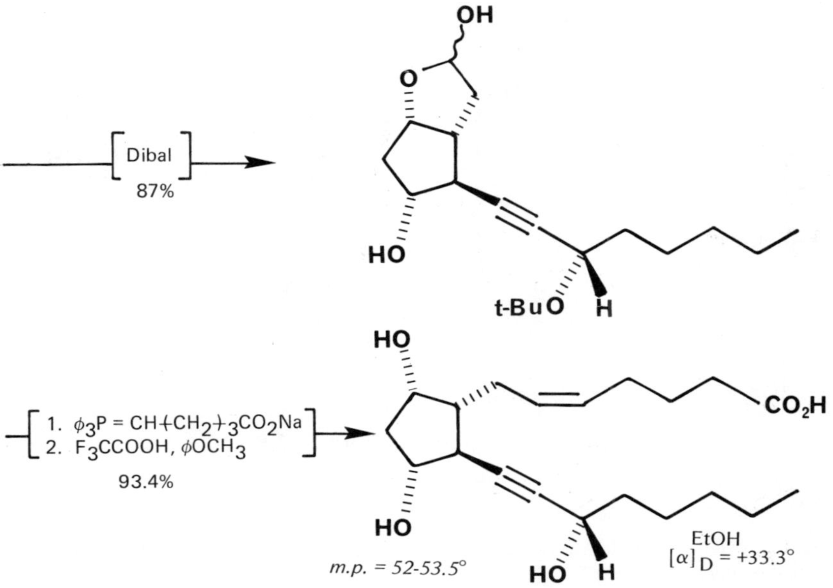

9. Unlike the dimethylalane which attacks both the C_{11} & C_{12} positions to give the C_{11} and C_{12} alkylated products (in ratios varying from 1:1 to 1:4 respectively), the methoxymethylalane opens the epoxide [3] regiospecifically to give the C_{12} alkylated product only. J. Fried & J. C. Sih, *Tet. Lett.*, 3899 (1973).
10. The regiospecificity of the epoxide opening has been explained by the authors on the following basis. A slower rate of alkynylation as compared to the rate of bond formation between the primary hydroxyl group in [3] and the methoxymethyl alane assures a transition state which favors the intramolecular alkylation regiospecifically.

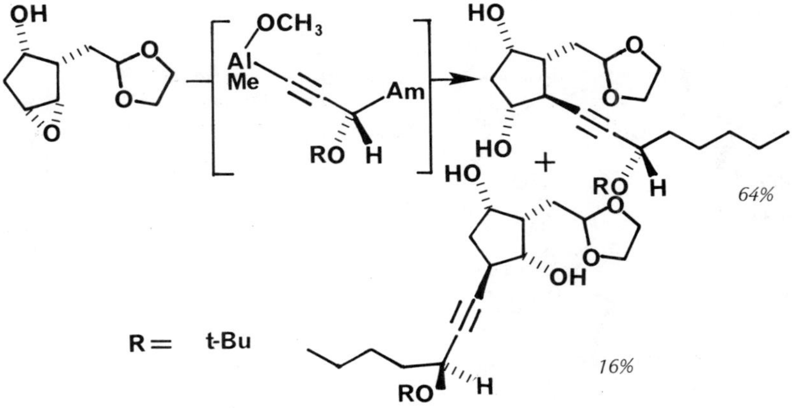

The *ent*-13-dehydro-15-epi-PGF$_{2\alpha}$ [5] was made in a similar way from the enantiomeric epoxide [4].

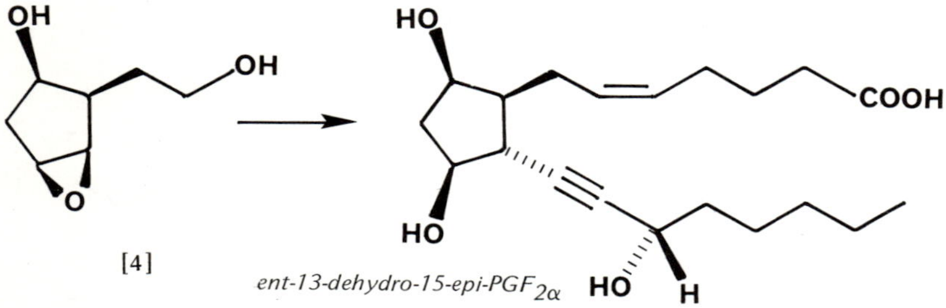

[4]

ent-13-dehydro-15-epi-PGF$_{2\alpha}$

[5]

13-DEHYDRO-16-FLUORO-PGF$_{2\alpha}$

The 16-fluoro-PGF$_{2\alpha}$ [7] derivatives were made by the opening of the epoxide [3] with the fluoro-methoxymethylalane.

Synthesis of the Fluoro-Acetylene [6]

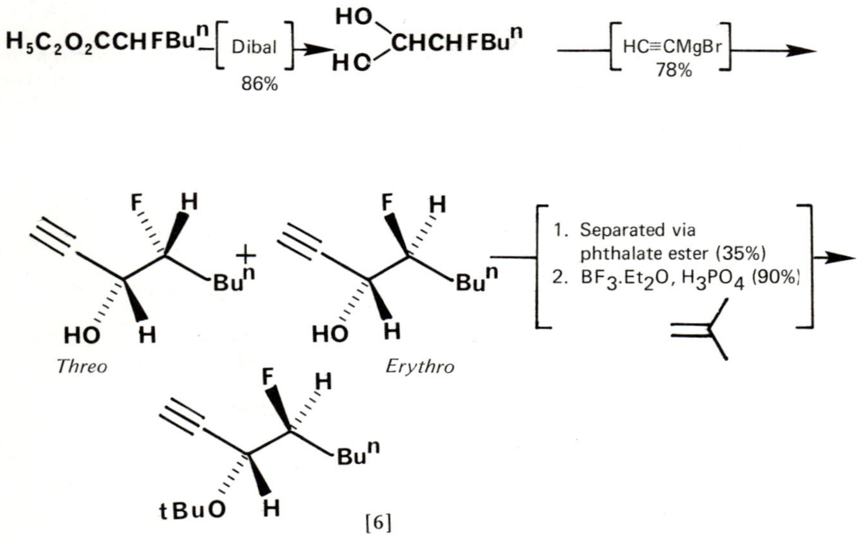

Threo *Erythro*

[6]

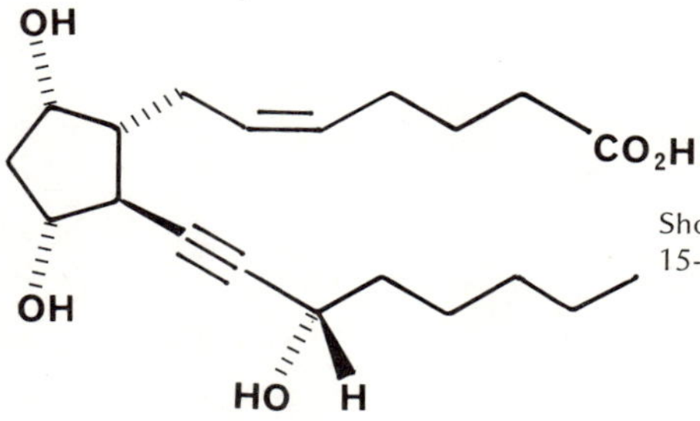

Shows activity similar to PGF$_{2\alpha}$. Inert to 15-hydroxyprostaglandin dehydrogenase.

13-dehydro-PGF$_{2\alpha}$

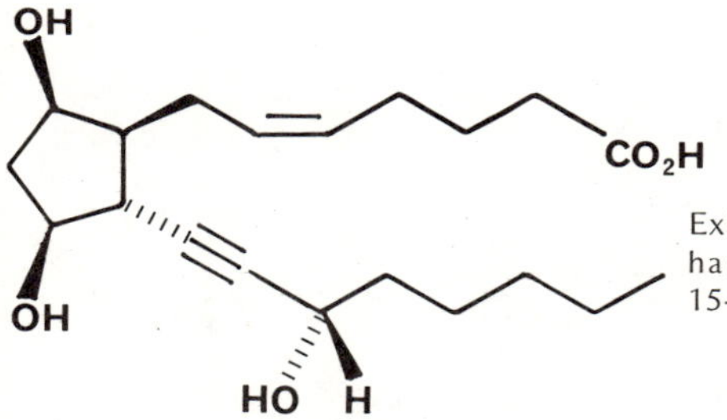

Exhibits unexpectedly high activity in the hamster antifertility assay. Inert to 15-hydroxyprostaglandin dehydrogenase.

Ent-13-Dehydro-PGF$_{2\alpha}$

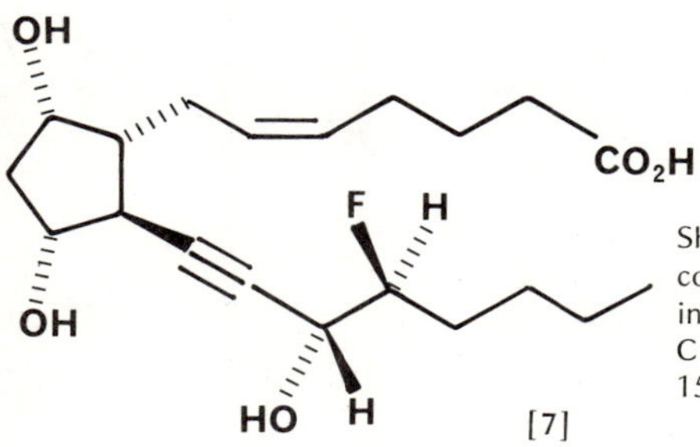

[7]

Shows similar activity as the nonfluorinated compound, with respect to antifertility activity in hamster and luteolytic activity in sheep. Completely inert to placental 15-hydroxyprostaglandin dehydrogenase.

(15R, 16S)-16-fluoro-13-dehydro-PGF$_{2\alpha}$

15-METHYL-PGE$_2$

SYNTHETIC PLAN[1]

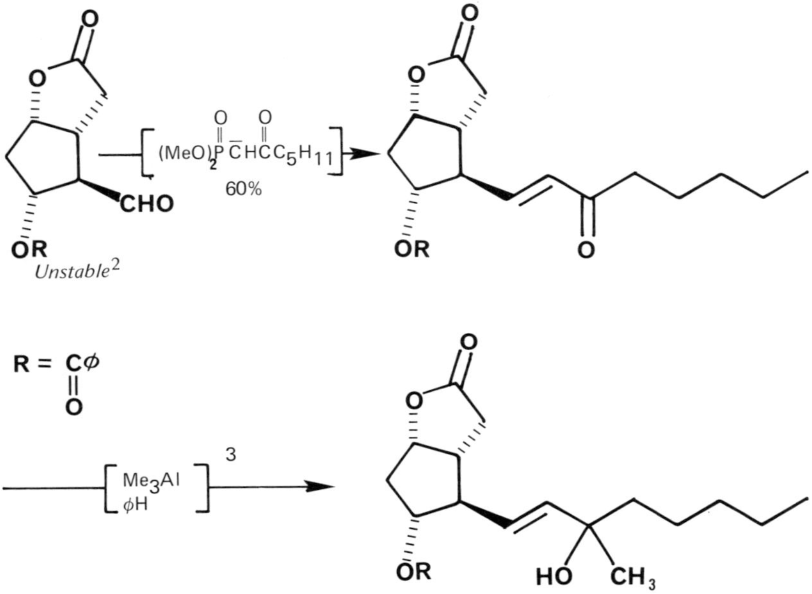

1. E. W. Yankee, U. Axen & G. L. Bundy, *J. Am. Chem. Soc.*, **96**, 5865 (1974).
2. The aldehyde is unstable and gives the unsaturated aldehyde.

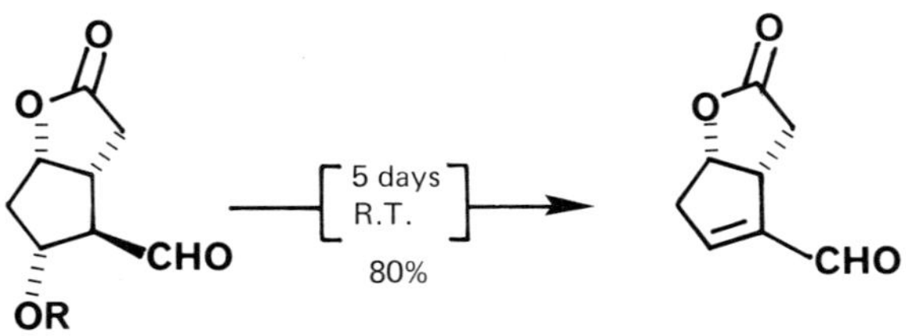

3. For a study of the mechanism of this reaction see H. M. Neumann, J. Laemmle & E. C. Ashby, *J. Am. Chem. Soc.*, **95**, 2597 (1973).

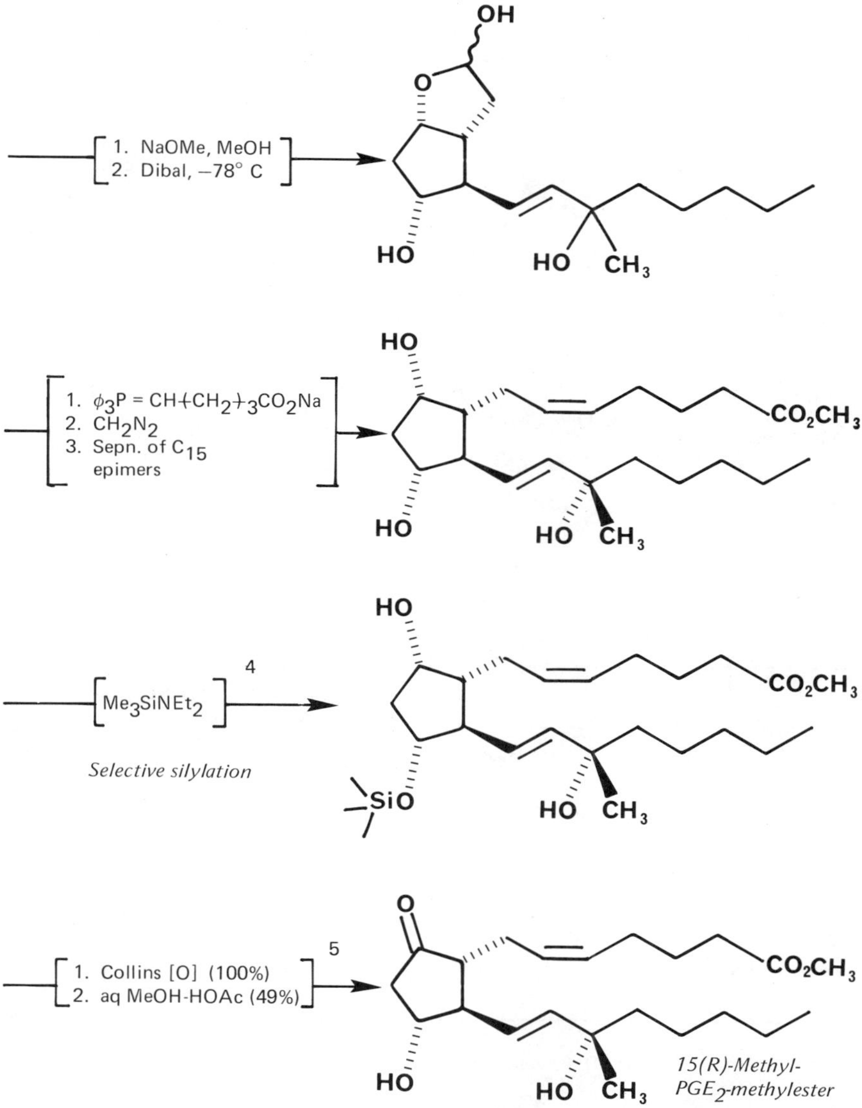

4. The silylation with this reagent is very sensitive to the steric environment of the hydroxyl group. I. Weisz, K. Felfoldi & K. Kovacs, *Acta. Chim. Acad. Sci. Hung.*, **58**, 189 (1968).
5. The trimethylsilylether survives Collins oxidation.

16-SUBSTITUTED $PGF_{2\alpha}$

Several 16-substituted analogs have been made by using substituted phosphonate reagents. These 16-substituted analogs are highly active.

SYNTHETIC PLAN[1]

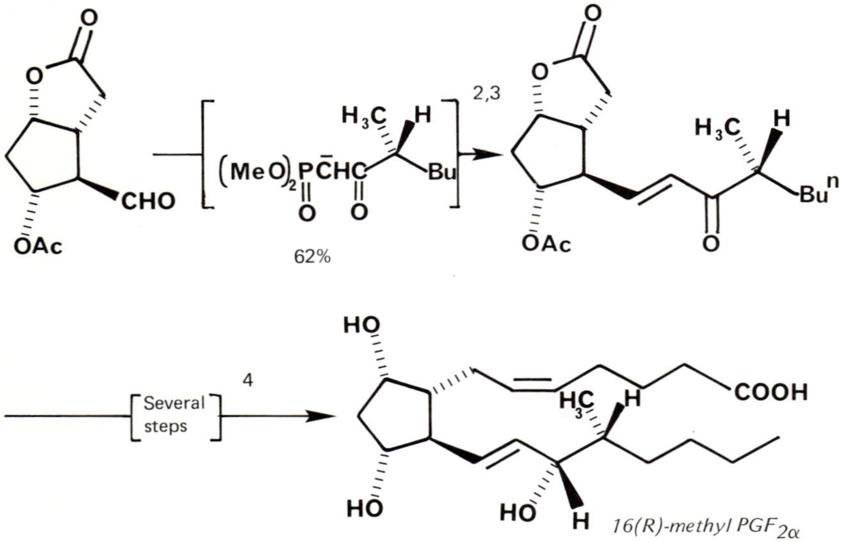

16(R)-methyl $PGF_{2\alpha}$

16(*R*) and 16(*S*)-methyl prostaglandins show much stronger prostaglandin-like activity than the natural prostaglandins.

16(*R*)-methyl-PGE_2 is 100-200 times more active than PGE_2 in gastric juice inhibition (rat).

Compounds with different C_{15} stereochemistry show similar activity.

---

1. M. Hayashi, H. Miyake, T. Tanouchi, S. Iguchi, Y. Iguchi & F. Tanouchi, *J. Org. Chem.*, **38**, 1250 (1973).
2. P. A. Levene & L. A. Mikeska, *J. Biol. Chem.*, **84**, 584 (1929).
3. It is interesting to note that there is no epimerization of the C_{16} chiral center under the basic conditions of the Wittig reaction.
4. E. J. Corey, T. K. Schaaf, W. Huber, U. Koelliker & N. M. Weinshenker, *J. Am. Chem. Soc.*, **92**, 397 (1970).

SYNTHETIC PLAN[5]

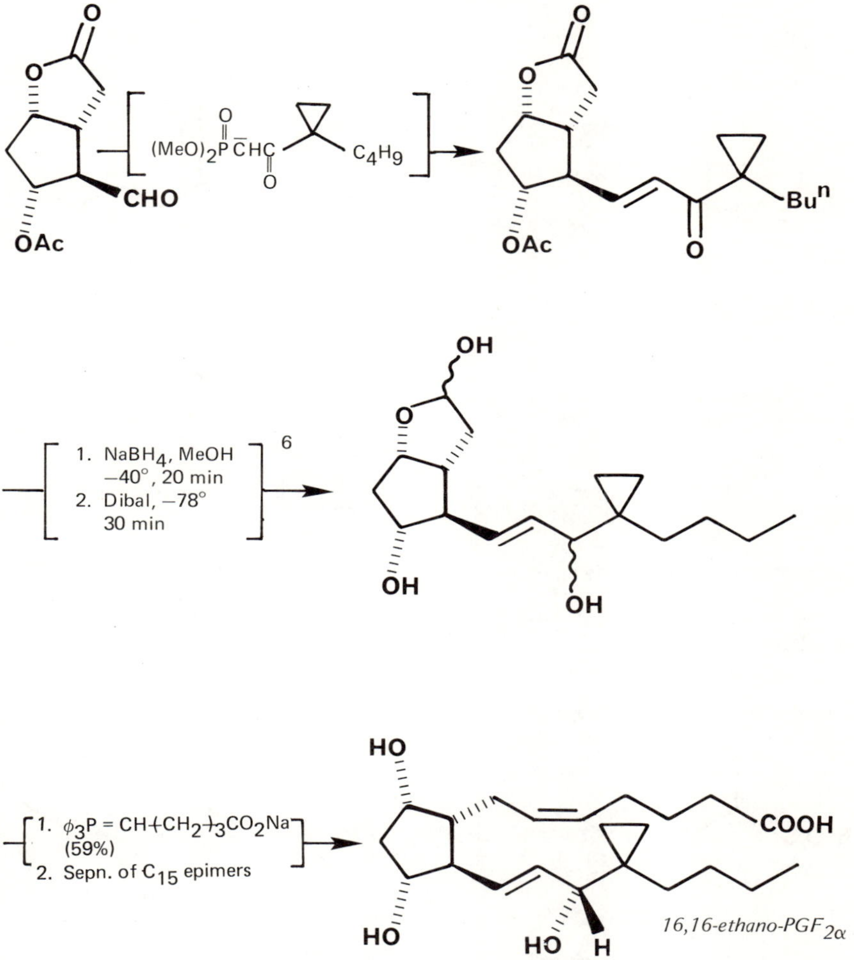

16,16-ethano-PGF$_{2\alpha}$

80 times more active than PGE_2 in the inhibitory action on pentagastrin induced gastric acid secretion in rats.

1/9 times as active as 16(*R*)-Methyl PGE_2 in diarrhea producing activity in mice after oral administration.

---

5. H. Miyake, S. Iguchi, S. Kori & M. Hayashi, *Chem. Lett.*, 211 (1976).
6. Dibal reduces the acetate, also, to the secondary alcohol.

SYNTHETIC PLAN[5]

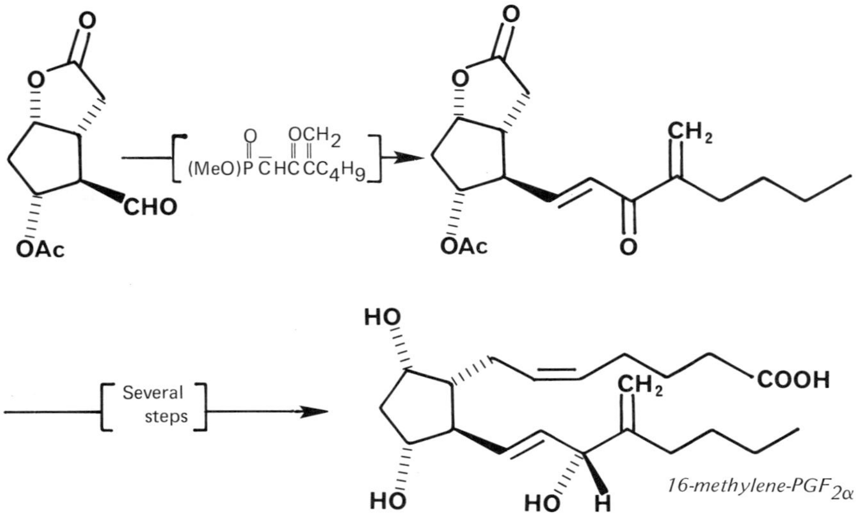

16-methylene-PGF$_{2\alpha}$

35 times more active than PGE_2 in the inhibitory action on pentagastrin induced secretion in rats.

1/30 times as active as 16-(*R*)-methyl PGE_2 in diarrhea producing activity in mice after oral administration.

Synthesis of the Phosphonate Reagents[5]

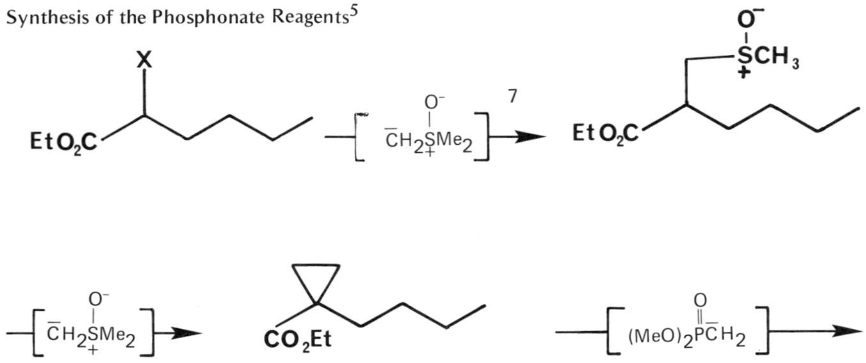

7. P. Bravo, G. Gaudiano, C. Ticozzi & A. Umani-Ronchi, *Tet. Lett.*, 4481 (1968).
8. P. E. Pfeffer, E. Kinsel & L. S. Silbert, *J. Org. Chem.*, **37**, 1256 (1972).

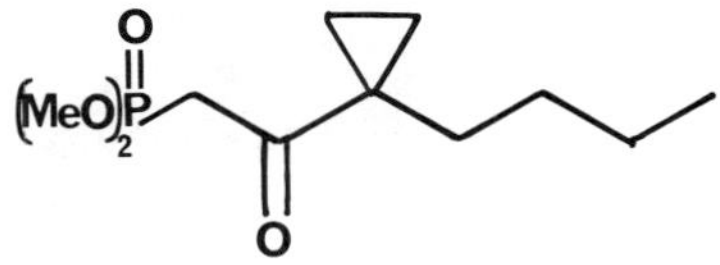

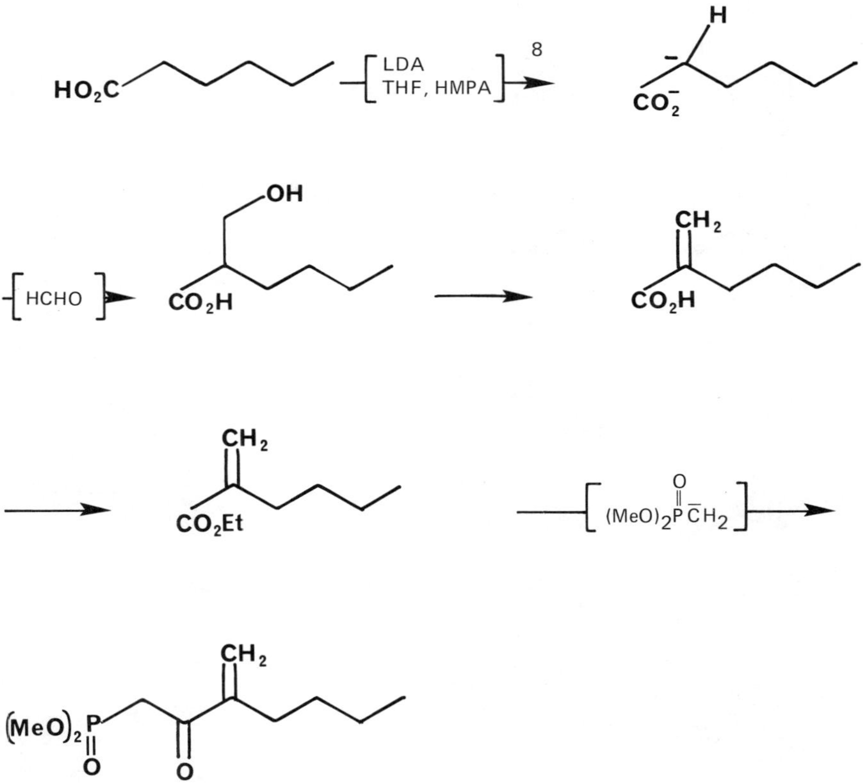
LDA
THF, HMPA
8
HCHO
$(MeO)_2\overset{O}{\overset{\|}{P}}\bar{C}H_2$

4,5-DIENYL $PGF_{2\alpha}$

The synthesis of 4,5-dienyl-PGE_2 derivative[1] is based on the original observation by Crabbe[2] that propargylic acetates react with dialkyl cuprates to give allenes.

SYNTHETIC PLAN[1]

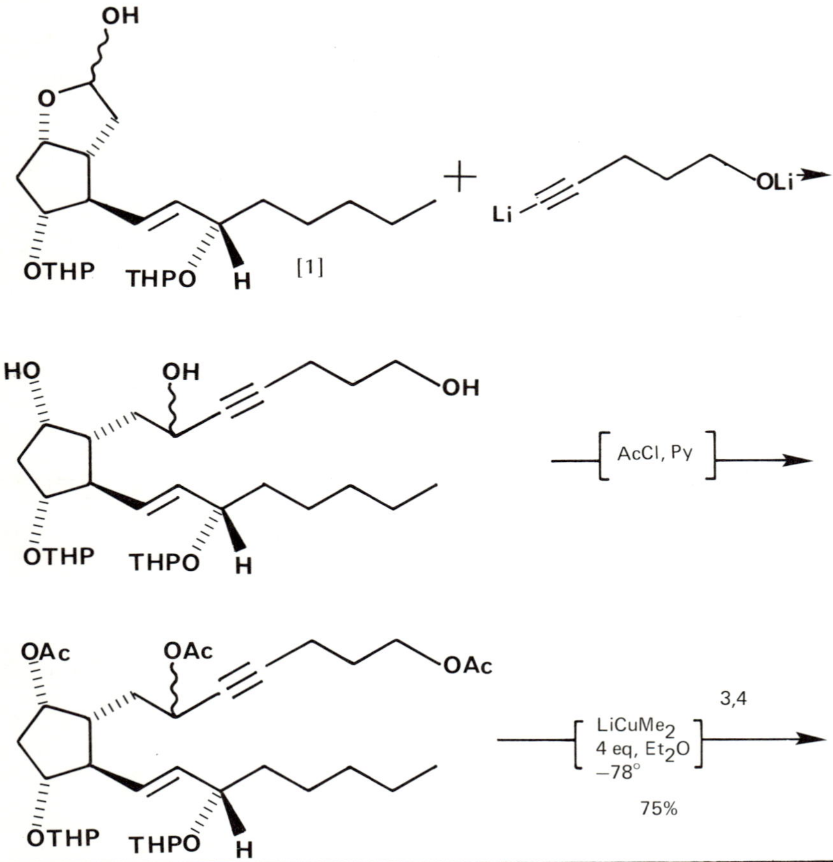

1. P. Crabbe & H. Carpio, *Chem. Commun.*, 904 (1972).
2. P. Rona & P. Crabbe, *J. Am. Chem. Soc.*, **91**, 3289 (1969).

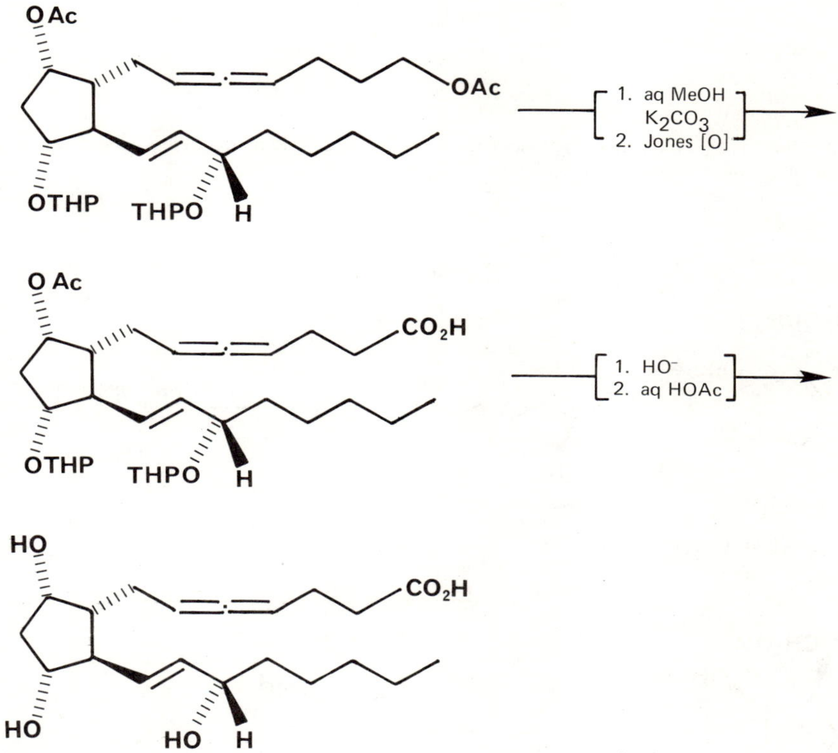

3. An isomeric mixture of allenes is obtained since the alkylation of the lactol [1] with the acetylide ion is not stereospecific.
4. For a discussion of the mechanism of this reaction see:
   J. L. Luche, E. Barreiro, J. M. Dollat & P. Crabbe, *Tet. Lett.*, 4615 (1975).
   J. K. Crandall, P. Battioni, J. T. Wehlacz & R. Bindra, *J. Am. Chem. Soc.*, **97**, 7171 (1975).
   P. Crabbe, E. Barreiro, J. M. Dollat & J. L. Luche, *Chem. Commun.*, 183 (1976).

7-OXA-PGF$_{2\alpha}$

The opening of cyclopentane epoxides with suitable organoaluminum derivative of the β- chain was first applied to the synthesis of 7-oxa-PGS.[1,2,3,4]

SYNTHETIC PLAN[1]

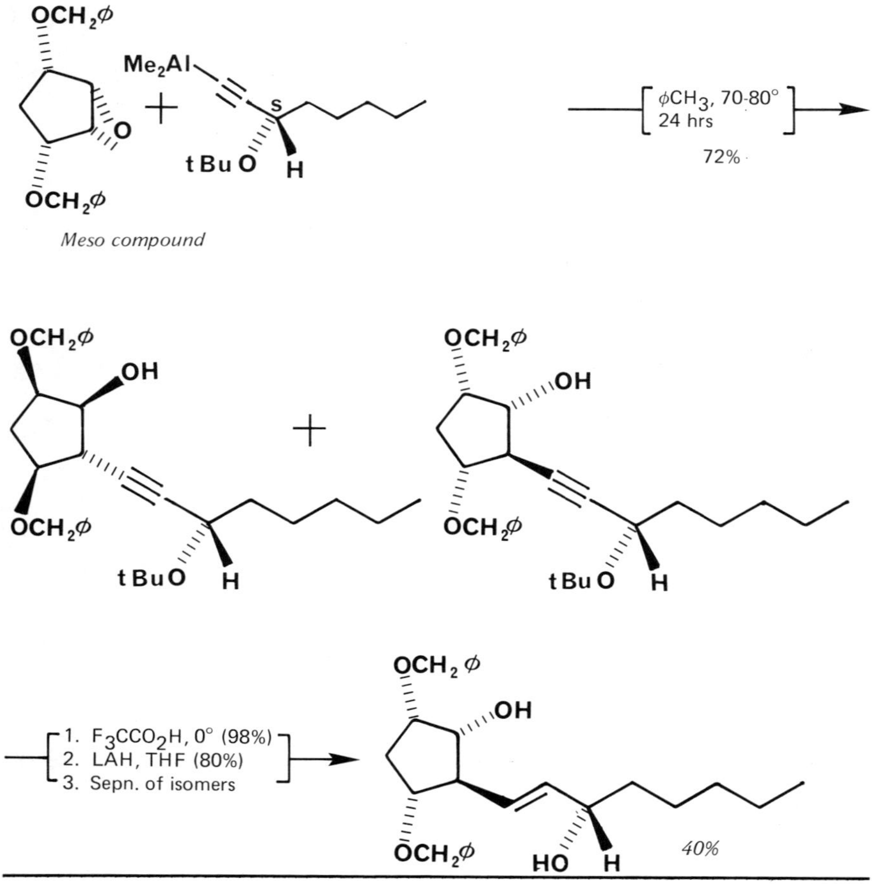

1. J. Fried, M. M. Mehra & W. L. Kao, *J. Am. Chem. Soc.*, **93**, 5594 (1971).

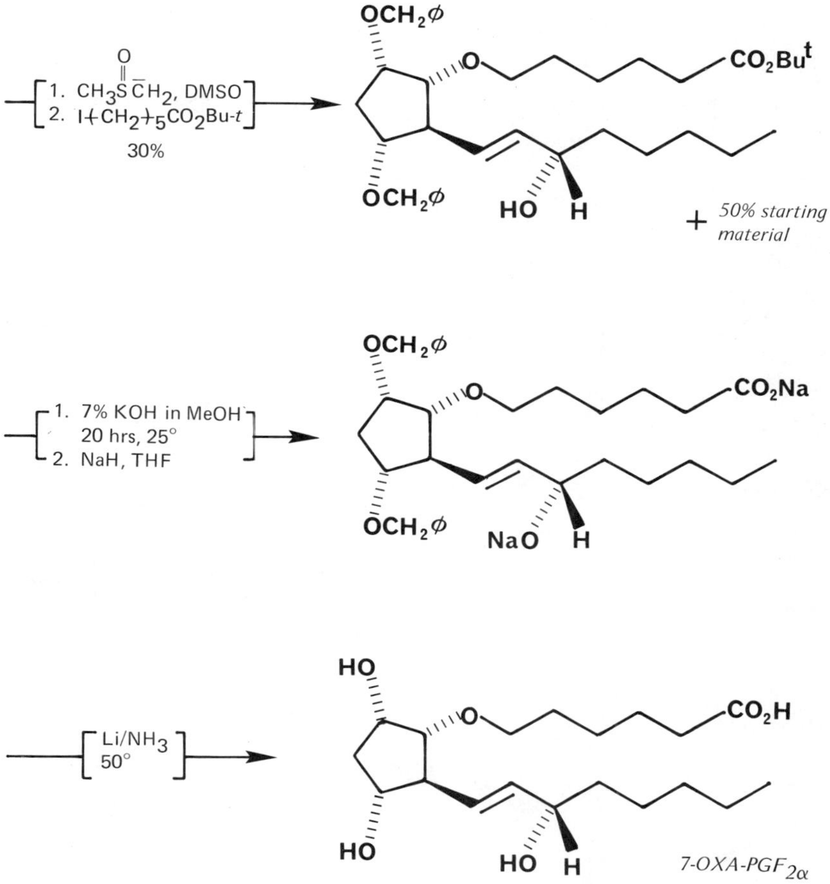

Exhibits 5% of the activity of PGF$_{1\alpha}$ in the gerbil colon assay.

Stimulates cAMP formation in mouse ovary (0.1 times PGF$_{1\alpha}$).

A substrate for the highly specific PG-15-dehydrogenase from swine lung.

---

2. J. Fried, S. Heim, S. J. Etheredge, P. Sunder-Plassmann, T. S. Santhanakrishnan, J. Himizu & C. H. Lin, *Chem. Commun.*, 634 (1968).
3. J. Fried, T. S. Santhanakrishnan, J. Himizu, C. H. Lin, S. H. Ford, B. Rubin & E. O. Grigas, *Nature* (Lond.), **223**, 208 (1969).
4. J. Fried, M. M. Mehra, W. L. Kao & C. H. Lin, *Tet. Lett.*, 2695 (1970).

7-THIA-PGF$_{2\alpha}$

The opening of the cyclopentane epoxide [1] with the thiol derivative of the α- chain leads to the synthesis of 7-thia-PGs.[1]

SYNTHETIC PLAN[1]

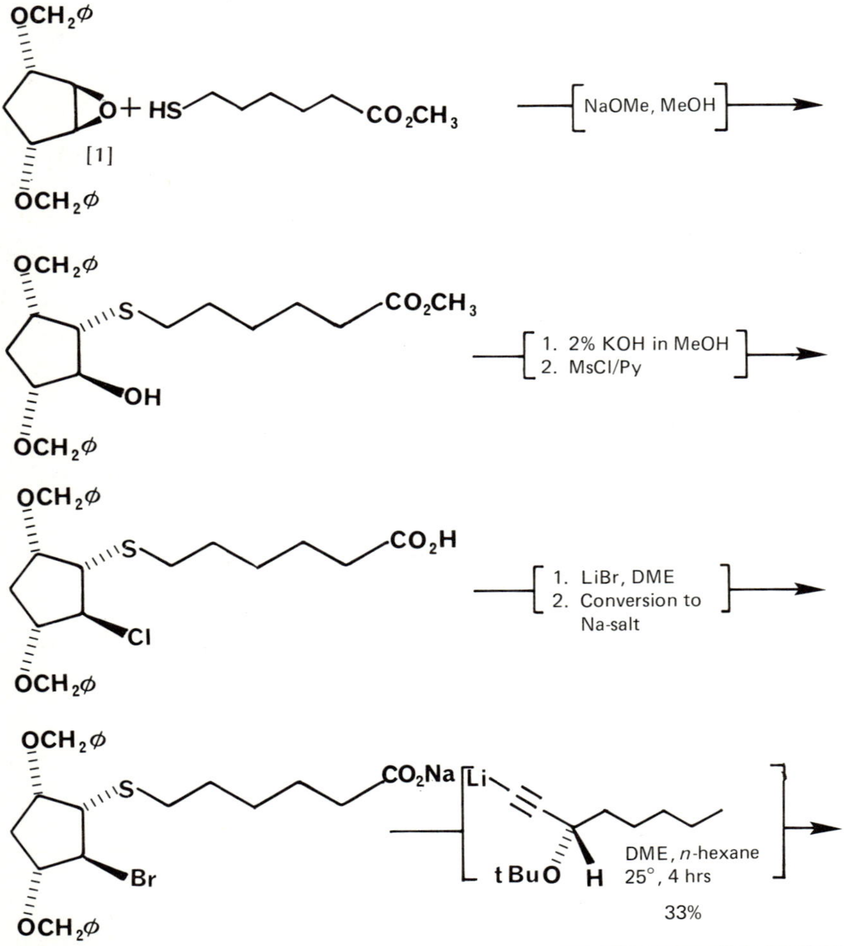

1. J. Fried, M. M. Mehra & Y. Y. Chan, *J. Am. Chem. Soc.*, **96**, 6759 (1974).

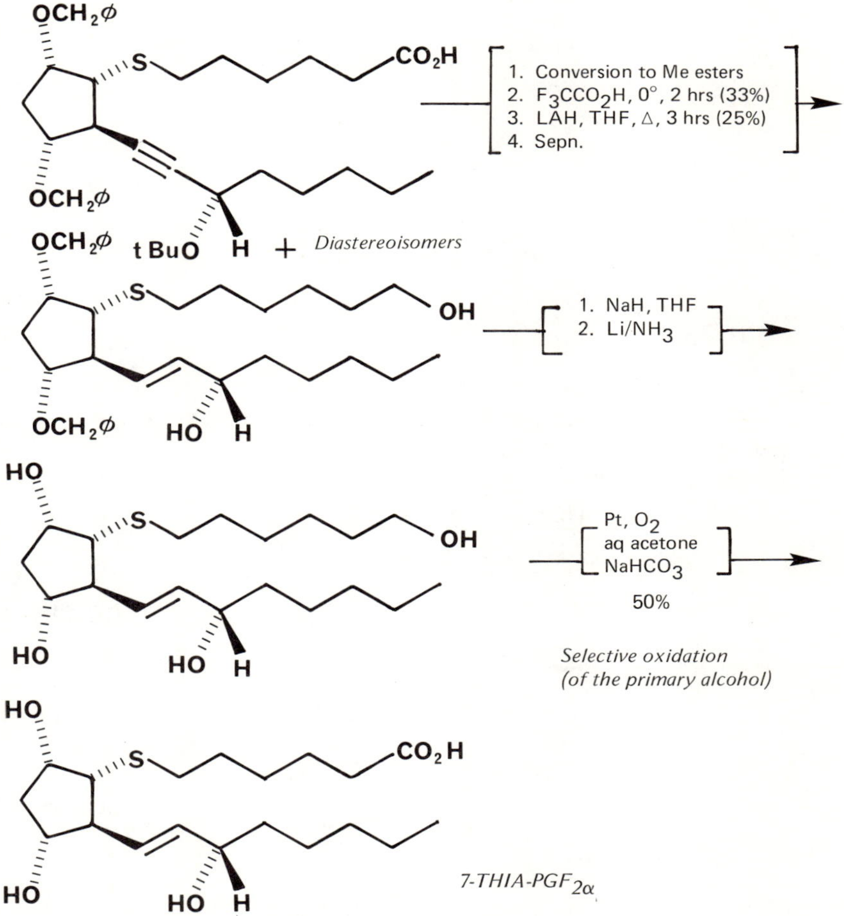

7-THIA-PGF$_{2\alpha}$

Stimulates cAMP synthesis in the mouse-ovary (threefold over control).

Shows binding to a bovine corpus luteum "receptor" with 1/10th the affinity of PGF$_{1\alpha}$

Inhibitor of placental PG-15-dehydrogenase.

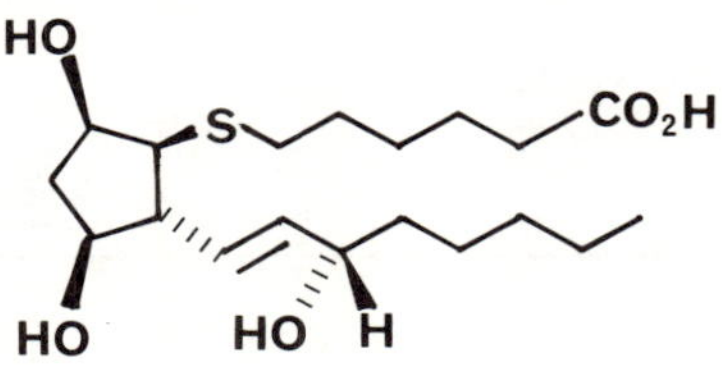

Shows no activity.

9,11-DIOXA-PG_1

SYNTHETIC PLAN[1]

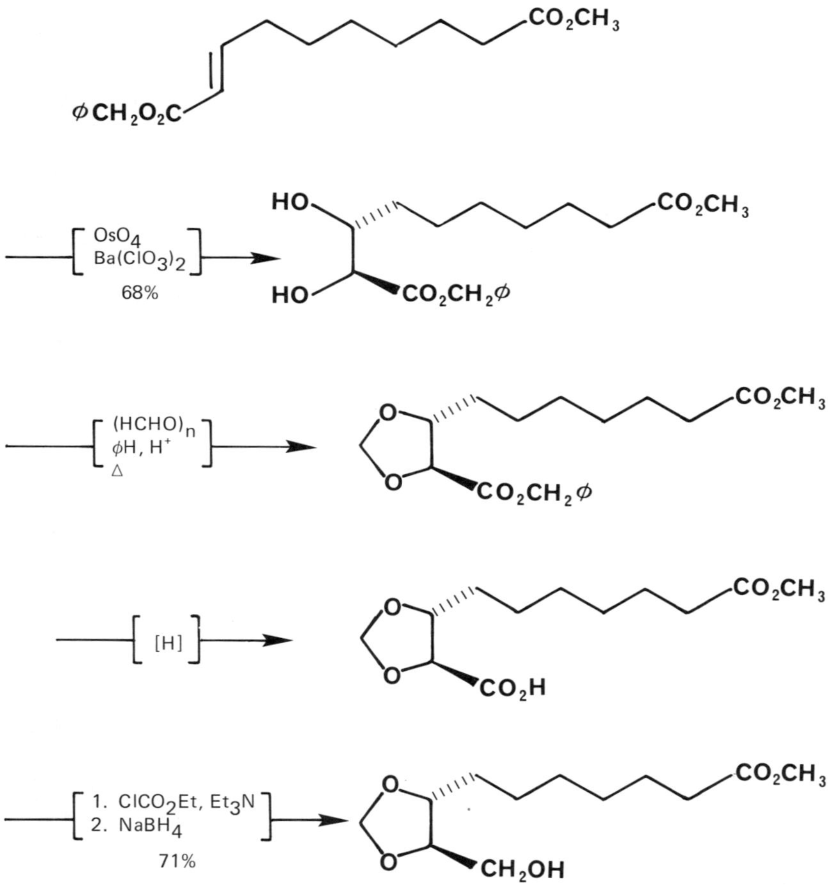

---

1. I. T. Harrison & V. R. Fletcher, *Tet. Lett.*, 2729 (1974).

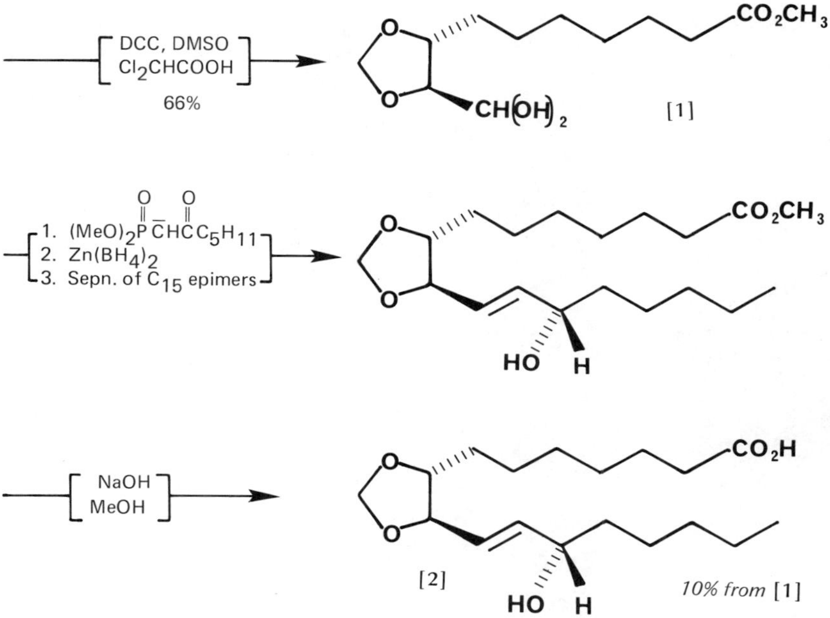

Active in gerbil colon assay (0.005 × PGE$_2$)

The corresponding carbonate analog was made by reaction of the diol [3] with phosgene followed by further elaboration.

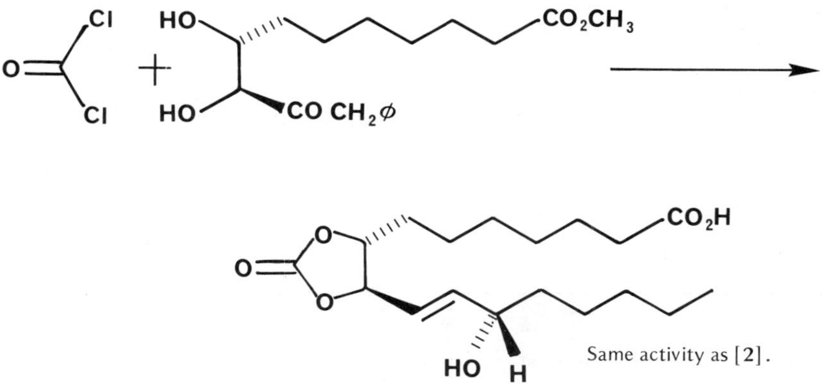

Same activity as [2].

9-AZA-11-DEOXY-PG

SYNTHETIC PLAN[1,2]

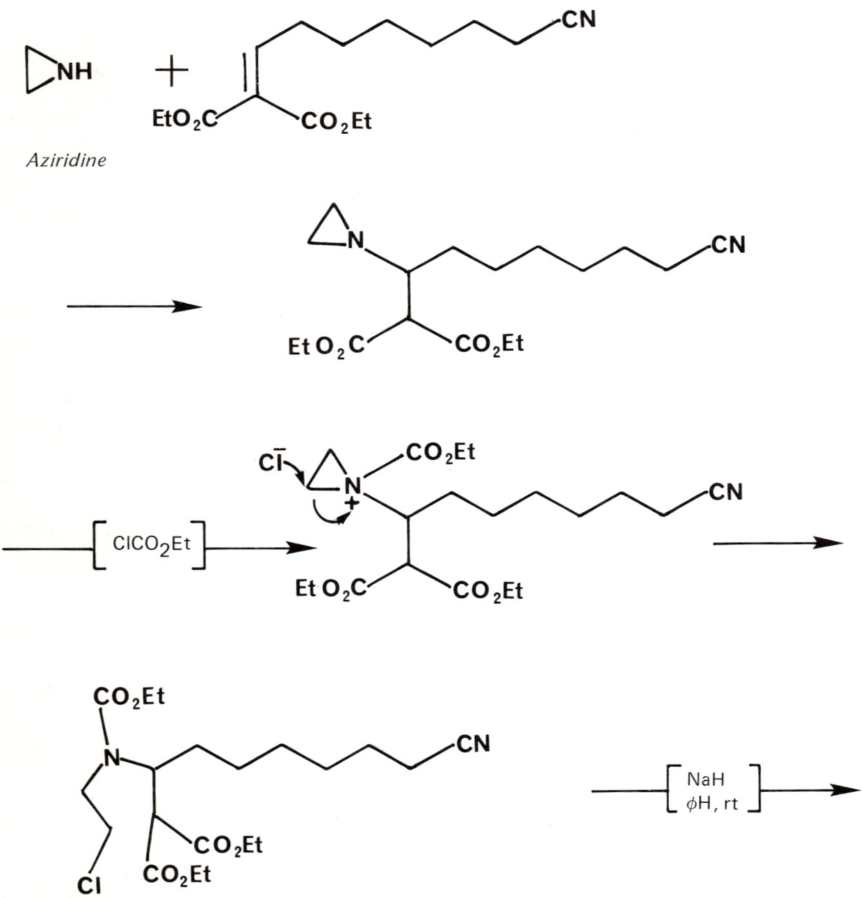

---

1. G. P. Rozing, T. J. H. Moinat, H. de Honing & H. O. Huisman, *Heterocycles,* **4**, 719 (1976).
2. Taken in part from the forthcoming thesis of G. P. Rozing, University of Amsterdam.
3. K. E. Pfitzner & J. G. Moffatt, *J. Am. Chem. Soc.,* **87**, 5661, 5670 (1965).

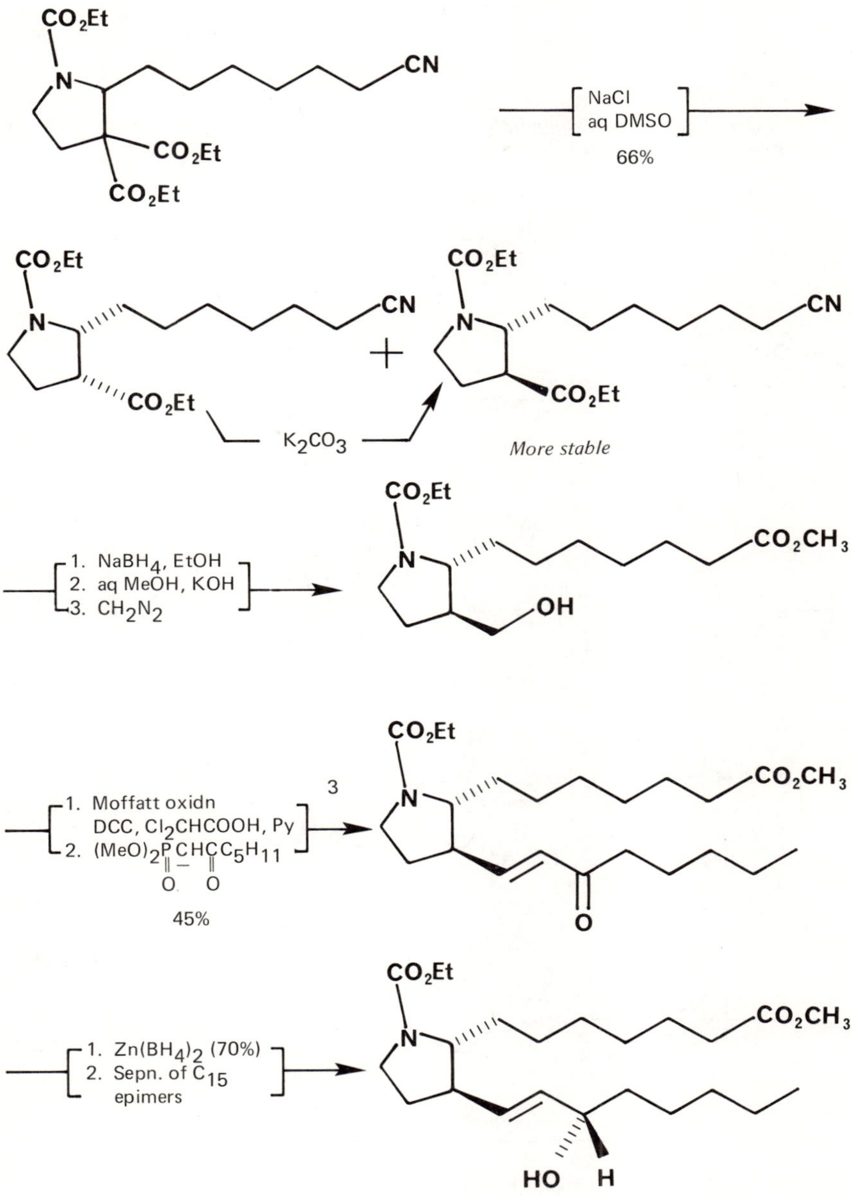
CO2Et
CN
CO2Et
CO2Et
NaCl
aq DMSO
66%
CO2Et
CN
CO2Et
K2CO3
CO2Et
CN
CO2Et
More stable
1. NaBH4, EtOH
2. aq MeOH, KOH
3. CH2N2
CO2Et
CO2CH3
OH
1. Moffatt oxidn
DCC, Cl2CHCOOH, Py
2. (MeO)2PCHCC5H11
O O
45%
3
CO2Et
CO2CH3
O
1. Zn(BH4)2 (70%)
2. Sepn. of C15
epimers
CO2Et
CO2CH3
HO H

8-AZA-11-DEOXY-PGE₁

The 8-aza-PG analog has been synthesized by the N-alkylation of methyl-pyroglutamate with the α-chain bromide. Subsequent steps follow the usual reaction sequence.[1]

SYNTHETIC PLAN[1]

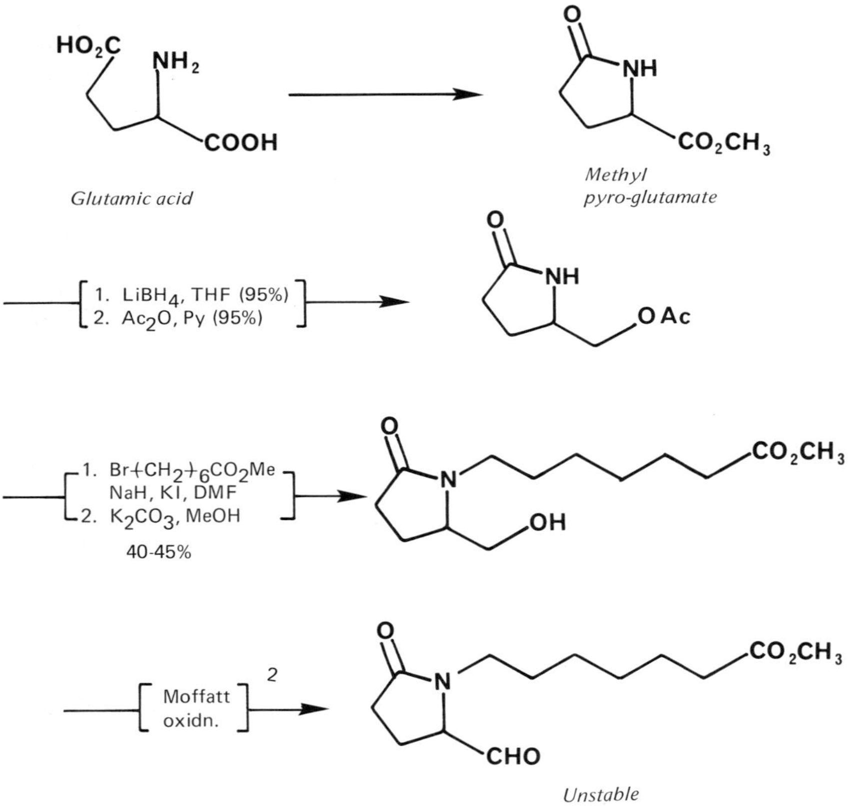

---

1. J. W. Bruin, H. de Koning & H. O. Huisman, *Tet. Lett.*, 4599 (1975).
2. K. E. Pfitzner & J. G. Moffatt, *J. Am. Chem. Soc.*, **88**, 5661, 5670 (1965).

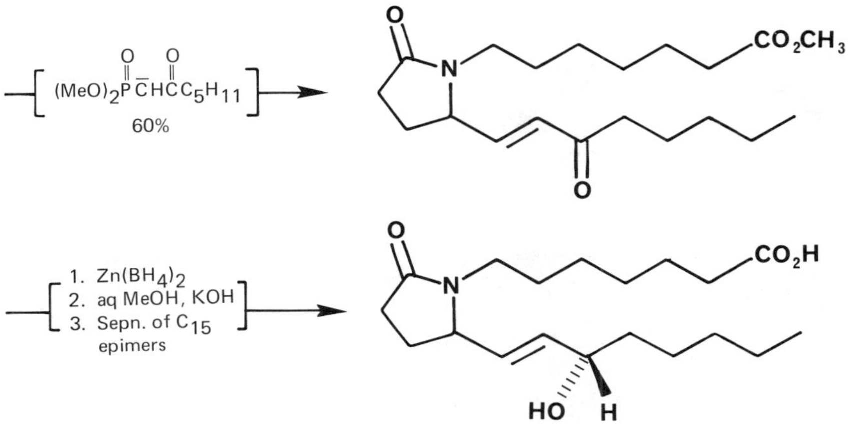

8-aza-PGE$_1$[3,4,5]

Substrate for 15-hydroxyprostaglandin dehydrogenase.

The corresponding C_{15}- epimer was not a substrate for 15-hydroxyprostaglandin dehydrogenase.

The methyl ester was more active in inhibition of gastric ulcers and decrease of blood pressure.

The 8-aza-PGE$_2$ showed similar activity as the 8-aza-PGE$_1$ derivative.

---

3. A similar synthesis has been reported by G. Bolliger & J. M. Muchowski, *Tet. Lett.*, 2931 (1975).
4. The 8-aza-PGE$_2$ was made by alkylation with the bromoheptynoate.

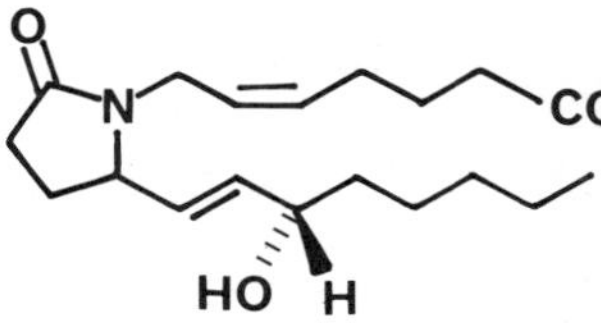

8-AZA-PGE$_2$

5. For another synthesis of 10-aza-PGE$_1$ see P. A. Zoretic,& F. Barcelos, *Tet. Lett.*, 529 (1977). For other synthesis of 8-aza-PGs see:
   P. A. Zoretic, N. D. Sinha & B. Branchaud, *Syn. Commun.*, in press (1977).
   P. A. Zoretic, B. Branchaud & N. D. Sinha, *J. Org. Chem.*, in press (1977).
   P. A. Zoretic & J. Chiang, *J. Org. Chem.*, in press (1977).

8-THIA-PG

SYNTHETIC PLAN[1]

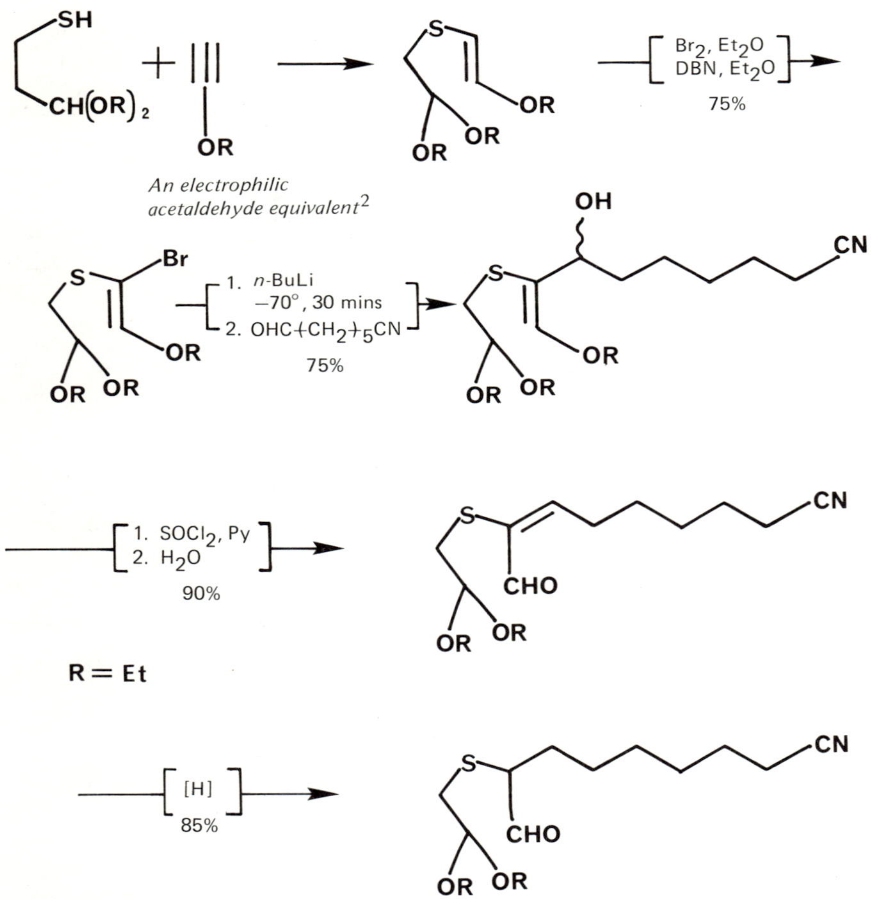

1. I. Vlattas, L. Della Vecchia & A. O. Lee, *J. Am. Chem. Soc.*, **98**, 2008 (1976).
2. J. F. Arens, A. G. Hermans & J. H. Sperna Weiland, *Proc. K. Ned. Acad. Wet., Ser. B,* **58**, 59 (1955).

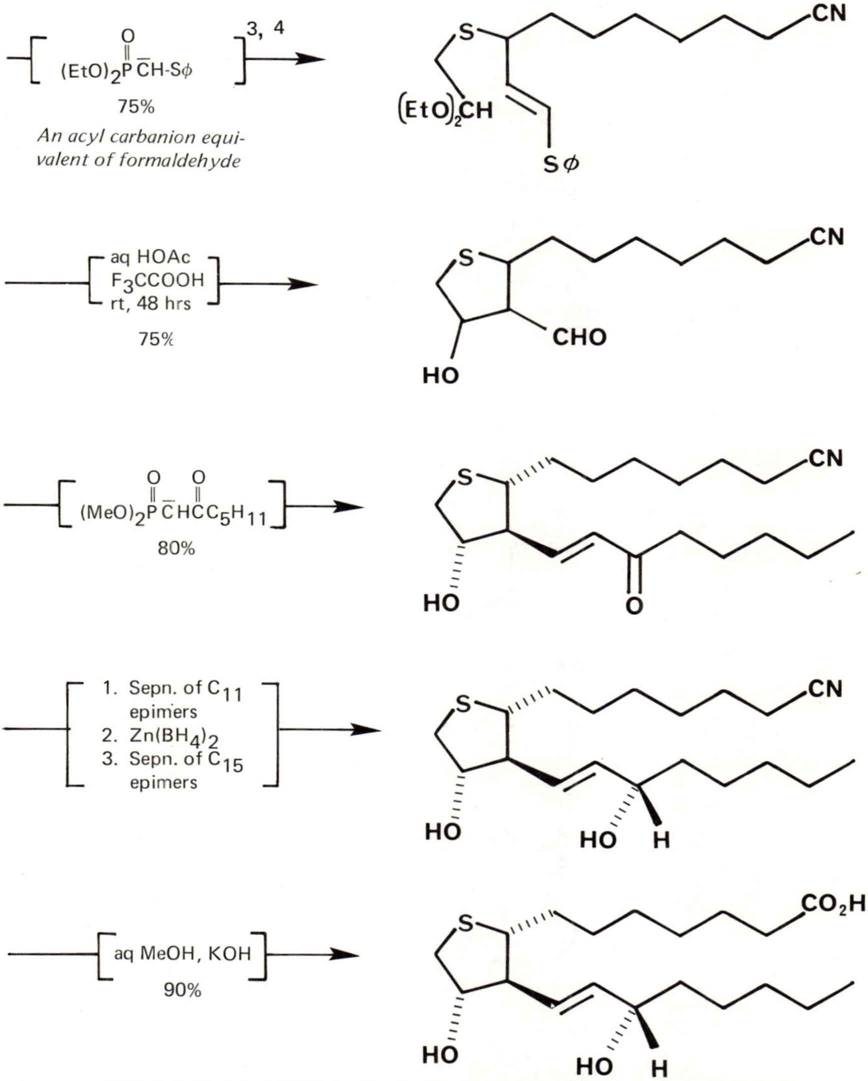

3. For similar synthesis of carbonyl compounds via vinylsulfides (formed by Horner-Emmons reaction) see E. J. Corey & J. I. Schulman, *J. Org. Chem.*, 35, 777 (1970).

4. $(EtO)_2\overset{O}{\overset{\|}{P}}\bar{C}H{-}S\phi Li^+$ in DMSO gives a mixture of *cis* and *trans* vinylsulfides.

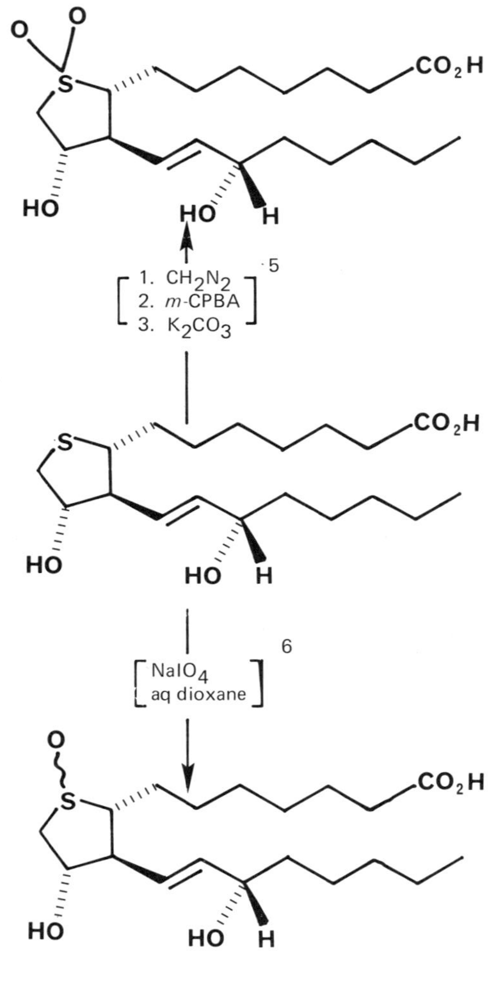

5. I. Vlattas & L. Della Vecchia, *Tet. Lett.*, 4267 (1974).
6. I. Vlattas & L. Della Vecchia, *Tet. Lett.*, 4459 (1974).

9-OXA-PG

SYNTHETIC PLAN[1]

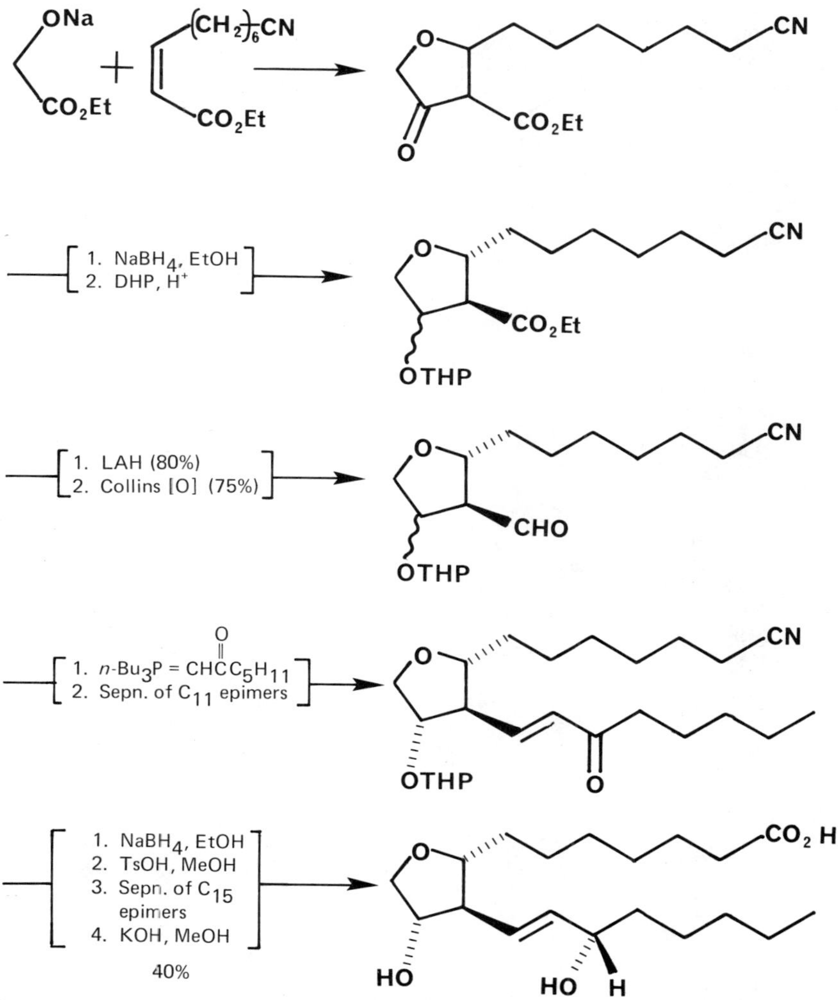

1. I. Vlattas & L. Della Vecchia, *Tet. Lett.*, 4455 (1974).

11-OXA-PGF$_{2\alpha}$

SYNTHETIC PLAN[1]

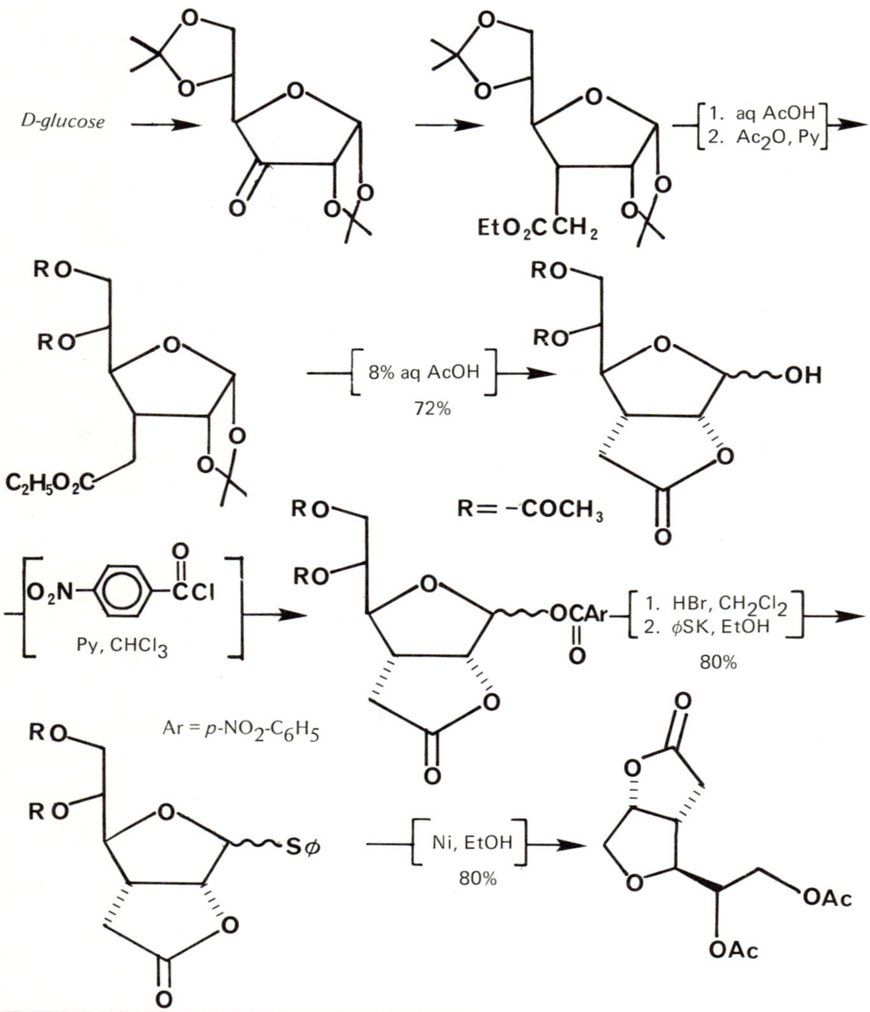

1. G. J. Lourens & J. M. Koekemoer, *Tet. Lett.*, 3719 (1975).

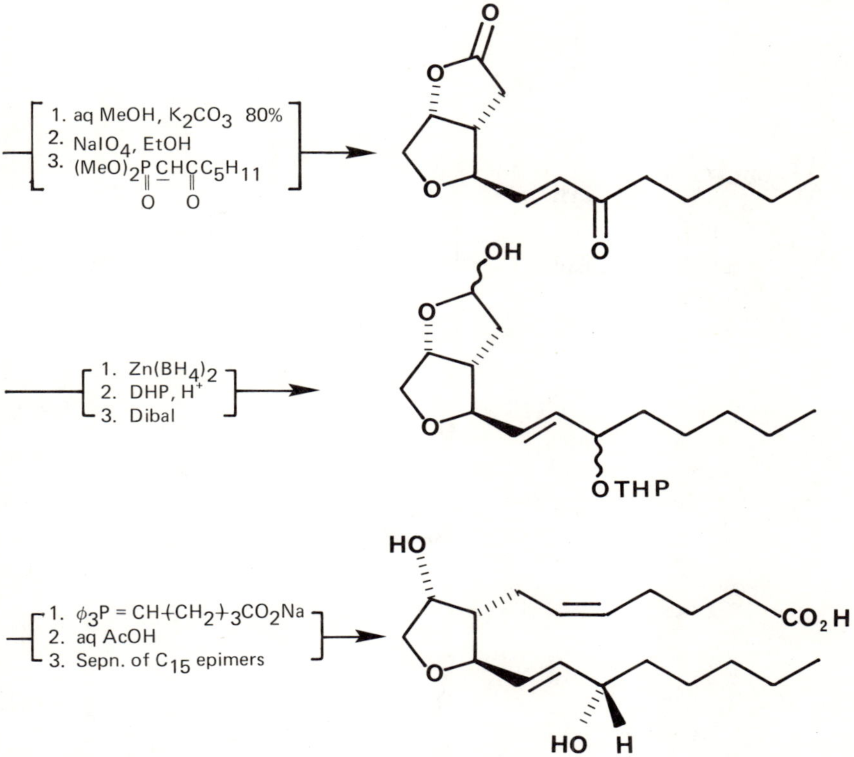

A 10-substituted 11-oxa-PG has also been made.[2]

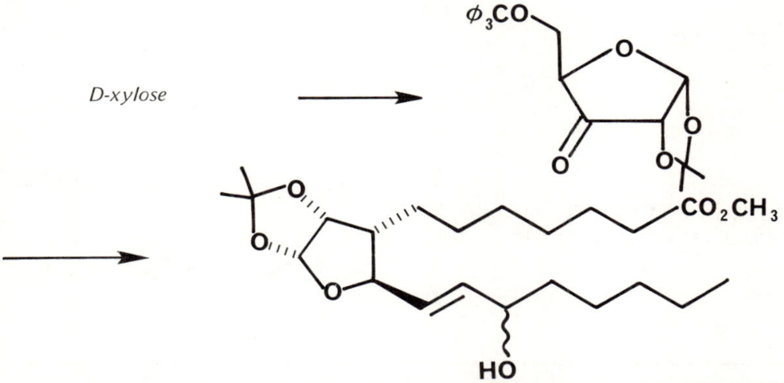

2. G. J. Lourens & J. M. Koekemoer, *Tet. Lett.*, 3715 (1975).

11-THIA-PGE$_1$

SYNTHETIC PLAN[1]

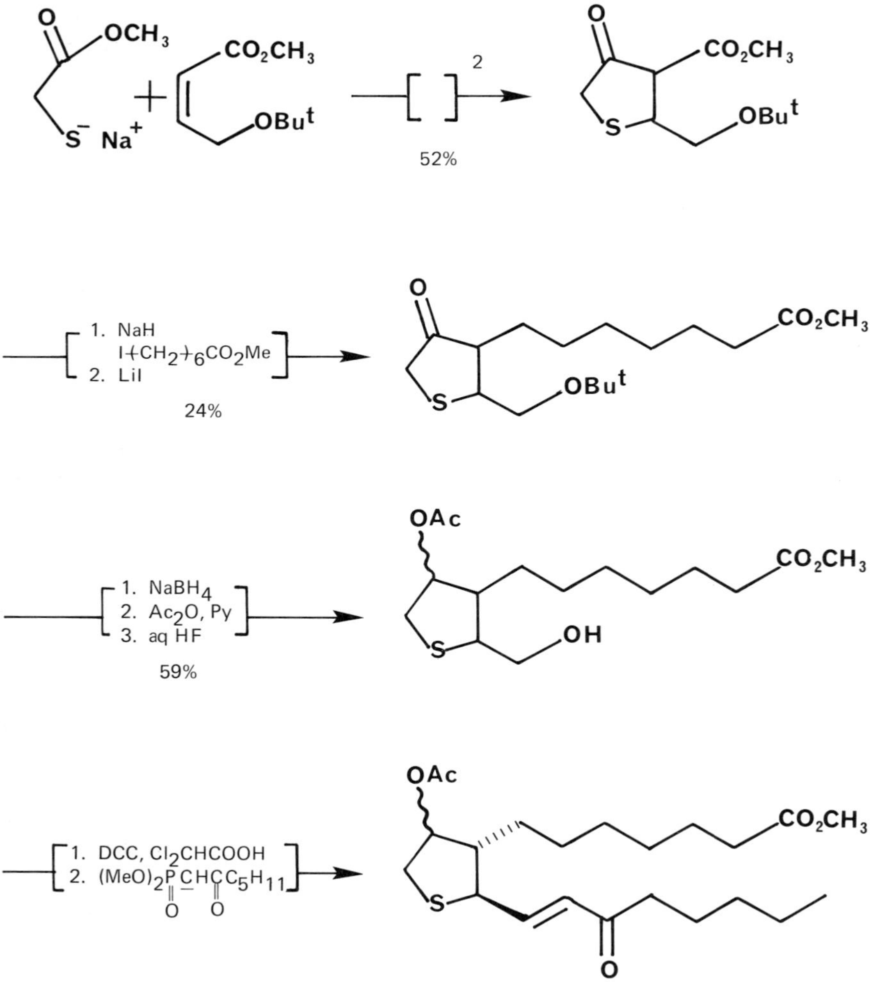

---

1. I. T. Harrison, R. J. K. Taylor & J. H. Fried, *Tet. Lett.*, 1165 (1975).
2. M. A. Gianturco, P. Friedel & A. S. Giammarino, *Tet. Lett.*, **20**, 1763 (1964).

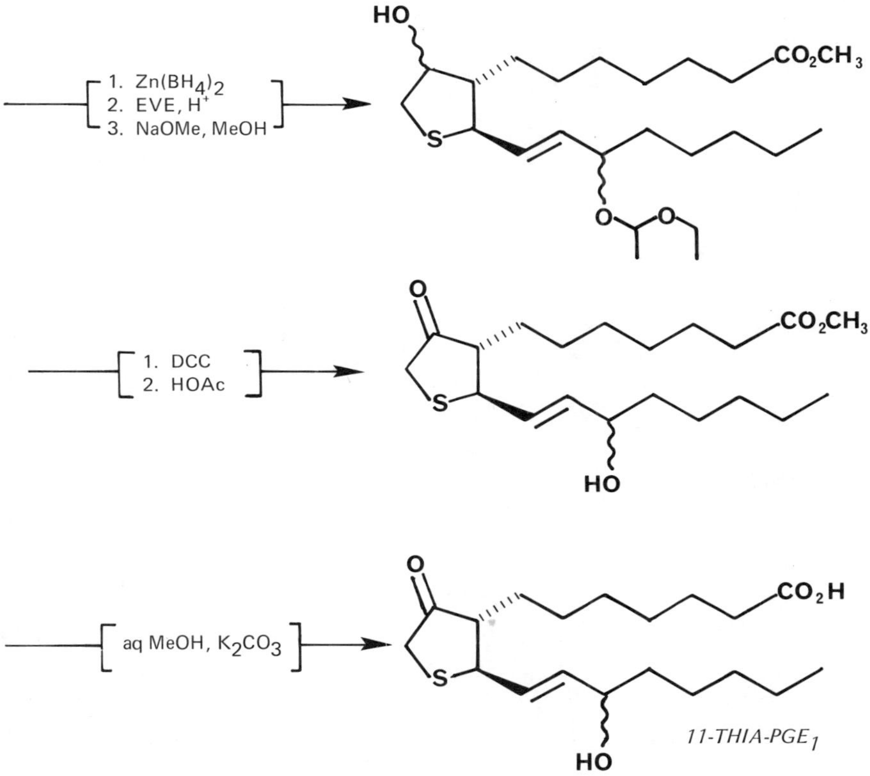

11-THIA-PGE$_1$

Active in gerbil colon assay (0.005 × PGE$_2$)

The corresponding 11-oxa-PGE$_1$ was made from the corresponding anion of methyl glycolate.[3]

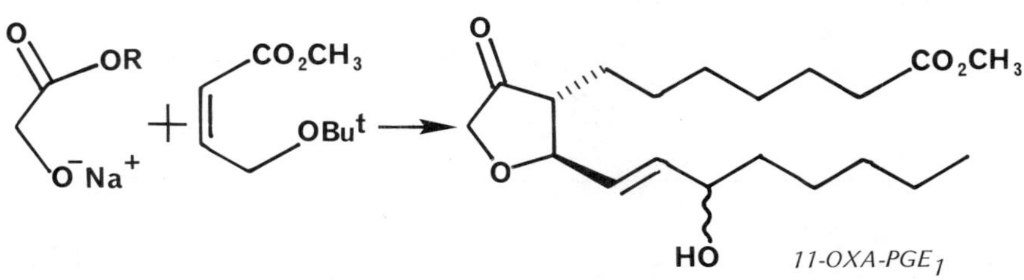

11-OXA-PGE$_1$

3. I. T. Harrison, V. R. Fletcher & J. H. Fried, *Tet. Lett.*, 2733 (1974).

9,11-AZO-PG

SYNTHETIC PLAN[1]

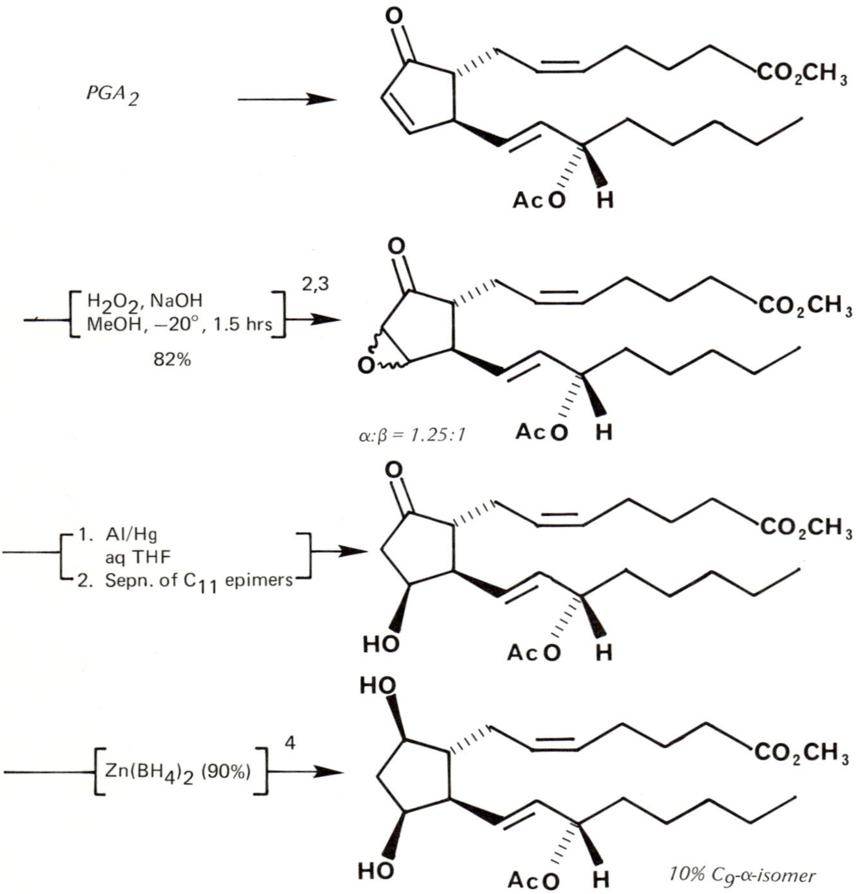

1. E. J. Corey, K. C. Nicolaou, M. Yoshimasa, C. L. Malmsten & B. Samuelsson, *Proc. Natl. Acad. Sci. USA*, **72**, 3355 (1975).
2. W. P. Schneider, R. D. Hamilton, L. E. Rhuland, *J. Am. Chem. Soc.*, **94**, 2122 (1973).
3. For a stereoselective method of epoxidation of PGA_2 using a remotely placed exogeneous group see E. J. Corey & H. E. Ensley, *J. Org. Chem.*, **38**, 3187 (1973).

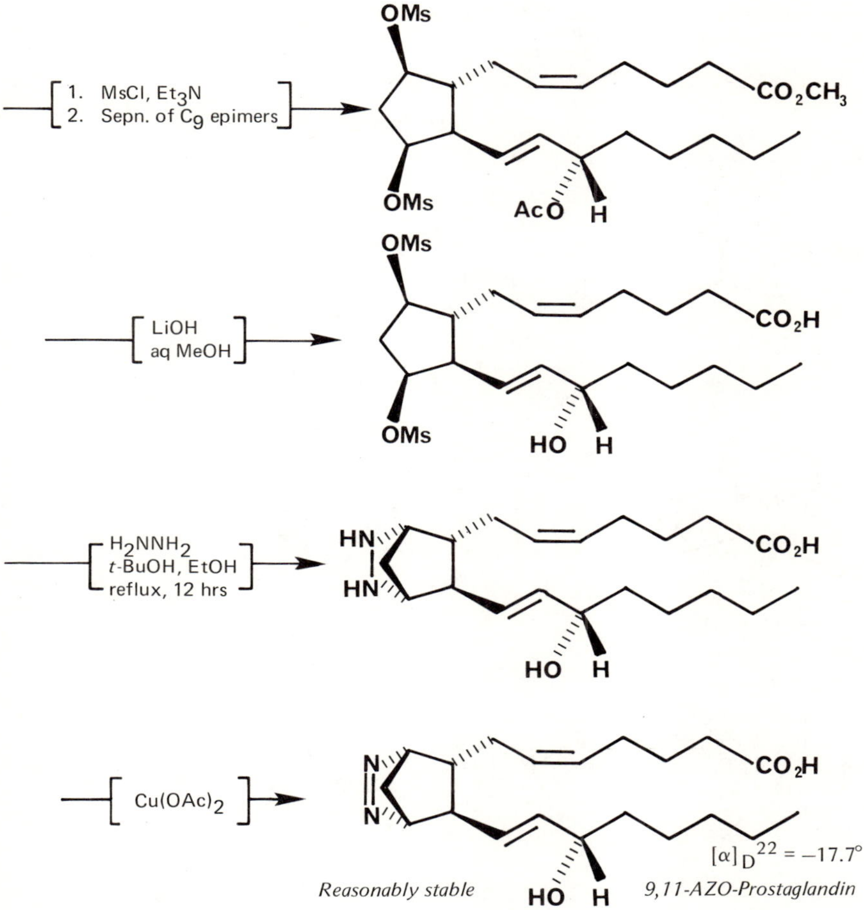

Reasonably stable

$[\alpha]_D^{22} = -17.7°$

9,11-AZO-Prostaglandin

7.9 times more active than PGG_2 with respect to aggregation of platelets in human platelet-rich plasma (PRP).

6 times more active than PGG_2 in the release of $[^{14}C]$serotonin from prelabeled platelets. It is metabolically more stable than PGG_2 and continues the release of serotonin.

1450 times more active than PGE_2 and 7 times more active than PGH_2 in the contraction of isolated rabbit-aorta strip.

---

4. $NaBH_4$ reduction of the C_9 ketone gives an equal mixture of the epimeric C_9 alcohols. But the reduction with $ZnBH_4$ gives predominantly the C_9-β-alcohol as the major isomer.

Another stereocontrolled synthesis of the 9,11-azo analog has been reported.[5] This route is not dependent on the availability of PGA_2.

SYNTHETIC PLAN[5]

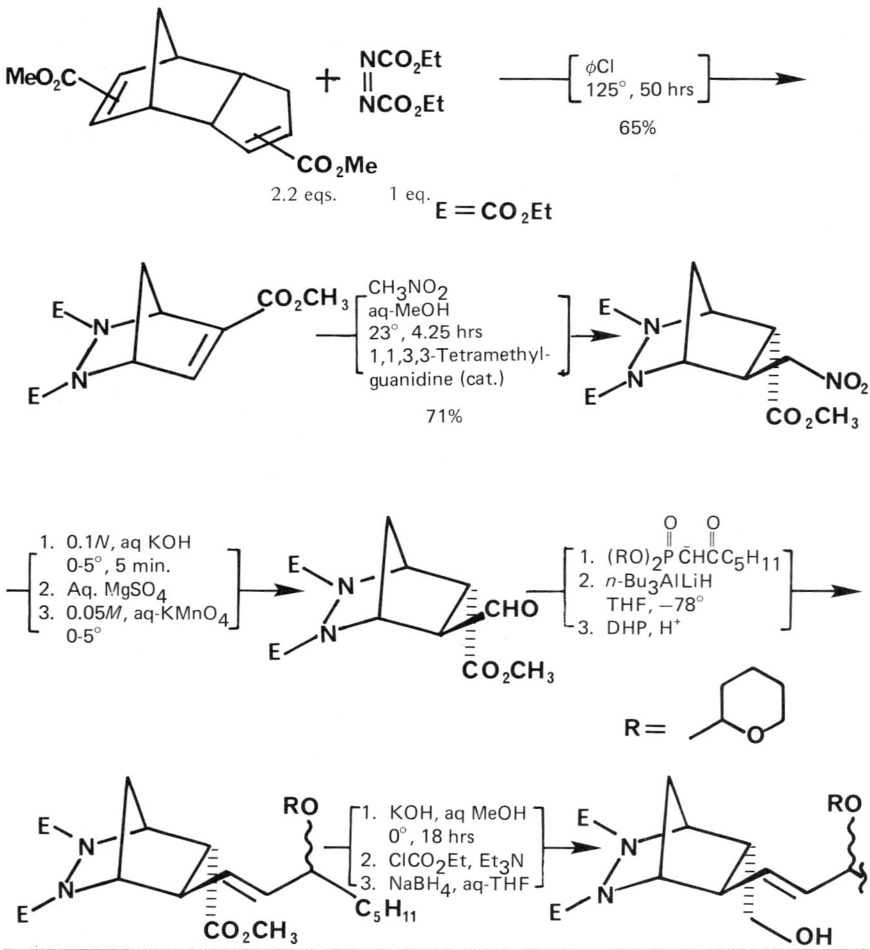

5. E. J. Corey, K. Narasaka & M. Shibasaki, *J. Am. Chem. Soc.*, **98**, 6417 (1976).
6. The conjugate addition had to be carried out under closely defined conditions.

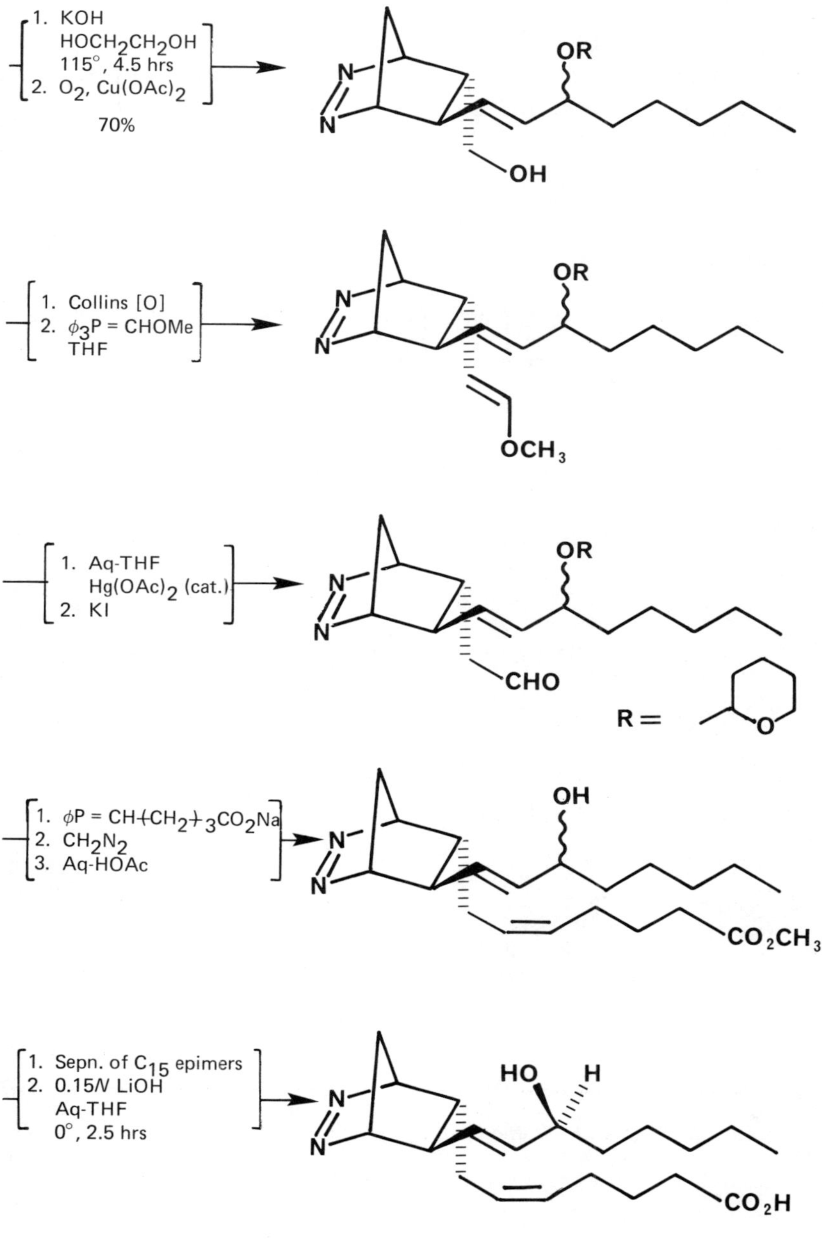
1. KOH
HOCH2CH2OH
115°, 4.5 hrs
2. O2, Cu(OAc)2
70%
OR
N
N
OH
1. Collins [O]
2. φ3P = CHOMe
THF
OR
OCH3
1. Aq-THF
Hg(OAc)2 (cat.)
2. KI
OR
CHO
R =
O
1. φP = CH(CH2)3CO2Na
2. CH2N2
3. Aq-HOAc
OH
CO2CH3
1. Sepn. of C15 epimers
2. 0.15N LiOH
Aq-THF
0°, 2.5 hrs
HO
H
CO2H

CARBOCYCLIC ANALOGS OF THE ENDOPEROXIDE

The carbocyclic analog of the enoperoxides (PGH_2 and PGG_2) have been by the 1,4-addition to the bicyclo[2.2.1]heptadiene derivative [1] followed by a one carbon homologation to get the aldehyde necessary for the elaboration of the α-chain.[1]

SYNTHETIC PLAN[1]

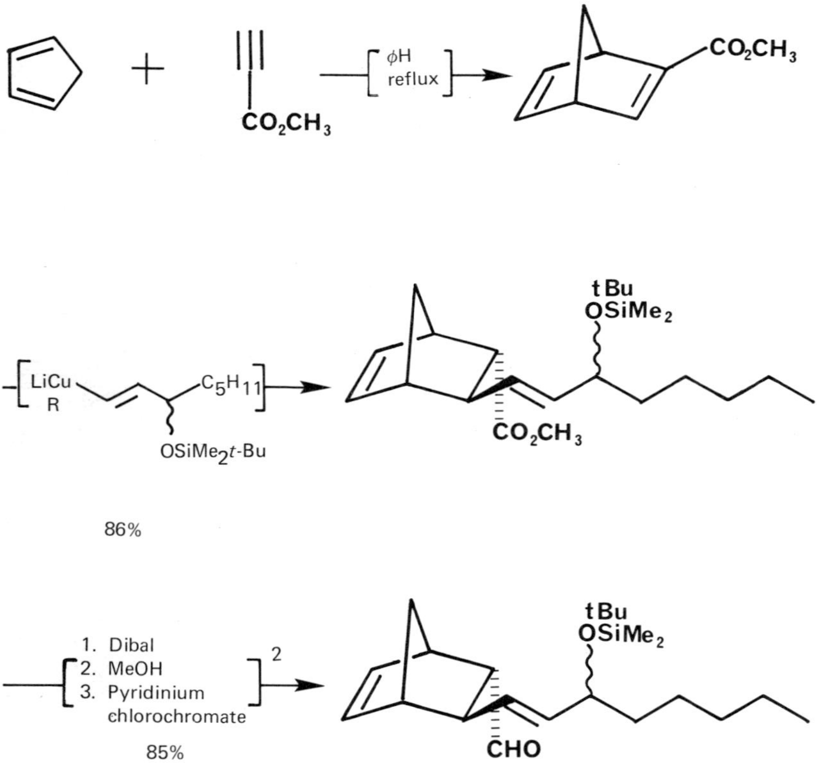

1. E. J. Corey, M. Shibasaki, K. C. Nicolaou, C. Malmsten & B. Samuelsson, *Tet. Lett.*, 737 (1976).
2. Pyridinium chlorochromate is a new oxidizing agent. E. J. Corey & J. W. Suggs, *Tet. Lett.*, 2647 (1975).

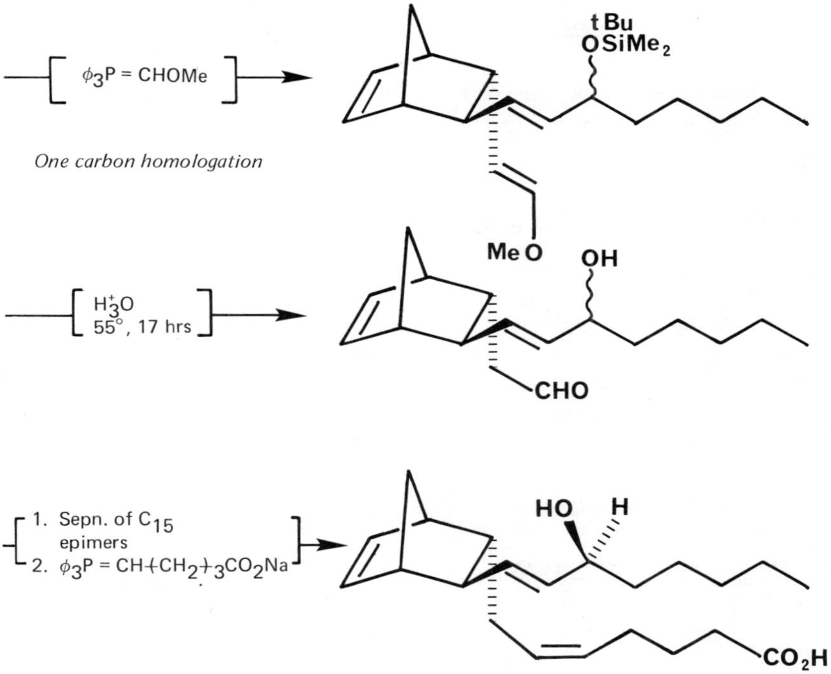

Induces aggregation in human platelet rich plasma (PRP).

Induces release of ^{14}C serotonin.

The corresponding C_{15} epimer neither induced nor inhibited aggregation.

---

3. The 15(R)-hydroxy derivative has been converted to the 15(*S*)-hydroxy derivative by displacement of the mesylate with K-superoxide.

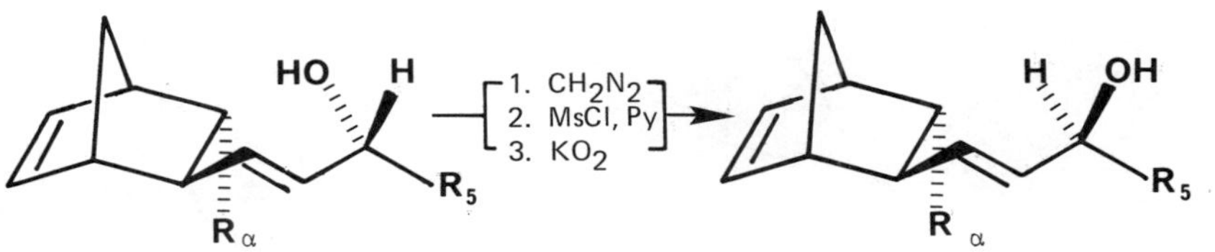

4. The carbocyclic analog has also been made by H. Shimomura, A. Sugie, J. Katsube & H. Yamamoto, *Tet. Lett.*, 4099 (1976).

9,11-BISHYDROXYMETHYL-PG

The 9,11-bishydroxymethyl PG analogs have been made from the bicyclo[2.2.1]heptene derivative by the oxidative cleavage of the norbornene double bond.[1]

SYNTHETIC PLAN[1]

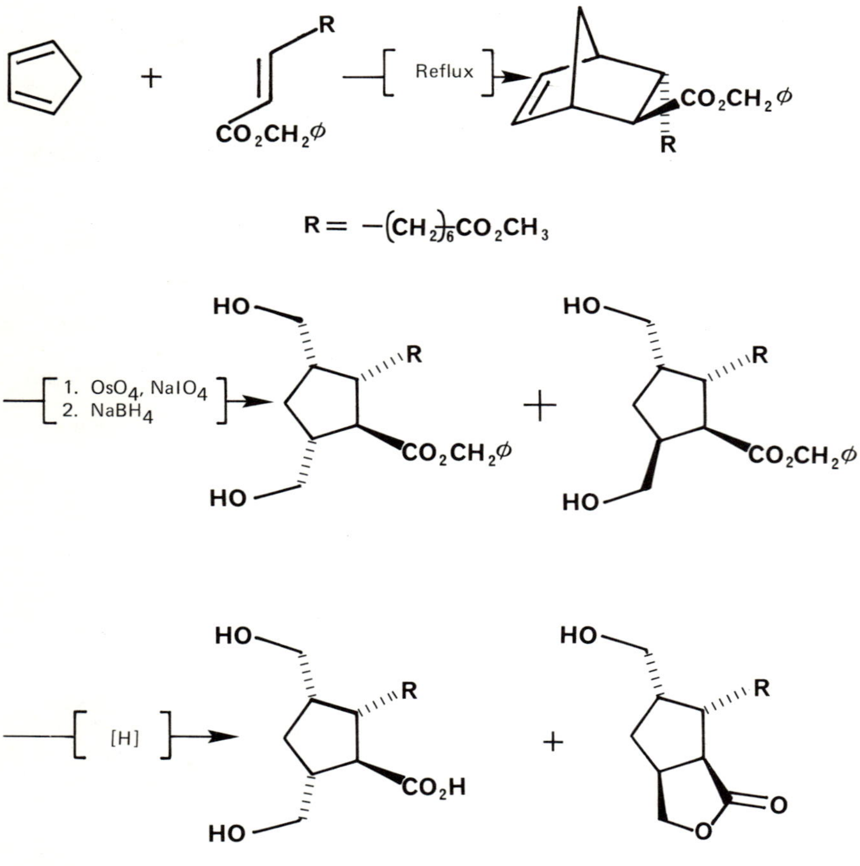

---

1. I. T. Harrison, R. Gayshan, T. Williams, A. Semenovski & J. H. Fried, *Tet. Lett.*, 5151 (1972).

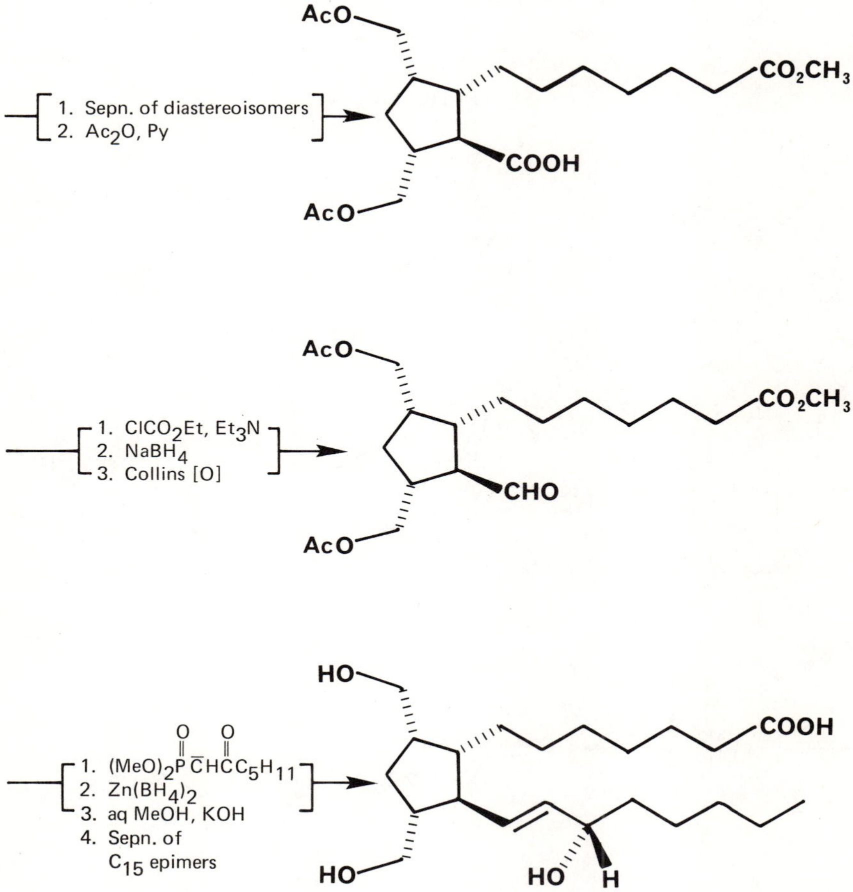

9,11-dideoxy-9,11-bishydroxymethyl-PGE$_1$

Weakly active in smooth muscle relaxation assays.

CYCLOBUTANE ANALOG OF PG

SYNTHETIC PLAN[1]

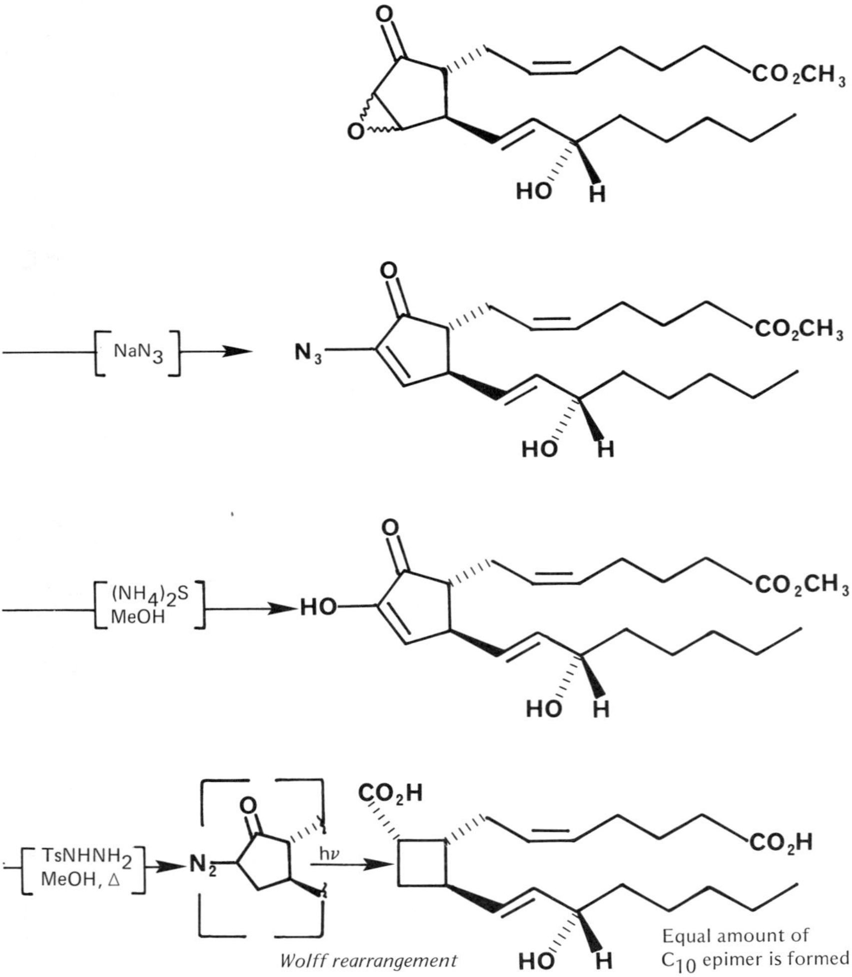

1/10th as active as $PGF_{2\alpha}$ in hamster antifertility assay.

---

1. A. Guzman, J. M. Muchowski & M. A. Vera, *Chem. & Indu.*, 884 (1975).

Another synthesis of 11-nor-prostaglandin has been reported.[2,3]

SYNTHETIC PLAN[2]

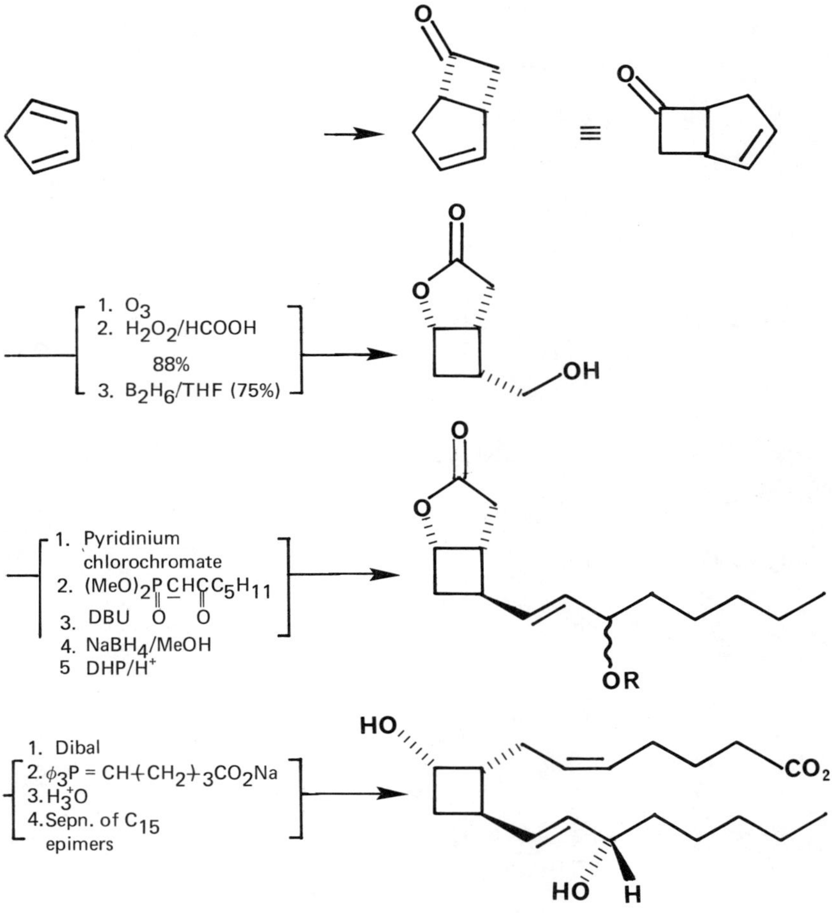

---

2. A. E. Greene, J. P. Depres, M. C. Meana & P. Crabbe, *Tet. Lett.*, 3755 (1976).
3. A similar synthesis has been reported by D. Reuschling, K. Kuhlein & A. Lukies, *Tet. Lett.*, 17 (1977).

CYCLOHEXANE ANALOG OF PG

SYNTHETIC PLAN[1,2]

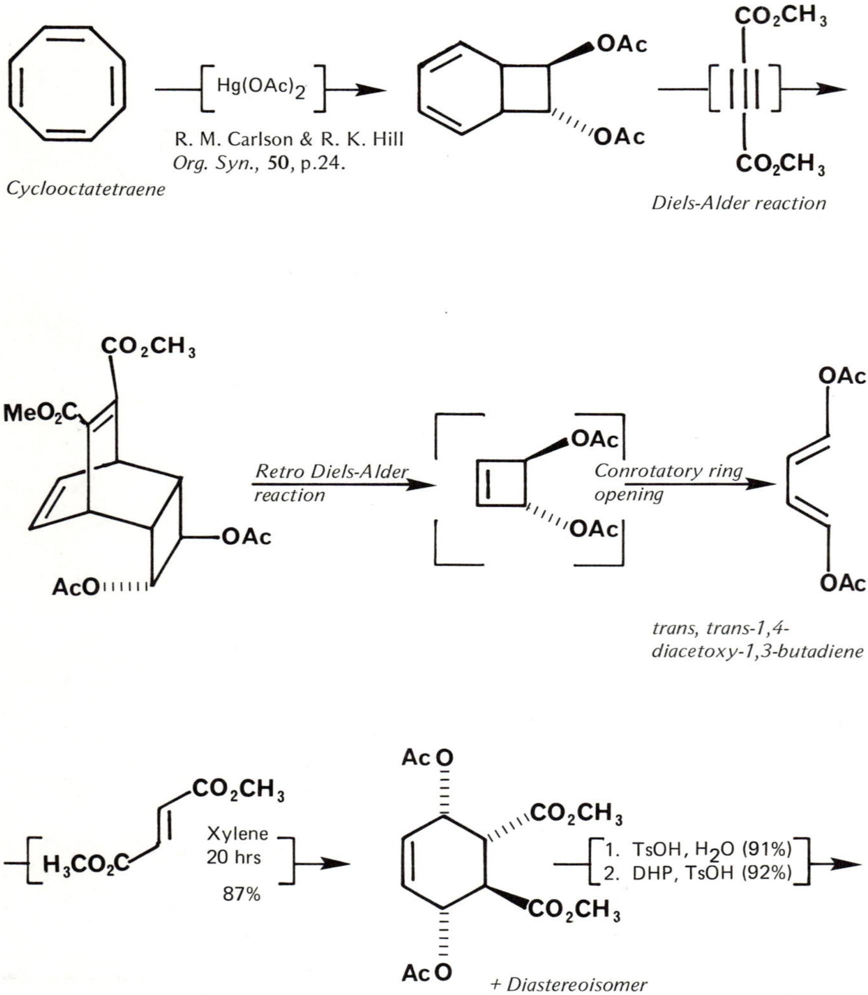

---

1. T. A. Elggelte, Ph.D. Dissertation Thesis, University of Amsterdam (1975).
2. Personal communication

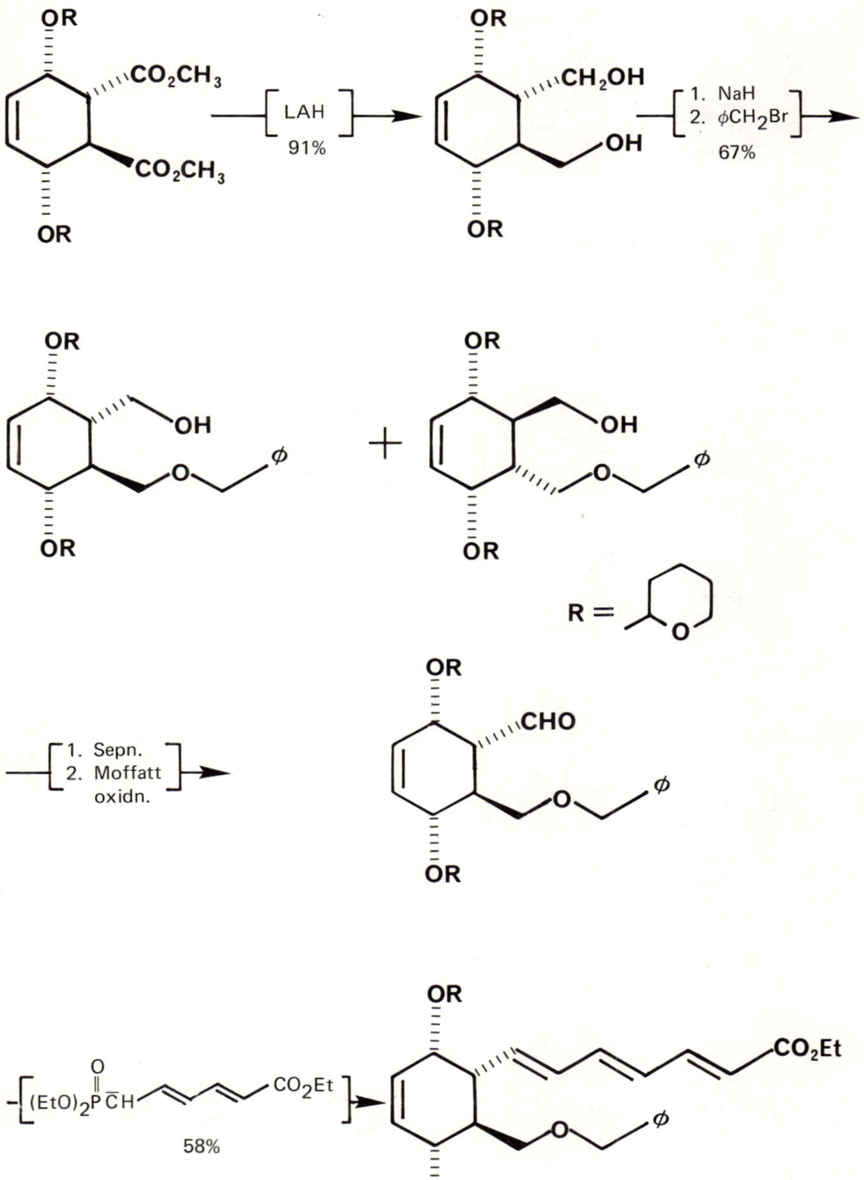
OR
CO_2CH_3
CO_2CH_3
LAH
91%
CH_2OH
OH
1. NaH
2. ϕCH_2Br
67%
OH
O
ϕ
R =
O
1. Sepn.
2. Moffatt oxidn.
CHO
$(EtO)_2\overset{O}{\parallel}{P}\bar{C}H$
CO_2Et
58%

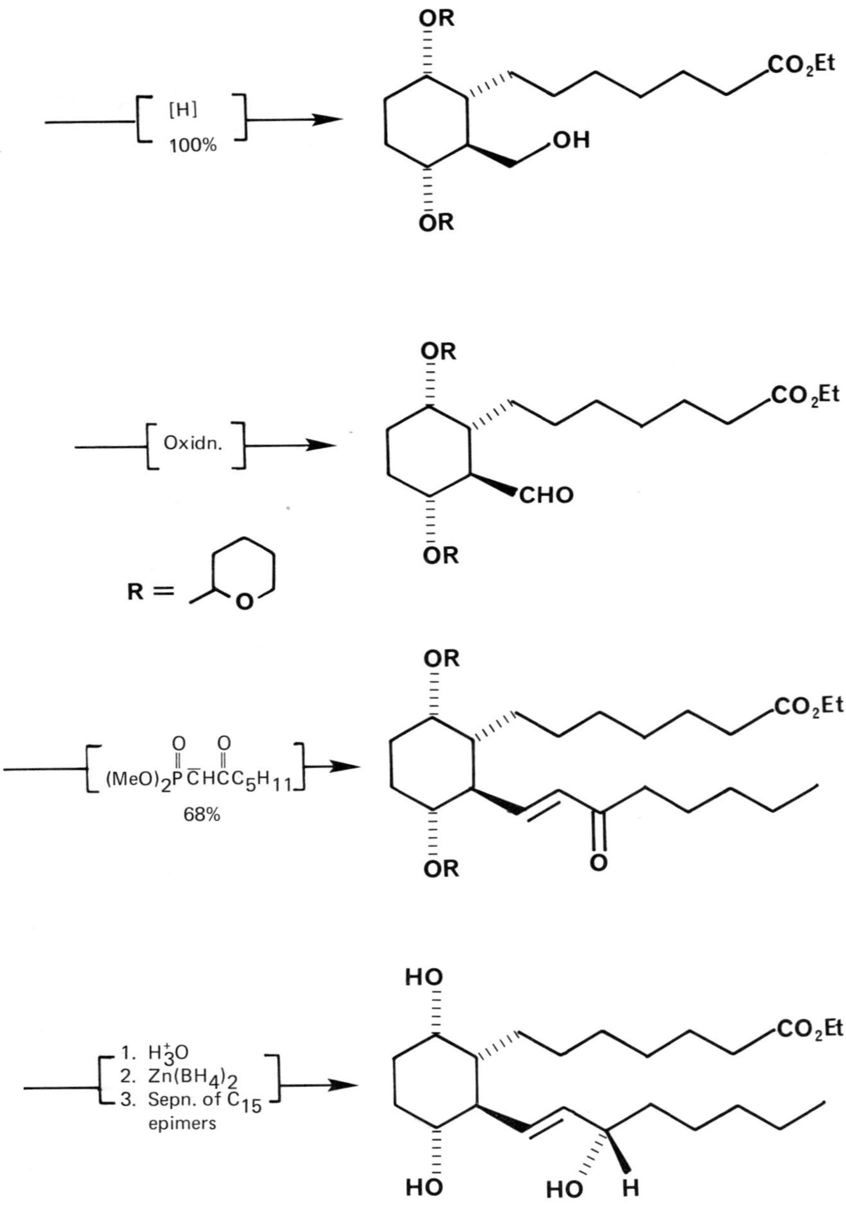
[H]
100%
OR
CO2Et
OH
OR
Oxidn.
OR
CO2Et
CHO
OR
R =
O
OR
CO2Et
(MeO)2P CHCC5H11
68%
OR
O
1. H3+O
2. Zn(BH4)2
3. Sepn. of C15 epimers
HO
CO2Et
HO
HO
H

Author Index

Subject Index